Anticancer Drug Discovery Based on Natural Products: From Computational Approaches to Clinical Studies

Anticancer Drug Discovery Based on Natural Products: From Computational Approaches to Clinical Studies

Guest Editors

Rajeev K. Singla
Anupam Bishayee

MDPI

Basel • Beijing • Wuhan • Barcelona • Belgrade • Novi Sad • Cluj • Manchester

Guest Editors
Rajeev K. Singla
West China Hospital
Sichuan University
Chengdu
China

Anupam Bishayee
College of Osteopathic
Medicine
Lake Erie College of
Osteopathic Medicine
Bradenton, FL
USA

Editorial Office
MDPI AG
Grosspeteranlage 5
4052 Basel, Switzerland

This is a reprint of the Special Issue, published open access by the journal *Cancers* (ISSN 2072-6694), freely accessible at: https://www.mdpi.com/journal/cancers/special_issues/1T6DNKD24N.

For citation purposes, cite each article independently as indicated on the article page online and as indicated below:

Lastname, A.A.; Lastname, B.B. Article Title. *Journal Name* **Year**, *Volume Number*, Page Range.

ISBN 978-3-7258-5277-2 (Hbk)
ISBN 978-3-7258-5278-9 (PDF)
https://doi.org/10.3390/books978-3-7258-5278-9

Contents

About the Editors

Rajeev K. Singla

Rajeev K. Singla Ph.D. is an assistant researcher at the Institutes for Systems Genetics, West China Hospital, Sichuan University, China. He has extensive experience in the fields of natural products, metabolic disorders, neurological diseases, infectious diseases, cheminformatics, and public health. Dr. Singla is the Editor-in-Chief of *Indo Global Journal of Pharmaceutical Sciences*, Associate Editor of *Journal of Alzheimer's Disease*, *Frontiers in Pharmacology*, and *Frontiers in Nutrition*, and an editorial board member of *Heliyon*, *BMC Complementary Medicine and Therapies* and *CNS & Neurological Disorders—Drug Targets*. He is among the top 2% of scientists according to Stanford University, Scopus, and Elsevier reports (based on publications in 2022, 2023, and 2024). He has published more than 140 papers in journals, including *International Journal of Surgery*, *Phytomedicine*, *Neuroscience and Biobehavioral Reviews*, *Critical Reviews in Food Science and Nutrition*, *Pharmacological Research*, *Aging Research Reviews*, *iMeta*, *npj Digital Medicine*, *Drugs*, *Comprehensive Reviews in Food Science and Food Safety*, and *Autoimmunity Reviews*. According to Scopus, he has published papers with 780 co-authors from 40 countries so far. To date, he has published 4 books and 19 chapters. He serves as an expert reviewer for the Sichuan University Innovation Training Program Academy and participates in co-guiding the College Students Innovation and Entrepreneurship Competition. In addition, he was awarded the 2024 Sichuan Province Foreign High-level Talent Certificate this year and won the second prize for the 2022–2023 Suzhou Natural Science Excellent Academic Paper Award. In 2024, he successfully applied for a Sichuan Provincial Science and Technology Department project to find alternative therapies extracted from coconut shells to the fight infections with Pseudomonas aeruginosa.

Anupam Bishayee

Anupam Bishayee is a Professor of Pharmacology and Director of Research at the Lake Erie College of Osteopathic Medicine (Bradenton, FL, USA). He received a Ph.D. (cancer prevention) from Jadavpur University, Kolkata, India, and performed post-doctoral research at Rutgers University, Newark, NJ. Dr. Bishayee's primary research interest encompasses natural products and dietary agents in health and disease. His laboratory is involved in investigating the cancer preventive and therapeutic effects of medicinal plants, natural products, and dietary agents using several pre-clinical models of cancer and underlying mechanisms of action. Dr. Bishayee received research funding from the National Institutes of Health and various pharmaceutical and biotechnological companies. Dr. Bishayee has been awarded a United States patent for the development of a potential drug for breast cancer prevention and treatment. Dr. Bishayee has published more than 325 peer-reviewed research papers and review articles, mostly in high-impact journals, 22 book chapters, and around 90 conference abstracts, and delivered at least 40 invited presentations at various national and international conferences. Dr. Bishayee has been serving various reputed journals as Section Editor-in-Chief, Consulting Editor, Editorial Board Member, and reviewer. Dr. Bishayee edited an Elsevier book *Epigenetics of Cancer Prevention* and several journal special issues on natural products and cancer published by leading publishers, such as Elsevier, Springer Nature, Multidisciplinary Digital Publishing Institute, and Bentham. Dr. Bishayee received the recognition of World's Top 2% Scientists—Clinical Medicine (Standford University/Elsevier, 2020–present). Dr. Bishayee is a "Highly Cited Researcher" and his papers rank in the top 1% by citations for a field or fields (Clarivate, Web of Science). His Scopus h-index is 85 and scholars from all over the world have cited Dr. Bishayee's published work more than 33,000 times.

cancers

Editorial

Anticancer Drug Discovery Based on Natural Products: From Computational Approaches to Clinical Studies

Rajeev K. Singla [1,2,*] and Anupam Bishayee [3,*]

1 Department of Pharmacy and Institutes for Systems Genetics, Center for High Altitude Medicine, Frontiers Science Center for Disease-Related Molecular Network, West China Hospital, Sichuan University, Chengdu 610041, China
2 School of Pharmaceutical Sciences, Lovely Professional University, Phagwara 144 411, Punjab, India
3 Department of Pharmacology, College of Osteopathic Medicine, Lake Erie College of Osteopathic Medicine, Bradenton, FL 34211, USA
* Correspondence: rajeevkumar@scu.edu.cn or rajeevsingla26@gmail.com (R.K.S.); abishayee@lecom.edu or abishayee@gmail.com (A.B.)

1. Introduction

Cancer represents a major public health, societal, and economic challenges in the 21st century. According to the data published by the International Agency for Research on Cancer/GLOBOCAN, close to 20 million new cases of cancer and 9.7 million deaths from this disease occurred in 2022 [1]. Furthermore, it has been estimated that approximately one in five men or women develop cancer in their lifetime [1]. In the United States alone, more than 2 million new cancer cases and 618,120 cancer deaths are expected to occur in 2025 [2]. All these data provide a strong impetus to explore novel agents for the prevention and treatment of cancer. Natural products have been an expansive source of new anticancer drugs. During the last several decades, a plethora of natural agents, especially bioactive phytocompounds, have been investigated based on cell culture assays, animal tumor models, and human subjects, to understand their potential for cancer prevention and treatment [3]. Figure 1 illustrates the multimodal target-based advancement required for anticancer drug discovery. Moreover, recent developments in cheminformatics and bioinformatics—such as network-pharmacology-based studies, pharmacokinetics and toxicity prediction, molecular docking, molecular dynamics simulations, artificial intelligence (AI)- and machine learning (ML)-based models—have contributed to accelerating anticancer drug development. Considering such progress, we are pleased to introduce this Special Issue, which documents recent advances in our knowledge of cancer preventive and the therapeutic efficacy of natural substances, with a view to understanding cellular and molecular mechanisms of action.

2. An Overview of Published Articles

This thematic issue contains five original research papers, four narrative reviews and one systematic review article which capture the translational aspects of preclinical anticancer studies to clinical development.

Gupta and colleagues (Contribution 1) investigated the cytotoxic activity of the mechanisms of action of two bioactive triterpenoids, namely oleanolic acid and ursolic acid, individually and in combination using MCF-7 (estrogen receptor-positive) and MDA-MB-231 (triple-negative) breast cancer cells. The results of this study indicated that both phytocompounds were equally effective against two cell lines. Interestingly, a combination of phytochemicals was more effective than ursolic acid alone. Mechanistic studies revealed

https://doi.org/10.3390/cancers17152507

that the phytochemical combination induced excessive autophagy via inhibition of phosphoinositide 3-kinase (phosphoinositide 3-kinase)-mediated phosphorylation of Akt and mammalian target of rapamycin (mTOR). These results underscore the potential of the tested natural compounds for cancer therapy, especially in adjuvant or neoadjuvant settings.

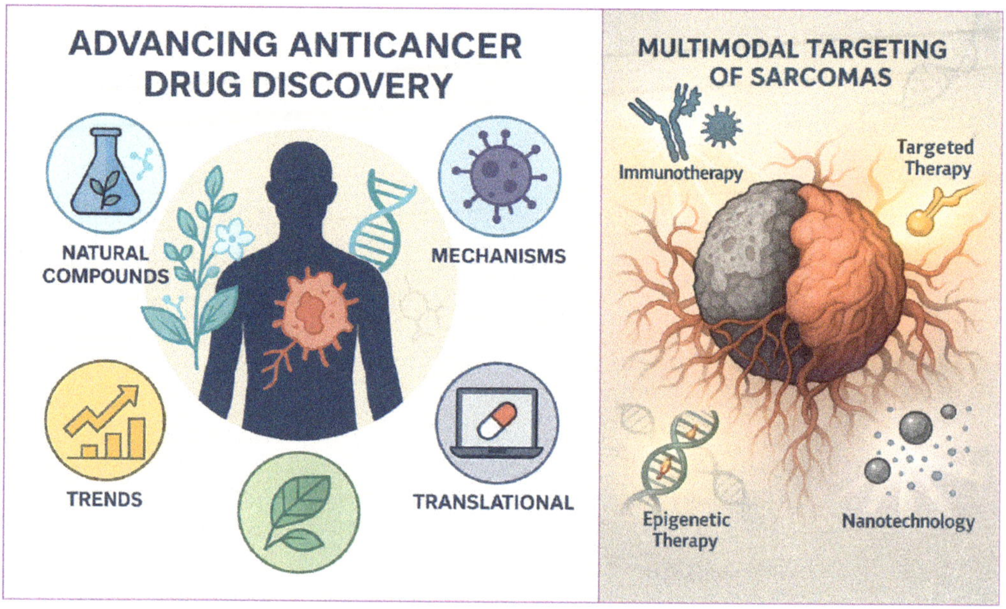

Figure 1. Multimodal strategies must be adopted while targeting various stages of cancers. Figure was generated with assistance of large-language models (LLMs) ChatGPT 4o, OpenAI's DALL·E, and Deepseek.

The study of Campanelli et al. (Contribution 2) established a genetically engineered mouse model which mimics advanced prostate cancer due to overexpression of prostate-specific metastasis-associated protein 1 (MTA1) and a loss of phosphatase and tensin homolog (PTEN) expression. Utilizing this tumor model, the authors showed that gnetin C, a stilbene family polyphenol, suppressed abnormal cell proliferation and angiogenesis and promoted apoptosis through efficient targeting of the MTA1/PTEN/Akt/mTOR pathway. This study provides a "proof-of-principle" that a novel natural compound, such as gnetin C, can target specific oncogenic signaling pathways for clinical management of advanced prostate cancer.

Mohamed and coinvestigators (Contribution 3) conducted a study to evaluate possible anticancer activities of naringin, a polyphenolic phytochemical, and naringin-dextrin nanocomposites (Nar-Dx-NCs) against diethylnitrosamine (DENA)/2-acetylaminofluorene (2-AAF)-induced lung carcinogenesis in rats. Naringin's chemopreventive action against the DEN/2-AAF lung tumor model was amplified by Nar-Dx-NCs as this novel formulation diminished lung carcinogenesis by decreasing tumor cell proliferation, activating apoptosis, and suppressing oxidative stress and inflammation. The encouraging results of this study may lead to additional research to understand the full potential of nanocomposites of naringin again human lung cancer.

Awad et al. (Contribution 4) investigated the therapeutic effect of crocin, a bioactive compound present in saffron, and its combination with sorafenib, a chemotherapeutic drug for hepatocellular carcinoma (HCC), against DENA-induced rat liver carcinogenesis. It was found that crocetin potentiated the anticancer effect of sorafenib. Further, a combined therapy also caused the highest level of apoptosis and a reduction in proliferation, as well as in β-catenin, cyclooxygenase, and nuclear factor-κB levels in tumor tissue, compared to monotreatment with each agent. These encouraging results present a potential strategy to optimize the anti-HCC effect of sorafenib by using a natural compound.

Boulos et al. (Contribution 5) tested the hypothesis that targeting c-MYC, a proto-oncogene, using adapalene, a third-generation retinoid, represents a novel treatment for hematological malignancies. Adapalene exhibited a potent cytotoxic effect through c-MYC inhibition, tubulin network suppression, and DNA damage in vitro and suppressed tumor growth via apoptotic and autophagic cell death in a xenograft zebrafish tumor model. The significance of this work lies in the fact that an adapalene-based design may lead to more effective and targeted therapies for multiple myeloma.

In this collection, four review articles present recent research developments on cancer prevention and anticancer therapeutic activities of various plant-based products and phytochemicals.

Pawłowski and colleagues (Contribution 6) have reviewed the potential anticancer properties of natural polyphenols, specifically curcumin, resveratrol, epigallocatechin-3-gallate, genistein, and quercetin, and related mechanisms of action, such as the inhibition of type IV collagenase enzymes, namely matrix metalloproteinase (MMP)-2 and MMP-9. Emerging evidence based on in vivo and in vitro studies highlighted the polyphenol's antioxidant, anti-inflammatory, pro-apoptotic, antiangiogenic, anti-invasive, and antimetastatic properties. Interestingly, authors have also highlighted various limitations, such as their low solubility and bioavailability, and suggested the utilization of advanced drug delivery systems to overcome these issues.

Jiménez-González and colleagues (Contribution 7) have focused on the anticancer potential of crude extracts and isolated bioactive compounds of the plants belonging to the *Euphorbiaceae* family. They have also covered nanoformulations of these natural products. Potential anticancer molecular mechanisms, such as the induction of apoptosis, modulation of oxidative stress, and interference with cancer cell signaling, highlighted the promising translational potential of *Euphorbiaceae*-derived bioactive compounds for future drug development.

Choudhary and colleagues (Contribution 8) have comprehensively reviewed the major contributing signaling pathways involved in the pathophysiology of lung cancer, currently available treatment options, and the anti-lung cancer potential of naturally occurring bioactive agents, such as alkaloids, terpenoids, phenolics, and sulfur-containing compounds. These phytochemicals were found to target important signaling cascades, including RAF/mitogen-activated protein kinase kinase (MEK)/extracellular signal-regulated kinase (ERK), PI3K/Akt/mTOR, and Janus kinase/signal transducer and activator of transcription (JAK/STAT). Credible evidence based on in vitro, in vivo, and emerging clinical data highlighted the possible translational potential of various natural compounds.

Another comprehensive review article, by Pal and colleagues (Contribution 9), focused on histone deacetylase inhibitors (HDACis), both natural as well as synthetic compounds, for the treatment and management of hematological malignancies, such as acute myeloid leukemia, B-cell lymphoma, and multiple myeloma. The modulation of histone acetylation results in gene expression associated oxidative stress, DNA damage, apoptosis, and autophagy; these are possible mechanisms underlying the anticancer potential of HDACis, with enhanced outcomes, particularly in combination therapies.

In their systematic review and meta-analysis, Odeniran and colleagues (Contribution 10) evaluated the efficacy and safety of camptothecin-derived chemotherapeutics, such as irinotecan and topotecan, combined with other chemotherapeutic agents based on phase

II and III clinical trials. This work covered various cancers, including lung, esophageal, gastric and colorectal cancers. It has been observed that irinotecan in combination with cisplatin could significantly improve response rate and progression-free survival in non-small cell lung cancer. However, irinotecan in combination with bevacizumab yielded superior outcomes in colorectal cancer.

Figure 2 illustrates the frequency mapping of various terminologies presented in the abstracts of the 10 articles of this Special Issue. Various frequently occurring terms were apoptosis, HDACis, naringin, MTA1, adapalene, mTOR, 2-AAF, among others. These articles featured a wide range of information where natural products have been evaluated and targeted against various kind of cancer, including but not limited to breast cancer, prostate cancer, lung cancer, hematological cancers, colorectal cancer, gastric cancer, and hepatocellular carcinoma. All these studies indicate that PI3K/Akt/mTOR, NF-κB, and MMP-related ECM pathways are the most commonly targeted pathways. Moreover, c-MYC, TP53, HDACs, and Bcl-2/Bax were the most studied gene targets in these studies. Gnetin C, oleanolic acid, ursolic acid, naringin, adapalene, and crocin were the promising translational natural agents, discussed repeatedly in these papers. Furthermore, cytotoxic autophagy, natural HDAC inhibitors, and bioavailability-improving nanotechnologies are emerging areas of focus.

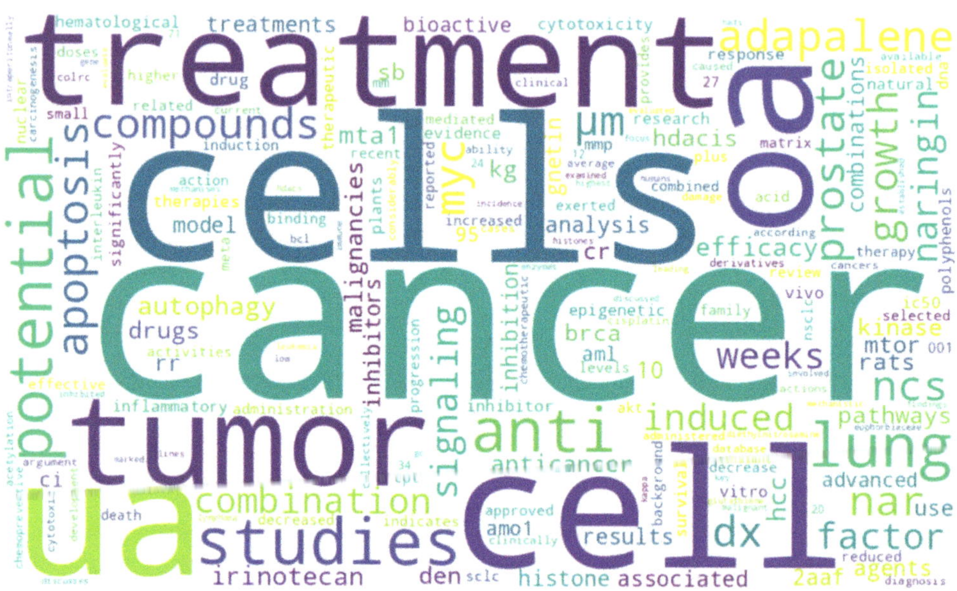

Figure 2. Word cloud with frequency mapping for important cancer and natural product terminology in the abstracts of these papers. This figure was generated with assistance of large-language models (LLMs) ChatGPT 4o, OpenAI's DALL·E, and Deepseek.

Historically, natural product-based drug discovery has been hindered by many concerns, involving a lack of systematic evaluations, unclear molecular targets and signaling networks, translational barriers, and limited synergy with modern tools. The articles published in our Special Issue tackle some of these concerns by conducting comprehensive meta-analyses, elucidating molecular mechanisms, utilizing advanced in silico and 3D modeling approaches, and exploring combination therapies.

3. Future Directions and Perspectives

Although this Special Issue advances knowledge in the domain of natural product-based anticancer drug discovery, the field is growing at a fast pace. Some of the avenues which remains underexplored and where researchers can place more focus in the future are thus listed below:

AI-guided compound screening: AI and ML can rationally expedite natural product screening by filtering out large datasets, such as PubChem, based on the prediction of efficacy, synergy, and toxicity [4,5].

Personalized medicine and biomarker integration: Focus should be on the genomic/molecular stratification to guide natural product-based therapies [6].

A. Emerging trends of natural products in immunotherapy and resistance: Exploration of natural products influencing immune checkpoints, tumor microenvironment, and host–tumor interactions [7,8].

B. Overcoming limitations of natural products: Natural products are not devoid of limitations, and limitations, such as bioavailability and supply, along with other factors limit their translational potential [9–11].

C. Clinical translation pathways: Focused studies with concerted efforts in pharmacokinetics, toxicology, and formulation optimization, so as to bridge gap between pre-clinical and clinical utility [12,13].

D. Microbiome and cancer: Role of microbiota in cancer development, progression, and therapeutic response [14,15].

4. Conclusions

In conclusion, this Special Issue highlights the growing significance of natural products as potential anticancer agents. Through the publication of a collection of original articles and comprehensive reviews, we underscore the therapeutic values and translational potential of bioactive phytochemicals. We urge continued multidisciplinary research and collaboration in advancing modern oncology. Finally, we would like to thank all the editorial team members, authors, and the reviewers for contributing to this Special Issue and advancing anticancer drug discovery and development based on natural products.

Funding: This work of RKS was supported by the Sichuan Science and Technology Program (Grant No. 2025YFHZ0213).

Acknowledgments: The authors have utilized the assistance of large-language models (LLMs) ChatGPT, OpenAI's DALL·E, and DeepSeek for data visualization and interpretation.

Conflicts of Interest: The authors declare no conflicts of interest.

List of Contributions:

1. Gupta, K.B.; Gao, J.; Li, X.; Thangaraju, M.; Panda, S.S.; Lokeshwar, B.L. Cytotoxic Autophagy: A Novel Treatment Paradigm against Breast Cancer Using Oleanolic Acid and Ursolic Acid. *Cancers* **2024**, *16*, 3367. https://doi.org/10.3390/cancers16193367.
2. Campanelli, G.; Francois, E.; Parupathi, P.; Devarakonda, L.S.; Yang, C.; Kumar, A.; Levenson, A.S. The Therapeutic Efficacy and Mechanism of Action of Gnetin C, a Natural Compound from the Melinjo Plant, in a Preclinical Mouse Model of Advanced Prostate Cancer. *Cancers* **2024**, *16*, 1344. https://doi.org/10.3390/cancers16071344.
3. Mohamed, E.E.; Ahmed, O.M.; Zoheir, K.M.A.; El-Shahawy, A.A.G.; Tamur, S.; Shams, A.; Burcher, J.T.; Bishayee, A.; Abdel-Moneim, A. Naringin-Dextrin Nanocomposite Abates Diethylnitrosamine/Acetylaminofluorene-Induced Lung Carcinogenesis by Modulating Oxidative Stress, Inflammation, Apoptosis, and Cell Proliferation. *Cancers* **2023**, *15*, 5102. https://doi.org/10.3390/cancers15205102.

4. Awad, B.; Hamza, A.A.; Al-Maktoum, A.; Al-Salam, S.; Amin, A. Combining Crocin and Sorafenib Improves Their Tumor-Inhibiting Effects in a Rat Model of Diethylnitrosamine-Induced Cirrhotic-Hepatocellular Carcinoma. *Cancers* **2023**, *15*, 4063. https://doi.org/10.3390/cancers15164063.
5. Boulos, J.C.; Chatterjee, M.; Shan, L.; Efferth, T. In Silico, In Vitro, and In Vivo Investigations on Adapalene as Repurposed Third Generation Retinoid against Multiple Myeloma and Leukemia. *Cancers* **2023**, *15*, 4136. https://doi.org/10.3390/cancers15164136.
6. Pawlowski, W.; Caban, M.; Lewandowska, U. Cancer Prevention and Treatment with Polyphenols: Type IV Collagenase-Mediated Mechanisms. *Cancers* **2024**, *16*, 3193. https://doi.org/10.3390/cancers16183193.
7. Jimenez-Gonzalez, V.; Kowalczyk, T.; Piekarski, J.; Szemraj, J.; Rijo, P.; Sitarek, P. Nature's Green Potential: Anticancer Properties of Plants of the Euphorbiaceae Family. *Cancers* **2023**, *16*, 114. https://doi.org/10.3390/cancers16010114.
8. Choudhary, N.; Bawari, S.; Burcher, J.T.; Sinha, D.; Tewari, D.; Bishayee, A. Targeting Cell Signaling Pathways in Lung Cancer by Bioactive Phytocompounds. *Cancers* **2023**, *15*, 3980. https://doi.org/10.3390/cancers15153980.
9. Pal, D.; Raj, K.; Nandi, S.S.; Sinha, S.; Mishra, A.; Mondal, A.; Lagoa, R.; Burcher, J.T.; Bishayee, A. Potential of Synthetic and Natural Compounds as Novel Histone Deacetylase Inhibitors for the Treatment of Hematological Malignancies. *Cancers* **2023**, *15*, 2808. https://doi.org/10.3390/cancers15102808.
10. Odeniran, P.O.; Madlala, P.; Mkhwanazi, N.P.; Soliman, M.E.S. Camptothecin and Its Derivatives from Traditional Chinese Medicine in Combination with Anticancer Therapy Regimens: A Systematic Review and Meta-Analysis. *Cancers* **2024**, *16*, 3802. https://doi.org/10.3390/cancers16223802.

References

1. Bray, F.; Laversanne, M.; Sung, H.; Ferlay, J.; Siegel, R.L.; Soerjomataram, I.; Jemal, A. Global cancer statistics 2022: GLOBOCAN estimates of incidence and mortality worldwide for 36 cancers in 185 countries. *CA Cancer J. Clin.* **2024**, *74*, 229–263. [CrossRef] [PubMed]
2. Siegel, R.L.; Kratzer, T.B.; Giaquinto, A.N.; Sung, H.; Jemal, A. Cancer statistics, 2025. *CA Cancer J. Clin.* **2025**, *75*, 10–45. [CrossRef]
3. Singla, R.K.; Ielciu, I.; Hanganu, D.; Frederich, M. Editorial: Reviews in ethnopharmacology: 2023. *Front. Pharmacol.* **2025**, *16*, 1589249. [CrossRef] [PubMed]
4. Stokes, J.M.; Yang, K.; Swanson, K.; Jin, W.; Cubillos-Ruiz, A.; Donghia, N.M.; MacNair, C.R.; French, S.; Carfrae, L.A.; Bloom-Ackermann, Z.; et al. A Deep Learning Approach to Antibiotic Discovery. *Cell* **2020**, *180*, 688-702.e613. [CrossRef] [PubMed]
5. Zhavoronkov, A.; Ivanenkov, Y.A.; Aliper, A.; Veselov, M.S.; Aladinskiy, V.A.; Aladinskaya, A.V.; Terentiev, V.A.; Polykovskiy, D.A.; Kuznetsov, M.D.; Asadulaev, A.; et al. Deep learning enables rapid identification of potent DDR1 kinase inhibitors. *Nat. Biotechnol.* **2019**, *37*, 1038–1040. [CrossRef] [PubMed]
6. Schilsky, R.L. Personalized medicine in oncology: The future is now. *Nat. Rev. Drug Discov.* **2010**, *9*, 363–366. [CrossRef] [PubMed]
7. O'Donnell, J.S.; Teng, M.W.L.; Smyth, M.J. Cancer immunoediting and resistance to T cell-based immunotherapy. *Nat. Rev. Clin. Oncol.* **2018**, *16*, 151–167. [CrossRef] [PubMed]
8. Sharma, P.; Allison, J.P. The future of immune checkpoint therapy. *Science* **2015**, *348*, 56–61. [CrossRef] [PubMed]
9. Atanasov, A.G.; Zotchev, S.B.; Dirsch, V.M.; Orhan, I.E.; Banach, M.; Rollinger, J.M.; Barreca, D.; Weckwerth, W.; Bauer, R.; Bayer, E.A.; et al. Natural products in drug discovery: Advances and opportunities. *Nat. Rev. Drug Discov.* **2021**, *20*, 200–216. [CrossRef] [PubMed]
10. Atanasov, A.G.; Waltenberger, B.; Pferschy-Wenzig, E.-M.; Linder, T.; Wawrosch, C.; Uhrin, P.; Temml, V.; Wang, L.; Schwaiger, S.; Heiss, E.H.; et al. Discovery and resupply of pharmacologically active plant-derived natural products: A review. *Biotechnol. Adv.* **2015**, *33*, 1582–1614. [CrossRef] [PubMed]
11. Paddon, C.J.; Westfall, P.J.; Pitera, D.J.; Benjamin, K.; Fisher, K.; McPhee, D.; Leavell, M.D.; Tai, A.; Main, A.; Eng, D.; et al. High-level semi-synthetic production of the potent antimalarial artemisinin. *Nature* **2013**, *496*, 528–532. [CrossRef] [PubMed]
12. Newman, D.J.; Cragg, G.M. Natural Products as Sources of New Drugs over the Nearly Four Decades from 01/1981 to 09/2019. *J. Nat. Prod.* **2020**, *83*, 770–803. [CrossRef] [PubMed]
13. Lipinski, C.A.; Lombardo, F.; Dominy, B.W.; Feeney, P.J. Experimental and computational approaches to estimate solubility and permeability in drug discovery and development settings. *Adv. Drug Deliv. Rev.* **2001**, *46*, 3–26. [CrossRef] [PubMed]

14. El Boukhari, R.; Matin, M.; Bouissane, L.; Ławiński, M.; Lushchak, O.; Singla, R.K.; Mickael, M.E.; Mayneris-Perxachs, J.; Grafakou, M.E.; Xu, S.; et al. Enhancing human gut health: Global innovations in dysbiosis management. *iMeta* **2025**, *4*, e70028. [CrossRef] [PubMed]
15. Garrett, W.S. Cancer and the microbiota. *Science* **2015**, *348*, 80–86. [CrossRef] [PubMed]

cancers

MDPI

Article

Cytotoxic Autophagy: A Novel Treatment Paradigm against Breast Cancer Using Oleanolic Acid and Ursolic Acid

Kunj Bihari Gupta [1], Jie Gao [1,2], Xin Li [1,3], Muthusamy Thangaraju [4], Siva S. Panda [4,5] and Bal L. Lokeshwar [1,*]

1 Georgia Cancer Center, Augusta University, Augusta, GA 30912, USA; kugupta@augusta.edu (K.B.G.); gaoj@uab.edu (J.G.); xli@cau.edu (X.L.)

2 Department of Clinical and Diagnostic Science, University of Alabama at Birmingham, Birmingham, AL 35233, USA

3 The Center for Cancer Research and Therapeutic Development, Clark Atlanta University, Atlanta, GA 30314, USA

4 Department of Biochemistry and Molecular Biology, Medical College of Georgia, Augusta University, Augusta, GA 30912, USA; mthangaraju@augusta.edu (M.T.); sipanda@augusta.edu (S.S.P.)

5 Department of Chemistry and Biochemistry, College of Science and Mathematics, Augusta University, Augusta, GA 30912, USA

* Correspondence: blokeshwar@augusta.edu

Simple Summary: Cancer chemotherapy is dominated by cytotoxic drugs that non-selectively kill proliferating cells by blocking DNA replication and inducing apoptosis. Some natural anticancer products are less toxic to normal, slow-replicating cells but kill aggressive tumor cells. The combination of two structural isomers of pentacyclic triterpenes, oleanolic acid and ursolic acid, showed potent cytotoxic activity in human breast cancer cells in vitro by inducing cytotoxic autophagy at a significantly lower dose than previously reported. They were nontoxic to breast epithelial cells. Their activity was mainly due to the inhibition of AKT-mediated cell survival and the inhibition of the mammalian target of rapamycin (mTOR) signaling pathway, a central regulator of cell metabolism, growth, and proliferation. The compounds were equally effective against ER+ and triple-negative breast cancer cells. Combining low doses of nontoxic inhibitors of PI3k kinase increased the activities of these compounds. In contrast, inhibition of autophagy by 3-methyl adenine annulled their activity, demonstrating that cytotoxic autophagy may be the dominant mechanism of cell death. These compounds have potential for cancer therapy in neoadjuvant or adjuvant settings.

Abstract: Background: Oleanolic acid (OA) and Ursolic acid (UA) are bioactive triterpenoids. Reported activities vary with the dose used for testing their activities in vitro. Studies using doses of ≥20 µM showed apoptosis activities in cancer cells. However, reported drug levels in circulation achieved by oral administration of UA and OA are ≤2 µM, thus limiting their use for treatment or delivering a combination treatment. Materials and Methods: The present report demonstrates the efficacy of OA, UA, and OA + UA on tumor cell-specific cytotoxicity at low doses (5 µM to 10 µM) in breast cancer (BrCa) cell lines MCF7 and MDA-MB231. Results: The data show that both OA and UA killed BrCa cells at low doses, but were significantly less toxic to MCF-12A, a non-tumorigenic cell line. Moreover, OA + UA at ≤10 µM was lethal to BrCa cells. Mechanistic studies unraveled the significant absence of apoptosis, but their cytotoxicity was due to the induction of excessive autophagy at a OA + UA dose of 5 µM each. A link to drug-induced cytotoxic autophagy was established by demonstrating a lack of their cytotoxicity by silencing the autophagy-targeting genes (ATGs), which prevented OA-, UA-, or OA + UA-induced cell death. Further, UA or OA + UA treatment of BrCa cells caused an inhibition of PI3 kinase-mediated phosphorylation of Akt/mTOR, the key pathways that regulate cancer cell survival, metabolism, and proliferation. Discussion: Combinations of a PI3K inhibitor (LY294002) with OA, UA, or OA + UA synergistically inhibited BrCa cell survival. Therefore, the dominance of cytotoxic autophagy by inhibiting PI3K-mediated autophagy may be the primary mechanism of PTT-induced anticancer activity in BrCa cells. Conclusion: These results suggest it would be worthwhile testing combined OA and UA in clinical settings.

Keywords: bioactive triterpenoids; triple-negative breast cancer; PI3 kinase inhibition; mitophagy; combination therapy

1. Introduction

Globally, breast cancer (BrCa) ranks second in incidence and mortality among women with cancer. The American Cancer Society reports about 310,720 women are likely to be diagnosed with invasive BrCa, with an estimated 42,250 deaths in the USA [1]. These grim data portray a dire situation where, despite the multiple modalities of treatment and therapy with multiple anticancer drugs approved by agencies such as the FDA, BrCa is a significant health concern in women. More potent, yet less toxic treatment must be developed for therapies against BrCa.

The patient's BrCa treatment depends on the patients' tumor stage and age [2]. The common initial treatment for localized disease is surgery or non-invasive high-beam radiation therapy. The non-surgical or post-surgical treatment options for BrCa patients vary, but most rely on cytotoxic chemotherapy drugs for post-surgical or radiation treatment to eliminate residual tumor cells in lymph node-positive BrCa patients. However, many women who receive adjuvant chemotherapy for early-stage breast cancer do not benefit significantly [3]. The cytotoxic chemotherapeutic (drugs) can cause systemic toxicity due to non-selective targets and the emergence of more aggressive drug-resistant BrCa that further require multiple treatment regimens. Chemo-hormonal therapies are increasingly used to combat disease progression and prolong therapeutic efficacy in patients with tumor biopsies showing cells with estrogen receptor (ER), progesterone receptor (PR), and human EGF receptor 2 (HER2) positivity [4,5]. However, patients with disease progression to the ER, PR, and HER2-negative (triple receptor-negative) stage of BrCa (TNBC) are given broader options, but with limited efficacy. TNBC is generally a disseminated disease with limited access to targeting specific therapy (e.g., metastasis to brain and bones) and highly aggressive proliferation.

Recently, more specific, molecularly targeted drugs have been developed that block specific tumor cell survival pathways, such as mTOR-mediated pathway inhibitors [6,7], targeting the cell cycle and metabolism [8,9], and those affecting the tumor microenvironment, such as immunotherapies. Treatment efficacy with all these agents suffers the same fate as chemotherapy drugs, namely, progression of therapy-resistant disease or significant systemic toxicity experienced by a sizable fraction of patients who opt for immunotherapies [10,11]. Anticancer agents that enhance cytotoxic drugs' therapeutic efficacy without significantly increasing systemic toxicity should improve the effectiveness and therapeutic index. Synthetic inhibitors of critical signaling molecules that trigger tumor cell proliferation, metastasis, and development of resistance have been extensively developed, yet much is needed to eliminate cancer deaths. Bioactive phytochemicals, identified by serendipity or empirical research, have been constantly evolving and tested for potential application in BrCa treatment. Several candidate phytochemicals have been investigated to treat BrCa, including many forms of curcumin, triterpenes, antiestrogens (e.g., genistein), polyphenols, and others. However, most of these compounds are seldom used in the clinic, as they do not meet the rigors of sufficient clinical efficacy [12]. However, natural compounds with unique bioactivities as anti-inflammatory and antiproliferative agents may offer significant advantages in treating patients alone or in a neoadjuvant or adjuvant setting.

The pentacyclic triterpenoids, such as ursolic acid (UA) and oleanolic acid (OA), are triterpenoids that function similarly to plant steroid hormones that are bioactive in human cells [13]. These compounds and betulinic acid are the most studied among triterpenes for human health [14,15]. Due to their abundance and ubiquitous presence in many edible plant products, UA and OA have been extensively investigated for their bioactivities in multiple ailments, including cancer [16–18], and their mechanisms of action in cancer cells [19,20]. However, in nature, OA and UA exist as structural isomers and their yields vary extensively from various natural sources, such as olives and apple peels [21,22]. Despite the molecular equivalency, there have been studies on a combination of OA and UA against cancer cells [23–26]. We saw significant potential for combining OA and UA to enhance the bioactivity, as both compounds have shown minimum systemic toxicity in the limited toxicological studies in humans [27]. In this study, we investigated the bioactivity and mechanism of OA and UA individually and in combination at various ratios to identify any advantage of using a specific combination of OA and UA to enhance bioactivity in BrCa cells. We report that the combination of OA and UA shows higher cancer cell-specific toxicity at lower doses than when used individually.

2. Materials and Methods

2.1. Chemicals of Certified Highest Quality from the Manufacturers Used in This Study

They were purchased from laboratory suppliers based in the USA, and details of these specific chemicals and kits are listed below in Table 1.

Table 1. List of fine chemicals used in this study.

Fine Chemicals	CAS No.	Manufacturer and Catalogue No.
Oleanolic acid (OA)	508-02-1	TCI America (Portland, OR, USA) O0317
Ursolic acid (UA)	77-52-1	Sigma-Aldrich U6753
LY294002	154447-36-6	LC Laboratories (Woburn, MA, USA) L-7988
Rapamycin	53123-88-9	LC Laboratories R-5000
Staurosporine	62996-74-1	Fisher Scientific/MedChem Express (Monmouth Junction, NJ, USA) NC1401148
TUNEL assay kit		Roche (Indianapolis, IN, USA) 11684795910

2.2. Cell Culture Methods

The human BrCa cell lines MCF7 and MDA-MB231 and non-malignant breast epithelial cell line MCF-12A were purchased from the ATCC (Manassas, VA, USA). All studies reported here were from cell cultures derived from aliquots frozen during the first five passages of ATCC stocks, as described before [28]. Periodically, cells were authenticated by Lab Corp Cell Line Authentication Lab, Burlington, NC. All cell lines were routinely cultured in the media recommended by ATCC (ATCC.Org, Manassas, VA, USA). Briefly, we maintained cells in RPMI 1640 medium supplemented with fetal bovine serum (10%, Bio-West USA Inc., Bradenton, FL, USA) and 0.2 mg/L gentamycin solution (IBI Scientific, Dubuque, IA, USA) with passaging every 5–7 days. All drug treatments were performed in cells cultured in multiwell plates with a seeding density of ~3–6 × 10^3 cells/cm^2 or as indicated for each experiment. Cultures were maintained in water-jacketed incubators with sterile air with 5% CO_2 and maintained at 37 °C.

2.3. Cell Viability Assay

The viability of cells treated with several doses of OA, UA, and their combination were estimated using a colorimetric assay, the 3-[4,5-dimethylthiazol-2-yl]-2,5-diphenyl-tetrazolium bromide (MTT) reduction assay. Briefly, cells were cultured in 96-well plates at a density of 2000 cells per well, and overnight-cultured cells were treated with the appropriate doses of OA, UA, and both for 72 h. Following incubation, the viability of surviving cells was determined by incubating with MTT solution (0.5 mg/mL) at 37 °C for three hours. The precipitated purple formazan crystals were dissolved in DMSO, and absorbance was read at 570/640 nm with a spectrophotometer. The fraction of viable cells is expressed as a percentage of viable cells from the ratio of the OD of treated wells divided by the OD of diluent-only treated cultures (control) [29,30].

2.4. Clonogenic Survival (Colony-Forming) Assay

The BrCa cells were cultured in replicate 35 mm-diameter 6-well plates at a density of ~1000 cells per well. The cell cultures were incubated with various doses of OA, UA, and both for 72 h. The culture medium was changed to remove drugs, and surviving cells were left to form colonies for the next 7–10 days. Emerged cell colonies after incubation were fixed with methanol and stained with 0.5% crystal violet for 30 min. Then, they were washed gently to remove excess dye solution and air-dried before manually counting the number of visible colonies by at least two investigators [31].

2.5. Target Identification by Immunoblotting

We prepared cell lysates from cultured cells treated with several doses of OA and UA and estimated total proteins in the lysates. Required sample lysates were boiled in SDS–polyacrylamide gel electrophoresis (SDS-PAGE) sample buffer, fractionated by SDS-PAGE under chemically reduced conditions, and blotted onto PVDF membranes for Western blot analysis as reported before [32]. The blots were incubated with indicated primary and secondary antibodies (see Table 2) and developed to visualize protein bands using an enhanced chemiluminescence detection kit [31] Blot images were captured using the Bio-Rad ChemiDoc™ Touch imaging system. Unless indicated otherwise, blots of β-actin in each sample were used as an internal loading control [31].

Table 2. List of antibodies used in this study.

Name of Antibody	Manufacturer and Catalogue No.	RRID
PARP	Cell Signaling Technology (Danvers, MA, USA) 9542	AB_2160739
mTOR	Cell Signaling Technology 2983	AB_2105622
p-mTOR (Ser2481)	Cell Signaling Technology 2974	AB_2262884
LC3B	ABclonal (Woburn, MA, USA) A7198	AB_2863546
P62/SQSTM1	Cell Signaling Technology 5114	AB_10624872
ULK-1	Cell Signaling Technology 4773	AB_2288252
pULK-1 (Ser757)	Cell Signaling Technology 6888	AB_10829226
P70S6 Kinase	ABclonal A2190	AB_2749844
p-P70S6 Kinase (Ser371)	Cell Signaling Technology 9208	AB_330990
4EBP1	Cell Signaling Technology 9644	AB_2097841
p-4EBP1 (Thr37/46)	Cell Signaling Technology 2855	AB_560835
AKT (Pan)	Cell Signaling Technology 9272	AB_329827
p-AKT (Thr308)	Epitomics (Burlingame, CA, USA) 2214	
p-AKT (Ser473)	Cell Signaling Technology 4060	AB_2315049
ATG-5	Cell Signaling Technology 2630	AB_2062340
ATG-7	Cell Signaling Technology 2631	AB_2227783
β-Actin	Proteintech (Rosemont, IL, USA) HRP-60008	AB_2819183
Anti-rabbit Secondary	Cell Signaling Technology 7074	AB_2099233
Fluorescence-labeled Secondary Antibody	Goat anti-Rabbit IgG (H + L) Alexa Fluor™ 488 A11008	AB_143165

2.6. Apoptotic DNA Fragmentation Assay: TUNEL Assay

Cells undergoing apoptotic death were detected by fluorescence labeling of their DNA fragments using a terminal deoxynucleotidyl transferase dUTP nick-end labeling kit (TUNEL kit, Table 1) according to the manufacturer's instructions. Briefly, cells were cultured and treated with 0.05% DMSO (Control), 2.0 μM staurosporine as a positive control (Sigma Aldrich Inc., St. Louis, MO, USA), OA, UA, and both for 48 h. Treated cells were fixed with 4% paraformaldehyde (PFA) and permeabilized with 0.1% Triton X-100 solution.

The intracellular fragments of DNA were then labeled with TUNEL reaction mixture for 1 h at 37 °C in a humidified chamber in the dark. Labeled cells in culture chambers were washed twice and mounted with a coverslip before microscopy. The fluorescence images of labeled cells were captured using a Keyence inverted fluorescence microscope [33].

2.7. Localization of LC3B and LC3BII by Immunofluorescence

Subcellular localization and formation of LC3B puncta were examined by fluorescence microscopy of cells labeled with anti-LC3BII antibody and anti-Rb-Alexa fluor IgG-Fab2 and counterstained with DAPI [4]. Slides were observed, and the fluorescence images were captured on the Keyence fluorescence microscope.

2.8. Autophagy Flux Determination

We used a dual-label fluorescence quench assay with cells transfected with a plasmid containing mCherry-GFP-LC3B genes in tandem sequence (Addgene Inc., Cambridge MA, USA), as reported in previous studies [4,34]. Briefly, cells were seeded in 35 mm culture dishes with glass coverslips placed in the bottom (MatTek catalogue number P35G) in an antibiotic-free media. Cultured cells were transfected with mCherry-GFP-LC3B plasmid using Lipofectamine™ 2000 (Life Technologies) as per the provider's instructions. Transfected cells were used for subsequent treatment with drugs 48 h after transfection. After completion of treatment (24 h), cells were labeled with DAPI DNA-binding dye and observed under the fluorescence microscope without formalin fixation. Fluorescence images of live cells were captured.

2.9. Alteration of ATG5 and ATG7 Levels Using siRNA-Mediated Gene Silencing

Human-specific small interfering RNA (siRNA) for ATG5 and ATG7 and scrambled siRNA were purchased from a vendor (Dharmacon, Thermo Fisher Scientific Inc., Waltham, MA, USA). The MCF7 andMDA-MB231 cells were cultured in 6-well plates and transfected with siRNAs using Lipofectamine™ 2000. Transfected cells were treated with UA, OA, and both for 48 h. Treated and control cultures with or without specific ATG siRNA were harvested to make cell lysates and assess viability following OA and UA treatment. Protein expression for ATG5 and ATG7 in control siRNA and specific siRNA transfectants was determined by Western blotting. An MTT-reduction assay was used to estimate cell viability after silencing these genes.

2.10. Statistical Analysis

All quantitative assays were conducted with triplicate samples in each experiment, and the experiments were repeated at least three times. Data are presented as means ± SD from the repeated experiments. We used Student's *t*-test or one-way ANOVA to determine statistical significance for all quantitative experiments. The comparison of combined data with a value of $p < 0.05$ against the null hypothesis was considered statistically significant. GraphPad Prism 9 (GraphPad Inc., San Diego, CA, USA) program was used for rapid analyses.

3. Results

3.1. OA and UA Specifically Inhibit the Growth and Colony-Forming Capacity of BrCa Cells, but Are Nontoxic to Normal Breast Epithelial Cells

Established BrCa cell lines and normal breast epithelial cells were treated with multiple doses of UA and OA separately and in combination to determine their effect on the viability of the incubated cells. The surviving cell fractions following 72 h incubation with the drugs were determined by MTT colorimetric assay, and the dose required to reduce the surviving fractions by 50% (IC50) was calculated. The IC50 of UA, OA, and OA + UA combination varied widely between the drugs and the cells tested. As listed in Figure 1A, OA and UA were weakly toxic to the non-tumorigenic MCF12A cells (IC50 > 50 μM), whereas they were toxic to tumorigenic MCF7 and MDA-MB231 cell lines. However, when cells were treated with UA and OA in a 1:1 ratio, the viability of MCF7 and MB231 cells significantly decreased, although this combination was weakly toxic to MCF-12A cells (Figure 1B).

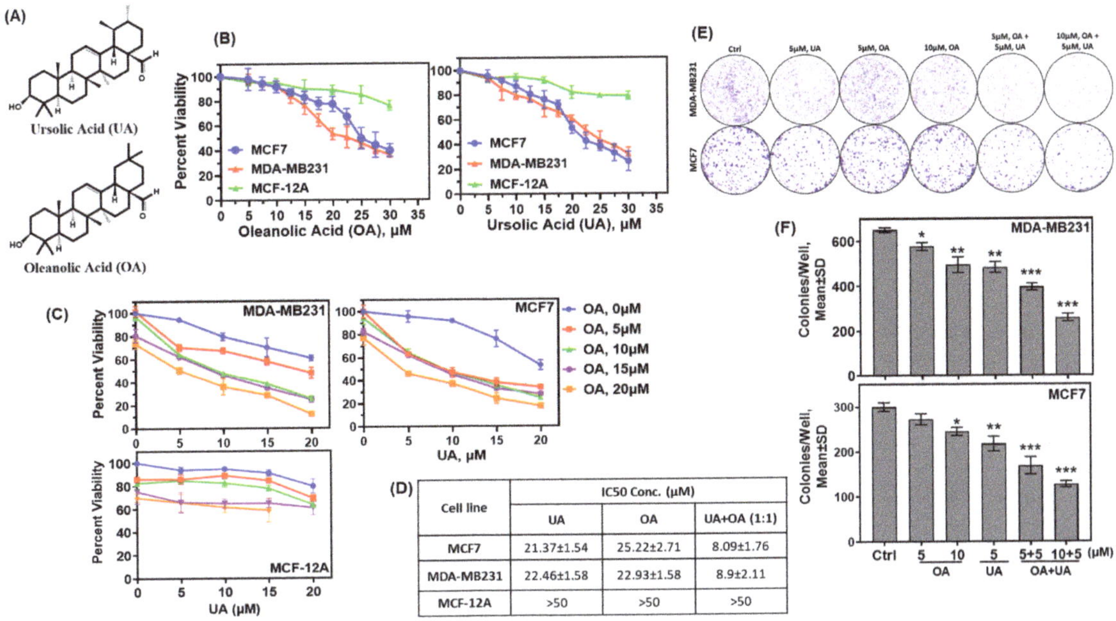

Cell line	IC50 Conc. (μM)		
	UA	OA	UA+OA (1:1)
MCF7	21.37±1.54	25.22±2.71	8.09±1.76
MDA-MB231	22.46±1.58	22.93±1.58	8.9±2.11
MCF-12A	>50	>50	>50

Figure 1. Pentacyclic triterpenes (PTTs) UA and OA induced cytotoxicity in normal breast epithelial cells and BrCa cells. (**A**) Chemical structure of UA and OA. (**B**) Cytotoxicity of OA and UA on MCF-12A (normal mammary epithelial cell line), MCF7, and MDA-MB231 cells. Surviving fractions after 72 h incubation with OA (**left** panel) and UA (**right** panel) were estimated by MTT-reduction colorimetric assay. (**C**) Surviving fractions (%) of BrCa cells and MCF-12A cells at various combinations of OA and UA. (**D**) Summary of IC50 of OA and UA on BrCa and MCF-12A cells. (**E**) Inhibition of clonogenic potential of BrCa cells treated with OA, UA, and both: colonies of surviving cells formed in 7 to 10 days following treatment with UA, OA, and both for three days. (**F**) Quantitative analysis of colonies/well (mean ± SD, n = 3) for MDA-MB231 and MCF7 cells. Pairwise *t*-tests were used to determine significance: * $p < 0.05$, ** $p < 0.005$, or *** $p < 0.001$ with untreated cell colonies as control.

Colorimetric assays to determine cytotoxicity using compounds such as MTT do not distinguish between the cytostatic versus cytotoxic effect of a drug or a drug's potential to diminish the clonogenic potential of the tumor cells if the cells are cultured in the absence of drugs following treatment. We opted to evaluate the cytotoxicity of OA, UA, and OA + UA combinations following a 72 h treatment rather than the commonly used 48 h, as the tested cell lines, including the non-transformed MCF-12A, had different rates of population doubling compared to MDA-MB231. Clonogenic survival or colony-formation assays provide a more accurate determination of tumor cells' survival potential, even after termination of therapy. We determined the activity of OA and UA and their combination to destroy the colony-forming potential without the drug. Cells were incubated with OA and UA at several doses alone or in combination for three days, followed by incubation in a drug-free growth medium for the next 7 to 10 days or until the surviving cells formed visible colonies in the culture dishes. Results of colony counts from each treatment group are shown in Figure 1B,D, showing a significant decline in colony numbers in UA- and OA-treated groups. As estimated by MTT assays in Figure 1A, colony numbers declined at all doses of UA and OA, but were significantly higher in the OA + UA treatment

(Figure 1D). These results demonstrate UA- and OA-induced cytotoxicity, but not reversible cytostatic activity.

We determined whether the cytotoxic effects of combination OA and UA treatment were additive, synergistic, or non-additive by the combination effect equation of Chou and Talalay [35]. The analysis performed using the program CompusSyn (PD Science, Paramus, NJ, USA) showed the combination index (C.I) < 1.0 in all combinations of OA and UA on both BrCa cells (Supplementary Figure S1). The normalized isobologram for the OA + UA combination was <1.0 at all doses tested. These results indicate the potential to increase the efficacy of UA and OA in small combinations and reduce the dose of either drug for treatment without affecting the efficacy.

3.2. *OA and UA Do Not Induce Programmed Cell Death (Apoptosis) in BrCa Cells*

Multiple publications have reported apoptosis as the principal mechanism of cell death in UA-treated cells. However, these studies used high doses of UA (>25 μM) in such demonstrations. Since we observed significant lethality of UA on BrCa cells at <10 μM of UA, we investigated whether apoptosis is the major mechanism of cell death at low doses of UA. We determined cleaved poly-adenosine ribose phosphorylase (PARP) levels and cellular DNA fragmentation (TUNEL) levels as markers of apoptosis in the control and PPT-treated cells. We attempted to detect both intact (116 kDa) and cleaved (89 kDa) PARP proteins in cells treated with PPTs and untreated control cells by Western blotting (Figure 2A). We found cleaved fragments of PARP only in cell lysates prepared from cells treated with the protein kinase C inhibitor staurosporine (Sta, 2.0 μM) for the same duration as other drugs in both MCF7 and MB231 cells (Figure 2A). The intact status of PARP detected in Western blots showed a lack of significant apoptosis.

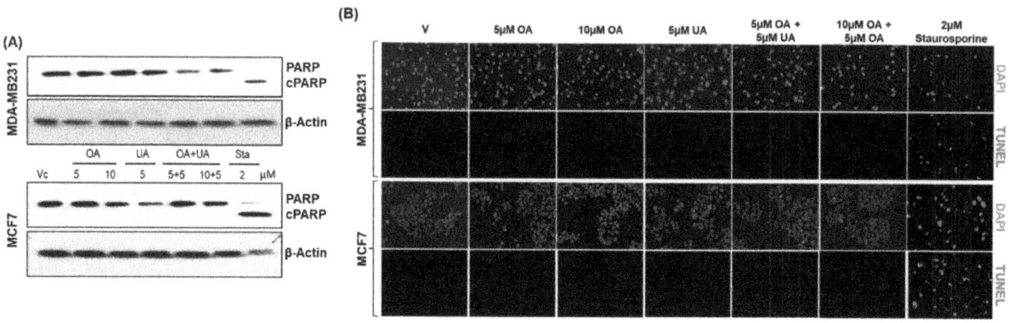

Figure 2. Lack of apoptotic activity in OA- and UA-treated BrCa cells. (**A**). Apoptotic activity visualized as changes in cleaved PARP by immunoblotting analysis showed a lack of cleaved PARP (c-PARP) in MDA-MB231 and MCF7 cells treated with OA, UA, and both. However, cells treated with 2 μM staurosporine (Sta) showed cPARP. β-actin bands reference the uniform loading of cell lysates in all electrophoretic blot lanes. Original images of western blots are shown in Supplementary Materials File S1. (**B**). DNA fragmentation levels in situ due to apoptosis were analyzed in BrCa cells by the TUNEL (terminal deoxynucleotidyl transferase dUTP nick-end labeling) assay. DNA fragmentation fluoresced red, and cells with intact nuclei did not. Cells treated with PTTs did not fluoresce, but those treated with staurosporine did, indicating an absence of apoptosis in PTT-treated cell cultures (Magnification: 100×).

Next, we examined the presence of DNA fragmentation in OA- and UA-treated cells. We used a fluorescence in situ terminal deoxynucleotidyl transferase dUTP nick-end labeling (TUNEL) assay with Texas red-labeled uridine nucleotide mix [36]. As shown in Figure 2B, Texas red-labeled TUNEL-positive fluorescence was found only in cells treated with 2 μM staurosporine, but not in cells treated with UA, OA, or UA + OA at doses $\leq$ 10 μM. These two results convinced us that apoptosis is not a likely cell death mechanism in BrCa cells after OA and UA treatments. The potential for other forms of apoptosis, such as necroptosis or ferroptosis, was unlikely, as the TUNEL-positive cells or cleaved PARP were uniformly absent in all treated samples at the indicated drug concentrations. Next, we investigated other potential cell death mechanisms, such as cytotoxic autophagy.

3.3. OA- and UA-Induced Cell Death via Activation of Autophagy

Several researchers have reported autophagy as a potential cell death mechanism. It has been reported that UA and OA induce autophagy in BrCa cells [14], where their cytotoxicity may be attributed to both apoptosis and autophagy. We determined the levels of the LC-3B protein (microtubule-associated protein 1A/1B-light chain 3 (LC3)) and P62/SQSTM1, well-known autophagy markers. As shown in Figure 3A, the levels of LC3B and P62 expression increased in the cells upon treatment with OA, UA, their combination, and rapamycin (a known inducer of autophagy).

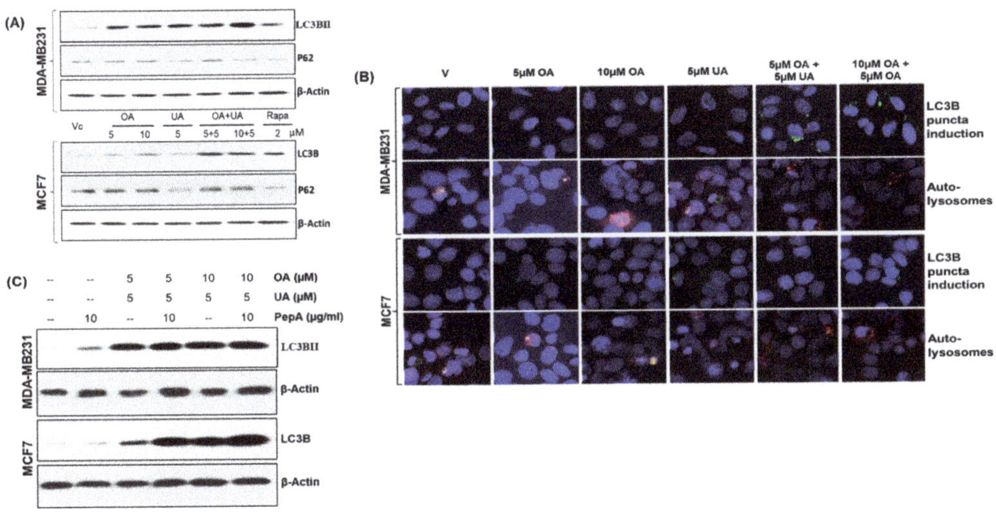

Figure 3. OA and UA combination treatment causes cell death in BrCa cells by cytotoxic autophagy. (**A**) Increased expression of two autophagy markers, LC3BII and P62 (SQSTM1), was found in the cells treated with OA, UA, and both in MDA-MB321 and MCF7 cells. The doses of the PTTs used for autophagy induction are shown in the middle or top panels. (**B**) The translocation of LC3B on the puncta of autophagosomes was made visible with FITC-labeled anti-rabbit antibodies against anti-LC3B antibodies, followed by counterstaining the cells with DAPI (top panel). Increased autophagic flux in PTT-treated BrCa cells was detected using differential localization of mCherry-GFP-LC3B-transfected cells treated with PTTs. The LC3B molecules exiting from neutral pH autophagosomes to acidic autolysosomes are shown. An increased level of autolysosomes in treated cells visualized by red fluorescence (mCherry) and quenching of GFP (green) in the acidic compartment of autophagosomes resulting from the fusion of autophagosomes and lysosomes. (**C**). Western blot analysis of LC3BII protein after treating both BrCa cell lines with OA, UA, and both with and without PepA (pepstatin A, an inhibitor of lysosomal proteases). The micrographs (magnification: 200×) shown are representative images from three replicate experiments. Original images of western blots are shown in Supplementary Materials File S1.

The expression of LC3B and its externalization as LC3BII in the puncta were observed following immunofluorescence labeling with anti-LC3B antibody. LC3BII localization in the puncta is an indicator of increased autophagic flux. The autophagosome formation seen in MCF7 and MDA-MD231 cell cultures treated with OA, UA, and OA + UA or rapamycin (Figure 3B, first and third panels) shows increased autophagy following drug treatment.

The cytoplasmic LC3B (LC3BI) is constitutively expressed, but the lighter chair, LC3BII, is associated with phagosome formation with characteristic puncta [4]. We determined the relative proportion of LC3B to LC3 using dual-autofluorescence protein labeled LC3 expression plasmid. A vital step of the autophagy process is the formation of an autolysosome. We utilized a selective in situ fluorescence quench assay to determine the dynamics of autophagy flux. For this, BrCa cells were transiently transfected with the mCherry-GFP-LC3 vector. The increase in autophagy (flux) resulted in the localization of LC3BII in acidic lysosomes, which quenched GFP. This quenching made only red (mCherry) fluorescence visible. If any drug treatment does not cause an increase in autophagy flux, the cells exhibit predominantly green fluorescence (GFP) or a mix of green and red (orange) fluorescence. As shown in Figure 3B (second panel for MDA-MB231 cells and fourth panel for MCF7 cells), a significant increase in overall autolysosomes was found, also predominantly displaying red fluorescence, indicating increased flux and thus rapid recycling of degraded proteins for catabolism. The flux was further enhanced in MDA-MB231 and MCF7 cells upon exposure to OA + UA. The autolysosome formation and red fluorescence were comparatively high in cells with OA + UA combination treatment.

We confirmed the increased occurrence of autophagy following exposure to OA and UA by treating the cells (or not) with pepstatin A (PepA), a known inhibitor of lysosomal proteases. Cell lysates were analyzed by immunoblotting for LC3BII. As presented in Figure 3C, the LC3BII levels did not decrease upon treatment with PepA in OA- or UA-treated cells, indicating the increased LC3BII levels were due to increased conversion of LC3BI to the autosomal puncta. These findings strongly support the occurrence of autophagy upon exposure to OA and UA.

3.4. Mechanism of Increased Autophagy in OA-, UA-, and OA + UA-Treated BrCa Cells

Autophagy constitutes an intricate biological process characterized by the orchestrated involvement of diverse proteins operating sequentially. We analyzed the cell lysates prepared from BrCa cells (MCF7 and MDA-MB231) treated with several doses and a combination of OA, UA, and rapamycin. The mammalian target of rapamycin (mTOR) is a crucial regulator of signals involved with protein synthesis, cell growth, and metabolism. It is also a master regulator of autophagy [37,38]. Under a normal state, mTOR is associated with other induction complexes (ULK1 and Atg13). It is reported that inhibition of mTOR phosphorylation (phospho-mTOR, p-mTOR) induces autophagy. As shown in Figure 4, the levels of p-mTOR (p-Ser2481) were significantly reduced in UA- and OA + UA-treated cells of both MCF7 and MB-231 lines, but OA did not inhibit p-mTOR.

Interestingly, the expression of ULK1 and phospho-ULK1 levels differentially varied in MCF7 and MDA-MB231 cells. ULK1 and p-ULK1 levels were low in control (0.1% DMSO, vehicle) MDA-MB231 cells, and p-ULK1 was increased with OA, UA, and OA + UA combination treatment (Figure 4, rows 3 and 4).

Ribosomal protein S6 kinase beta 1 (P70 S6 kinase) is a crucial regulator of the cell cycle, cellular proliferation, and autophagy process. The expression of P70 S6 kinase and P70 S6 kinase (Ser371) were high in treated cells compared with untreated, but its expression was higher following UA and OA + UA combination treatments (Figure 4) in both MCF7 and MDA-MB231 cells.

Eukaryotic translation initiation factor 4E-binding protein 1 (4EBP1) is a downstream effector of mTOR and negatively regulates autophagy. 4EBP1 was constitutively expressed in vehicle-only treated cells and cells treated with OA or UA alone. Still, its expression was drastically reduced in cells treated with OA + UA combination or rapamycin. The phosphorylated form of 4EBP1, 4EBP1Thr37/46 expression was minimal in MDA-MB231 cells following treatment but was higher in MCF7 cells. These results cumulatively indicate the initiation of phagophore formation in treated cells, especially with the OA + UA combination, and progression of the autophagosome, with ultimate induction of excessive autophagy-induced cell death.

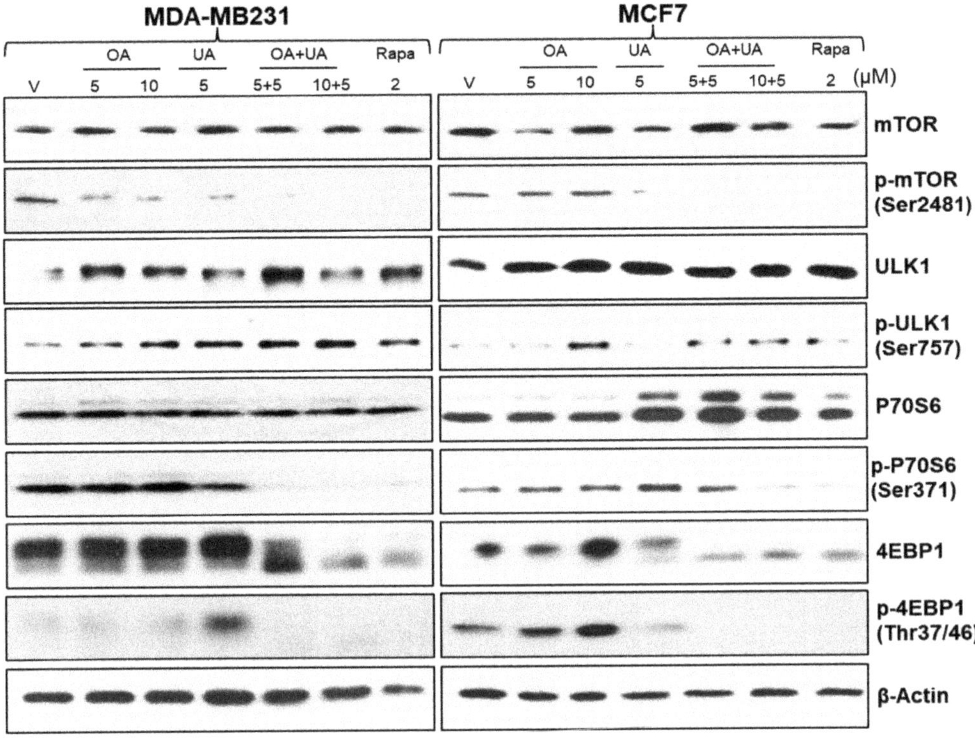

Figure 4. The molecular landmarks of autophagy-induced cell death in BrCa cells were analyzed by Western blotting of cell lysates from BrCa cells treated with OA, UA, and both. Molecular analysis of rapamycin-treated cells served as a positive control. β-actin was used as an internal loading control. Results were comparable from all three replicate experiments. Original images of western blots are shown in Supplementary Materials File S1.

3.5. *OA- and UA-Induced Autophagy Is Regulated by ATG5 and ATG7*

To understand the induction of autophagy cascade resulting from OA, UA, and OA + UA treatments, we investigated the role of two critical autophagy-regulating genes (ATGs) by transiently depleting ATG7 and ATG5 in both MCF7 and MDA-MB231 cells by siRNAs and measuring the viability of depleted cells when treated with OA, UA, and OA + UA. As shown in Figure 5A, ATG5, and ATG7 proteins were completely depleted using the on-target siRNA-transfected cells, whereas their expression was unaltered in cells transfected with scrambled siRNA (control). Furthermore, treating the transfected cells with UA, OA, and OA + UA did not increase the expression of these two ATGs in mRNA-depleted MCF7 or MDA-MB231 cells. The expression of LC3BII in ATG-mRNA-depleted cells was undetectable in both cell lines, irrespective of drug treatment (Figure 5B).

We next investigated if inhibition of autophagy regulators could reduce the cytotoxicity of OA, UA, or both in the two BrCa cell lines. We performed cell viability assays on the ATG knockdown cells after treating them with OA, UA, and OA + UA. The results presented in Figure 5C show increased viability by >50% in MB231 and >40% in MCF7 cells that did not express ATGs or LC3Bs compared to scrambled siRNA (control)-transfected cells. These observations indicated that inhibiting the ATG5 and ATG7 significantly, although not wholly, rescued OA- and UA induced cytotoxicity, further corroborating other related observations presented in this report.

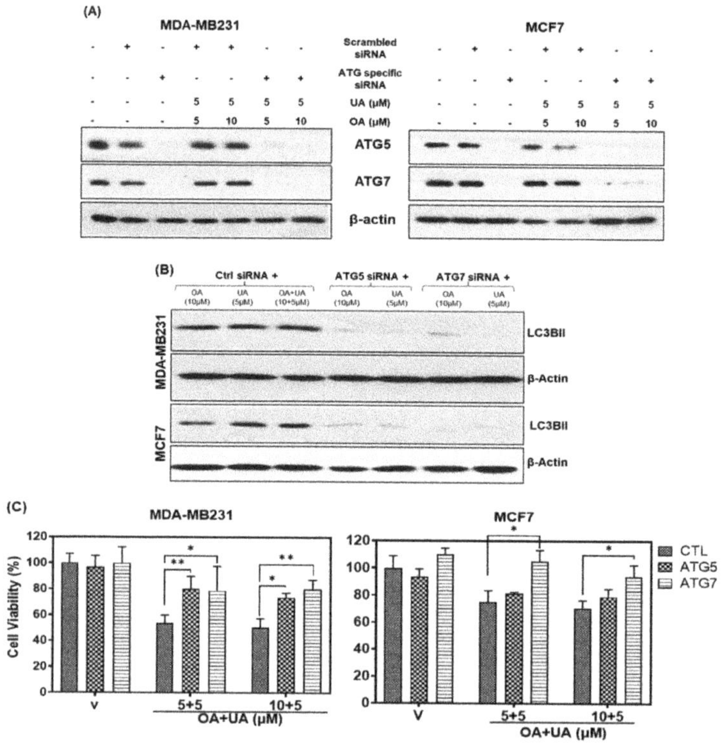

Figure 5. The knockdown of ATGs blocks the PTT-induced autophagy and cell death. (**A**) Immunoblotting after silencing of ATG7 and ATG5 by siRNA and treating with OA and UA in both BrCa cells (MDA-MB231 and MCF7). (**B**) Cell viability assay: increased cell viability in ATG knockdown BrCa cells compared to the control siRNA after OA and UA treatments. Results are expressed as mean ± SD (n = 3), and pairwise *t*-tests were used to determine the significance: $p < 0.05$ = * $p < 0.005$ = **. (**C**) Induction of autophagy (level of LC3BII) after treating the ATG knockdown BrCa cells with OA, UA, and both. β-actin was used as an internal loading control for all Western blots. Experiments were performed thrice with comparable results. Original images of western blots are shown in Supplementary Materials File S1.

3.6. OA and UA Inhibit AKT Signaling Pathway

Previous reports show that mTOR negatively regulates autophagy in a transcription independent manner, which is tightly controlled downstream of AKT activation-induced signaling, where AKT is phosphorylated at Thr308 (by PDK1) and Ser473 (by PDK2). The AKT and phosphorylated AKT expression in both BrCa cells were examined after treating the cells with OA, UA, and OA + UA. Cell lysates were prepared and analyzed following a fixed period of drug exposure. We used a well-established inhibitor of AKT activation, LY294002 (LY; a broad-acting reversible PI3K inhibitor), as a positive control for this experiment. As shown in Figure 6, the pAKT (Thr308) level decreased after 48 h of exposure, but in the case of combination treatment, its decrease was more acute. Nearly the same trend was observed in the case of pAKT (Ser473), but its decrease in expression was more prominent than pAKT (Thr308). However, the expression of total AKT did not show a significant change as the time of exposure increased (Figure 6).

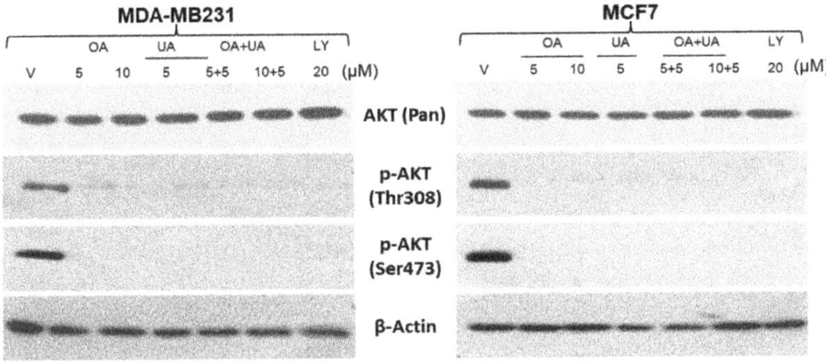

Figure 6. PTTs downregulate AKT activation. Western blotting analyses were performed to estimate the extent of activated AKT (phosphorylated (Thr308) and Ser473) and total AKT in whole-cell lysates of MDA-MB231 and MCF7 cells. The cells were treated with OA, UA, and both with or without LY94002 (PI3K inhibitor). β-actin is used as an internal loading control. Original images of western blots are shown in Supplementary Materials File S1.

We next examined whether autophagy inhibitors would negatively regulate OA-, UA-, and OA + UA-induced autophagic death. We used a low dose of 3-methyladenine (3MA), which inhibits autophagosome formation and promotes autophagy progression. Regarding cell viability in the presence and absence of 0.1 μM 3MA and various OA, UA, and OA + UA doses, we observed that co-incubation of OA, UA, and both in the presence of 3MA nearly abolished the cytotoxic lethality of OA, UA, and OA + UA (Figure 7). Although the common dose of 3MA used in such experiments was ≥5 mM, 3MA was able to inhibit autophagy-induced cell death completely in both MDA-MB231 and MCF7 cells.

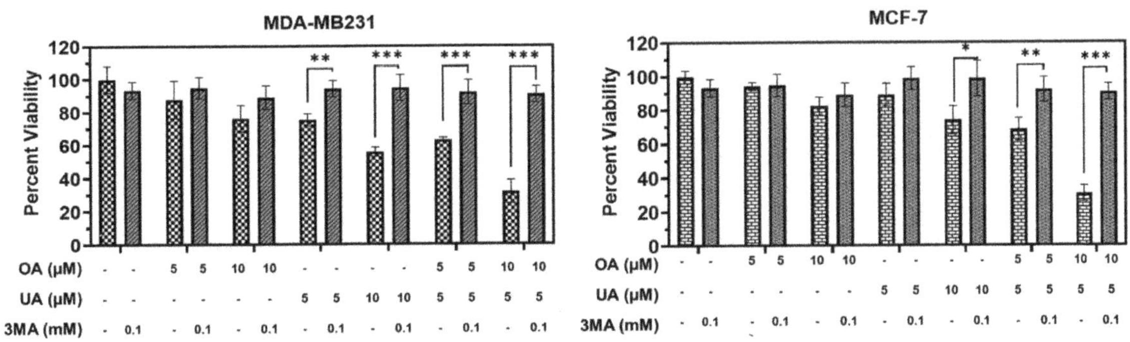

Figure 7. Treatment with 3-methyladenine (3MA) attenuates PTT-induced cytotoxicity. Cell viability recovered significantly following simultaneous incubation with 3MA and PTTs in MDA-MF231 and MCF7 cell cultures, indicating the cells were solely dependent on cytotoxic autophagy as PTT-induced autophagy. Results are expressed as means ± standard deviation (SD) (n = 3), and pairwise *t*-tests were used to determine significance: $p < 0.05$ = *, $p < 0.005$ = **, $p < 0.001$ = ***.

Most inducers of cytoprotective autophagy do so by inhibiting PI3K, a critical step in MTORC1 signaling. However, cytotoxic autophagy involves the use of drugs that inhibit PI3K as well. Usually, nontoxic PI3K inhibitors, such as LY294002, may help the cytotoxic drug induce a more robust additive or synergistic response. We found that co-incubation of LY294002 was not significantly cytotoxic to MCF7 or MDA-MB231 cells as measured by MTT assay (Figure 8); however, co-incubation with the TTPs significantly decreased cell viability at lower doses of both OA and UA in both BrCa cell lines (Figure 8).

The dose–effect combined cytotoxicity of OA, UA, or OA + UA with 5 μM of LY294002 was synergistic.

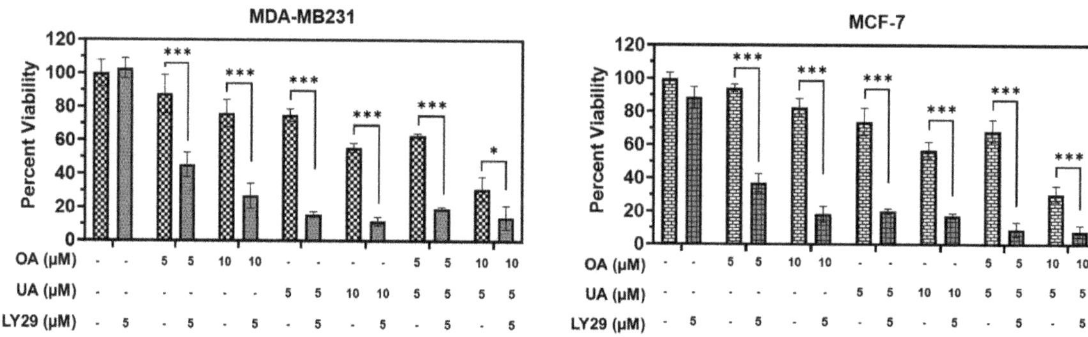

Figure 8. The PI3K inhibitor LY294002 enhances the cell death induced by pentacyclic triterpenes (PTTs). MTT assay-based cell viability was measured after treatment with OA, UA, and both with and without LY294002 (LY29); a specific inhibitor of PI3K) in both the BrCa cell lines. LY29 boosted the cytotoxicity induced by the PTTs. Results are expressed as means ± standard deviation (SD) (n = 3), and pairwise *t*-tests were used to determine significance: $p < 0.05$ = *, $p < 0.001$ = ***.

4. Discussion

The data presented in this study establish that OA and UA have cytotoxic effects against human BrCa cells at significantly lower doses when combined. The combination treatment synergistically (combination index (C.I.) < 1.0) inhibited cell viability at ≤10 μM, including at a dose of 5 μM each. Based on our cell viability and colony-forming assays, we found that OA is less effective than UA. Still, these two PTTs are more effective in combination treatment, especially against MDA-MB231 (TNBC) cells (Figure 1B–E), which may point to their potential clinical application in BrCa patients with terminal stages of the disease. TNBC is the terminal stage of breast cancer for which only palliative treatments exist. Cytotoxic chemotherapy is predominantly administered, or a combination of chemoradiation and hyperthermia, or even combined chemoradiation therapy ("hot chemotherapy"), with a survival advantage of no more than a few months [39].

Our results showed that select PTTs were differentially toxic to tumorigenic cells, eliminated the clonogenic potential of treated cells at a reasonable dose (<7 μM), and did not kill non-tumorigenic breast epithelial cells that grew at a similar rate and in a similar growth medium. The cancer-specific toxicity of UA or OA + UA was more than 400% at UA 10 μM and OA + UA 5 + 5 μM, calculated from dose-equivalent toxicity between tumorigenic (MDA-MB231, MCF7) and non-tumorigenic (MCF-12A) cells.

In contrast to the shared mechanism of cell death induced by cytotoxic chemotherapy drugs used in BrCa therapy, such as doxorubicin, paclitaxel, and docetaxel, the PTTs did not kill BrCa cells by apoptotic mechanisms, as we were unable to identify any markers of apoptosis in PTT-treated cells (Figure 2A,B). Although when cells are treated with staurosporine, a positive inducer of apoptosis by its potent inhibition of several protein kinases [40], cleaved PARP bands and increased TUNEL signal showing DNA fragmentation were seen in both BrCa cell lines, indicating that apoptosis may not be a significant mechanism of cell death. This finding is supported by previous reports [14,41–43]. We could not find significant evidence for OA + UA-induced necroptosis or ferroptosis, as shown by the complete absence of any apoptosis markers in OA-, UA-, or OA + UA-treated cells (Figure 2). However, others have reported UA-induced apoptosis at higher concentrations (e.g., >30 μM) [42,44].

The other mechanism of the cell death pathway, predominantly autophagy (Figure 3A), was significant. The expression of LC3BII and P62/SQSTM1 (both molecular markers of autophagy) was high after OA and UA treatment, indicating that autophagy may be the primary mechanism of cell death in both ER+ and TNBC cells (MCF7 and MB231, respectively). Along with the expression of LC3BII, the formation of autolysosomes and induction of LC3B puncta are molecular indicators of autophagy [45]. As shown in Figure 3B, in both BrCa cell lines, LC3BII-containing puncta and autolysosome formation was high in UA-treated cells, indicating autophagy cell death because of UA or OA + UA treatment. This was further confirmed by increased LC3BII levels in cells simultaneously treated with UA and pepstatin A, a potent inhibitor of lysosomal protein degradation (Figure 3C) [14,41–43]. Previous studies have shown that the AKT/mTOR pathway is critical for the regulation of autophagy and site-specific phosphorylation/dephosphorylation of many proteins that are involved in autophagic pathways, such as ULK1 (Unc-51-like autophagy-activating kinase 1; homologue of ATG1 in mammals), P70S6 (ribosomal protein S6 kinase beta 1), 4EBP1 (eukaryotic translation initiation factor 4E-binding protein 1), etc., play critical roles in the execution of autophagy [46–48].

Autophagy-related proteins (ATGs) are essential for initiating phagophores, sequestration, autophagosome formation, and overall autophagy regulation. Approximately 40 types of ATGs have been identified that regulate or coordinate the formation of autophagosomes. Out of these, ATG5 and ATG7 are essential regulators of autophagy. We demonstrated their role in the PTT-induced execution of autophagy that progressed through ATG5/ATG7, which was reversed and increased the survival of tumor cell populations by silencing them [49]. As previously mentioned, the regulation of autophagy involves the AKT/mTOR pathways and the site-specific phosphorylation of AKT and mTOR. Treatment with OA and UA (in MDA-MB231 cells) significantly suppressed mTOR phosphorylation (as shown in Figure 4) and site-specific AKT phosphorylation in a time-dependent manner (shown in Figure 6) in both BrCa cell lines. Moreover, OA and UA reduced AKT phosphorylation at Thr308, associated with mTORC1 activation, and AKT phosphorylation at the Ser473 site, which plays a role in the phosphorylation and activation of mTORC2. Therefore, OA and UA treatment significantly decrease AKT's activity by inhibiting both sites [50]. This inhibition, escorted by the decrease in phosphorylation of P70S6K and increase in phosphorylation of 4EBP1 (as shown in Figure 4), ultimately leads to mTORC1 and mTORC2 becoming inactivated, which leads to activation of autophagy [4,6].

OA and UA have shown activity in several cell systems at high doses ($\geq$50 μM to 0.4 mM). UA has anticancer, antidiabetic, and antiobesity activities at 150–500 mg/kg/day [16,51]. Administration of UA in feed (1% *w/w*) for up to 36 weeks did not show toxicity and achieved a serum level of $\geq$3 μM [52]. In limited human studies, OA and UA have shown tolerable toxicity profiles at an oral dose of 0.45 g to 3 g once daily for up to 8 weeks [27]. However, none of these studies tested the efficacy of the OA + UA combination, although they are structural isomers and are likely to coexist in variable ratios among edible plants. A sole chemodietary combination of OA + UA by themselves or in a neoadjuvant and adjuvant setting for patients with TNBC may benefit them by increasing their life span in terms of disease-free survival or reduced disease severity.

5. Conclusions

In conclusion, this study demonstrates the therapeutic potential of OA and UA in breast cancers when used at low doses, and these are equally elective on both TNBC and ER+ BrCa, represented by MDA-MB231 and MCF7 cells, respectively. The results also demonstrate that the combination of OA + UA is more effective than UA alone, although OA at the tested dose alone did not promote cytotoxicity. The study provides valuable insights into the underlying mechanisms of PTT-induced cell death and highlights its future potential as a nontoxic adjuvant therapy for BrCa patients.

Supplementary Materials: The following supporting information can be downloaded at https://www.mdpi.com/article/10.3390/cancers16193367/s1. Figure S1: Isobologram analysis of UA- and OA-treated BrCa cells. File S1: Original images of western blots.

Author Contributions: Study conceptualization, initial manuscript draft, and illustrations, B.L.L., K.B.G., J.G., X.L. and S.S.P.; methodology: K.B.G., J.G., X.L., M.T. and B.L.L.; software, GraphPad Prism (v. 9.1) validation, built-in statistical programs in Prism software, K.B.G. and B.L.L. All authors have read and agreed to the published version of the manuscript.

Funding: This work was partially supported by USAMRAA-HT9425-23-1-0761 (B. Lokeshwar), J. Harold Harrison, M.D., Endowment of Medical College of Georgia (B. Lokeshwar), and Salary On Grant and Start-Up funds from Georgia Cancer Center, Augusta University.

Institutional Review Board Statement: Not applicable.

Informed Consent Statement: Not applicable.

Data Availability Statement: Data are shown in the Section 3, along with Supplementary Materials details. Also, they are available upon request from the corresponding author.

Acknowledgments: The authors are grateful to Vinata B. Lokeshwar and the past members of Bal Lokeshwar's Laboratory for their technical support. The authors are also grateful for the support of Georgia Cancer Center's instrument core facilities. Resources, core instrumentation and facilities services of Georgia Cancer Center, Augusta University and core resources, Department of Chemistry and Biochemistry, College of Science and Mathematics, Augusta University.

Conflicts of Interest: The authors declare no potential conflicts of interest.

References

1. Siegel, R.L.; Miller, K.D.; Wagle, N.S.; Jemal, A. Cancer statistics, 2023. *CA Cancer J. Clin.* **2023**, *73*, 17–48. [CrossRef] [PubMed]
2. Li, S.; Goins, B.; Hrycushko, B.A.; Phillips, W.T.; Bao, A. Feasibility of eradication of breast cancer cells remaining in postlumpectomy cavity and draining lymph nodes following intracavitary injection of radioactive immunoliposomes. *Mol. Pharm.* **2012**, *9*, 2513–2522. [CrossRef] [PubMed]
3. Bedard, P.L.; Cardoso, F. Can some patients avoid adjuvant chemotherapy for early-stage breast cancer? *Nat. Rev. Clin. Oncol.* **2011**, *8*, 272–279. [CrossRef] [PubMed]
4. Zhang, L.; Shamaladevi, N.; Jayaprakasha, G.K.; Patil, B.S.; Lokeshwar, B.L. Polyphenol-rich extract of Pimenta dioica berries (Allspice) kills breast cancer cells by autophagy and delays growth of triple negative breast cancer in athymic mice. *Oncotarget* **2015**, *6*, 16379–16395. [CrossRef] [PubMed]
5. Varghese, E.; Samuel, S.M.; Líšková, A.; Samec, M.; Kubatka, P.; Büsselberg, D. Targeting Glucose Metabolism to Overcome Resistance to Anticancer Chemotherapy in Breast Cancer. *Cancers* **2020**, *12*, 2252. [CrossRef]
6. Meric-Bernstam, F.; Gonzalez-Angulo, A.M. Targeting the mTOR signaling network for cancer therapy. *J. Clin. Oncol.* **2009**, *27*, 2278–2287. [CrossRef]
7. Markman, B.; Dienstmann, R.; Tabernero, J. Targeting the PI3K/Akt/mTOR pathway—Beyond rapalogs. *Oncotarget* **2010**, *1*, 530–543. [CrossRef]
8. Lim, S.O.; Li, C.W.; Xia, W.; Lee, H.H.; Chang, S.S.; Shen, J.; Hsu, J.L.; Raftery, D.; Djukovic, D.; Gu, H.; et al. EGFR Signaling Enhances Aerobic Glycolysis in Triple-Negative Breast Cancer Cells to Promote Tumor Growth and Immune Escape. *Cancer Res.* **2016**, *76*, 1284–1296. [CrossRef]
9. Schwartz, G.K.; Shah, M.A. Targeting the cell cycle: A new approach to cancer therapy. *J. Clin. Oncol.* **2005**, *23*, 9408–9421. [CrossRef]
10. Obidiro, O.; Battogtokh, G.; Akala, E.O. Triple Negative Breast Cancer Treatment Options and Limitations: Future Outlook. *Pharmaceutics* **2023**, *15*, 1796. [CrossRef]
11. Mediratta, K.; El-Sahli, S.; D'Costa, V.; Wang, L. Current Progresses and Challenges of Immunotherapy in Triple-Negative Breast Cancer. *Cancers* **2020**, *12*, 3529. [CrossRef] [PubMed]
12. Rushing, B.R.; Wiggs, A.; Molina, S.; Schroder, M.; Sumner, S. Metabolomics Analysis Reveals Novel Targets of Chemosensitizing Polyphenols and Omega-3 Polyunsaturated Fatty Acids in Triple Negative Breast Cancer Cells. *Int. J. Mol. Sci.* **2023**, *24*, 4406. [CrossRef] [PubMed]
13. Zhu, Z.; Qian, Z.; Yan, Z.; Zhao, C.; Wang, H.; Ying, G. A phase I pharmacokinetic study of ursolic acid nanoliposomes in healthy volunteers and patients with advanced solid tumors. *Int. J. Nanomed.* **2013**, *8*, 129–136.
14. Leng, S.; Hao, Y.; Du, D.; Xie, S.; Hong, L.; Gu, H.; Zhu, X.; Zhang, J.; Fan, D.; Kung, H. Ursolic acid promotes cancer cell death by inducing Atg5-dependent autophagy. *Int. J. Cancer* **2013**, *133*, 2781–2790. [CrossRef]
15. Bishayee, A.; Ahmed, S.; Brankov, N.; Perloff, M. Triterpenoids as potential agents for the chemoprevention and therapy of breast cancer. *Front. Biosci. Landmark Ed.* **2011**, *16*, 980–996. [CrossRef]
16. Shanmugam, M.K.; Ong, T.H.; Kumar, A.P.; Lun, C.K.; Ho, P.C.; Wong, P.T.H.; Hui, K.M.; Sethi, G. Ursolic acid inhibits the initiation, progression of prostate cancer and prolongs the survival of TRAMP mice by modulating pro-inflammatory pathways. *PLoS ONE* **2012**, *7*, e32476. [CrossRef]

17. Kornel, A.; Nadile, M.; Retsidou, M.I.; Sakellakis, M.; Gioti, K.; Beloukas, A.; Sze, N.S.K.; Klentrou, P.; Tsiani, E. Ursolic Acid against Prostate and Urogenital Cancers: A Review of In Vitro and In Vivo Studies. *Int. J. Mol. Sci.* **2023**, *24*, 7414. [CrossRef]
18. Yin, M.C.; Lin, M.C.; Mong, M.C.; Lin, C.Y. Bioavailability, distribution, and antioxidative effects of selected triterpenes in mice. *J. Agric. Food Chem.* **2012**, *60*, 7697–7701. [CrossRef]
19. Deng, S.; Shanmugam, M.K.; Kumar, A.P.; Yap, C.T.; Sethi, G.; Bishayee, A. Targeting autophagy using natural compounds for cancer prevention and therapy. *Cancer* **2019**, *125*, 1228–1246. [CrossRef]
20. Lewinska, A.; Adamczyk-Grochala, J.; Kwasniewicz, E.; Deregowska, A.; Wnuk, M. Ursolic acid-mediated changes in glycolytic pathway promote cytotoxic autophagy and apoptosis in phenotypically different breast cancer cells. *Apoptosis* **2017**, *22*, 800–815. [CrossRef]
21. Pérez-Camino, M.C.; Cert, A. Quantitative determination of hydroxy pentacyclic triterpene acids in vegetable oils. *J. Agric. Food Chem.* **1999**, *47*, 1558–1562. [CrossRef] [PubMed]
22. He, X.; Wang, Y.; Hu, H.; Zhang, Z. In vitro and in vivo antimammary tumor activities and mechanisms of the apple total triterpenoids. *J. Agric. Food Chem.* **2012**, *60*, 9430–9436. [CrossRef] [PubMed]
23. Piet, M.; Paduch, R. Ursolic and oleanolic acids in combination therapy inhibit migration of colon cancer cells through down-regulation of the uPA/uPAR-dependent MMPs pathway. *Chem. Biol. Interact.* **2022**, *368*, 110202. [CrossRef] [PubMed]
24. Oprean, C.; Ivan, A.; Bojin, F.; Cristea, M.; Soica, C.; Drăghia, L.; Caunii, A.; Paunescu, V.; Tatu, C. Selective in vitro anti-melanoma activity of ursolic and oleanolic acids. *Toxicol. Mech. Methods* **2018**, *28*, 148–156. [CrossRef]
25. Hsu, H.Y.; Yang, J.J.; Lin, C.C. Effects of oleanolic acid and ursolic acid on inhibiting tumor growth and enhancing the recovery of hematopoietic system postirradiation in mice. *Cancer Lett.* **1997**, *111*, 7–13. [CrossRef]
26. Balanehru, S.; Nagarajan, B. Intervention of adriamycin induced free radical damage. *Biochem. Int.* **1992**, *28*, 735–744.
27. Seo, D.Y.; Lee, S.R.; Heo, J.-W.; No, M.-H.; Rhee, B.D.; Ko, K.S.; Kwak, H.-B.; Han, J. Ursolic acid in health and disease. *Korean J. Physiol. Pharmacol.* **2018**, *22*, 235–248. [CrossRef]
28. Salazar, N.; Muñoz, D.; Kallifatidis, G.; Singh, R.K.; Jordà, M.; Lokeshwar, B.L. The chemokine receptor CXCR7 interacts with EGFR to promote breast cancer cell proliferation. *Mol. Cancer* **2014**, *13*, 198. [CrossRef]
29. Gupta, K.B.; Mantha, A.K.; Dhiman, M. Mitigation of Gliadin-Induced Inflammation and Cellular Damage by Curcumin in Human Intestinal Cell Lines. *Inflammation* **2021**, *44*, 873–889. [CrossRef]
30. Shamaladevi, N.; Lyn, D.A.; Escudero, D.O.; Lokeshwar, B.L. CXC receptor-1 silencing inhibits androgen-independent prostate cancer. *Cancer Res.* **2009**, *69*, 8265–8274. [CrossRef]
31. Seremak, J.R.; Gupta, K.B.; Bonigala, S.; Liu, E.; Marshall, B.; Zhi, W.; Bokhtia, R.M.; Panda, S.S.; Lokeshwar, V.B.; Lokeshwar, B.L. Targeting Chemoresistance in Advanced Bladder Cancers with a Novel Adjuvant Strategy. *Mol. Cancer Ther.* **2024**, OF1–OF15. [CrossRef] [PubMed]
32. Smith, D.K.; Hasanali, S.L.; Wang, J.; Kallifatidis, G.; Morera, D.S.; Jordan, A.R.; Terris, M.K.; Klaassen, Z.; Bollag, R.; Lokeshwar, V.B.; et al. Promotion of epithelial hyperplasia by interleukin-8-CXCR axis in human prostate. *Prostate* **2020**, *80*, 938–949. [CrossRef] [PubMed]
33. Li, Z.; Sturm, S.; Stuppner, H.; Schraml, E.; Moser, V.A.; Siegl, V.; Pfragner, R. The dichloromethane fraction of Stemona tuberosa Lour inhibits tumor cell growth and induces apoptosis of human medullary thyroid carcinoma cells. *Biologics* **2007**, *1*, 455–463. [PubMed]
34. Hundeshagen, P.; Hamacher-Brady, A.; Eils, R.; Brady, N.R. Concurrent detection of autolysosome formation and lysosomal degradation by flow cytometry in a high-content screen for inducers of autophagy. *BMC Biol.* **2011**, *9*, 38. [CrossRef] [PubMed]
35. Chou, T.C.; Talalay, P. Quantitative analysis of dose-effect relationships: The combined effects of multiple drugs or enzyme inhibitors. *Adv. Enzyme Regul.* **1984**, *22*, 27–55. [CrossRef]
36. Mirzayans, R.; Murray, D. Do TUNEL and Other Apoptosis Assays Detect Cell Death in Preclinical Studies? *Int. J. Mol. Sci.* **2020**, *21*, 9090. [CrossRef]
37. Lum, J.J.; DeBerardinis, R.J.; Thompson, C.B. Autophagy in metazoans: Cell survival in the land of plenty. *Nat. Rev. Mol. Cell Biol.* **2005**, *6*, 439–448. [CrossRef]
38. Xie, Y.; Lei, X.; Zhao, G.; Guo, R.; Cui, N. mTOR in programmed cell death and its therapeutic implications. *Cytokine Growth Factor. Rev.* **2023**, *71–72*, 66–81. [CrossRef]
39. Zhang, X.; Yeung, K.T. Metastatic Triple-Negative Breast Cancer. *Curr. Breast Cancer Rep.* **2023**, *15*, 288–297. [CrossRef]
40. Gani, O.A.; Engh, R.A. Protein kinase inhibition of clinically important staurosporine analogues. *Nat. Prod. Rep.* **2010**, *27*, 489–498. [CrossRef]
41. Wang, Z.; Zhang, P.; Jiang, H.; Sun, B.; Luo, H.; Jia, A. Ursolic Acid Enhances the Sensitivity of MCF-7 and MDA-MB-231 Cells to Epirubicin by Modulating the Autophagy Pathway. *Molecules* **2022**, *27*, 3399. [CrossRef] [PubMed]
42. Zhao, C.; Yin, S.; Dong, Y.; Guo, X.; Fan, L.; Ye, M.; Hu, H. Autophagy-dependent EIF2AK3 activation compromises ursolic acid-induced apoptosis through upregulation of MCL1 in MCF-7 human breast cancer cells. *Autophagy* **2013**, *9*, 196–207. [CrossRef] [PubMed]
43. Castrejón-Jiménez, N.S.; Leyva-Paredes, K.; Baltierra-Uribe, S.L.; Castillo-Cruz, J.; Campillo-Navarro, M.; Hernández-Pérez, A.D.; Luna-Angulo, A.B.; Chacón-Salinas, R.; Coral-Vázquez, R.M.; Estrada-García, I.; et al. Ursolic and Oleanolic Acids Induce Mitophagy in A549 Human Lung Cancer Cells. *Molecules* **2019**, *24*, 3444. [CrossRef] [PubMed]

44. Kim, K.H.; Seo, H.S.; Choi, H.S.; Choi, I.; Shin, Y.C.; Ko, S.G. Induction of apoptotic cell death by ursolic acid through mitochondrial death pathway and extrinsic death receptor pathway in MDA-MB-231 cells. *Arch. Pharm. Res.* **2011**, *34*, 1363–1372. [CrossRef] [PubMed]
45. Klionsky, D.J.; Abdel-Aziz, A.K.; Abdelfatah, S.; Abdellatif, M.; Abdoli, A.; Abel, S.; Abeliovich, H.; Abildgaard, M.H.; Abudu, Y.P.; Acevedo-Arozena, A.; et al. Guidelines for the use and interpretation of assays for monitoring autophagy (4th edition)(1). *Autophagy* **2021**, *17*, 1–382.
46. Liu, L.; Yan, L.; Liao, N.; Wu, W.Q.; Shi, J.L. A Review of ULK1-Mediated Autophagy in Drug Resistance of Cancer. *Cancers* **2020**, *12*, 352. [CrossRef]
47. Heinonen, H.; Nieminen, A.; Saarela, M.; Kallioniemi, A.; Klefström, J.; Hautaniemi, S.; Monni, O. Deciphering downstream gene targets of PI3K/mTOR/p70S6K pathway in breast cancer. *BMC Genom.* **2008**, *9*, 348. [CrossRef]
48. Rutkovsky, A.C.; Yeh, E.S.; Guest, S.T.; Findlay, V.J.; Muise-Helmericks, R.C.; Armeson, K.; Ethier, S.P. Eukaryotic initiation factor 4E-binding protein as an oncogene in breast cancer. *BMC Cancer* **2019**, *19*, 491. [CrossRef]
49. Niklaus, N.J.; Tokarchuk, I.; Zbinden, M.; Schläfli, A.M.; Maycotte, P.; Tschan, M.P. The Multifaceted Functions of Autophagy in Breast Cancer Development and Treatment. *Cells* **2021**, *10*, 1447. [CrossRef]
50. Mahajan, K.; Mahajan, N.P. PI3K-independent AKT activation in cancers: A treasure trove for novel therapeutics. *J. Cell. Physiol.* **2012**, *227*, 3178–3184. [CrossRef]
51. Liu, J. Pharmacology of oleanolic acid and ursolic acid. *J. Ethnopharmacol.* **1995**, *49*, 57–68. [CrossRef] [PubMed]
52. Bang, H.S.; Seo, D.Y.; Chung, Y.M.; Oh, K.-M.; Park, J.J.; Arturo, F.; Jeong, S.-H.; Kim, N.; Han, J. Ursolic Acid-induced elevation of serum irisin augments muscle strength during resistance training in men. *Korean J. Physiol. Pharmacol.* **2014**, *18*, 441–446. [CrossRef] [PubMed]

cancers MDPI

Article

The Therapeutic Efficacy and Mechanism of Action of Gnetin C, a Natural Compound from the Melinjo Plant, in a Preclinical Mouse Model of Advanced Prostate Cancer

Gisella Campanelli [1], Ekniel Francois [2], Prashanth Parupathi [2], Lakshmi Sirisha Devarakonda [2], Ching Yang [1], Avinash Kumar [2,*] and Anait S. Levenson [1,*]

1 Department of Veterinary Biomedical Sciences, College of Veterinary Medicine, Long Island University, Brookville, NY 11548, USA; gisella.campanelli@liu.edu (G.C.); ching.yang@liu.edu (C.Y.)

2 Division of Pharmaceutical Sciences, Arnold & Marie Schwartz College of Pharmacy and Health Sciences, Long Island University, Brooklyn, NY 11201, USA; ekniel.francois@my.liu.edu (E.F.); prashanth.parupathi@my.liu.edu (P.P.); lakshmisirisha.devarakonda@my.liu.edu (L.S.D.)

* Correspondence: avinash.kumar@liu.edu (A.K.); anait.levenson@liu.edu (A.S.L.)

Simple Summary: Incidence and mortality rates for prostate cancer remain high due to advanced disease characterized by the heterogeneous activation of numerous molecular pathways. In the current study, utilizing a genetic mouse model of advanced prostate cancer with hyperactivated metastasis-associated protein 1/mammalian target of rapamycin (MTA1/mTOR) tumor-promoting pathway, we show for the first time that gnetin C, a natural compound from the melinjo plant, blocks the progression of prostate cancer by reducing cell proliferation and angiogenesis and promoting cell death through the efficient targeting of the MTA1/mTOR pathway. These data may provide a foundation from which to explore gnetin C as a monotherapy and/or combination therapy with approved drugs against advanced prostate cancer in patients with a loss of phosphatase and tensin homolog (PTEN) expression and activated MTA1/mTOR signaling.

Abstract: The metastasis-associated protein 1/protein kinase B (MTA1/AKT) signaling pathway has been shown to cooperate in promoting prostate tumor growth. Targeted interception strategies by plant-based polyphenols, specifically stilbenes, have shown great promise against MTA1-mediated prostate cancer progression. In this study, we employed a prostate-specific transgenic mouse model with MTA1 overexpression on the background of phosphatase and tensin homolog (*Pten*) null (*R26^{MTA1}*; *Pten$^{f/f}$*) and PC3M prostate cancer cells which recapitulate altered molecular pathways in advanced prostate cancer. Mechanistically, the MTA1 knockdown or pharmacological inhibition of MTA1 by gnetin C (dimer resveratrol) in cultured PC3M cells resulted in the marked inactivation of mammalian target of rapamycin (mTOR) signaling. In vivo, mice tolerated a daily intraperitoneal treatment of gnetin C (7 mg/kg bw) for 12 weeks without any sign of toxicity. Treatment with gnetin C markedly reduced cell proliferation and angiogenesis and promoted apoptosis in mice with advanced prostate cancer. Further, in addition to decreasing MTA1 levels in prostate epithelial cells, gnetin C significantly reduced mTOR signaling activity in prostate tissues, including the activity of mTOR-target proteins: p70 ribosomal protein S6 kinase (S6K) and eukaryotic translational initiation factor 4E (eIF4E)-binding protein 1 (4EBP1). Collectively, these findings established gnetin C as a new natural compound with anticancer properties against MTA1/AKT/mTOR-activated prostate cancer, with potential as monotherapy and as a possible adjunct to clinically approved mTOR pathway inhibitors in the future.

Keywords: natural products; plant-derived polyphenols; gnetin C; targeted therapeutics; anticancer effects; MTA1/mTOR; advanced prostate cancer

1. Introduction

Prostate cancer patients are a heterogeneous group with a prognosis ranging from full recovery to malignant and lethal disease. Between 2007 and 2014, the number of prostate cancers diagnosed declined due to changes in screening recommendations concerning the detection of prostate-specific antigen. Consequently, the incidence rate for advanced stage prostate cancer has increased by about 5% per year [1]. Therefore, an urgent need exists to better understand the biological basis for the progression to aggressive disease and metastasis. Prostate tumors begin from preinvasive lesions such as prostatic intraepithelial neoplasia (PIN), which eventually progress to adenocarcinoma and, in some cases, metastatic disease. Different phases of prostate cancer are characterized by a distinct molecular makeup, during which various signaling pathways are activated. While androgen receptor (AR) signaling is considered the most critical pathway in hormone-sensitive disease, hormone-refractory tumors, which emerge after failing hormone deprivation therapy, are governed by the activation of other tumor-promoting networks, such as the phosphatase and tensin homolog (PTEN) loss of function-associated activation of the protein kinase B/mammalian target of rapamycin (AKT/mTOR) cell survival signaling pathway [2–7]. Yet another pathway having major implications in advanced prostate cancer is metastasis-associated protein 1 (MTA1) signaling, which is strongly associated with clinically aggressive prostate cancer [8,9]. We have previously reported increased levels of MTA1 in *Pten*-deficient and *Pten*-loss mouse models of prostate cancer, which affected downstream inflammation and cell survival pathways [10]. Our initial finding that reduced levels of MTA1 were inversely correlated with PTEN acetylation and activation, which resulted in significantly inhibited disease progression partly through the inhibition of p-AKT, revealed a novel deregulated signaling network in prostate cancer: the MTA1/PTEN/AKT pathway [10,11]. Furthermore, our recent studies in a mouse model of premalignant high-risk prostate cancer (*R26^{MTA}; Pten$^{+/f}$; Pb-Cre^{+}*) demonstrated that targeting the MTA1/PTEN/AKT signaling pathway by diets supplemented with natural stilbenes, such as pterostilbene and gnetin C (dimer resveratrol), was effective in preventing prostate cancer progression from high-grade PIN to adenocarcinoma [12,13].

Despite significant advances in developing pharmacological inhibitors of PI3K/AKT/mTOR kinases, the results from clinical trials in prostate cancer demonstrated severe toxicity [14] and a lack of clinical benefit [15]. In the last two decades, there has been much interest in the potential health benefits of plant-based natural polyphenols as anti-inflammatory and anticancer agents [16–18]. Different classes of polyphenols have been shown to have anticancer effects through numerous signaling pathways including PI3K/AKT/mTOR [19–21]. Our group systematically reported on MTA1-mediated anticancer effects by members of the stilbene family of polyphenols, namely resveratrol, pterostilbene, and gnetin C [10,22]. We recently demonstrated gnetin C as a preclinical tumor growth inhibitor in prostate cancer xenografts and as a dietary interceptive agent in a transgenic mouse model of prostate cancer [13,23]. Based on our previous findings, we hypothesized that gnetin C might be effective as an MTA1-targeted therapeutic agent against advanced prostate cancer. Two major advantages will be gained: (1) new biomarkers such as MTA1 involved in the AKT/mTOR pathway may allow for the selection of a subpopulation of patients more likely to benefit from inhibitors of specific pathways that do not alter kinase activity; (2) safe natural compounds with the ability to inhibit this pathway through MTA1 may provide the rationale for novel combination approaches with low toxicity.

In the current study, we sought to (1) establish a genetically engineered mouse model which recapitulates advanced prostate cancer due to prostate-specific MTA1 overexpression and the loss of PTEN expression (*R26^{MTA1}; Pten$^{f/f}$; Pb-Cre^{+}*, hereafter *R26^{MTA1}; Pten$^{f/f}$*); (2) identify downstream pathways associated with an overexpression of MTA1 in PTEN-loss tumors and examine how these pathways contribute to the cooperative promotion of cancer progression; and (3) investigate the targeted efficacy of gnetin C on MTA1 downstream signaling in vivo.

2. Materials and Methods

2.1. Reagents and Cell Culture

Gnetin C was a generous gift from Hosoda SHC Co., Ltd. (Fukui, Japan). For in vitro and in vivo experiments, gnetin C was dissolved in dimethyl sulfoxide (DMSO, final concentration 0.1% for in vitro and 10% for in vivo) and stored in the dark at −20 °C until use.

PC3M cells were a gift from Dr. R. Bergman (University of Nebraska Medical Center, Omaha, NE, USA). PC3M cells were cultured in RPMI-1640 media containing 10% fetal bovine serum in an incubator at 37 °C with 5% CO_2. MTA1 knockdown PC3M cells were generated as described previously [24] using three different shRNAs and selecting clone #3 for demonstrating the most efficient knockdown for the current study (Supplementary Figure S1). Cells were certified as being mycoplasma-free using the Universal Mycoplasma Detection Kit (ATCC, Manassas, VA, USA).

2.2. RNA Sequencing

Prostate tissues of 18-week-old mice from the following four genotypes were used for RNA-Seq: (1) *R26^{MTA1}; Pb-Cre$^-$* (WT); (2) *R26^{MTA1}; Pb-Cre$^+$* (MTA1 OE); (3) *Pten$^{f/f}$; Pb-Cre$^+$* (Pten-null); and (4) *R26^{MTA1}; Pten$^{f/f}$; Pb-Cre$^+$* (Pten-null MTA1 OE). Genotypes were confirmed by PCR-based tail genomic DNA genotyping using primers previously described [12]. The total RNA was isolated using the miRNeasy Kit (Qiagen, Hilden, Germany) and sent to LC Sciences (Houston, TX, USA) for RNA sequencing. RNA-Seq libraries were generated from two biologically independent replicates per genotype (described above). The obtained sequencing reads were aligned to the GRCm39 mouse reference transcriptome from the Ensembl genome database (https://www.ensembl.org, accessed on 22 March 2023) and transcript abundance was aggregated to gene-level count using biomaRt (Bioconductor R-package, https://www.bioconductor.org/, accessed on 22 March 2023). Differentially expressed genes (DEGs) among the groups were identified using DESeq2 [25] and were defined using a cutoff of FDR < 0.05 and absolute $\log_2$ fold change set at 1. To determine the underlying potential signaling pathways enriched among groups, the DEGs were compared with gene sets curated in the Molecular Signatures Database (MSigDB) [26] for the "Hallmark gene sets" collection with FDR < 0.05 for multiple comparisons.

2.3. Western Blot Analysis

Protein lysates from cells and prostate tissues were separated using 6%, 10%, or 15% polyacrylamide gels and transferred onto polyvinylidene difluoride membranes as described previously [13]. Membranes were probed with primary antibodies for MTA1, AKT, p-AKT^{Ser473}, mTOR, p-mTOR^{S2448}, p-S6K^{T389}, p-4EBP1, and CyclinD1 from Cell Signaling Technology, Beverly, MA, USA. β-actin and HSP70 were used as loading controls (Santa Cruz Biotechnology, Dallas, TX, USA) (Supplementary Table S1). Signals were detected on ChemiDoc (Bio-Rad, Hercules, CA, USA) using enhanced chemiluminescence (Thermo Fisher Scientific, Somerset, NJ, USA). Densitometry was performed using Image J, v 1.54h (NIH, Bethesda, MD, USA). Quantitation was carried out using the ratio of the intensity of the phosphorylated protein to the total protein of interest versus loading control.

2.4. Animals and Study Design

All mice were housed in a pathogen-free facility, and all procedures were performed in accordance with policies and guidelines outlined by the Long Island University Institutional Animal Care and Use Committee (IACUC, approved protocol ID # 2022-011, 10 March 2022). Mice had free access to drinking water and food and were monitored daily for their general health.

Mouse Models: Mice with biallelic overexpression of MTA1 in the prostate (*R26^{MTA1}; Pb-Cre$^+$*) have been described previously by us [12]. *R26^{MTA1}; Pb-Cre$^+$* mice then interbred with C57BL/6J mice homozygous for the "floxed" allele of *Pten* gene (*Pten$^{f/f}$*) (Jackson

Laboratories, Nashville, TN, USA) to obtain *R26^{MTA1}; Pten$^{+/f}$; Pb-Cre^{+}* [12,13] and *R26^{MTA1}; Pten$^{f/f}$; Pb-Cre^{+}* male mice (hereafter *R26^{MTA1}; Pten$^{f/f}$*) for this study. Tail genotyping was performed using the following primers: MTA1 F: 5′-GCT GCT CTC ATC CTC AGA AAC C-3′; MTA1 R: 5′-CTC GAT GTT GTG GCG GAT CTT GAA GTT-3′ with a band of 715 bp; PTEN F: 5′-CAA GCA CTC TGC GAA CTG AG-3′; PTEN R: 5′-AAG TTT TTG AAG GCA AGA TGC-3′ with a wild-type band of 156 bp and mutant band of 328 bp; and Cre F: 5′-TCG CGA TTA TCT TCT ATA TCT TCA G-3′; Cre R: 5′-GCT CGA CCA GTT TAG TTA CCC-3′ with a band of 392 bp [12]. PCR was performed on an Eppendorf thermocycler. *R26^{MTA1}; Pb-Cre^{-}* mice with normal prostates (n = 3) served as a reference control group.

Experimental Design: Dose calculations: In our previous studies with transgenic mice and pterostilbene i.p. administration, we found that pterostilbene had anticancer effects at 10 mg/kg bw without any toxicity [10]. Given gnetin C's improved pharmacokinetic profile [27] and its reported safe dose in animal studies [28], we selected a gnetin C dose of 7 mg/kg bw per day. The dose translation formula used for the determination of equivalent human doses (HEDs) [HED (mg/kg) = Animal dose (mg/kg) × Km ratio, where Km = 0.081 for mice] [29] demonstrated clinical relevance at a 7 mg/kg bw dose. This dose translates to 39.69 mg per day (for an average human male of 70 kg bw), which is within the range of doses shown to be well tolerated and safe in human clinical trials with gnetin C [27,30–32].

For gnetin C treatment experiments, two groups of *R26^{MTA1}; Pten$^{f/f}$* mice were weaned at 3–4 weeks of age and treated with daily i.p. injections of either 10% DMSO vehicle (control, n = 7) or gnetin C at a 7 mg/kg bw dose (n = 11). The mice received their respective treatment for 5 consecutive days, with 2 days off for a period of 12 weeks. Mice were weighed daily and observed for signs of distress following treatment. At the conclusion of the study, mice were sacrificed in accordance with the approved IACUC protocol. Due to the small size of the mouse prostate, animals from the same treatment group were used either for UGS (prostate, seminal vesicles, and bladder) isolation and fixed in formalin and paraffin-embedded for histology and IHC, or prostate tissue protein extraction stored at −80 °C for Western blot analysis. Blood was collected by cardiac puncture upon sacrifice, and serum samples were stored at −80 °C.

2.5. Histology and Immunohistochemistry Analyses of Prostate Tissues

Formalin-fixed, paraffin-embedded sections (Reveal Biosciences, San Diego, CA, USA) were stained with hematoxylin and eosin (H&E) for independent histopathologic examination (GC and CY). The severity of prostatic intraepithelial neoplasia (PIN) and adenocarcinoma was scored by a board-certified veterinary pathologist (CY) using the following system: Score 0: No detectable PIN and prostate carcinoma; Score 1: Only PIN is present; Score 2: Both PIN and adenocarcinoma are present, where adenocarcinoma accounts for less than 50% of the prostate gland; Score 3: Both PIN and adenocarcinoma are present, where adenocarcinoma accounts for more than 50% of the prostate gland. A minimum of five random sections from different locations in the prostate tissues were examined for each mouse. The phenotype was scored based on the analyses of multiple sections per mouse.

Slides were subjected to IHC staining using antibodies for Ki67, MTA1, CD31, cleaved caspase 3 (CC3), p-mTOR, p-SK6, and p-4EBP1 (Supplementary Table S1). Briefly, tissues were deparaffinized, hydrated, and treated to exposed target proteins. Active sites were blocked with serum and endogenous peroxidases were quenched. Tissues were incubated in primary antibody overnight, followed by secondary antibody and avidin–biotin complex (Vectastain ABC Elite Kit, Vector Laboratories, Newark, CA, USA). Stain was developed using the ImmPACT DAB kit (Vector Laboratories). Images were taken using an EVOS XL Core microscope (Thermo Fisher Scientific, Somerset, NJ, USA). The staining intensity of the markers was evaluated and scored by GC. The percentage of positive nuclei was evaluated for Ki67. The total nuclear and cytoplasmic staining intensity was scored according to a four-tier system: 1 (weak staining), 2 (fair staining), 3 (moderate staining), and 4 (strong staining). Analyses of IHC staining were performed using at least five randomly selected areas for each sample in each group using Image J, v 1.54h (NIH, Bethesda, MD, USA) or QuPath v 0.5.0 automated bioimage analysis. Image J was used for cell counting and measuring the CD31 endothelial-stained vessel area in mm^2. QuPath was used to quantitate the presence and severity of PIN and adenocarcinoma.

2.6. ELISA

The levels of IL-2 in mice sera (50 μL samples) were determined by using a commercially available kit (Abcam, Boston, MA, USA) as previously described [12,13]. Briefly, samples and standards in duplicate wells were incubated with the antibody mix and detected by adding 3,3′, 5,5′-tetramethylbenzidine substrate. The reaction was read at 450 nm using a microplate reader (Tecan, Mannedorf, Switzerland). The concentration of IL-2 in samples was calculated from a standard curve.

2.7. Statistical Analysis

Statistical analyses were performed using GraphPad Prism v9 software (San Diego, CA, USA). The statistical significance of differences between groups was determined by either Student's *t*-test or one-way ANOVA as appropriate. Data are shown as mean value ± SEM; $p < 0.05$ was considered statistically significant.

3. Results

3.1. Prostate-Specific MTA1 Overexpression Makes $Pten^{f/f}$ Mice Progress with Invasive Adenocarcinoma

Based on previous studies showing that MTA1 overexpression in the prostate enhances and accelerates PIN development in $Pten^{+/f}$ mice [12,13], we hypothesized that MTA1 overexpression in the context of PTEN loss-of-function ($Pten^{f/f}$) would increase the aggressiveness of prostate cancer progression and might even result in metastasis. Therefore, we generated a prostate-specific $R26^{MTA1}$; $Pten^{f/f}$ mouse model, in which mice develop PIN that progresses to adenocarcinoma. The number of glands exhibiting adenocarcinoma versus PIN in $R26^{MTA1}$; $Pten^{f/f}$ and $Pten^{f/f}$ mice was comparable. Likewise, the prostate-specific upregulation of MTA1 did not significantly accelerate tumor progression in the context of the loss-of-function of PTEN, and no metastases were found in either renal or iliac lymph nodes of these mice even by 36 weeks of age. Histopathologically, MTA1 overexpression in prostate epithelial cells lacking PTEN expression was characterized by well to moderately differentiated invasive adenocarcinoma composed of neoplastic epithelial cells arranged in glandular structures associated with desmoplasia and variable numbers of inflammatory infiltrates composed of lymphocytes, plasma cells, and neutrophils. There was no evidence of lymphovascular invasion by the neoplastic cells. The neoplastic cells invading the basement membrane did not show a spindle-shaped morphology (Figure 1).

To identify molecular alterations affected by prostate-specific MTA1 overexpression, we performed RNA-Seq using mouse prostate tissues. A total of 867 genes were found to be significantly upregulated and 1088 genes downregulated (FDR < 0.05) in the $R26^{MTA1}$; $Pten^{f/f}$ compared to the $Pten^{f/f}$ group. A heatmap view of the gene clustering of $R26^{MTA1}$; $Pten^{f/f}$ compared to $Pten^{f/f}$ is shown in Figure 2A (Supplementary Table S2). The pathway most affected by MTA1 overexpression in the PTEN-loss prostate was the mTORC1 (hereafter mTOR) pathway (Figure 2B, Supplementary Table S3), which is known to be aberrantly activated in castration-resistant prostate cancer [33] and advanced prostate cancer with a reduced expression of PTEN [14]. The Principal Component Analysis (PCA) and Multidimensional Scaling (MDS) scatter plot are shown in Supplementary Figure S2. Therefore, our $R26^{MTA1}$; $Pten^{f/f}$ mice mimic a subtype of advanced prostate cancer that exhibits the involvement of mTOR signaling, suggesting that targeting the MTA1/mTOR pathway by natural stilbene gnetin C could be an effective means for blocking prostate cancer progression.

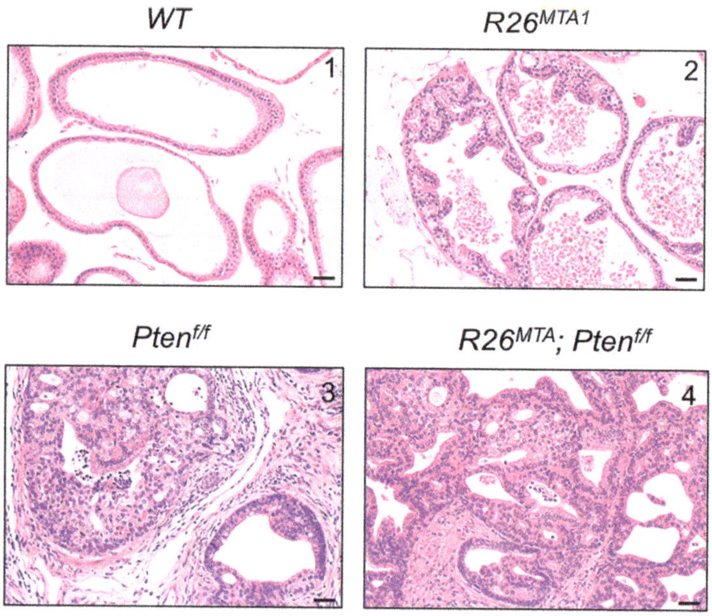

Figure 1. Representative photomicrographs of prostates from four prostate-specific genetic groups: (**1**) *R26*^{MTA1}; *Pb-Cre-negative* (WT), (**2**) *R26*^{MTA1}, (**3**) *Pten*$^{f/f}$, and (**4**) *R26*^{MTA1}; *Pten*$^{f/f}$ were evaluated using H&E staining (scale bar, 100 μm). The prostate in WT mice is unremarkable (**upper left**). In *R26*^{MTA1} mice, there is an occasional hyperplasia of the prostatic epithelium without nuclear or cellular atypia (**upper right**). In *Pten*$^{f/f}$ and *R26*^{MTA1}; *Pten*$^{f/f}$ mice, both PIN and prostatic adenocarcinoma are observed. The images (**lower left** and **right**) show well to moderately differentiated invasive prostatic adenocarcinoma with desmoplasia and inflammatory infiltrates.

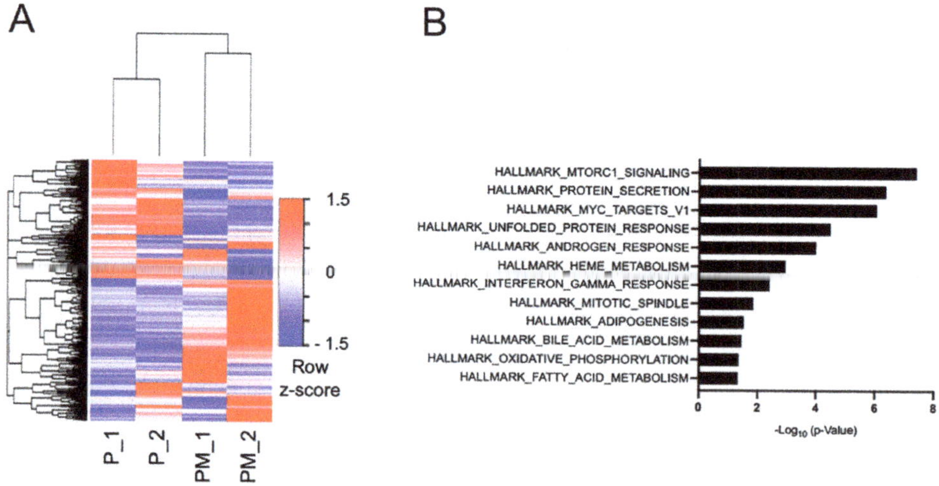

Figure 2. (**A**) Heatmap showing DEGs in the *R26*^{MTA1}; *Pten*$^{f/f}$ (PM_1 and PM_2) compared to the *Pten*$^{f/f}$; (P_1 and P_2) group. (**B**) Gene set enrichment analysis for the Hallmark gene sets from MSigDB for the DEGs in the *R26*^{MTA1}; *Pten*$^{f/f}$ compared to the *Pten*$^{f/f}$ group.

3.2. Inhibition of MTA1/mTOR Pathway by Gnetin C in Cell Culture

To gain initial insights regarding the mechanistic basis for targeting the MTA1/mTOR pathway, we first investigated the link between MTA1 and mTOR signaling in PC3M prostate cancer cells, which are known to have a PTEN-null status [34] and the highest MTA1 expression of all prostate cancer cell lines [8]. Oncogenic signaling via the AKT/mTOR pathway is mediated through both mTORC1 and mTORC2, with mTORC1 regulating cell growth by controlling the activity of p70 ribosomal protein S6 kinase (S6K) and eukaryotic translational initiation factor 4E (elF4E)-binding protein 1 (4EBP1), while mTORC2 phosphorylates AKT to promote cell survival [14,35]. Further, the activated mTOR pathway which results in phosphorylated 4EBP1 and S6K leads to higher levels of CyclinD1 [36–38], while the inhibition of PI3K/AKT/mTOR/S6K leads to decreased CyclinD1 expression in cancer cells [38,39].

A Western blot analysis of mTOR signaling revealed the marked downregulation of the p-AKT and p-mTOR pathway and its downstream target substrates p-S6K and p-4EBP1 as well as CyclinD1 in PC3M MTA1 knockdown cells compared to control NS cells, indicating that MTA1 acts as an upstream regulator of the mTOR pathway (Figure 3A,C). These data suggest that the MTA1-dependent activation of the mTOR/S6K/4EBP1/CyclinD1 pathway may represent a mechanism through which prostate cancer progresses under conditions of PTEN loss, which suggests a direct positive crosstalk between the MTA1 and mTOR pathway independent of the MTA1/PTEN link [11]. Gnetin C, which previously showed cytotoxicity in PC3M cells with IC_{50} = 8.7 μM [26,27], pharmacologically inhibited MTA1 and reduced the expression of p-mTOR, p-S6K, p-4EBP1, and CyclinD1 (Figure 3B,D) indicating the efficacy of gnetin C for suppressing the MTA1/mTOR pathway.

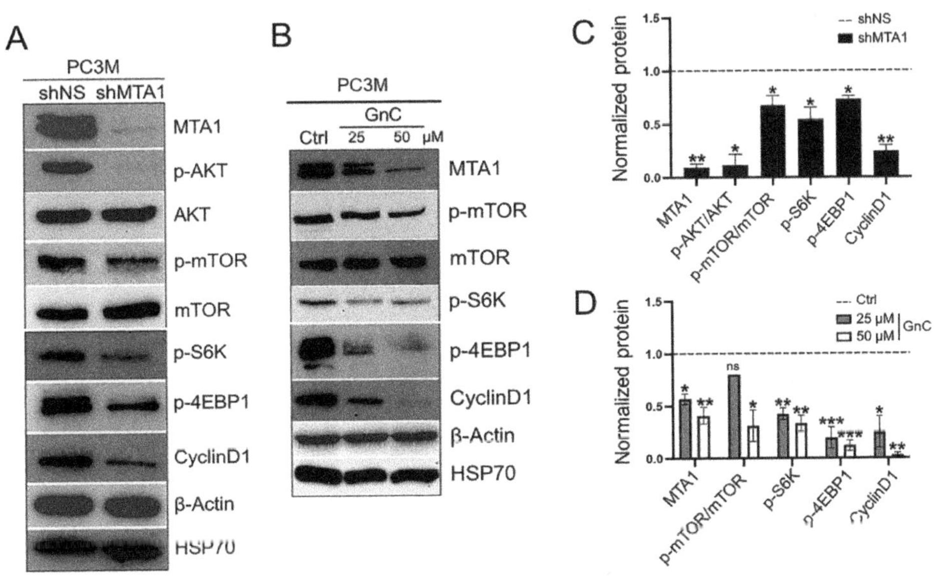

Figure 3. (**A**) Representative Western blot analysis and quantitation of molecular markers of MTA1/mTOR signaling pathway in PC3M MTA1-expressing (shNS) and MTA1 knockdown (shMTA1) cells. (**B**) Gnetin C inhibits MTA1/mTOR pathway markers in a dose-dependent manner. β-actin and HSP70 were used as loading controls. (**C**) Quantitation analysis of molecular markers in PC3M shNS and shMTA1 cells. (**D**) Quantitation analysis of molecular markers in PC3M cells treated with 25 and 50 μM of gnetin C (GnC). Quantitation represents mean ± SEM of three independent experiments. * $p < 0.05$; ** $p < 0.01$; *** $p < 0.001$; ns, non-significant (Student's t-test and one-way ANOVA). The uncropped blots are shown in File S1.

3.3. Gnetin C Treatment Diminishes Adenocarcinoma Progression in $R26^{MTA1}$; $Pten^{f/f}$ Mice

Upon the accumulation of 18 $R26^{MTA1}$; $Pten^{f/f}$ mice, we randomized 4-week-old mice into two groups: mice treated by intraperitoneal (i.p.) injection with vehicle (n = 7) or 7 mg/kg bw gnetin C (GnC, n = 11) for 12 weeks. Mice were sacrificed in week 13, and prostate tissues and blood were collected for analysis (Figure 4). We also had Cre-negative mice serving as the reference control. Body weight and health condition were monitored. No signs of toxicity were identified.

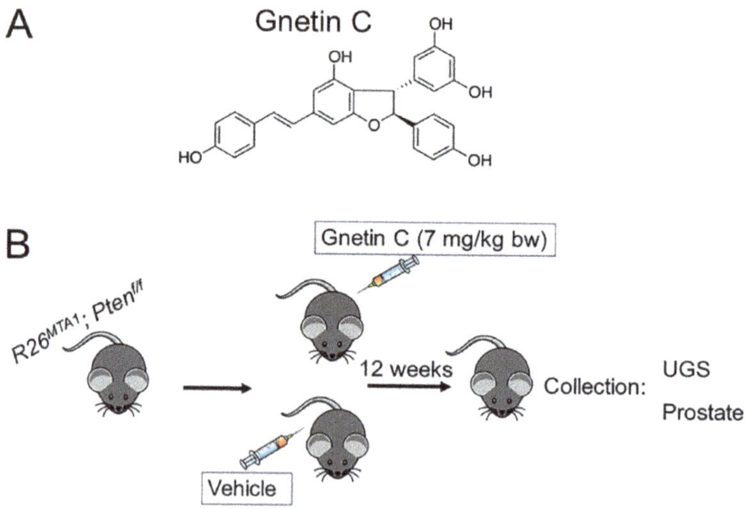

Figure 4. (**A**) Chemical structure of gnetin C. (**B**) Schematic of experimental design used for studying therapeutic effects of gnetin C in advanced prostate cancer murine model. $R26^{MTA1}$; $Pten^{f/f}$ mice were treated with vehicle (n = 7) or single daily dose of gnetin C (7 mg/kg bw), (n = 11) for 12 weeks, after which UGS or prostate tissues were collected for histopathological and molecular analysis, respectively.

Figure 5A (upper panel) shows that in the vehicle-treated group, mice predominantly exhibited adenocarcinoma characterized by the proliferation of the neoplastic glandular epithelium with the invasion of the basement membrane surrounded by desmoplastic reaction and moderate-to-large numbers of infiltrating inflammatory cells composed of neutrophils, lymphocytes, and plasma cells. There is no evidence of lymphovascular invasion by the neoplastic cells. The neoplastic cells invading the basement membrane did not show a spindle-shaped morphology. In contrast, mice treated with gnetin C demonstrated more areas of PIN characterized by the proliferation of glands without the invasion of the basement membrane into surrounding stroma and rare inflammatory cells. The IHC analysis of prostate tissues of mice treated with gnetin C showed a significantly reduced number of Ki67-positive cells and CD31 staining, indicating a significant decrease in proliferation and angiogenesis compared to vehicle-treated mice. Further, we detected increased apoptosis (CC3 staining) in prostates of mice treated with gnetin C compared to vehicle-treated mice (Figure 5A). We next explored the therapeutic potential of gnetin C in inhibiting the MTA1/mTOR pathway. Our finding revealed a significant decrease in MTA1 and the activated mTOR pathway (p-mTOR, p-S6K, and p-4EBP1) in mice treated with gnetin C compared to the vehicle-treated group (Figure 5B).

For further analysis, we evaluated the response to treatments by measuring levels of MTA1/mTOR pathway markers in prostate tissue lysates by Western blot (Figure 6A). Although demonstrating noticeable heterogeneity, MTA1 and associated activated mTOR-downstream targets (p-4EBP1 and CyclinD1) levels were significantly downregulated in the prostates of mice treated with gnetin C compared to the vehicle-treated group (Figure 6A). Curiously, the results of p-mTOR and mTOR levels in prostate tissues detected by Western blot were not associated with treatment benefits. This can be explained in part by the very low number of prostate tissues for our Western blot analysis but could also reflect the contradictory role of p-mTOR/mTOR found in prostate cancer patients whose elevated levels positively correlated with a favorable prognosis [40,41]. Existing ambiguity surrounding the biological role of p-mTOR/mTOR in prostate cancer could explain the limited clinical efficacy of PI3K/AKT/mTOR inhibitors [14,40,41]. Nevertheless, the inclusion of MTA1, p-4EBP1, and CyclinD1 in clinical studies may help select patients with high levels of MTA1 that are likely to benefit from gnetin C-targeted therapies.

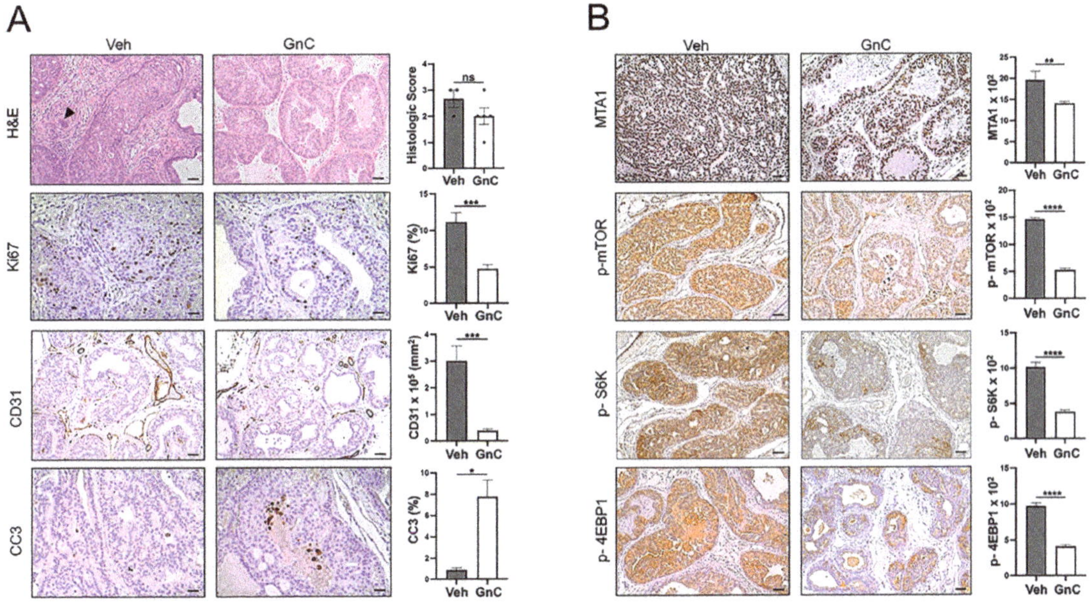

Figure 5. (**A**) **Left**: Representative images of H&E (scale bar, 50 μm). An island of neoplastic epithelial cells invading the adjacent fibrous connective tissue is present (arrowhead). The IHC staining of Ki67, CC3 (scale bar, 20 μm), and CD31 (scale bar, 50 μm) in the prostate tissues from vehicle-treated and gnetin C-treated mice. **Right**: The quantitation of prostate glands involved in PIN vs. adenocarcinoma and the quantitation analysis of Ki67, CD31, and CC3 staining. (**B**) **Left**: Representative images of molecular markers of the MTA1/mTOR pathway in the prostate tissues from vehicle (Veh)-treated and gnetin C (GnC)-treated mice. **Right**: The quantitation of MTA1, p-mTOR, p-S6K, and p-4EBP1 (scale bar, 50 μm) staining. Values are mean ± SEM analyzed from five to seven separate areas per sample (Veh, n = 3 and GnC, n = 5). * $p < 0.05$; ** $p < 0.01$; *** $p < 0.001$; **** $p < 0.0001$; ns, non-significant (Student's t-test).

Finally, we evaluated the anti-inflammatory response to gnetin C treatment in $R26^{MTA1}$; $Pten^{f/f}$ mice by determining the levels of pro-inflammatory IL-2 cytokine in murine sera (Figure 6B). Consistent with our previous observations using low doses of a gnetin C-supplemented diet in a high-risk PIN model of prostate cancer [13], our current study demonstrated that gnetin C was able to reduce the levels of IL-2 compared to the vehicle.

Taken together, our data demonstrated that gnetin C treatment restored favorable histopathology in $R26^{MTA1}$, $Pten^{f/f}$ mice with a statistically significant reduction in MTA1, accompanied by a reduced rate of cell proliferation and angiogenesis, increased levels of apoptosis, and the inhibition of MTA1-associated markers of activated mTOR signaling, as evidenced by IHC and Western blot analysis. These results suggest that gnetin C has several potent beneficial features, including anti-inflammatory and anticancer properties, defining its therapeutic efficacy in a preclinical mouse model of advanced prostate cancer.

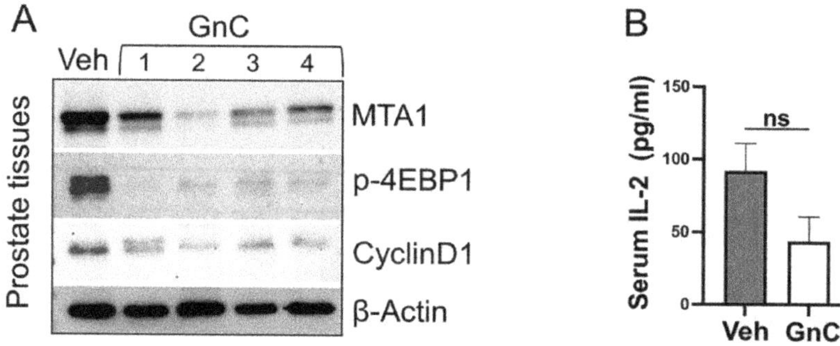

Figure 6. (**A**) Representative immunoblot images of the inhibitory effect of gnetin C (GnC) on molecular markers of the MTA1/mTOR pathway in the prostate tissues from mice in different treatment groups. β-actin was used as a loading control. (**B**) The effect of GnC on circulating IL-2 cytokine levels measured by ELISA in murine sera (n = 4 per group). Data represent the mean ± SEM of three independent experiments performed in duplicate. ns, non-significant. Veh, vehicle. The uncropped blots are shown in File S1.

4. Discussion

Although mTOR inhibitors are effective in many cancers [42–44], they have shown limited efficacy in the treatment of prostate cancer [14,45,46]. In addition, mTOR inhibitor-associated toxicity is a critical problem dictating the need for effective and safe targeted therapies [14,44].

In this study, to discover a novel natural mTOR pathway inhibitor in prostate cancer, we have established a clinically relevant mouse model to test the efficacy of gnetin C-targeted therapy. The prostate-specific *R26*^{MTA1}; *Pten*$^{f/f}$ genetically engineered mouse model recapitulates features of PTEN-loss advanced prostate cancer facilitated by the overexpression of MTA1.

In our previous studies of MTA1-associated prostate cancer progression, we found an inverse relationship between MTA1 overexpression and PTEN activation, which resulted in an aberrant activation of the AKT signaling pathway [10,11]. In the current study, we have investigated a direct link between the MTA1 and AKT kinase downstream effector, e.g., the mTOR signaling pathway, and found that MTA1 is an upstream regulator of mTOR that is independent of PTEN. Reassuringly, the same association between MTA1 and AKT/mTOR/4EBP1 was recently reported in endometrial cancer, in which miR-30c/MTA1 axes regulated cell proliferation, migration, and invasion via AKT/mTOR signaling defining MTA1 as a therapeutic target in endometrial cancer [47]. Importantly, for the first time, we have pharmacologically targeted the MTA1/mTOR pathway using the natural compound gnetin C both in vitro and in vivo. We report here that gnetin C effectively suppressed the MTA1/mTOR pathway indicated by the downregulated MTA1 and the associated reduced phosphorylation of AKT, mTOR, S6K, 4EBP1, and CyclinD1 in PC3M prostate cancer cells. In prostate tissues, despite the limitations due to a small number of samples, gnetin C showed a significant inhibition of MTA1 and associated p-4EBP1 and CyclinD1. Considering the intricacy of the mTOR signaling network in prostate cancer, it is understandable that preclinical studies would also reflect this complexity. Hence, it becomes important then that there are other biomarkers associated with mTOR that can be indicators of therapy response. Notably, targeting MTA1 by gnetin C consistently resulted in the downregulation of the activated mTOR pathway response markers p-S6K, p-4EBP1, and CyclinD1 detected either by IHC or Western blot analysis. Our data agree with previously reported gnetin C activity on AKT/mTOR signaling in leukemia cells, in which gnetin C's antitumor effects are demonstrated in cancer cell lines, patient samples, and in vivo through AKT/mTOR and ERK1/2 pathways. This study demonstrated that a combination of gnetin C with low doses of chemotherapeutic drugs leads to a synergistic antitumor effect against acute myeloid leukemia [28].

In the future, modifications of the chemical structure of gnetin C with improved pharmacokinetics could expand therapeutic outcomes when used as monotherapy. Moreover, gnetin C or its derivatives, with their chemosensitizing ability, could be used in combination with clinically approved drugs for synergistic efficacy. We recently demonstrated that gnetin C acts synergistically with enzalutamide to inhibit cell proliferation and angiogenesis and to promote apoptosis in a castrate-resistant xenograft model by the dual-targeting of AR-V7 and MTA1 [48]. While specific MTA1 inhibitors are not available, mTOR inhibitors such as rapamycin and its derivatives are commercially available and suitable for combination therapy in a reduced dose. Therefore, in the future, combinatorial targeted therapies can be beneficial to a biomarker-selected subpopulation of patients with MTA1/mTOR activation-mediated advanced prostate cancer. Further investigations are warranted to determine how MTA1-tumor heterogeneity impacts the effectiveness of treatment and whether target phospho-protein levels can be used as reliable biomarkers for combinatorial treatment response.

5. Conclusions

We conclude that *R26*^{MTA1}; *Pten*$^{f/f}$ mice recapitulate key features of MTA1/mTOR signaling pathway activation-associated advanced prostate cancer and represent a useful model for exploring novel therapeutic approaches to manage advanced disease. The discovery of a new mTOR inhibitor with decent efficacy and low toxicity increases the translational potential of the MTA1/mTOR pathway as a therapeutic target. Collectively, our data show that targeting the MTA1/mTOR pathway by the natural stilbene, gnetin C, is highly effective in a preclinical model of prostate cancer and suggests that it could be beneficial for blocking prostate cancer progression in a cohort of patients with a deregulated MTA1/PTEN/AKT/mTOR pathway (Figure 7). Novel natural compounds, such as gnetin C, that target specific biological pathways represent the future for the clinical management of advanced prostate cancer.

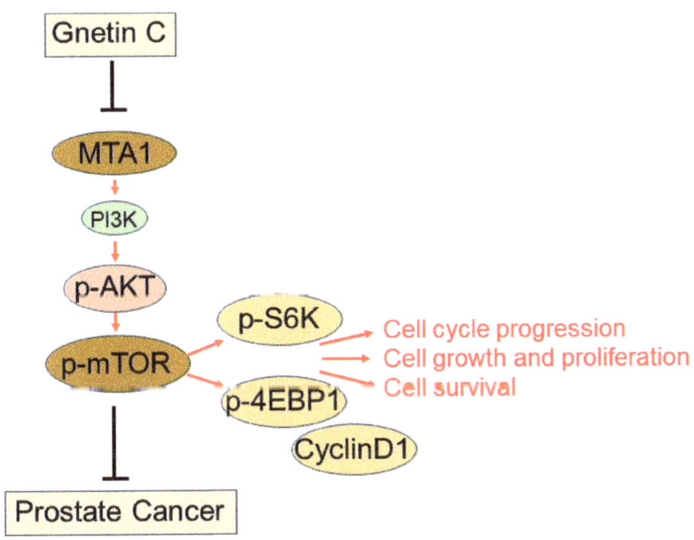

Figure 7. Schematic representation of MTA1/mTOR pathway in prostate cancer. MTA1 overexpression in *R26*^{MTA1}; *Pten*$^{f/f}$ preclinical model of prostate cancer leads to hyperactivation of mTOR resulting in phosphorylation of downstream target proteins such as S6K and 4EBP1 and CyclinD1. These changes promote cell growth, proliferation, and survival. Gnetin C, plant-derived stilbene, inhibits MTA1-associated mTOR pathway activation resulting in antitumor activity.

Supplementary Materials: The following supporting information can be downloaded at: https://www.mdpi.com/article/10.3390/cancers16071344/s1, Figure S1: Validation of MTA1 knockdown in PC3M cells; Figure S2: PCA and MDS scatter plot of gene expression; Table S1: Antibodies used for western blot and IHC; Table S2: Hallmark gene sets; Table S3: Heatmap-PMvP; File S1: Western blot information.

Author Contributions: Conceptualization, A.S.L.; methodology, A.K., G.C., E.F., P.P., L.S.D., C.Y., and A.S.L.; formal analysis, G.C., C.Y., A.K., E.F., and A.S.L.; investigation, G.C., P.P., E.F., and L.S.D.; resources, A.K. and A.S.L.; writing—original draft preparation, A.S.L.; writing—review and editing, G.C., C.Y., A.K., and A.S.L.; visualization, G.C., A.K., C.Y., and A.S.L.; supervision, A.K. and A.S.L.; data curation, A.S.L., project administration, A.S.L., funding acquisition, A.S.L. All authors have read and agreed to the published version of the manuscript.

Funding: This study was partly supported by the National Cancer Institute of the National Institutes of Health under Award Number R15CA216070 to A.S. Levenson. The content is solely the responsibility of the author and does not necessarily represent the official views of the National Institutes of Health.

Institutional Review Board Statement: The animal study protocol was approved by the Institutional Animal Care and Use Committee of the Long Island University Brooklyn (ID # 2022-011, 10 March 2022.

Informed Consent Statement: Not applicable.

Data Availability Statement: The data generated in this study are available upon request from the corresponding author.

Acknowledgments: The authors are grateful to S. Yoo and J. Zhu (Icahn School of Medicine, Mount Sinai, NY, USA) for their assistance with the RNA-Seq data analysis. The authors also thank Dicky Gunawan, Hosoda SHC Co., Ltd., Fukui, Japan for providing gnetin C for this study and students in the lab for their contribution.

Conflicts of Interest: The authors declare no conflicts of interest.

Abbreviations

AKT	v-akt murine thymoma viral oncogene (protein kinase B)
ANOVA	Analysis of variance
AR	Androgen receptor
bw	Body weight
CC3	Cleaved caspase 3
CD31	Cluster of differentiation 31
CRPC	Castration-resistant prostate cancer
DEGs	Differentially expressed genes
DMSO	Dimethyl sulfoxide
Ctrl	Control
ELISA	Enzyme-linked immunosorbent assay
ERK1/2	Extracellular signal-regulated kinase 1/2
FDR	False discovery rate
GAPDH	Glyceraldehyde 3-phosphate dehydrogenase
f/f	Pten gene flanked by two loxP sites in each allele
GnC	gnetin C
GRCm39	Genome reference consortium mouse build 39
H&E	Hematoxylin and eosin
HED	Human equivalent dose
HSP70	Heat shock protein 70
IACUC	Institutional Animal Care and Use Committee
IHC	Immunohistochemistry
IL-2	Interleukin 2
i.p.	Intraperitoneal
Ki67	Cellular protein marker of proliferation
LIU	Long Island University

mTOR	mammalian target of rapamycin
ns	Non-significant
NS	Non-silenced
OE	Overexpression
p-AKT^{S473}	Phosphorylation of serine 473 in C-terminus of AKT
p-4EBP1	Phosphorylated eukaryotic translational initiation factor 4E (elF4E)-binding protein 1
p-S6K	Phosphorylated p70 ribosomal protein S6 kinase
p-mTOR	Phosphorylated mammalian target of rapamycin
Pb-Cre+	Probasin promoter directing expression of epithelial Cre recombinase
PC3M	Human prostate cancer cell line
PCR	Polymerase chain reaction
PI3K	Phosphoinositide 3-kinase
PIN	Prostate intraepithelial neoplasia
PTEN	Phosphatase and tensin homolog
Pten+/f	Pten heterozygous mice
Ptenf/f	Pten homozygous, Pten-null
qRT-PCR	Quantitative reverse transcriptase polymerase chain reaction
RNA	Ribonucleic acid
RPMI-1640	Roswell Park Memorial Institute 1640 cell culture media
R26	Rosa26 loci in the mouse genome
SEM	Standard error of mean
shMTA1	short hairpin MTA1
shNS	short hairpin non-silence
UGS	Urogenital system
WT	Wild-type

References

1. Siegel, R.L.; Miller, K.D.; Wagle, N.S.; Jemal, A. Cancer statistics, 2023. *CA Cancer J. Clin.* **2023**, *73*, 17–48. [CrossRef]
2. Malik, S.N.; Brattain, M.; Ghosh, P.M.; Troyer, D.A.; Prihoda, T.; Bedolla, R.; Kreisberg, J.I. Immunohistochemical demonstration of phospho-Akt in high Gleason grade prostate cancer. *Clin. Cancer Res.* **2002**, *8*, 1168–1171. [PubMed]
3. Paweletz, C.P.; Charboneau, L.; Bichsel, V.E.; Simone, N.L.; Chen, T.; Gillespie, J.W.; Emmert-Buck, M.R.; Roth, M.J.; Petricoin, I.E.; Liotta, L.A. Reverse phase protein microarrays which capture disease progression show activation of pro-survival pathways at the cancer invasion front. *Oncogene* **2001**, *20*, 1981–1989. [CrossRef] [PubMed]
4. Kim, M.J.; Cardiff, R.D.; Desai, N.; Banach-Petrosky, W.A.; Parsons, R.; Shen, M.M.; Abate-Shen, C. Cooperativity of Nkx3.1 and Pten loss of function in a mouse model of prostate carcinogenesis. *Proc. Natl. Acad. Sci. USA* **2002**, *99*, 2884–2889. [CrossRef] [PubMed]
5. Grant, S. Cotargeting survival signaling pathways in cancer. *J. Clin. Investig.* **2008**, *118*, 3003–3006. [CrossRef]
6. Shorning, B.Y.; Dass, M.S.; Smalley, M.J.; Pearson, H.B. The PI3K-AKT-mTOR Pathway and Prostate Cancer: At the Crossroads of AR, MAPK, and WNT Signaling. *Int. J. Mol. Sci.* **2020**, *21*, 4507. [CrossRef]
7. Kinkade, C.W.; Castillo-Martin, M.; Puzio-Kuter, A.; Yan, J.; Foster, T.H.; Gao, H.; Sun, Y.; Ouyang, X.; Gerald, W.L.; Cordon-Cardo, C.; et al. Targeting AKT/mTOR and ERK MAPK signaling inhibits hormone-refractory prostate cancer in a preclinical mouse model. *J. Clin. Investig.* **2008**, *118*, 3051–3064. [CrossRef] [PubMed]
8. Dias, S.J.; Zhou, X.; Ivanovic, M.; Gailey, M.P.; Dhar, S.; Zhang, L.; He, Z.; Penman, A.D.; Vijayakumar, S.; Levenson, A.S. Nuclear MTA1 overexpression is associated with aggressive prostate cancer, recurrence and metastasis in African Americans. *Sci. Rep.* **2013**, *3*, 2331–2341. [CrossRef] [PubMed]
9. Hofer, M.D.; Kuefer, R.; Varambally, S.; Li, H.; Ma, J.; Shapiro, G.I.; Gschwend, J.E.; Hautmann, R.E.; Sanda, M.G.; Giehl, K.; et al. The role of metastasis-associated protein 1 in prostate cancer progression. *Cancer Res.* **2004**, *64*, 825–829. [CrossRef]
10. Dhar, S.; Kumar, A.; Zhang, L.; Rimando, A.M.; Lage, J.M.; Lewin, J.R.; Atfi, A.; Zhang, X.; Levenson, A.S. Dietary pterostilbene is a novel MTA1-targeted chemopreventive and therapeutic agent in prostate cancer. *Oncotarget* **2016**, *7*, 18469–18484. [CrossRef]
11. Dhar, S.; Kumar, A.; Li, K.; Tzivion, G.; Levenson, A.S. Resveratrol regulates PTEN/Akt pathway through inhibition of MTA1/HDAC unit of the NuRD complex in prostate cancer. *Biochim. Biophys. Acta* **2015**, *1853*, 265–275. [CrossRef] [PubMed]
12. Hemani, R.; Patel, I.; Inamdar, N.; Campanelli, G.; Donovan, V.; Kumar, A.; Levenson, A.S. Dietary Pterostilbene for MTA1-Targeted Interception in High-Risk Premalignant Prostate Cancer. *Cancer Prev. Res.* **2022**, *15*, 87–100. [CrossRef] [PubMed]
13. Parupathi, P.; Campanelli, G.; Deabel, R.A.; Puaar, A.; Devarakonda, L.S.; Kumar, A.; Levenson, A.S. Gnetin C Intercepts MTA1-Associated Neoplastic Progression in Prostate Cancer. *Cancers* **2022**, *14*, 6038. [CrossRef]
14. Choudhury, A.D. PTEN-PI3K pathway alterations in advanced prostate cancer and clinical implications. *Prostate* **2022**, *82* (Suppl. S1), S60–S72. [CrossRef] [PubMed]
15. Braglia, L.; Zavatti, M.; Vinceti, M.; Martelli, A.M.; Marmiroli, S. Deregulated PTEN/PI3K/AKT/mTOR signaling in prostate cancer: Still a potential druggable target? *Biochim. Biophys. Acta Mol. Cell Res.* **2020**, *1867*, 118731. [CrossRef] [PubMed]

16. Asensi, M.; Ortega, A.; Mena, S.; Feddi, F.; Estrela, J.M. Natural polyphenols in cancer therapy. *Crit. Rev. Clin. Lab. Sci.* **2011**, *10*, 197–216. [CrossRef] [PubMed]
17. Rudzinska, A.; Juchaniuk, P.; Oberda, J.; Wisniewska, J.; Wojdan, W.; Szklener, K.; Mandziuk, S. Phytochemicals in Cancer Treatment and Cancer Prevention-Review on Epidemiological Data and Clinical Trials. *Nutrients* **2023**, *15*, 1896. [CrossRef] [PubMed]
18. Swetha, M.; Keerthana, C.K.; Rayginia, T.P.; Anto, R.J. Cancer Chemoprevention: A Strategic Approach Using Phytochemicals. *Front. Pharmacol.* **2021**, *12*, 809308.
19. Tewari, D.; Patni, P.; Bishayee, A.; Sah, A.N.; Bishayee, A. Natural products targeting the PI3K-Akt-mTOR signaling pathway in cancer: A novel therapeutic strategy. *Semin. Cancer Biol.* **2022**, *80*, 1–17. [CrossRef]
20. Narayanankutty, A. Inhibitory Potential of Dietary Nutraceuticals on Cellular PI3K/Akt Signaling: Implications in Cancer Prevention and Therapy. *Curr. Top. Med. Chem.* **2021**, *21*, 1816–1831. [CrossRef]
21. Narayanankutty, A. Phytochemicals as PI3K/Akt/mTOR Inhibitors and Their Role in Breast Cancer Treatment. *Recent Pat. Anticancer Drug Discov.* **2020**, *15*, 188–199. [CrossRef] [PubMed]
22. Levenson, A.S. Metastasis-associated protein 1-mediated antitumor and anticancer activity of dietary stilbenes for prostate cancer chemoprevention and therapy. *Semin. Cancer Biol.* **2020**, *80*, 107–117. [CrossRef] [PubMed]
23. Gadkari, K.; Kolhatkar, U.; Hemani, R.; Campanelli, G.; Cai, Q.; Kumar, A.; Levenson, A.S. Therapeutic Potential of Gnetin C in Prostate Cancer: A Pre-Clinical Study. *Nutrients* **2020**, *12*, 3631. [CrossRef] [PubMed]
24. Kumar, A.; Dholakia, K.; Sikorska, G.; Martinez, L.A.; Levenson, A.S. MTA1-Dependent Anticancer Activity of Gnetin C in Prostate Cancer. *Nutrients* **2019**, *11*, 2096. [CrossRef] [PubMed]
25. Love, M.I.; Huber, W.; Anders, S. Moderated estimation of fold change and dispersion for RNA-seq data with DESeq2. *Genome Biol.* **2014**, *15*, 550. [CrossRef] [PubMed]
26. Liberzon, A.; Birger, C.; Thorvaldsdottir, H.; Ghandi, M.; Mesirov, J.P.; Tamayo, P. The Molecular Signatures Database (MSigDB) hallmark gene set collection. *Cell Syst.* **2015**, *1*, 417–425. [CrossRef] [PubMed]
27. Tani, H.; Hikami, S.; Iizuna, S.; Yoshimatsu, M.; Asama, T.; Ota, H.; Kimura, Y.; Tatefuji, T.; Hashimoto, K.; Higaki, K. Pharmacokinetics and safety of resveratrol derivatives in humans after oral administration of melinjo (*Gnetum gnemon* L.) seed extract powder. *J. Agric. Food Chem.* **2014**, *62*, 1999–2007. [CrossRef] [PubMed]
28. Espinoza, J.L.; Elbadry, M.I.; Taniwaki, M.; Harada, K.; Trung, L.Q.; Nakagawa, N.; Takami, A.; Ishiyama, K.; Yamauchi, T.; Takenaka, K.; et al. The simultaneous inhibition of the mTOR and MAPK pathways with Gnetin-C induces apoptosis in acute myeloid leukemia. *Cancer Lett.* **2017**, *400*, 127–136. [CrossRef] [PubMed]
29. Nair, A.B.; Jacob, S. A simple practice guide for dose conversion between animals and human. *J. Basic Clin. Pharm.* **2016**, *7*, 27–31. [CrossRef]
30. Nakagami, Y.; Suzuki, S.; Espinoza, J.L.; Vu Quang, L.; Enomoto, M.; Takasugi, S.; Nakamura, A.; Nakayama, T.; Tani, H.; Hanamura, I.; et al. Immunomodulatory and Metabolic Changes after Gnetin-C Supplementation in Humans. *Nutrients* **2019**, *11*, 1403. [CrossRef]
31. Konno, H.; Kanai, Y.; Katagiri, M.; Watanabe, T.; Mori, A.; Ikuta, T.; Tani, H.; Fukushima, S.; Tatefuji, T.; Shirasawa, T. Melinjo (*Gnetum gnemon* L.) Seed Extract Decreases Serum Uric Acid Levels in Nonobese Japanese Males: A Randomized Controlled Study. *Evid. Based Complement Altern. Med.* **2013**, *2013*, 589169. [CrossRef] [PubMed]
32. Espinoza, J.L.; An, D.T.; Trung, L.Q.; Yamada, K.; Nakao, S.; Takami, A. Stilbene derivatives from melinjo extract have antioxidant and immune modulatory effects in healthy individuals. *Integr. Mol. Med.* **2015**, *2*, 405–413.
33. Bitting, R.L.; Armstrong, A.J. Targeting the PI3K/Akt/mTOR pathway in castration-resistant prostate cancer. *Endocr. Relat. Cancer* **2013**, *20*, R83–R99. [CrossRef]
34. Sharrard, R.M.; Maitland, N.J. Regulation of protein kinase B activity by PTEN and SHIP2 in human prostate-derived cell lines. *Cell. Signal.* **2007**, *19*, 129–138. [CrossRef] [PubMed]
35. Hay, N.; Sonenberg, N. Upstream and downstream of mTOR. *Genes Dev.* **2004**, *18*, 1926–1945. [CrossRef]
36. Cai, Z.; Wang, J.; Li, Y.; Shi, Q.; Jin, L.; Li, S.; Zhu, M.; Wang, Q.; Wong, L.L.; Yang, W.; et al. Overexpressed Cyclin D1 and CDK4 proteins are responsible for the resistance to CDK4/6 inhibitor in breast cancer that can be reversed by PI3K/mTOR inhibitors. *Sci. China Life Sci.* **2023**, *66*, 94–109. [CrossRef] [PubMed]
37. Xu, Y.; Chen, S.Y.; Ross, K.N.; Balk, S.P. Androgens induce prostate cancer cell proliferation through mammalian target of rapamycin activation and post-transcriptional increases in cyclin D proteins. *Cancer Res.* **2006**, *66*, 7783–7792. [CrossRef]
38. Recchia, A.G.; Musti, A.M.; Lanzino, M.; Panno, M.L.; Turano, E.; Zumpano, R.; Belfiore, A.; Ando, S.; Maggiolini, M. A cross-talk between the androgen receptor and the epidermal growth factor receptor leads to p38MAPK-dependent activation of mTOR and cyclinD1 expression in prostate and lung cancer cells. *Int. J. Biochem. Cell Biol.* **2009**, *41*, 603–614. [CrossRef] [PubMed]
39. Gao, N.; Flynn, D.C.; Zhang, Z.; Zhong, X.S.; Walker, V.; Liu, K.J.; Shi, X.; Jiang, B.H. G1 cell cycle progression and the expression of G1 cyclins are regulated by PI3K/AKT/mTOR/p70S6K1 signaling in human ovarian cancer cells. *Am. J. Physiol. Cell Physiol.* **2004**, *287*, C281–C291. [CrossRef]
40. Stelloo, S.; Sanders, J.; Nevedomskaya, E.; de Jong, J.; Peters, D.; van Leenders, G.J.; Jenster, G.; Bergman, A.M.; Zwart, W. mTOR pathway activation is a favorable prognostic factor in human prostate adenocarcinoma. *Oncotarget* **2016**, *7*, 32916–32924. [CrossRef]

41. Barata, P.C.; Magi-Galluzzi, C.; Gupta, R.; Dreicer, R.; Klein, E.A.; Garcia, J.A. Association of mTOR Pathway Markers and Clinical Outcomes in Patients with Intermediate-/High-risk Prostate Cancer: Long-Term Analysis. *Clin. Genitourin. Cancer* **2019**, *17*, 366–372. [CrossRef]
42. Jerusalem, G.; Rorive, A.; Collignon, J. Use of mTOR inhibitors in the treatment of breast cancer: An evaluation of factors that influence patient outcomes. *Breast Cancer* **2014**, *6*, 43–57. [CrossRef]
43. Battelli, C.; Cho, D.C. mTOR inhibitors in renal cell carcinoma. *Therapy* **2011**, *8*, 359–367. [CrossRef] [PubMed]
44. Hua, H.; Kong, Q.; Zhang, H.; Wang, J.; Luo, T.; Jiang, Y. Targeting mTOR for cancer therapy. *J. Hematol. Oncol.* **2019**, *12*, 71. [CrossRef]
45. Edlind, M.P.; Hsieh, A.C. PI3K-AKT-mTOR signaling in prostate cancer progression and androgen deprivation therapy resistance. *Asian J. Androl.* **2014**, *16*, 378–386. [PubMed]
46. Armstrong, A.J.; Netto, G.J.; Rudek, M.A.; Halabi, S.; Wood, D.P.; Creel, P.A.; Mundy, K.; Davis, S.L.; Wang, T.; Albadine, R.; et al. A pharmacodynamic study of rapamycin in men with intermediate- to high-risk localized prostate cancer. *Clin. Cancer Res.* **2010**, *16*, 3057–3066. [CrossRef] [PubMed]
47. Xu, X.; Kong, X.; Liu, T.; Zhou, L.; Wu, J.; Fu, J.; Wang, Y.; Zhu, M.; Yao, S.; Ding, Y.; et al. Metastasis-associated protein 1, modulated by miR-30c, promotes endometrial cancer progression through AKT/mTOR/4E-BP1 pathway. *Gynecol. Oncol.* **2019**, *154*, 207–217. [CrossRef]
48. Campanelli, G.; Deabel, R.A.; Puaar, A.; Devarakonda, L.S.; Parupathi, P.; Zhang, J.; Waxner, N.; Yang, C.; Kumar, A.; Levenson, A.S. Molecular Efficacy of Gnetin C as Dual-Targeted Therapy for Castrate-Resistant Prostate Cancer. *Mol. Nutr. Food Res.* **2023**, *67*, e2300479. [CrossRef]

cancers

MDPI

Article

Naringin–Dextrin Nanocomposite Abates Diethylnitrosamine/Acetylaminofluorene-Induced Lung Carcinogenesis by Modulating Oxidative Stress, Inflammation, Apoptosis, and Cell Proliferation

Eman E. Mohamed [1], Osama M. Ahmed [1,*], Khairy M. A. Zoheir [2], Ahmed A. G. El-Shahawy [3], Shadi Tamur [4], Anwar Shams [5,6,7,*], Jack T. Burcher [8], Anupam Bishayee [8] and Adel Abdel-Moneim [1]

1 Physiology Division, Faculty of Science, Beni-Suef University, Beni-Suef 62521, Egypt; eman_ezzeldien@yahoo.com (E.E.M.); adel_men2020@yahoo.com or adel.hassan@science.bsu.edu.eg (A.A.-M.)
2 Cell Biology Department, Biotechnology Research Institute, National Research Centre, Cairo 12622, Egypt; khma25@gmail.com
3 Materials Science and Nanotechnology Department, Faculty of Postgraduate Studies for Advanced Sciences, Beni-Suef University, Beni-Suef 62521, Egypt; ahmedelshahawy382@yahoo.com
4 Departement of Pediatrics, College of Medicine, Taif University, Taif 21944, Saudi Arabia; shaditamur@tu.edu.sa
5 Departement of Pharmacology, College of Medicine, Taif University, Taif 21944, Saudi Arabia
6 Centre of Biomedical Sciences Research, Deanship of Scientific Research, Taif University, Taif 21974, Saudi Arabia
7 High Altitude Research Center, Taif University, Taif 21944, Saudi Arabia
8 College of Osteopathic Medicine, Lake Erie College of Osteopathic Medicine, Bradenton, FL 34211, USA; jburcher83447@med.lecom.edu (J.T.B.); abishayee@lecom.edu or abishayee@gmail.com (A.B.)
* Correspondence: osamamoha@yahoo.com or osama.ahmed@science.bsu.edu.eg (O.M.A.); a.shams@tu.edu.sa or anwar.shams@mail.mcgill.ca (A.S.)

Simple Summary: Despite advancements in the field, lung malignancies are the primary cause of cancer-attributable morbidity and mortality on a global scale. Recently, therapeutic agents have demonstrated improved efficacy when combined with nanocarriers to improve their delivery, bioavailability, and efficacy. Accordingly, the aim of this study is to evaluate the effects and mechanisms of action of naringin–dextrin nanocomposites (Nar-Dx-NCs) against diethylnitrosamine (DEN)/2-acetylaminofluorene (2AAF)-induced lung carcinogenesis in male Wistar rats. Naringin's preventive action against DEN/2AAF-induced lung cancer was amplified using Nar-Dx-NCs, which exerted heightened anti-carcinogenic effects by suppressing oxidative stress, inflammation, and cell proliferation and activating apoptosis.

Abstract: Nanotechnology has proven advantageous in numerous scientific applications, one being to enhance the delivery of chemotherapeutic agents. This present study aims to evaluate the mechanisms underlying the chemopreventive action of naringin–dextrin nanocomposites (Nar-Dx-NCs) against diethylnitrosamine (DEN)/2-acetylaminofluorene (2AAF)-induced lung carcinogenesis in male Wistar rats. DEN was administered intraperitoneally (i.p.) (150 mg/kg/week) for two weeks, followed by the oral administration of 2AAF (20 mg/kg) four times a week for three weeks. Rats receiving DEN/2AAF were concurrently treated with naringin or Nar-Dx-NCs orally at a dose of 10 mg/kg every other day for 24 weeks. Naringin and Nar-Dx-NCs treatments prevented the formation of tumorigenic cells within the alveoli of rats exposed to DEN/2AAF. These findings were associated with a significant decrease in lipid peroxidation, upregulation of antioxidant enzyme (glutathione peroxidase and superoxide dismutase) activity, and enhanced glutathione and nuclear factor erythroid 2–related factor 2 expression in the lungs. Naringin and Nar-Dx-NCs exerted anti-inflammatory actions manifested by a decrease in lung protein expression of tumor necrosis factor-α and interleukin-1β and mRNA expression of interleukin-6, interferon-γ, nuclear factor-κB, and inducible nitric oxide synthase, with a concurrent increase in interleukin-10 expression. The anti-inflammatory effect of Nar-Dx-NCs was more potent than naringin. Regarding the effect on apoptosis, both naringin and Nar-Dx-NCs significantly reduced Bcl-2 and increased Bax and P53 expressions. Moreover, naringin or Nar-Dx-NCs induced a significant decrease in the expression of the proliferator marker, Ki-67, and the effect of Nar-Dx-NCs was more marked. In conclusion, Nar-Dx-NCs improved naringin's preventive action against DEN/2AAF-induced lung cancer and exerted anticarcinogenic effects by suppressing oxidative stress and inflammation and improving apoptotic signal induction and propagation.

Keywords: diethylnitrosamine; acetylaminofluorene; lung cancer; naringin; naringin–dextrin nanocomposite; anticancer; anti-inflammatory; antioxidant; apoptosis

1. Introduction

Malignancies of the lung are among the most frequently diagnosed types of cancer in both sexes, affecting 11.6% of the population. Due to its aggressive nature, lung cancer has a high mortality rate worldwide, with over 18% of patients ultimately succumbing to cancer-related complications [1,2]. Risk factors include tobacco use, radiation to the thorax, and exposure to secondhand smoke, radon gas, asbestos, and other carcinogens. Diethylnitrosamine (DEN), for example, is frequently used as a carcinogenic agent in in vivo analyses; it has been reported that rodents exposed to DEN develop lung, liver, skin, and gastrointestinal cancers [3,4]. The metabolism of DEN via the metabolic activation of cytochrome P450 (CYP450)-dependent monooxygenase system results in oxidative stress, leading to cytotoxicity, mutagenicity, and carcinogenesis [5,6]. The lungs are perhaps most sensitive to these effects, as DEN has been established to most frequently cause lung cancer compared to other primary tumors [7]. Reactive oxygen species (ROS) produced during the metabolism of DEN may be a major factor in the emergence of cancer. An imbalance between ROS production and antioxidant capacities leads to DNA damage and oxidative stress, ultimately triggering carcinogenesis [8,9]. Another genotoxic carcinogen, 2-acetylaminofluorene (2AAF), forms covalent interactions between metabolic derivatives of 2AAF and DNA to initiate tumorigenesis in many species [10].

Inflammation plays a significant role as an innate broad defense mechanism against injury and generalized infection [11]. During this process, macrophages produce pro-inflammatory cytokines, including interferon-γ (IFN-γ), tumor necrosis factor-alpha (TNF-α), interleukin-6 (IL-6), as well as other inflammatory proteins, including inducible nitric oxide synthase (iNOS) [12]. Cytokines are essential regulators of the immune and inflammatory responses via intricate networks and, therefore, serve as biomarkers for disease [13]. Key pro-inflammatory cytokines implicated in tumorigenesis include TNF-α, interleukin-1β (IL-1β), and IL-6 [14,15]. Tumorigenesis and inflammation are closely related, and much effort pertaining to cancer research is focused on this topic [16]. For example, the crucial importance of nuclear factor erythroid 2-related factor 2 (Nrf2) was recently shown to control the antioxidant response element (ARE), which protects against oxidative stress [17].

Natural sources of antioxidants are an increasingly attractive option for chemoprevention due to their relatively nontoxic side effect profiles [18]. Naringin, a polyphenolic phytochemical belonging to the flavonoid subclass, has already been reported to possess antioxidant, anti-inflammatory, and antitumor effects [19,20]. Targeted drug delivery systems have been substantially advanced in recent years, allowing drugs to be delivered to specific locations to treat a variety of diseases with greater efficacy and, in theory, reduced toxicity [21]. Compared to native formulations, the solubility, release profiles, and bioavailability of nanoscale drugs, in conjunction with their nano-based delivery systems, have proven beneficial for cancer treatment. The use of targeted nano-based drug delivery systems permits a more appropriate route of administration, fewer adverse effects, diminished toxicity, greater diffusivity, and a longer half-life of anticancer drugs [22]. Previous research has demonstrated that nanomaterials can selectively enter organs, tissues, and cells to release treatments at precise locations previously considered to be inaccessible without great difficulty [23,24]. Combining nanodrug formulations with natural products may further reduce drug toxicity and augment the therapeutic properties of both conventional agents and natural compounds [25–29]. Newly published in vitro and in vivo data are already in support of naringin–dextrin nanocomposites (Nar-Dx-NCs) exhibiting anti-inflammatory and anticancer effects against hepatocellular carcinoma, but information regarding the effects of Nar-Dx-NCs in the context of lung cancer is lacking [30,31]. Therefore, the purpose of our study is to report the anticarcinogenic effects and mechanisms of action of Nar-Dx-NCs in DEN/2AAF-induced lung carcinogenesis in male Wistar rats.

2. Materials and Methods

2.1. Chemicals

DEN (Cat. #049K1613V), 2AAF (Cat. #A7015), naringin (Cat. #BCBT3477), and dextrin (Cat. # D2006) were obtained from Sigma-Aldrich (St. Louis, MO, USA). All other chemicals and solvents utilized were of analytical grade.

2.2. Synthesis of Nar-Dx-NCs

Nar-Dx-NCs were prepared according to the method described by Manchu et al. [32]. Briefly, a 5% (*w*/*w* or 0.2 mg/mL) aqueous nanoemulsion of dextrin and naringin was produced by continuous ultrasonication for 1 min. Formaldehyde was then added in exact molar ratios to dextrin, homogenized via ultrasonication at high pressure for 30 min, and stirred at room temperature for 12 h. After precipitating with ethanol 99% (*v*/*v*), the crosslinked dextrin–naringin nanocomposite was centrifuged at 14,000 rpm for 45 min at 4 °C before being frozen for 48 h. The nanoemulsion was stored as a powder at 4 °C. In our earlier publication [30], we outlined the techniques utilized to characterize the Nar-Dx-NCs, including X-ray diffraction (XRD), Fourier transformation infrared (FTIR) spectroscopy, transmission electron microscopy (TEM), zetasizer and zeta potential studies, and ultraviolet-visible (UV-Vis) spectrometry. Additionally, Nar-Dx-NCs were evaluated according to entrapment effectiveness (EE) and the release of naringin from dextrin.

2.3. Animal Experimentation

Wistar male adult rats weighing 100–120 g and aged 7–8 weeks were utilized in this study. The animals were purchased from the Animal House Facility of the Egyptian Organization for Biological Products and Vaccines (VACSERA, Cairo, Egypt). Rats were observed for 7 days prior to the start of experimental procedures to allow acclimation to their new environment and monitor for infection. The rats were kept in a controlled environment with a 12/12 h light/dark cycle, a standard diet, and unrestricted access to water. The temperature was kept between 20 and 25 °C. All procedures involving animals conducted in this present study were approved by the Animal Ethics Committee of the Faculty of Science at Beni-Suef University in Egypt (Approval Number: BNS:020-91).

2.4. Experimental Design

Adult male Wistar rats were divided into four groups, each comprising 12 rats. Group 1 served as an untreated normal group, while groups 2, 3, and 4 received 150 mg/kg of DEN intraperitoneally (i.p.) twice a week for two weeks plus 20 mg/kg 2AAF via oral gavage four times a week for three weeks [33,34]. Group 2 served as the positive control group and received no further interventions. Groups 3 and 4 received naringin or Nar-Dx-NCs, respectively, at a dose of 10 mg/kg every other day from the start of carcinogenesis for the duration of this study (24 weeks), according to a previously established protocol [35]. Groups 1 and 2 received the same volume of the vehicle (5 mL 1% carboxymethyl cellulose), in which naringin and Nar-Dx-NCs were dissolved. After 24 weeks, the animals were anesthetized with diethyl ether before being sacrificed (Figure 1).

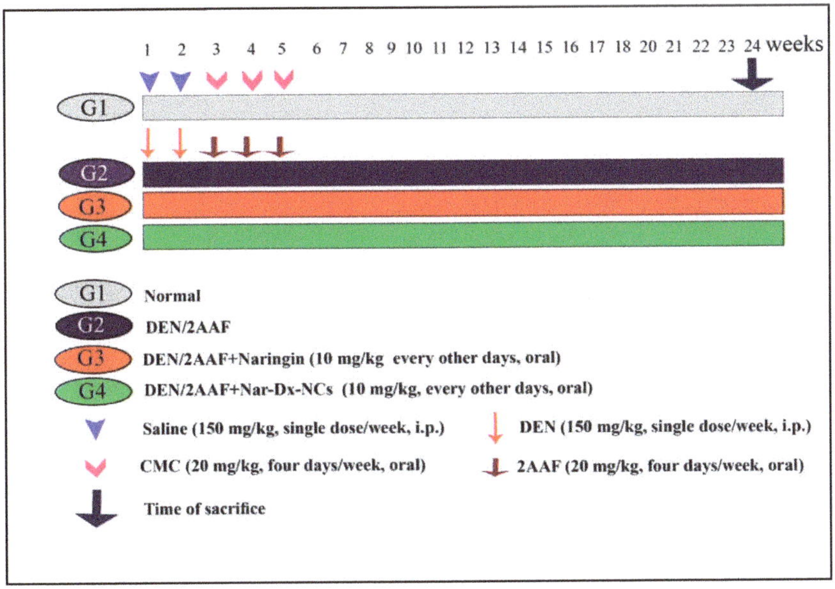

Figure 1. Schematic of the experimental design. Abbreviations: 2AAF, 2-acetylaminofluorene; CMC, carboxymethyl cellulose; DEN, diethylnitrosamine; Nar-Dx-NCs, naringin–dextrin nanocomposites.

2.5. Lung Sampling and Analysis

The lung parenchyma of euthanized rats was resected and washed with cold sterile saline. Each lung was cut into four pieces (3 mm^3). After one day of fixation in 10% neutral buffered formalin, one lung piece was cut into sections for histological analysis. Another lung sample was mixed with phosphate buffer at 25% w/v and centrifuged at 3000 rpm for 15 min at 4 °C. The supernatants were stored at −30 °C until they were used to investigate antioxidant activities, oxidative stress, and biomarker levels, including TNF-α, IL-1β, and Nrf2. The third portion of the lung tissue was kept at −70 °C in sterilized tubes and used for RNA isolation and real-time polymerase chain reaction (PCR) assays. A fourth lung tissue sample was kept at −30 °C and was used for Western blot analysis of proliferator marker, Kiel-67 (Ki-67). Various experimental endpoints are illustrated in Figure 2.

2.6. Histopathological Examination

Additional samples of lung tissue fixed for 24 h in 10% neutral buffered formalin were dehydrated with ethyl alcohol and embedded in paraffin. The lung sections (5 mm^3) were then stained with hematoxylin and eosin (H&E) according to the method described by Bancroft and Gamble [36] and examined under a light microscope. The histopathological lesions of lung sections stained with H&E were evaluated via histomorphometric analysis using ImageJ 1.46r software (Leica Qwin 500 image system, Cambridge, UK) [37]. The mean area of alveoli space and mean area percentages of inflammation and hemorrhage were measured.

2.7. Biochemical Assays

Lung lipid peroxide (LPO), reduced glutathione (GSH), glutathione peroxidase (GPx), and superoxide dismutase (SOD) were analyzed using kits from Bio-Diagnostic (Dokki, Giza, Egypt) according to the manufacturer's instructions. Antibodies against TNF-α, IL-1β, and Nrf2 were used on the lung tissue obtained from rats using Enzyme-Linked Immunosorbent Assay (ELISA) kits following the guidelines of the manufacturer (R&D Systems, Minneapolis, MN, USA).

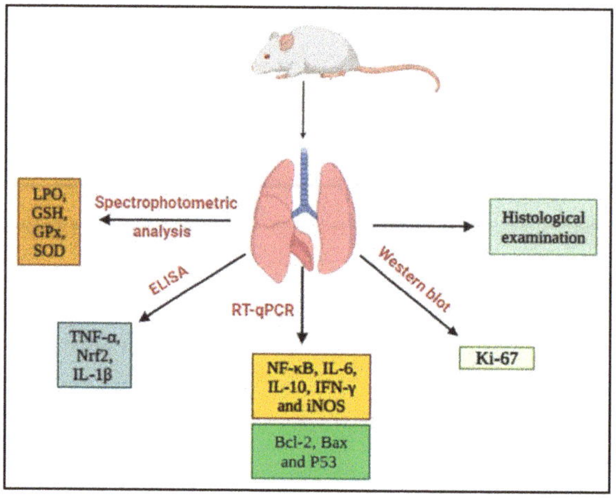

Figure 2. Schematic diagram of analyses performed on lung samples and endpoints recorded. Abbreviations: Bax, Bcl-2-associated X protein; Bcl-2, B-cell lymphoma-2; ELISA, enzyme-linked immunosorbent assay; GSH, glutathione; GPx, glutathione peroxidase; Ki-67, Kiel-67; IFN-γ, interferon-γ; IL-1β, interleukin-1β; IL-6, interleukin-6; IL-10, interleukin-10; iNOS, inducible nitric oxide synthase; LPO, lipid peroxidation; NF-κB, nuclear factor-κB; Nrf2, nuclear factor erythroid 2-related factor 2; RT-qPCR, reverse transcription–quantitative polymerase chain reaction; SOD, superoxide dismutase.

2.8. Isolation of Total RNA and Reverse Transcription–Quantitative PCR (RT-qPCR)

Total RNA was extracted from homogenates of lung tissue using the TRIzol reagent (Cat. # 15596018, Invitrogen; Eugene, OR, USA) according to the manufacturer's instructions. RNA absorbance was measured at 260 nm using the method described by Sthoeger et al. [38]. The RNA quality was ascertained by measuring the ratio of the absorbance at 260 and 280 nm (260/280 ratio). The first strand of cDNA was synthesized using the high-capacity cDNA reverse transcription kit (Cat. # 4368814) from Applied Biosystems® (Foster City, CA, USA). Quantitative analyses of the target genes' mRNA expression were performed via quantitative PCR using the ABI Prism 7500 System (Biosystems, Foster City, CA, USA) and 96-well optical reaction plates. In brief, the cDNA was amplified via PCR (Applied Biosystems, Foster City, CA, USA) using a 25-μL reaction mixture, including 0.1 μL of 10 μM forward primer and 0.1 μL of 10 μM reverse primer each (final concentration of each primer: 40 nM), 11.05 μL of nuclease-free water, 12.5 μL of SYBR Green Universal Master mix, and 1.25 μL of cDNA sample. Table 1 contains a list of the primers used in this present study. The primers were obtained from Santa Cruz Biotechnology, Inc., Heidelberg, Germany. Results are displayed as a fold change in the gene expression normalized to that of the reference gene β-actin using the $2^{-\Delta\Delta CT}$ method.

Table 1. Primer sequences for RT-qPCR assays.

Genes	GenBank Accession Number	Sequence (5′–3′)
NF-κB	NM_001276711.1	F: TTCAACATGGCAGACGACGA R: TGCTCTAGTATTTGAAGGTATGGG
Bcl-2	NM_016993.1	F: TAAGCTGTCACAGAGGGGCT R: TGAAGAGTTCCTCCACCACC
Bax	NM_007527.3	F: CTGGATCCAAGACCAGGGTG R: CCTTTCCCCTTCCCCCATTC
P53	NM_030989.3	F: GTTTTTGTTCCTGAGCCCCG R: GAGCAAGGGGTGACTTTGGG

Table 1. *Cont.*

Genes	GenBank Accession Number	Sequence (5′–3′)
iNOS	NM_012611	F: CTATGGCCGCTTTGATGTGC R: CAACCTTGGTGTTGAAGGCG
IFN-γ	NM_138880.2	F: ACAACCCACAGATCCAGCAC R: CCAGAATCAGCACCGACTCC
IL-6	NM_012589.2	F: CACTTCACAAGTCGGAGGCT R: AGCACACTAGGTTTGCCGAG
IL-10	NM_012854	F: TTGAACCACCCGGCATCTAC R: CCAAGGAGTTGCTCCCGTTA
β-actin	NM_031144.3	F: TCACTATCGGCAATGTGCGG R: GCTCAGGAGGAGCAATGATG

Abbreviations: Bax, Bcl-2-associated X protein; Bcl-2, B-cell lymphoma-2; IFN-γ, interferon-γ; IL-6, interleukin-6; IL-10, interleukin-10; iNOS, inducible nitric oxide synthase; P53 tumor suppressor protein 53; NF-κB, nuclear factor-κB.

2.9. Western Blot Analysis

Lung tissues were homogenized in radioimmunoprecipitation assay (RIPA) buffer and centrifuged to obtain clear supernatants. The total protein content was measured using the Bradford reagent (SK3041) (Bio Basic Inc., Markham, ON, Canada). Afterward, 30 μg of proteins were separated using sodium dodecyl sulfate–polyacrylamide gel electrophoresis (SDS–PAGE) (Cat. # 161-0181; Bio-Rad Laboratories, Inc., Hercules, CA, USA) and then transferred to nitrocellulose membranes. After blocking in tris-buffered saline with Tween 20 (TBST) containing 5% non-fat milk powder, the membranes were incubated with primary antibodies against Ki-67 (Cat. # AB9260; EMD Millipore Corporation, Temecula, CA, USA) and β-actin (Sc-8432). The membranes were developed with the help of the chemiluminescent substrate (Cat. # 170-5060) (ClarityTM Western ECL substrate, Bio-Rad Laboratories, Inc., Hercules, CA, USA) and then examined with the corresponding horseradish peroxidase (HRP)-conjugated secondary antibodies (goat anti-rabbit IgG-HRP-1 mg goat monoclonal antibody) (Novus Biologicals, Littleton, CO, USA). Finally, the intensity ratio in the control sample was compared with the band intensities of the target proteins using image analysis (ChemiDoc MP Imaging system, Bio-Rad, Hercules, CA, USA) normalized to that of the housekeeping protein β-actin.

2.10. Statistical Analysis

The data are shown as means ± standard errors (SE). A one-way analysis of variance was performed using SPSS version 20 software (Chicago, IL, USA) to identify statistical differences between groups. Duncan's test was then used to compare various groups, with significance set at $p < 0.05$.

3. Results

3.1. Naringin and Nar-Dx-NCs Abrogated Histopathological Changes in Lung Parenchyma of Rats Administered DEN/2AAF

The histopathological examination of lung sections from the normal group revealed normal histology with thin and delicate walls in the alveolar area. The alveoli were well-aerated and contained only occasional pulmonary macrophages (Figure 3A). In contrast, rats receiving DEN/2AAF presented histological abnormalities consistent with carcinogenesis, including aggregation of tumor cells and diffuse thickening in interstitial tissues, with hemorrhage and congested blood vessels (Figure 3B). Tumor cells grew within the alveoli following lepidic and papillary growth patterns. Additionally, macrophages and other myeloid cells invaded adjacent alveolar air spaces. Tumor cells also displayed an acinar pattern of invasive adenocarcinoma. The invasion of a vessel via tumor cells was also observed (Figure 3C,D).

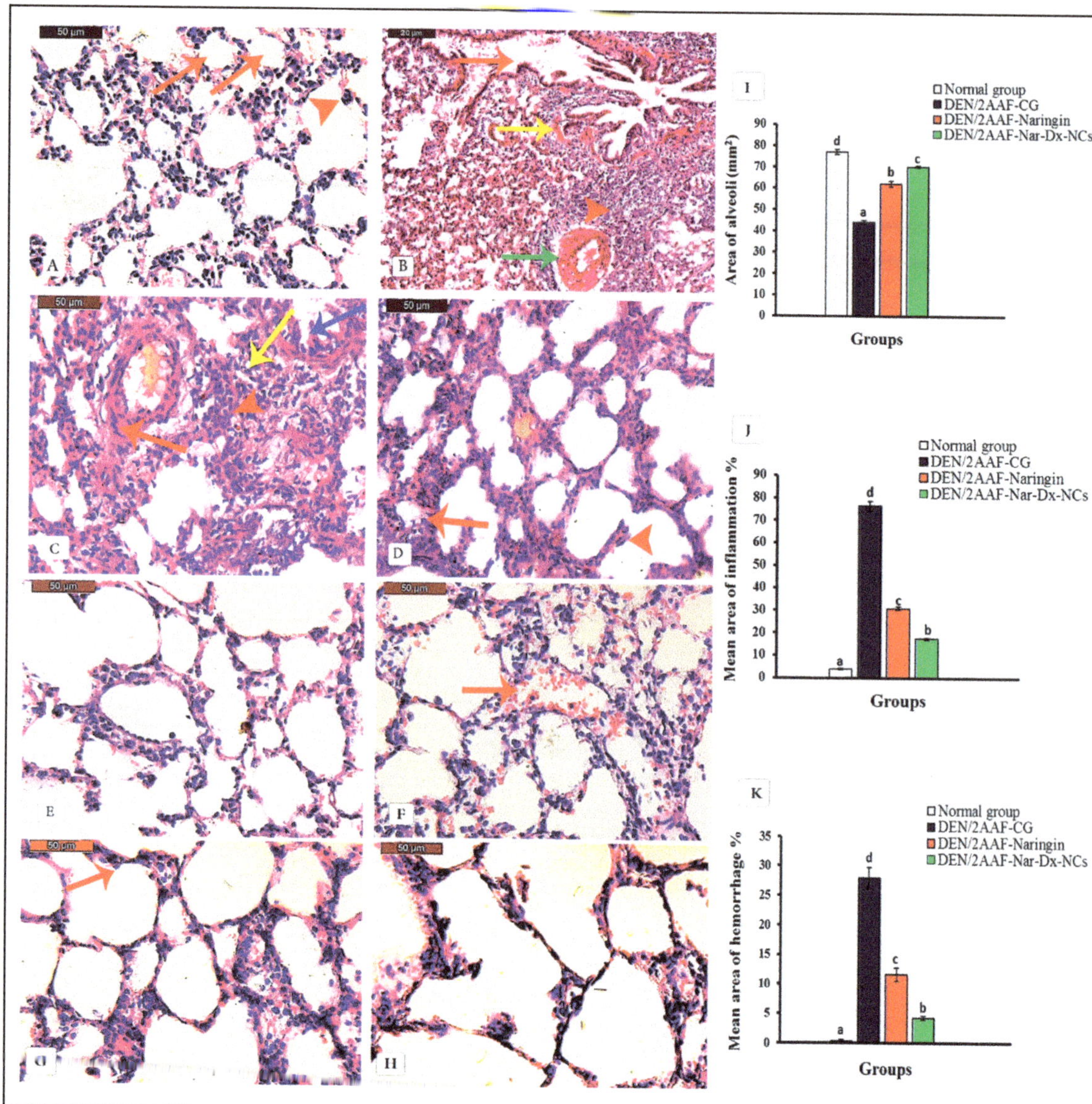

Figure 3. (**A**) Photomicrographs of sections of the lungs from control rats showing normal histology of the alveolar area, including thin and delicate walls (red arrow). The alveoli were well aerated and contained only an occasional pulmonary macrophage (red arrowhead) (hematoxylin and eosin [H&E] staining, scale bar: 50 µm). (**B**) Photomicrograph of lung section from DEN/2AAF-administered rat showing lung cancerous injuries including aggregation of tumor cells (red arrowhead) diffuse thickening in interstitial tissues (red arrow), hemorrhage (yellow arrow), and congested blood vessel (green arrow) (H&E staining, scale bar: 20 µm). (**C**) Photomicrograph of lung section from DEN/2AAF-administered rat displays invasive adenocarcinoma with an acinar pattern. Tumor is seen invading into a vessel (red arrow). Typical lepidic (blue arrow) and papillary (yellow arrow) growth patterns of tumor cells within alveoli. Macrophages and other myeloid cells infiltrated adjacent alveolar air spaces (red arrowhead) (H&E staining, scale bar: 50 µm). (**D**) Photomicrograph

of lung section from DEN/2AAF-administered rat showing lepidic (red arrow) and papillary (red arrowhead) growth patterns of tumor cells within alveoli. Macrophages and other myeloid cells infiltrated adjacent alveolar air spaces (red arrow) (H&E staining, scale bar: 50 μm). (**E**,**F**) Photomicrographs of lung sections of DEN/2AAF-administered rats treated with naringin showing a relatively normal structure of the alveolar walls. A hemorrhage was found in the lumen of some alveoli (red arrow) (H&E staining, scale bar: 50 μm). (**G**,**H**) Photomicrographs of lung sections of DEN/2AAF-administered rats treated with Nar-Dx-NCs showing a near-normal structure of the alveolar walls. Occasional pulmonary macrophages (arrow) were observed (H&E staining, scale bar: 50 μm). (**I–K**) Graphs displaying the mean area of alveoli to determine tumor cells within alveoli and mean area percentages of inflammation and hemorrhage, respectively, in each group studied. Means for each group are represented at the top of each bar. Different symbols (a–d) within the same graph are significantly different at $p < 0.05$. Abbreviations: 2AAF, 2-acetylaminofluorene; CG, control group; DEN, diethylnitrosamine; Nar-Dx-NCs, naringin–dextrin nanocomposites.

The structure of the alveolar walls of the lungs of DEN/2AAF-administered rats treated with naringin was relatively similar to that of healthy controls (Figure 3E). A hemorrhage was found in the lumen of some alveoli (Figure 3F). The structure of the alveolar walls of the lungs of DEN/2AAF-administered rats treated with Nar-Dx-NCs also appeared nearly normal. Occasional pulmonary macrophages were observed (Figure 3G,H). The statistical analysis of the mean area of alveoli space to determine tumor cells within alveoli, mean area percentages of inflammation, and hemorrhage confirmed an improvement in DEN/2AAF-administered groups treated with native or nanocomposite naringin compared to those not receiving concurrent chemoprophylaxis. These findings were more pronounced in Group IV, which received Nar-Dx-NCs, compared to native naringin (Group III) (Figure 3I–K).

3.2. *Effect of Naringin and Nar-Dx-NCs on Oxidative Stress and Antioxidant Defense System in Lung Tissues*

DEN/2AAF administration significantly ($p < 0.05$) elevated lung LPO and reduced the lung GSH content as well as GPx and SOD activities compared with those of normal rats. Free naringin or Nar-Dx-NCs treatment significantly ($p < 0.05$) reduced lung LPO and could increase GSH content and GPx and SOD activities compared with the values obtained in rats receiving DEN/2AAF alone (Table 2).

Table 2. Effect of naringin and Nar-Dx-NCs on lung LPO, GSH content, and GPx and SOD activities in lungs of DEN/2AAF-administered rats.

Groups	LPO (nmole MDA/100 mg Tissue/h)	GSH (nmole /100 mg Tissue)	GPx (mU/100 mg Tissue)	SOD (U/g Tissue)
Normal group	65.06 ± 0.084^{a}	85.86 ± 1.03^{d}	214.40 ± 1.40^{c}	16.76 ± 0.51^{c}
DEN/2AAF	134.45 ± 0.83^{c}	44.00 ± 0.75^{a}	85.61 ± 0.77^{a}	3.11 ± 0.02^{a}
DEN/2AAF + Naringin	75.28 ± 1.06^{b}	67.30 ± 0.98^{b}	205.51 ± 0.97^{b}	9.26 ± 0.12^{b}
DEN/2AAF + Nar-Dx-NCs	62.73 ± 0.55^{a}	75.73 ± 0.91^{c}	212.53 ± 2.52^{c}	11.03 ± 0.37^{b}

Data are expressed as mean ± SE ($n = 6$). Means with different superscript symbols (a–d) within the same column are significantly different at $p < 0.05$. Abbreviations: GSH, glutathione; GPx, glutathione peroxidase; LPO, lipid peroxidation; SOD, superoxide dismutase.

3.3. *Effects of Naringin and Nar-Dx-NCs on TNF-α, IL-1β, and Nrf2 Levels in Lung Tissues*

TNF-α and IL-1β levels in lung tissues were higher in DEN/2AAF-administered rats, whereas Nrf2 levels were lower ($p < 0.05$) compared to normal rats. In DEN/2AAF-administered rats, treatment with naringin or Nar-Dx-NCs reversed this effect (Figure 4).

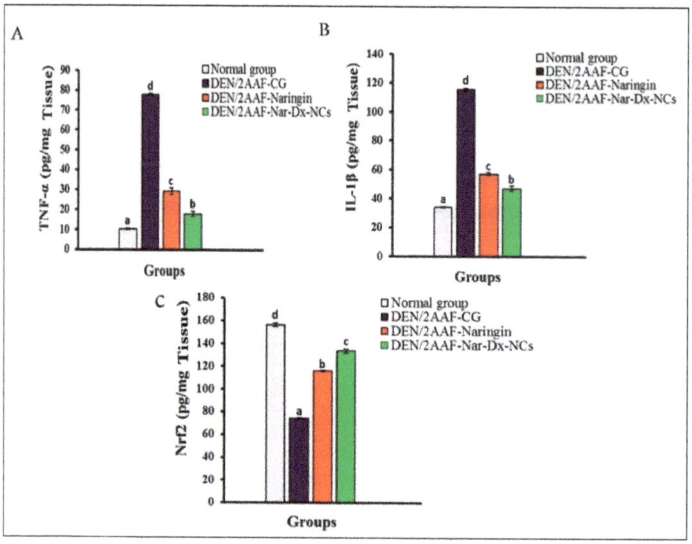

Figure 4. Effect of naringin or Nar-Dx-NCs on (**A**) TNF-α, (**B**) IL-1β, and (**C**) Nrf2 levels in the lungs of DEN/2AAF-administered rats. Data are expressed as means ± SE ($n = 6$). Means for each group are represented at the top of each bar. Different symbols (a–d) within the same graph are significantly different at $p < 0.05$. Abbreviations: 2AAF, 2-acetylaminofluorene; CG, control group; DEN, diethylnitrosamine; IL-1β, interleukin-1β; Nar-Dx-NCs, naringin–dextrin nanocomposites; Nrf2, nuclear factor erythroid 2-related factor 2; TNF-α, tumor necrosis factor-α.

3.4. Effects of Naringin and Nar-Dx-NCs on IL-6, IL-10, NF-κB, IFN-γ, and iNOS mRNA Expression in Lung Tissues

DEN/2AAF-administered rats exhibited greater IL-6, NF-κB, IFN-γ, and iNOS levels in lung tissues and a significant decrease in IL-10 expression compared with normal rats. The treatment of DEN/2AAF-administered rats with free naringin or Nar-Dx-NCs had a significant effect on the increase in IL-6, NF-κB, IFN-γ, and iNOS mRNA expressions and decreased IL-10 mRNA levels compared with those in DEN/2AAF rats (Figure 5).

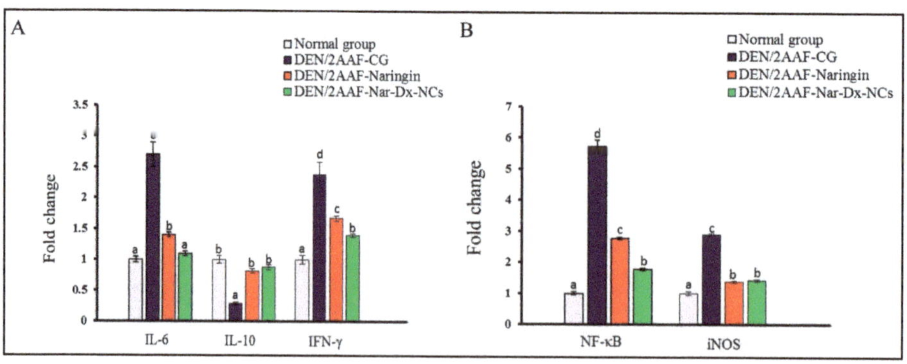

Figure 5. Effect of naringin and Nar-Dx-NCs on (**A**) IL-6, IL-10, and IFN-γ mRNA expressions as well as (**B**) NF-κB and iNOS mRNA levels in the lung of DEN2AAF-administered rats. Data are expressed as means ± SE ($n = 6$). Means for each group are represented at the top of each bar. Different symbols (a–d) within the same graph are significantly different at $p < 0.05$. Abbreviations: IFN-γ, interferon-γ; IL-10, interleukin-10; IL-6, interleukin-6; iNOS, inducible nitric oxide synthase; NF-κB, nuclear factor-κB.

3.5. *Effects of Naringin and Nar-Dx-NCs on mRNA Expression of Antiapoptotic and Proapoptotic Biomarkers*

DEN/2AAF-administered rats produced a significant elevation in the lung expression of antiapoptotic protein B-cell lymphoma-2 (Bcl-2) and significantly reduced levels of the proapoptotic factors Bcl-2-associated X protein (Bax) and P53 compared with those in normal rats. The cotreatment of DENA/2AAF plus free naringin or Nar-Dx-NCs significantly suppressed Bcl-2 expression and elevated Bax and P53 levels (Figure 6).

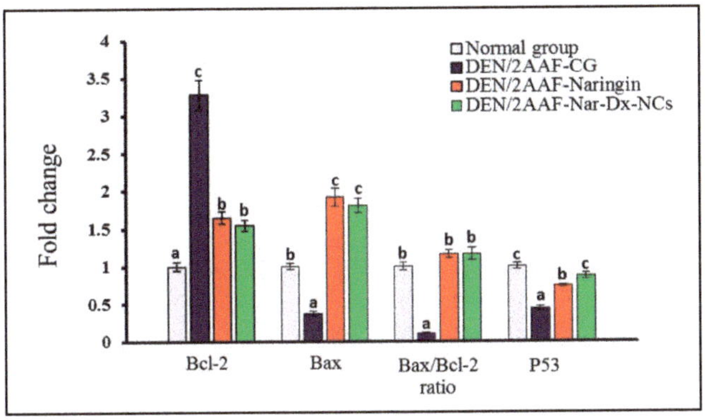

Figure 6. Effect of naringin and Nar-Dx-NCs on Bcl-2 and Bax mRNA levels, Bax/Bcl-2 ratio, and P53 mRNA levels in the lungs of DEN/2AAF-administered rats. Data are expressed as means ± SE (n = 6). Means for each group are represented at the top of each bar. Different symbols (a–c) within the same graph are significantly different at $p < 0.05$. Abbreviations: 2AAF, 2-acetylaminofluorene; Bax, Bcl-2-associated X protein; Bcl-2, B-cell lymphoma-2; CG, control group; DEN, diethylnitrosamine; Nar-Dx-NCs, naringin–dextrin nanocomposites.

3.6. *Effects of Naringin and Nar-Dx-NCs on Ki-67 Protein Expression*

Ki-67 protein expression was significantly ($p < 0.05$) upregulated in the lung parenchyma of DEN/2AAF-administered rats. Naringin or Nar-Dx-NCs significantly downregulated lung Ki-67 expression levels compared with those measured after DEN/2AAF administration alone, suggesting an inhibition of cell proliferation (Figure 7).

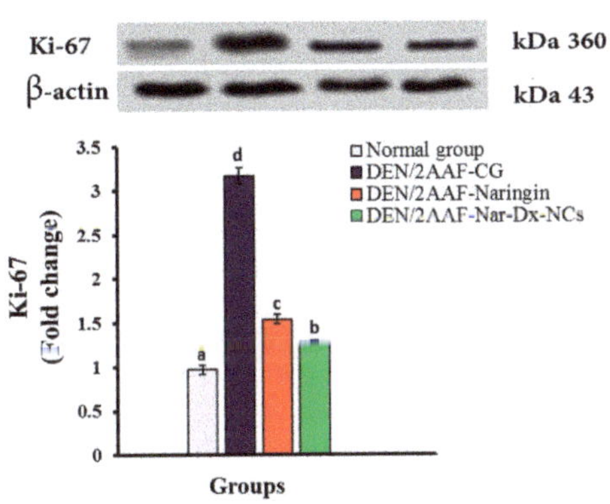

Figure 7. Effect of naringin and Nar-Dx-NCs on Ki-67 levels in the lungs of DEN/2AAF-administrated rats. Data are expressed as means ± SE (n = 3). Means, which are represented as different symbols (a–d) at the top of each bar, were considered significantly different for $p < 0.05$. Abbreviations: 2AAF, 2-acetylaminofluorene; Bax, Bcl-2-associated X protein; Bcl-2, B-cell lymphoma-2; CG, control group; DEN, diethylnitrosamine; Ki-67, Kiel-67; Nar-Dx-NCs, naringin–dextrin nanocomposites. The uncropped blots are shown in Figure S1 and S2.

4. Discussion

Lung cancer is a common neoplasm with high incidence and mortality worldwide [2]. DEN is a chemical compound widely utilized to cause lung, liver, and esophageal cancers in experimental animals [39] and may be used alone or in conjunction with a cancer promoter, such as 2AAF [34]. Naringin is the primary bioactive polyphenol found in citrus fruits, and its consumption has been beneficial to human health since ancient times. Numerous preclinical and clinical findings have documented its antioxidant activity and capacity to protect against inflammation and various organ- or system-specific cancers [40]. In this work, we have prepared naringin–dextrin nanocomposites (Nar-Dx-NCs) and investigated the chemopreventive role of this nanoformulation against DEN/2AAF-induced lung cancer and related mechanisms of action compared to free naringin in a Wistar rat model.

The histopathological analysis revealed various lung cancerous injuries, including aggregation of tumor cells, diffuse thickening in interstitial tissues, and tumor cell growth in lepidic and papillary patterns within the alveoli in the lungs of rats given DEN/2AAF. Moreover, there was an invasion of macrophages and other myeloid cells in adjacent alveolar air spaces and a display of invasive adenocarcinoma with an acinar pattern. Based on these observations, it has been demonstrated that lung adenocarcinoma is predominantly caused by DEN, as described by Sivalingam et al. [39] and Abdel-Moneim et al. [34]. This present study revealed an improvement in tissue dysplasia and several biomarkers resulting from cotreatment with naringin or Nar-Dx-NCs, which can minimize the production of ROS induced via DEN injection, thus mitigating tissue damage and cancer-related tissue injury. Compared to free naringin, Nar-Dx-NCs were more effective in exerting anticarcinogenic effects.

DEN treatment increased ROS and LPO levels and decreased SOD, GPx, and GSH activities. These effects were similar to those of Sivalingam et al. [39] and Abdel-Moneim et al. [34], who indicated that DEN increased LPO levels and decreased GPx and SOD activities as well as GSH content in the lungs of rats exposed to DEN. Enzymatic and non-enzymatic antioxidants, like GPx, SOD, and GSH, scavenge ROS and decrease LPO levels. Many studies [31,34,41] found a significant decrease in SOD, GPx, and GSH activities in rat lung and liver cancers, along with increased free radicals and specific humoral factors. LPO levels increase during the development of cancer and are regarded as a strong carcinogen and mutagen [42]. Naringin or Nar-Dx-NCs treatment reduced high LPO levels and increased SOD and GPx activities and GSH content in the lungs. Our data are parallel with the findings of Kim et al. [43]. Naringin, a naturally occurring flavonoid, displays protective effects and increases the activity of antioxidant enzymes in the lungs [44]. The antioxidant defense system in the rat was improved using Nar-Dx-NCs [30]. Dietary antioxidants may help to reduce oxidative stress and cellular damage in addition to supporting the body's natural antioxidant defense system. There is proof that naringin scavenges free radicals and prevents oxidative DNA damage [45]. Nar-Dx-NCs improved the antioxidant defense system in the rat lungs compared with the effects of crude naringin at the same dose, mainly by increasing naringin concentration and enhancing naringin protective activity.

Inflammation is the primary response to infections and injuries, but tissue damage may result from an uncontrolled prolongation of the inflammatory repertoire [46]. Recent studies have focused on the cytokines involved in the induction and maintenance of inflammation. TNF-α, IL-1β, IL-6, and INF-γ, as well as the anti-inflammatory IL-10, are the chief mediators of inflammation [47,48]. Our results showed an elevation in TNF-α, IL-1β, NF-κB, and IL-6 expressions, in addition to decreased Nrf2 and IL-10 levels, in lung tissues of DEN/AAF2-administered rats compared to unexposed controls. These results corroborate the findings of previous studies by Man et al. [49], Wu et al. [50], and Cicek et al. [51]. In this current study, the amounts of TNF-α, IL-1β, and IL-6 increased after treating rats with DEN/2AAF but were abrogated using both free naringin and Nar-Dx-NCs [52–54]. The DEN/2AAF-induced production of ROS, which activates oxidative stress, may be a contributing factor to the chronic inflammation developing in lung tissues. Lung cancer is also caused by chronic inflammation, and many pro-inflammatory genes, including TNF-α and

IL-6, are crucial for apoptosis, proliferation, angiogenesis, and metastasis inhibition [55]. Importantly, the present data indicated that the Nar-Dx-NC formula was significantly more potent than free naringin in mediating this inflammatory response.

Nrf2 is essential for lung cancer cell protection because it is responsible for compensatory mechanisms responsible for attenuating oxidative stress (Figure 6). Additionally, it also controls the inflammatory response within the tumor microenvironment by reducing the expression levels of TNF-α, IL-1β, and IL-6 [56]. Nrf2 is inhibited in malignant lung tumors [57]. IL-10 facilitates immunosuppressive actions and is produced in a variety of solid tumors and hematopoietic tumors. Moreover, it inhibits the synthesis of a number of cytokines, including different inflammatory and growth factors, and promotes the release of anti-inflammatory factors in the body [58]. The levels of IL-10 were effectively restored to near-normal levels via treatment with free naringin or Nar-Dx-NC. In this present study, rats treated with DEN/2AAF also showed a significant elevation in IFN-γ expression compared to rats receiving no interventions. IFN-γ plays a significant role in the contribution of inflammation to carcinogenesis [59], and there is a long history of IFN-γ use as a pro-tumor factor [60]. Chronic uncontrolled inflammation continuously generates harmful ROS, which can change the genome and cause DNA damage, consequently initiating the growth of tumors. Inflammatory mediators such as TNF-α, IL-1β, IL-6, and IFN-γ promote an increase in blood supply to the tumor [61,62].

NF-κB is a transcription factor that regulates the cell cycle, inflammation, and cell survival. NF-κB expression was found to be significantly increased in DEN/2AAF-induced animals relative to that of the control group. These results agree with those of Hamza et al. [63], who suggested that, under oxidative stress, NF-κB becomes activated and translocates to the nucleus to activate inflammatory genes, ultimately facilitating an oncogenic environment. Inflammation has been shown to be stimulated via the upregulation of inflammatory-related genes, such as NF-κB [64]. The pro-inflammatory mediators are primarily controlled via NF-κB, which is induced via chemical carcinogens and is constitutively active in most tumors [65]. When NF-κB is activated, the expression of many genes, including those involved in the production of pro-inflammatory cytokines TNF-α, IFN-γ, IL-1β, and IL-6, is upregulated [66,67]. DEN/2AAF significantly increased these pro-inflammatory cytokines, whereas naringin and Nar-Dx-NCs suppressed this phenomenon. The NF-κB pathway is essential for the survival of cancer cells and their resistance to apoptosis. Naringin inhibits the growth, promotion, and spread of cancer via a variety of mechanisms, including the modulation of numerous uncontrolled signaling pathways related to inflammation, apoptosis, proliferation, angiogenesis, autophagy, invasion, and metastasis [68].

In this present study, iNOS gene expression significantly increased in lung tissue samples of rats administered DEN/2AAF compared to unexposed controls. This finding is supported by the conclusions of Unsal and Kurutaş [69], who found that DEN cytotoxicity and carcinogenicity were attributed to their ability to cause oxidative stress and toxicity. During the inflammatory response, macrophages produce a large amount of nitric oxide (NO), an inflammatory mediator, thanks to the catalytic activity of iNOS. Moreover, excessive NO can cause severe oxidative stress and exacerbate tissue injury [70]. When iNOS is activated via DEN, endogenous NO is produced and causes damage and inflammation. Superoxide anion (O2) and NO interact non-enzymatically to form the reactive nitrogen species peroxynitrite ($ONOO^-$). $ONOO^-$ causes protein oxidation when it interacts with amino acids. Additionally, $ONOO^-$ oxidizes nuclear tyrosine, DNA, and other aromatic amino acids. The nitration of tyrosine produces 3-nitrotyrosine (3-NT), which is a biomarker of oxidative damage and inflammation [71]. The expression of iNOS is affected by endogenous pro-inflammatory mediators like IFN-γ, TNF-α, IL-1β, and IL-6, and iNOS induced via inflammatory stimuli contributes to a large amount of NO production [72].

Treatment with naringin and Nar-Dx-NCs might protect rats from DEN/2AAF-induced inflammation via the downregulation of pro-inflammatory cytokines, such as TNF-α, IL-1β, IL-6, and INF-γ, and by increasing IL-10 and Nrf2 levels compared to those of rats treated with DEN/2AAF alone. Naringin treatment may minimize tissue damage by lowering pro-inflammatory biomarkers levels and stimulating anti-inflammatory mediator production in lung tissue [73]. Naringin reduces inflammation in the rat lungs by decreasing iNOS and TNF-α levels via NF-κB signaling inhibition [74]. Additionally, evidence suggests that naringin is effective at reducing the expression of a number of signaling molecules involved in the inflammatory response other than NF-κB, iNOS, and TNF-α, including IL-6 and Nrf2 [75]. The levels of pro-inflammatory mediators were decreased after treatment with naringin and Nar-Dx-NCs. Thus, naringin and Nar-Dx-NCs treatments inhibit the release of cytokines and are extremely effective against DEN/2AAF-induced lung cancer. The mechanisms triggered by naringin for its anti-inflammatory action might include the inhibition of iNOS and NF-κB signaling pathways [76,77].

Apoptosis results from the activation of the intrinsic and/or extrinsic pathways. The tumor suppressor p53 is a powerful apoptosis regulator that controls the expression of apoptosis-related genes, such as Bax and Bcl-2 [78,79]. Our data showed that exposure to DEN/2AAF elevated Bcl-2 expression while reducing Bax and P53 expression in the lung tissues of Wistar rats. The upregulation of lung Bcl-2 and the reduction in Bax expression in DEN/2AAF-administered animals agrees with the observations of Sivalingam et al. [39]. Campbell and Tait [80] previously demonstrated that the Bcl-2 family, when unbalanced, can act as a barrier to apoptosis and facilitate tumor development and resistance to cancer therapy. The antiapoptotic Bcl-2 negatively regulates apoptosis by inhibiting the activity of the proapoptotic Bax [81]. Bax, Bcl-2, and cytochrome *c* control the apoptotic pathway, which culminates in the activation of caspases [82]. The Bax/Bcl-2 ratio regulates the activation of caspase [83] and thus controls the cell's decision toward survival or apoptosis.

The present data showed that when DEN/2AAF was administered, lung P53 expression was significantly reduced compared to that of unexposed controls. This finding is supported by the work of Abdel-Moneim et al. [34]. Two functions of P53 are involved in the regulation of oxidative stress; it has prooxidant activity that causes oxidative damage, but it also acts as an antioxidant factor to prevent oxidative stress. Thus, numerous variables, including the absence of a functional P53, contribute to the overproduction of ROS [84]. Human tumors with genetic mutations were found to have inactivated p53, which contributes to the development of tumors from normal cells [85]. Here, treatment with naringin or Nar-Dx-NCs enhanced apoptosis in lung cancer. On the other hand, elevated levels of Bax and P53 and reduced Bcl-2 expression were detected in the lung tissue of DEN/2AAF-administered animals receiving naringin or Nar-Dx-NCs. Naringin has previously been shown to inhibit tumor cell growth, promote apoptosis of tumor cells, and have great potential as a cytotoxic anticancer agent [86,87]. Flavonoids like naringin affecting oxidative stress and apoptosis were shown to stimulate Bax and P53 expression and inhibit Bcl-2 expression in past works [40,88]

Ki-67 is a nuclear marker associated with tumor cell proliferation that has been linked to the progression, metastasis, and prognosis of many cancers [89]. Numerous studies have suggested that patients harboring lung adenocarcinoma with high tumor Ki-67 expression have a worse prognosis, and Ki-67 expression may be an important prognostic factor in advanced lung cancer cases [90,91]. The present findings demonstrate a significant increase in Ki-67 expression levels in the lungs of rats exposed to DEN/2AAF, a finding that has also been reported by Abdel-Moneim et al. [34]. DEN/2AAF-administered rats treated with naringin and Na-Dx-NCs expressed less Ki-67 than DEN/2AAF-administered rats. Naringin is a prooxidant and may inhibit the growth of cancer cells by blocking NF-κB signaling [40]. Thus, the anticancer effects of Nar-Dx-NCs might involve both the inhibition of cancerous cell proliferation and stimulation of apoptosis [30]. Nar-Dx-NCs were significantly more potent than free naringin. Additional efforts are required to clarify the mechanisms involved in the preventive effect of Nar-Dx-NCs on lung cancer and identify other related factors.

The prolonged-release properties of naringin may be responsible for Nar-Dx-NCs potent anticancer properties, indicating dextrin's consistency as an effective nanocarrier for long-term naringin delivery [30]. The nanocarriers enable a controlled (sustained) drug release from the matrix. Enhanced transport to, or uptake by, target cells may be another reason the nanocomposite impact is superior in addition to sustained release [92]. Nar-Dx-NCs is more potent than free naringin against oxidative stress, inflammation, and cell proliferation may be due to the same reasons.

This present study has several limitations. In particular, additional apoptosis, cell signaling, and proliferation biomarkers might be assessed, and other techniques, such as Western blot and immunohistochemistry, might prove useful in measuring protein levels and confirming the efficacy of Nar-Dx-NCs against lung cancer. Moreover, further studies are required to assess the naringin and Nar-Dx-NCs dose–response effects on DEN/2AAF-induced lung carcinogenesis and other experimental lung cancer models, such as benzo[a]pyrene-induced lung carcinogenesis in rodents.

5. Conclusions

The present findings demonstrate that dextrin served as an effective nanocarrier for naringin. This is the first research to document the inhibitory effects of Nar-Dx-NCs on lung cancer. This new formulation diminished lung carcinogenesis induced via DEN/2AAF in different pathways, including the suppression of oxidative stress and inflammation, increasing apoptosis, and decreasing tumor cell proliferation (summarized in Figure 8). Notably, our data reveal Nar-Dx-NCs significantly enhances the anticarcinogenic effects of naringin, thus improving its protective effects against lung cancer. The two important limitations of this study were to assess the effects of Nar-Dx-NCs on normal rats and to compare the anticancer effects of different doses of Nar-Dx-NCs with other existing chemotherapeutic agents. Moreover, although the anticarcinogenic effects of Nar-Dx-NC were confirmed in the lungs of male Wistar rats of this present study, additional preclinical investigations using other animal species and genders, as well as clinical studies, are necessary to confirm the effectiveness of nanocomposites of naringin against human lung cancer.

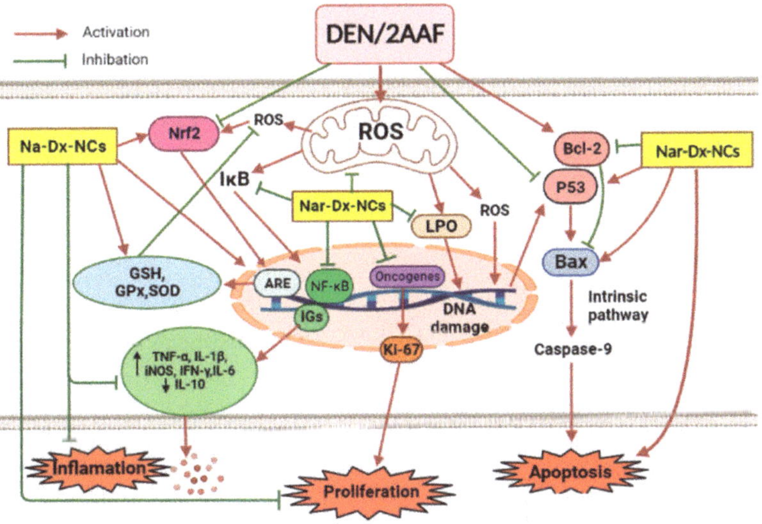

Figure 8. Schematic diagram showing the mechanism of actions of Nar-Dx-NCs against DEN/2AAF-induced lung carcinogenesis, including the suppression of oxidative stress, inflammation, proliferation, and upregulation of apoptosis. Abbreviations: ARE, antioxidant response element; Bax, Bcl-2-associated X protein; Bcl-2, B-cell lymphoma-2; IFN-γ, interferon- γ; IGs, inflammatory genes; IL-6, interleukin-6; IL-10, interleukin-10; iNOS, inducible nitric oxide synthase; NF-κB, nuclear factor-kappa-B; ROS, reactive oxygen species.

Supplementary Materials: The following supporting information can be downloaded at: https://www.mdpi.com/article/10.3390/cancers15205102/s1, Figure S1: Original Immunoblot Ki-67 replicate 1. Figure S2: Original Immunoblot Ki-67 replicates 2 and 3.

Author Contributions: Conceptualization, O.M.A., K.M.A.Z., A.A.G.E.-S. and A.A.-M.; methodology, E.E.M., O.M.A. and K.M.A.Z.; software, E.E.M.; validation, E.E.M., O.M.A., K.M.A.Z., A.A.G.E.-S., S.T., A.S., A.B. and A.A.-M.; formal analysis, E.E.M., O.M.A., K.M.A.Z., A.A.G.E.-S., S.T., A.S., A.B. and A.A.-M.; investigation, E.E.M., O.M.A., K.M.A.Z. and A.A.G.E.-S.; resources, E.E.M., S.T. and A.S.; data curation, E.E.M., O.M.A., K.M.A.Z., A.A.G.E.-S. and A.A.-M.; writing—original draft preparation, O.M.A., K.M.A.Z. and A.A.-M.; writing—review and editing, E.E.M., O.M.A., K.M.A.Z., A.A.G.E.-S., S.T., A.S., J.T.B., A.B. and A.A.-M.; supervision, O.M.A., K.M.A.Z., A.A.G.E.-S. and A.A.-M.; project administration, O.M.A., K.M.A.Z., A.A.G.E.-S. and A.A.-M.; funding acquisition, E.E.M., S.T. and A.S. All authors have read and agreed to the published version of the manuscript.

Funding: This research received no external funding.

Institutional Review Board Statement: The experimental work was approved by the Faculty of Science Experimental Animal Ethics Committee (Ethical Approval number: 020-91), Beni-Suef University, Egypt.

Informed Consent Statement: Not applicable.

Data Availability Statement: All data are available from corresponding authors upon reasonable request.

Acknowledgments: The authors would like to acknowledge the Deanship of Scientific Research, Taif University, for funding this work. The authors would like also to extend their sincere thanks to the High Altitude Research Center at Taif University, Saudi Arabia. The authors are also grateful to Abdel Razik H. Farrag, Department of Pathology, National Research Centre, Dokki, Cairo, Egypt, for his help in the examination and identification of histopathological changes in the lung histological sections and to Dina Sabry, Faculty of Medicine, Cairo University, Cairo, Egypt for performing the Western blot analysis.

Conflicts of Interest: The authors declare no conflict of interest.

Abbreviations

2AAF	2-acetylaminofluorene
3-NT	3-nitrotyrosine
ARE	antioxidant response element
Bax	Bcl-2-associated X protein
Bcl-2	B-cell lymphoma-2
CMC	carboxymethyl cellulose
CYP450	cytochrome P450
DEN	diethylnitrosamine
EE	entrapment effectiveness
ELISA	enzyme-linked immunosorbent assay
FTIR	Fourier transformation infrared
GPx	glutathione peroxidase
GSH	glutathione
H&E	hematoxylin and eosin
HRP	horseradish peroxidase
i.p.	Intraperitoneally
IFN-γ	interferon-γ
IGs	inflammatory genes
IL-10	interleukin-10
IL-1β	interleukin-1β
IL-6	interleukin-6
iNOS	inducible nitric oxide synthase
LPO	lipid peroxidation
Nar-Dx-NCs	naringin-dextrin nanocomposite

NF-κB	nuclear factor-κB
NO	nitric oxide
Nrf2	nuclear factor erythroid 2-related factor 2
O2	superoxide anion
ONOO−	peroxynitrite
P53	tumor suppressor protein 53
PCR	polymerase chain reaction
RIPA	radioimmunoprecipitation assay
ROS	reactive oxygen species
RT-qPCR	reverse transcription–quantitative polymerase chain reaction
SDS–PAGE	sodium dodecyl sulfate–polyacrylamide gel electrophoresis
SE	standard error
SOD	superoxide dismutase
TBST	tris-buffered saline with Tween 20
TEM	transmission electron microscopy
TNF-α	tumor necrosis factor-α
UV-Vis	ultraviolet-visible
XRD	X-ray diffraction

References

1. Bray, F.; Ferlay, J.; Soerjomataram, I.; Siegel, R.L.; Torre, L.A.; Jemal, A. Global cancer statistics 2018: GLOBOCAN estimates of incidence and mortality worldwide for 36 cancers in 185 countries. *CA Cancer J. Clin.* **2018**, *68*, 394–424. [CrossRef] [PubMed]
2. Siegel, R.L.; Miller, K.D.; Fuchs, H.E.; Jemal, A. Cancer statistics. *CA Cancer J. Clin.* **2021**, *71*, 7–33. [CrossRef]
3. Saber, S.; Mahmoud, A.; Helal, N.; El-Ahwany, E.; Abdelghany, R. Liver protective effects of renin-angiotensin system inhibition have no survival benefits in hepatocellular carcinoma induced by repetitive administration of diethylnitrosamine in mice. *Maced. J. Med. Sci.* **2018**, *6*, 955–968. [CrossRef] [PubMed]
4. Zhang, H.E.; Henderson, J.M.; Gorrell, M.D. Animal models for hepatocellular carcinoma. *Biochim. Biophy. Acta-Mol. Basis Dis.* **2019**, *1865*, 993–1002. [CrossRef]
5. Farombi, E.O.; Shrotriya, S.; Surh, Y.J. Kolaviron inhibits dimethyl nitrosamine-induced liver injury by suppressing COX-2 and iNOS expression via NF-kappaB and AP-1. *Life Sci.* **2009**, *8*, 149–155. [CrossRef]
6. Pradeep, K.; Raj Mohan, C.V.; Gobianand, K.; Karthikeyan, S. Protective effect of *Cassia fistula* Linn. on diethylnitrosamine induced hepatocellular damage and oxidative stress in ethanol pretreated rats. *Biol. Res.* **2010**, *43*, 113–125. [CrossRef] [PubMed]
7. Mervai, Z.; Egedi, K.; Kovalszky, I.; Baghy, K. Diethylnitrosamine induces lung adenocarcinoma in FVB/N mouse. *BMC Cancer* **2018**, *18*, 157. [CrossRef]
8. Geiger-Maor, A.; Guedj, A.; Even-Ram, S. Macrophages regulate the systemic response to DNA damage by a cell nonautonomous mechaism. *Cancer Res.* **2015**, *75*, 2663–2673. [CrossRef]
9. Kishida, N.; Matsuda, S.; Itano, O.; Shinoda, M.; Kitago, M.; Yagi, H.; Abe, Y.; Hibi, T.; Masugi, Y.; Aiura, K.; et al. Development of a novel mouse model of hepatocellular carcinoma with nonalcoholic steatohepatitis using a high-fat, choline-defcient diet and intraperitoneal injection of diethylnitrosamine. *BMC Gastroenterol.* **2016**, *16*, 61. [CrossRef] [PubMed]
10. Downs, T.R.; Arlt, V.M.; Barnett, B.C.; Posgai, R.; Pfuhler, S. Effect of 2-acetylaminofluorene and its genotoxic metabolites on DNA adduct formation and DNA damage in 3D reconstructed human skin tissue models. *Mutagenesis* **2021**, *36*, 63–74. [CrossRef]
11. Tu, X.; Ma, S.; Gao, Z.; Wang, J.; Huang, S.; Chen, W. One-Step Extraction and Hydrolysis of Flavonoid Glycosides in Rape Bee Pollen Based on Soxhlet-Assisted Matrix Solid Phase Dispersion. *Phytochem. Anal.* **2017**, *28*, 505–511. [CrossRef] [PubMed]
12. Li, H.; Zhu, F.; Chen, H.; Cheng, K.W.; Zykova, T.; Oi, N.; Lubet, R.A.; Bode, A.M.; Wang, M.; Dong, Z. 6-C-(E-phenylethenyl)-Naringenin Suppresses Colorectal Cancer Growth by Inhibiting Cyclooxygenase-1. *Cancer Res.* **2014**, *74*, 243–252. [CrossRef] [PubMed]
13. Liu, C.; Chu, D.; Kalantar-Zadeh, K.; George, J.; Young, H.A.; Liu, G. Cytokines: From clinical significance to quantification. *Adv. Sci.* **2021**, *8*, 2004433. [CrossRef] [PubMed]
14. Van Gorp, H.; Lamkanfi, M. The emerging roles of inflammasome-dependent cytokines in cancer development. *EMBO Rep.* **2019**, *20*, e47575. [CrossRef] [PubMed]
15. Quintanilla, M.; Montero-Montero, L.; Renart, J.; Martin-Villar, E. Podoplanin in inflammation and cancer. *Int. J. Mol. Sci.* **2019**, *20*, 707. [CrossRef] [PubMed]
16. Qian, S.; Golubnitschaja, O.; Zhan, X. Chronic inflammation: Key player and biomarker-set to predict and prevent cancer development and progression based on individualized patient profiles. *Epma J.* **2019**, *10*, 365–381. [CrossRef]
17. Liu, Q.; Gao, Y.; Ci, X. Role of Nrf2 and its activators in respiratory diseases. *Oxidative Med. Cell. Longev.* **2019**, *2019*, 7090534. [CrossRef] [PubMed]
18. Abouzed, T.K.; Althobaiti, F.; Omran, A.F.; Eldomany, E.B.; El-Shazly, S.A.; Alharthi, F.; Elkattawy, A.M.; Kahilo, K.A.; Dorghamm, D.A. The chemoprevention of spirulina platensis and garlic against diethylnitrosamine induced liver cancer in rats via amelioration of inflammatory cytokines expression and oxidative stress. *Toxicol. Res.* **2022**, *11*, 22–31. [CrossRef] [PubMed]

19. Sharma, P.; Kumar, V.; Guleria, P. Naringin: Biosynthesis and pharmaceutical applications. *Indian J. Pharm. Sci.* **2019**, *81*, 988–999. [CrossRef]
20. Ghanbari-Movahed, M.; Jackson, G.; Farzaei, M.H.; Bishayee, A.A. systematic review of the preventive and therapeutic effects of naringin against human malignancies. *Front. Pharmacol.* **2021**, *12*, 639840. [CrossRef]
21. Mintz, K.J.; Leblanc, R.M. The use of nanotechnology to combat liver cancer: Progress and perspectives. *Biochim. Biophys. Acta Rev. Cancer* **2021**, *1876*, 188621. [CrossRef] [PubMed]
22. Palazzolo, S.; Bayda, S.; Hadla, M.; Caligiuri, I.; Corona, G.; Toffoli, G.; Rizzolio, F. The clinical translation of organic nanomaterials for cancer therapy: A focus on polymeric nanoparticles, micelles, liposomes and exosomes. *Curr. Med. Chem.* **2018**, *25*, 4224–4268. [CrossRef] [PubMed]
23. Yang, Z.; Shi, J.; Xie, J.; Wang, Y.; Sun, J.; Liu, T.; Zhao, Y.; Zhao, X.; Wang, X.; Ma, Y.; et al. Large-scale generation of functional mRNA-encapsulating exosomes via cellular nanoporation. *Nat. Biomed. Eng.* **2020**, *4*, 69–83. [CrossRef] [PubMed]
24. Wu, Z.; Ma, X.; Ma, Y.; Yang, Z.; Yuan, Y.; Liu, C. Core/Shell PEGS/HA hybrid nanoparticle via micelle-coordinated mineralization for tumor-specific therapy. *ACS Appl. Mater. Interfaces* **2020**, *12*, 12109–12119. [CrossRef]
25. Milewska, S.; Niemirowicz-Laskowska, K.; Siemiaszko, G.; Nowicki, P.; Wilczewska, A.Z.; Car, H. Current trends and challenges in pharmacoeconomic aspects of nanocarriers as drug delivery systems for cancer treatment. *Int. J. Nanomed.* **2021**, *16*, 659344. [CrossRef]
26. Ghanbari-Movahed, M.; Mondal, A.; Farzaei, M.H.; Bishayee, A. Quercetin-and rutin-based nano-formulations for cancer treatment: A systematic review of improved efficacy and molecular mechanisms. *Phytomedicine* **2022**, *97*, 153909. [CrossRef] [PubMed]
27. Ghanbari-Movahed, M.; Kaceli, T.; Mondal, A.; Farzaei, M.H.; Bishayee, A. Recent advances in improved anticancer efficacies of camptothecin nano-formulations: A systematic review. *Biomedicines* **2021**, *9*, 480. [CrossRef]
28. Kashyap, D.; Tuli, H.S.; Yerer, M.B.; Sharma, A.; Sak, K.; Srivastava, S.; Pandey, A.; Garg, V.K.; Sethi, G.; Bishayee, A. Natural product-based nanoformulations for cancer therapy: Opportunities and challenges. *Semin. Cancer Biol.* **2021**, *69*, 5–23. [CrossRef]
29. Lagoa, R.; Silva, J.; Rodrigues, J.R.; Bishayee, A. Advances in phytochemical delivery systems for improved anticancer activity. *Biotech. Adv.* **2020**, *38*, 107382. [CrossRef]
30. Mohamed, E.E.; Abdel-Moneim, A.; Ahmed, O.M.; Zoheir, K.M.; Eldin, Z.E.; El-Shahawy, A.A. Anticancer activity of a novel naringin-dextrin nanoformula: Preparation, characterization, and in vitro induction of apoptosis in human hepatocellular carcinoma cells by inducing ROS generation, DNA fragmentation, and cell cycle arrest. *J. Drug Deliv. Sci. Technol.* **2022**, *75*, 103677. [CrossRef]
31. Mohamed, E.E.; Ahmed, O.M.; Abdel-Moneim, A.; Zoheir, K.M.; Elesawy, B.H.; Al Askary, A.; El-Shahawy, A.A. Protective Effects of Naringin–Dextrin Nanoformula against Chemically Induced Hepatocellular Carcinoma in Wistar Rats: Roles of Oxidative Stress, Inflammation, Cell Apoptosis, and Proliferation. *Pharmaceuticals* **2022**, *15*, 1558. [CrossRef]
32. Manchun, S.; Dass, C.R.; Sriamornsak, P. Designing nanoemulsion templates for fabrication of dextrin nanoparticles via emulsion cross-linking technique. *Carbohydr. Polym.* **2014**, *101*, 650–655. [CrossRef] [PubMed]
33. Morsy, H.M.; Ahmed, O.M.; Zoheir, K.M.A.; Abdel-Moneim, A. The anticarcinogenic effect of eugenol on lung cancer induced by diethylnitrosamine/2-acetylaminofluorene in Wistar rats: Insight on the mechanisms of action. *Apoptosis* **2023**, *28*, 1184–1197. [CrossRef] [PubMed]
34. Abdel-Moneim, A.; Ahmed, O.M.; El-Twab, A.; Sanaa, M.; Zaky, M.Y.; Bakry, L.N. Prophylactic effects of *Cynara scolymus* L. leaf and flower hydroethanolic extracts against diethylnitrosamine/acetylaminoflourene-induced lung cancer in Wistar rats. *Environ. Sci. Pollut. Res.* **2021**, *28*, 43515–43527. [CrossRef]
35. Camargo, C.A.; Gomes-Marcondes, M.C.; Wutzki, N.C.; Aoyama, H. Naringin inhibits tumor growth and reduces interleukin-6 and tumor necrosis factor α levels in rats with Walker 256 carcinosarcoma. *Anticancer Res.* **2012**, *32*, 129–133. [PubMed]
36. Bancroft, J.D.; Gamble, M. (Eds.) *Theory and Practice of Histological Techniques*, 6th ed.; Elsevier Health Sciences; Churchill Livingstone: Beijing, China, 2008.
37. Abràmoff, M.D.; Magalhes, P.J.; Ram, S.J. Image processing with imageJ. *Biophoton Int.* **2004**, *11*, 36–42.
38. Sthoeger, Z.; Zinger, H.; Sharabi, A.; Asher, I.; Mozes, E. The tolerogenic peptide, hCDR1, down-regulates the expression of interferon-α in murine and human systemic lupus erythematosus. *PLoS ONE* **2013**, *8*, e60394. [CrossRef]
39. Sivalingam, K.; Amirthalingam, V.; Ganasan, K.; Huang, C.Y.; Viswanadha, V.P. Neferine suppresses diethylnitrosamine-induced lung carcinogenesis in Wistar rats. *Food Chem. Toxicol.* **2019**, *123*, 385–398. [CrossRef]
40. Stabrauskiene, J.; Kopustinskiene, D.M.; Lazauskas, R.; Bernatoniene, J. Naringin and naringenin: Their mechanisms of action and the potential anticancer activities. *Biomedicines* **2022**, *10*, 1686. [CrossRef]
41. Ahmed, O.M.; Fahim, H.I.; Mohamed, E.E.; Abdel-Moneim, A. Protective effects of *Persea americana* fruit and seed extracts against chemically induced liver cancer in rats by enhancing their antioxidant, anti-inflammatory, and apoptotic activities. *Environ. Sci. Pollut. Res.* **2022**, *4*, 43858–43873. [CrossRef]
42. Barrera, G. Oxidative stress and lipid peroxidation products in cancer progression and therapy. *Int. Sch. Res. Not.* **2012**, *2012*, 137289. [CrossRef] [PubMed]
43. Kim, J.K.; Park, J.H.; Ku, H.J.; Kim, S.H.; Lim, Y.J.; Park, J.W.; Lee, J.H. Naringin protects acrolein-induced pulmonary injuries through modulating apoptotic signaling and inflammation signaling pathways in mice. *J. Nutr. Biochem.* **2018**, *59*, 10–16. [CrossRef] [PubMed]

44. Akintunde, J.K.; Abioye, J.B.; Ebinama, O.N. Potential protective effects of naringin on oculo-pulmonary injury induced by PM10 (wood smoke) exposure by modulation of oxidative damage and acetylcholine esterase activity in a rat model. *Curr. Ther. Res. Clin. Exp.* **2020**, *92*, 100586. [CrossRef]
45. Cavia-Saiz, M.; Busto, M.D.; Pilar-Izquierdo, M.C.; Ortega, N.; Perez-Mateos, M.; Muniz, P. Antioxidant properties, radical scavenging activity and biomolecule protection capacity of flavonoid naringenin and its glycoside naringin: A comparative study. *J. Sci. Food Agric.* **2010**, *90*, 1238–1244. [CrossRef]
46. Askari, V.R.; Shafiee-Nick, R. Promising neuroprotective effects of β-caryophyllene against LPS-induced oligodendrocyte toxicity: A mechanistic study. *Biochem. Pharmacol.* **2018**, *159*, 154–171. [CrossRef] [PubMed]
47. Jawa, R.S.; Anillo, S.; Huntoon, K.; Baumann, H.; Kulaylat, M. Interleukin-6 in surgery, trauma, and critical care part II: Clinical implications. *J. Intensive Care Med.* **2011**, *26*, 73–87. [CrossRef]
48. Janakiram, N.B.; Valerio, M.S.; Goldman, S.M.; Dearth, C.L. The role of the inflammatory response in mediating functional recovery following composite tissue injuries. *Int. J. Mol. Sci.* **2021**, *22*, 13552. [CrossRef]
49. Man, S.; Li, J.; Qiu, P.; Liu, J.; Liu, Z.; Ma, L.; Gao, W. Inhibition of lung cancer in diethylnitrosamine-induced mice by *Rhizoma paridis* saponins. *Mol. Carcinog.* **2017**, *56*, 1405–1413. [CrossRef]
50. Wu, Y.; Sreeharsha, N.; Sharma, S.; Mishra, A.; Singh, A.K.; Gubbiyappa, S.K. Anticancer effect of rosiglitazone, a PPAR-γ agonist against Diethylnitrosamine-induced lung carcinogenesis. *ACS Omega* **2020**, *5*, 5334–5339. [CrossRef]
51. Cicek, B.; Hayme, S.; Kuzucu, M.; Cetin, A.; Yeni, Y.; Genc, S.; Yildirim, S.; Bolat, I.; Kantarci, M.; Gul, M.; et al. Sorafenib Alleviates Inflammatory Signaling of Tumor Microenvironment in Lung Cancer. *Res. Sq.* **2022**. [CrossRef]
52. Lin, X.; Ju, Y.N.; Gao, W.; Li, D.M.; Guo, C.C. Desflurane attenuates ventilator-induced lung injury in rats with acute respiratory distress syndrome. *BioMed. Res. Int.* **2018**, *2018*, 7507314. [CrossRef] [PubMed]
53. Liu, W.; Liu, K.; Zhang, S.; Shan, L.; Tang, J. Tetramethylpyrazine showed therapeutic effects on sepsis-induced acute lung injury in rats by inhibiting endoplasmic reticulum stress protein kinase RNA-like endoplasmic reticulum kinase (PERK) signaling-induced apoptosis of pulmonary microvascular endothelial cells. *Med. Sci. Monit. Int. Med. J. Exp. Clin. Res.* **2018**, *24*, 1225–1231.
54. Yang, Y.; Huang, Z.; Li, J.; Mo, Z.; Huang, Y.; Ma, C.; Wang, W.; Pan, X.; Wu, C. PLGA porous microspheres dry powders for codelivery of afatinib-loaded solid lipid nanoparticles and paclitaxel: Novel therapy for EGFR tyrosine kinase inhibitors resistant nonsmall cell lung cancer. *Adv. Healthc. Mater.* **2019**, *8*, 1900965. [CrossRef]
55. Aggarwal, B.B.; Shishodia, S.; Sandur, S.K.; Pandey, M.K.; Sethi, G. Inflammation and cancer: How hot is the link? *Biochem. Pharmacol.* **2006**, *72*, 1605–1621. [CrossRef]
56. Rojo de la Vega, M.; Chapman, E.; Zhang, D.D. NRF2 and the Hallmarks of Cancer. *Cancer Cell* **2018**, *34*, 21–43. [CrossRef]
57. Sánchez-Ortega, M.; Carrera, A.C.; Garrido, A. Role of NRF2 in lung cancer. *Cells* **2021**, *10*, 1879. [CrossRef]
58. Hamzavi, M.; Tadbir, A.A.; Rezvani, G.; Ashraf, M.J.; Fattahi, M.J.; Khademi, B.; Sardari, Y.; Jeirudi, N. Tissue expression, serum and salivary levels of IL-10 in patients with head and neck squamous cell carcinoma. *Asian Pac. J. Cancer Prev.* **2013**, *14*, 1681–1685. [CrossRef]
59. Kobelt, D.; Zhang, C.; Clayton-Lucey, I.A.; Glauben, R.; Voss, C.; Siegmund, B.; Stein, U. Pro-inflammatory TNF-α and IFN-γ Promote Tumor Growth and Metastasis via Induction of MACC1. *Front. Immunol.* **2020**, *11*, 980. [CrossRef]
60. Jorgovanovic, D.; Song, M.; Wang, L.; Zhang, Y. Roles of IFN-γ in tumor progression and regression: A review. *Biomark. Res.* **2020**, *8*, 49. [CrossRef] [PubMed]
61. Todoric, J.; Antonucci, L.; Karin, M. Targeting Inflammation in Cancer Prevention and Therapy. *Cancer Prev. Res.* **2016**, *9*, 895–905. [CrossRef] [PubMed]
62. Ginwala, R.; Bhavsar, R.; Chigbu, D.G.; Jain, P.; Khan, Z.K. Potential role of flavonoids in treating chronic inflammatory diseases with a special focus on the anti-inflammatory activity of apigenin. *Antioxidants* **2019**, *8*, 35. [CrossRef] [PubMed]
63. Hamza, A.A.; Heeba, G.H.; Elwy, H.M.; Murali, C.; El-Awady, R.; Amin, A. Molecular characterization of the grape seeds extract's effect against chemically induced liver cancer: In vivo and in vitro analyses. *Sci. Rep.* **2018**, *8*, 1270–1276. [CrossRef]
64. Rashid, S.; Ali, N.; Nafees, S.; Ahmad, T.; Hasan, S.K.; Sultana, S. Abrogation of 5-flourouracil induced renal toxicity by bee propolis via targeting oxidative stress and inflammation in Wistar rats. *J. Pharm. Res.* **2013**, *7*, 189–194. [CrossRef]
65. Zhao, Y.; Xu, Y.; Li, Y.; Xu, W.; Luo, F.; Wang, B.; Pang, Y.; Xiang, Q.; Zhou, J.; Wang, X.; et al. NF-κB-mediated inflammation leading to EMT via miR-200c is involved in cell transformation induced by cigarette smoke extract. *Toxicol. Sci.* **2013**, *135*, 265–276. [CrossRef] [PubMed]
66. Atiq, A.; Shal, B.; Naveed, M.; Khan, A.; Ali, J.; Zeeshan, S.; Al-Sharari, S.D.; Kim, Y.S.; Khan, S. Diadzein ameliorates 5-fluorouracil-induced intestinal mucositis by suppressing oxidative stress and inflammatory mediators in rodents. *Eur. J. Pharmacol.* **2019**, *843*, 292–306. [CrossRef]
67. Hayaza, S.; Darmanto, W.; Wahyuningsih, S.P.A.; Susilo, R.J.K.; Husen, S.A.; Winarni, D.; Doong, R.A. Immunomodulatory activity of Okra raw polysaccharide extract by regulating TNF-A, IFN-G Levels, and cell apoptosis in DEN-induced mice. *Res. J. Pharm. Technol.* **2022**, *15*, 546–550. [CrossRef]
68. Zhang, H.W.; Hu, J.J.; Fu, R.Q.; Liu, X.; Zhang, Y.H.; Li, J.; Liu, L.; Li, Y.N.; Deng, Q.; Luo, Q.S.; et al. Flavonoids inhibit cell proliferation and induce apoptosis and autophagy through downregulation of PI3Kγ mediated PI3K/AKT/mTOR/p70S6K/ULK signaling pathway in human breast cancer cells. *Sci. Rep.* **2018**, *8*, 11255. [CrossRef]
69. Unsal, V.; Kurutaş, E.B. Experimental Hepatic Carcinogenesis: Oxidative Stress and Natural Antioxidants. *Maced. J. Med. Sci.* **2017**, *5*, 686–691. [CrossRef]

70. Pacher, P.; Beckman, J.S.; Liaudet, L. Nitric oxide and peroxynitrite in health and disease. *Physiol. Rev.* **2007**, *87*, 315–324. [CrossRef]
71. Bishayee, A.; Barnes, K.F.; Bhatia, D.; Darvesh, A.S.; Carroll, R.T. Resveratrol suppresses oxidative stress and inflammatory response in diethylnitrosamine-initiated rat hepatocarcinogenesis. *Cancer Prev. Res.* **2010**, *3*, 753–763. [CrossRef]
72. Yu, X.; Ge, L.; Niu, L.; Lian, X.; Ma, H.; Pang, L. The dual role of inducible nitric oxide synthase in myocardial ischemia/reperfusion injury: Friend or foe? *Oxidative Med. Cell. Longev.* **2018**, *2018*, 8364848. [CrossRef]
73. Ahmad, S.F.; Attia, S.M.; Bakheet, S.A.; Zoheir, K.M.; Ansari, M.A.; Korashy, H.M.; Abdel-Hamied, H.E.; Ashour, A.E.; Abd-Allah, A.R. Naringin attenuates the development of carrageenan-induced acute lung inflammation through inhibition of NF-κb, STAT3 and pro-inflammatory mediators and enhancement of IκBα and anti-inflammatory cytokines. *Inflammation* **2015**, *38*, 846–857. [CrossRef]
74. Liu, Y.; Wu, H.; Nie, Y.C.; Chen, J.L.; Su, W.W.; Li, P.B. Naringin attenuates acute lung injury in LPS-treated mice by inhibiting NF-κB pathway. *Int. Immunopharmacol.* **2011**, *11*, 1606–1612. [CrossRef]
75. Habauzit, V.; Sacco, S.M.; Gil-Izquierdo, A.; Trzeciakiewicz, A.; Morand, C.; Barron, D.; Pinaud, S.; Offord, E.; Horcajada, M.N. Differential effects of two citrus flavanones on bone quality in senescent male rats in relation to their bioavailability and metabolism. *Bone* **2011**, *49*, 1108–1116. [CrossRef] [PubMed]
76. Chtourou, Y.; Aouey, B.; Kebieche, M.; Fetoui, H. Protective role of naringin against cisplatin induced oxidative stress, inflammatory response and apoptosis in rat striatum via suppressing ROS-mediated NF-κB and P53 signaling pathways. *Chem. Biol. Interact.* **2015**, *239*, 76–86. [CrossRef] [PubMed]
77. Lv, Z.; Wu, W.; Ge, S.; Jia, R.; Lin, T.; Yuan, Y.; Kuang, H.; Yang, B.; Wu, L.; Wei, J.; et al. Naringin protects against perfluorooctane sulfonate-induced liver injury by modulating NRF2 and NF-κB in mice. *Int. Immunopharmacol.* **2018**, *65*, 140–147. [CrossRef] [PubMed]
78. Purvis, J.E.; Karhohs, K.W.; Mock, C.; Batchelor, E.; Loewer, A.; Lahav, G. p53 dynamics control cell fate. *Science* **2012**, *336*, 1440–1444. [CrossRef] [PubMed]
79. Ou, X.; Lu, Y.; Liao, L.; Li, D.; Liu, L.; Liu, H.; Xu, H. Nitidine chloride induces apoptosis in human hepatocellular carcinoma cells through a pathway involving p53, p21, Bax and Bcl-2. *Oncol. Rep.* **2015**, *33*, 1264–1274. [CrossRef]
80. Campbell, K.J.; Tait, S.W. Targeting BCL-2 regulated apoptosis in cancer. *Open Biol.* **2018**, *8*, 180002. [CrossRef]
81. Kang, M.H.; Reynolds, C.P. Bcl-2 inhibitors: Targeting mitochondrial apoptotic pathways in cancer therapy. *Clin. Cancer Res.* **2009**, *15*, 1126–1132. [CrossRef]
82. Zhu, L.; Han, M.B.; Gao, Y.; Wang, H.; Dai, L.; Wen, Y.; Na, L.X. Curcumin triggers apoptosis via upregulation of Bax/Bcl-2 ratio and caspase activation in SW872 human adipocytes. *Mol. Med. Rep.* **2015**, *12*, 1151–1156. [CrossRef]
83. Liu, Z.; Ding, Y.; Ye, N.; Wild, C.; Chen, H.; Zhou, J. Direct activation of Bax protein for cancer therapy. *Med. Res. Rev.* **2016**, *36*, 313–341. [CrossRef]
84. Liu, X.; Fan, L.; Lu, C.; Yin, S.; Hu, H. Functional role of p53 in the regulation of chemical-induced oxidative stress. *Oxidative Med. Cell. Longev.* **2020**, *2020*, 6039769. [CrossRef] [PubMed]
85. Qi, F.; Li, A.; Inagaki, Y. Induction of apoptosis by cinobufacini preparation through mitochondria- and Fas-mediated caspase-dependent pathways in human hepatocellular carcinoma cells. *Food Chem. Toxicol.* **2012**, *20*, 295–302. [CrossRef] [PubMed]
86. Chen, R.; Qi, Q.L.; Wang, M.T.; Li, Q.Y. Therapeutic potential of naringin: An overview. *Pharm. Biol.* **2016**, *54*, 3203–3210. [CrossRef]
87. Abotaleb, M.; Samuel, S.M.; Varghese, E.; Varghese, S.; Kubatka, P.; Liskova, A.; Büsselberg, D. Flavonoids in cancer and apoptosis. *Cancers* **2018**, *11*, 28. [CrossRef]
88. Raina, R.; Hussain, A.; Sharma, R. Molecular insight into apoptosis mediated by flavones in cancer. *World Acad. Sci. J.* **2020**, *2*, 6. [CrossRef]
89. Tramm, T.; Kyndi, M.; Sørensen, F.B.; Overgaard, J.; Alsner, J. Influence of intra-tumoral heterogeneity on the evaluation of BCL2, E-cadherin, EGFR, EMMPRIN, and Ki-67 expression in tissue microarrays from breast cancer. *Acta Oncol.* **2018**, *57*, 102–106. [CrossRef]
90. Wen, S.; Zhou, W.; Li, C.M.; Hu, J.; Hu, X.M.; Chen, P.; Shao, G.L.; Guo, W.H. Ki-67 as a prognostic marker in early-stage non-small cell lung cancer in Asian patients: A meta-analysis of published studies involving 32 studies. *BMC Cancer* **2015**, *15*, 520. [CrossRef]
91. Wang, D.; Ye, W.; Shi, Q. Prognostic Value of Ki-67 Expression in Advanced Lung Squamous Cell Carcinoma Patients Treated with Chemotherapy. *Cancer Manag. Res.* **2021**, *13*, 6429. [CrossRef]
92. De Jong, W.H.; Borm, P.J. Drug delivery and nanoparticles: Applications and hazards. *Int. J. Nanomed.* **2008**, *3*, 133–149. [CrossRef] [PubMed]

cancers MDPI

Article

In Silico, In Vitro, and In Vivo Investigations on Adapalene as Repurposed Third Generation Retinoid against Multiple Myeloma and Leukemia

Joelle C. Boulos [1], Manik Chatterjee [2], Letian Shan [3] and Thomas Efferth [1,*]

1 Department of Pharmaceutical Biology, Institute of Pharmaceutical and Biomedical Sciences, Johannes Gutenberg University, Staudinger Weg 5, 55128 Mainz, Germany; joboulos@uni-mainz.de
2 Translational Oncology, Comprehensive Cancer Center Mainfranken, University Hospital Würzburg, 97080 Würzburg, Germany; chatterjee_m@ukw.de
3 The First Affiliated Hospital, Zhejiang Chinese Medical University, Hangzhou 310053, China; letian.shan@foxmail.com
* Correspondence: efferth@uni-mainz.de; Tel./Fax: +49-6131-3925751

Simple Summary: Hematological neoplasms afflict millions of children and adults yearly and are often uncurable due to refractory illness and recurrence. Therefore, new treatment approaches are required. The proto-oncogene c-MYC has been linked to carcinogenesis, particularly in hematological malignancies. Consequently, to develop new and effective therapies for blood cancers, it is essential to target c-MYC, specifically that c-MYC inhibitors have not yet received clinical approval. In this research, the verification of adapalene as a c-MYC inhibitor may be a glimmer of hope, especially that it is an already Food and Drug Administration (FDA)-approved drug, and its toxicity profiles, pharmacokinetics, and pharmacodynamics are well established. Our study presents a rationale that the discovery of adapalene as a c-MYC inhibitor may significantly lower the drug development costs of new anticancer medications. It also provides further insights in the future of adapalene-based designs that could result in more effective and targeted innovative therapies for multiple myeloma.

Abstract: The majority of hematopoietic cancers in adults are incurable and exhibit unpredictable remitting-relapsing patterns in response to various therapies. The proto-oncogene c-MYC has been associated with tumorigenesis, especially in hematological neoplasms. Therefore, targeting c-MYC is crucial to find effective, novel treatments for blood malignancies. To date, there are no clinically approved c-MYC inhibitors. In this study, we virtually screened 1578 Food and Drug Administration (FDA)-approved drugs from the ZINC15 database against c-MYC. The top 117 compounds from PyRx-based screening with the best binding affinities to c-MYC were subjected to molecular docking studies with AutoDock 4.2.6. Retinoids consist of synthetic and natural vitamin A derivatives. All-trans-retinoic acid (ATRA) were highly effective in hematological malignancies. In this study, adapalene, a third-generation retinoid usually used to treat acne vulgaris, was selected as a potent c-MYC inhibitor as it robustly bound to c-MYC with a lowest binding energy (LBE) of −7.27 kcal/mol, a predicted inhibition constant (pKi) of 4.69 μM, and a dissociation constant (K_d value) of 3.05 μM. Thus, we examined its impact on multiple myeloma (MM) cells in vitro and evaluated its efficiency in vivo using a xenograft tumor zebrafish model. We demonstrated that adapalene exerted substantial cytotoxicity against a panel of nine MM and two leukemic cell lines, with AMO1 cells being the most susceptible one (IC_{50} = 1.76 ± 0.39 μM) and, hence, the focus of this work. Adapalene (0.5 × IC_{50}, 1 × IC_{50}, 2 × IC_{50}) decreased c-MYC expression and transcriptional activity in AMO1 cells in a dose-dependent manner. An examination of the cell cycle revealed that adapalene halted the cells in the G_2/M phase and increased the portion of cells in the sub-G_0/G_1 phase after 48 and 72 h, indicating that cells failed to initiate mitosis, and consequently, cell death was triggered. Adapalene also increased the number of p-H3(Ser10) positive AMO1 cells, which is a further proof of its ability to prevent mitotic exit. Confocal imaging demonstrated that adapalene destroyed the tubulin network of U2OS cells stably transfected with a cDNA coding for α-tubulin-GFP, refraining the migration of malignant cells. Furthermore, adapalene induced DNA damage in AMO1 cells. It also induced apoptosis and autophagy, as demonstrated by flow cytometry and western blotting. Finally, adapalene impeded tumor growth in a xenograft tumor zebrafish model. In summary, the discovery of the vitamin A derivative adapalene as a c-MYC inhibitor reveals its potential as an avant-garde treatment for MM.

Keywords: drug repurposing; hematological malignancies; microtubules; programmed cell death; targeted chemotherapy; third-generation retinoid; xenograft tumor zebrafish model

1. Introduction

Cancers affecting lymph nodes, bone marrow, and blood are collectively known as hematological malignancies. This category comprises lymphoma (Hodgkin and non-Hodgkin types), multiple myeloma (MM), and different kinds of leukemia such as chronic myeloid (CML), acute myeloid (AML), chronic lymphocytic (CLL), and acute lymphocytic (ALL). All together, these hematopoietic neoplasms constitute about 9% of all cancers that are newly diagnosed, with lymphomas (particularly non-Hodgkin's) being more prevalent than MM or leukemia. Blood cancers often increase with age, with the exception of Hodgkin's lymphoma and ALL [1].

MM is a rare blood malignancy that accounts for 1% of all cancers and 10% of hematological cancers. It is the second most frequent blood cancer in industrialized countries. A hallmark of MM is the invasion of the bone marrow by monoclonal plasma cells which produce and discharge monoclonal immunoglobulin into the blood and urine [2]. The amassment of these immunoglobulins causes organ malfunction such as bone lesions, anemia, renal insufficiency, and hypercalcemia. At this point, patients begin to develop symptoms. MM generally starts as an asymptomatic precursor malignancy. Monoclonal gammopathy of undetermined significance (MGUS) and smoldering undetermined significance (MGUS) are the diseases that manifest at this stage in which genetic defects, such as hyperdiploidy and the involvement of immunoglobulin heavy chain in translocations, are initiated [3]. A translocation adjoining an oncogene next to an immunoglobulin enhancer occurs in the plasma cells of around half of individuals with MGUS [4]. These translocations might serve as a starting point for later oncogenic processes that eventually engender MM. Malignant cell gene expression profiling revealed diverse disease subgroups, likely attributable to the activation of several oncogenic pathways in various patients [5].

c-MYC deregulation may contribute to the progression of MGUS to MM [6]. Several processes, including mutation, translocation, and gene amplification, result in c-MYC overexpression. Numerous MM cell lines and, to a certain extent, primary MM cells (15–46%) harbor c-MYC chromosomal rearrangements [7]. Additionally, 40% of all c-MYC translocations in human MM cells do not affect immunoglobulin genes. Contrarily, patients overexpressing c-MYC have been delineated in a greater portion than the ones with c-MYC translocations [8]. Importantly, the experimental c-MYC knockdown was lethal to MM cells, implying that MM may be addicted for c-MYC activity to survive, and targeting c-MYC may improve the treatment outcome of MM [9].

Even with recent medical advancements such as monoclonal antibodies, histone deacetylase inhibitors, immunomodulatory drugs, proteasome inhibitors, anthracyclines, alkylating agents, corticosteroids, stem cell transplantation, radiotherapy, bisphosphonate treatment, and combination therapies [10], patients with MM frequently experience multiple relapses following one or more treatment procedures, or evolve into a refractory state, primarily as a result of drug resistance. Having in mind the impending negative effects of the available hematopoietic treatments and given that c-MYC dysregulation is a distinct feature in the genetic profile of MM, alternative approaches were forged to identify novel drugs targeting c-MYC, especially because such therapies are not yet available [11,12]. To date, numerous approaches have been developed to specifically target c-MYC in MM. Nevertheless, the pharmacokinetic characteristics and the efficacy of many of these strategies are subpar. Moreover, finding ligands that directly inhibit c-MYC is still challenging [13].

Despite improvements in technology and the advanced perception of human diseases, the development of new therapeutic approaches has proceeded far slower than anticipated. Drug repurposing, often referred to as drug reprofiling, repositioning, or re-tasking, could be an alternate method for discovering new applications for approved or experimental drugs that go beyond the limits of the typical medical prescription [14]. This strategy has significant advantages over developing a brand-new medication for a specific indication because the toxicity profiles, pharmacokinetics, and pharmacodynamics of commercially available drugs are well established. If repurposing is successful, it is possible to significantly save time and financial outlays on a drug's preclinical and clinical testing [15].

Adapalene (Figure 1A), also known as CD271 and differin, belongs to the third generation of retinoids that were approved by the Food and Drug Administration (FDA) in 1996 to treat acne vulgaris [16]. Adapalene is a naphthoic acid derivative known to bind to retinoic acid nuclear receptors [17]. There are several documented actions of adapalene, including immunomodulatory, anti-proliferative, anti-inflammatory, comedolytic, anti-bacterial, and neuroprotective activities [18]. Regarding anticancer studies, adapalene promoted G1 cell cycle arrest and inhibited CDK2 in colorectal cancer cells. It also prompted apoptotic cell death in hepatoma cells by modulating the ratio of Bax and Bcl-2 [17,19]. Furthermore, adapalene inhibited the proliferation of melanoma cells through S-phase arrest of the cell cycle, and subsequently induced apoptosis through DNA damage [20]. Adapalene suppressed the proliferation of ES-2 ovarian cancer cells by inhibiting glutamicoxaloacetic transaminase 1 (GOT1) [21]. It also reduced the growth of prostate cancer cells by triggering DNA damage, halting the cell cycle in the S phase, and evoking apoptosis [22]. Finally, adapalene arrested triple-negative breast cancer cells in the S-phase, inhibiting their proliferation [23]. All these findings proved that repurposing adapalene for cancer treatment represents a promising approach.

The aim of the present study is to locate prospective FDA-approved drugs that target the oncogenic transcription factor c-MYC using in silico tools (virtual screening by PyRx and molecular docking by AutoDock) to examine the molecular interaction of the preeminent FDA-approved drug adapalene and c-MYC using microscale thermophoresis (MST), and to confirm that adapalene is an effective c-MYC inhibitor by a MYC reporter assay. Given that MM cells depend on c-MYC for their survival, and since there are currently no reports on the application of adapalene for the treatment of hematological malignancies, we were further interested in investigating the effect of adapalene against a panel of MM cell lines, determining its mechanism of action and its cell death modality through in vitro studies. Finally, we verified its growth inhibitory efficacy in vivo using a T-ALL zebrafish model.

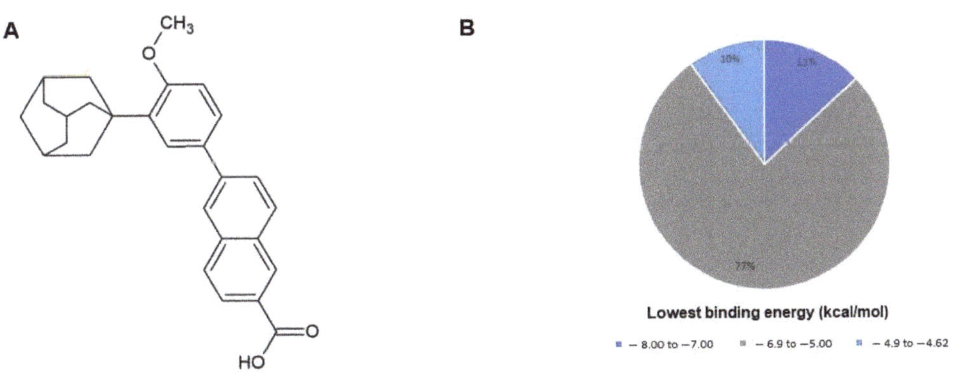

Figure 1. *Cont.*

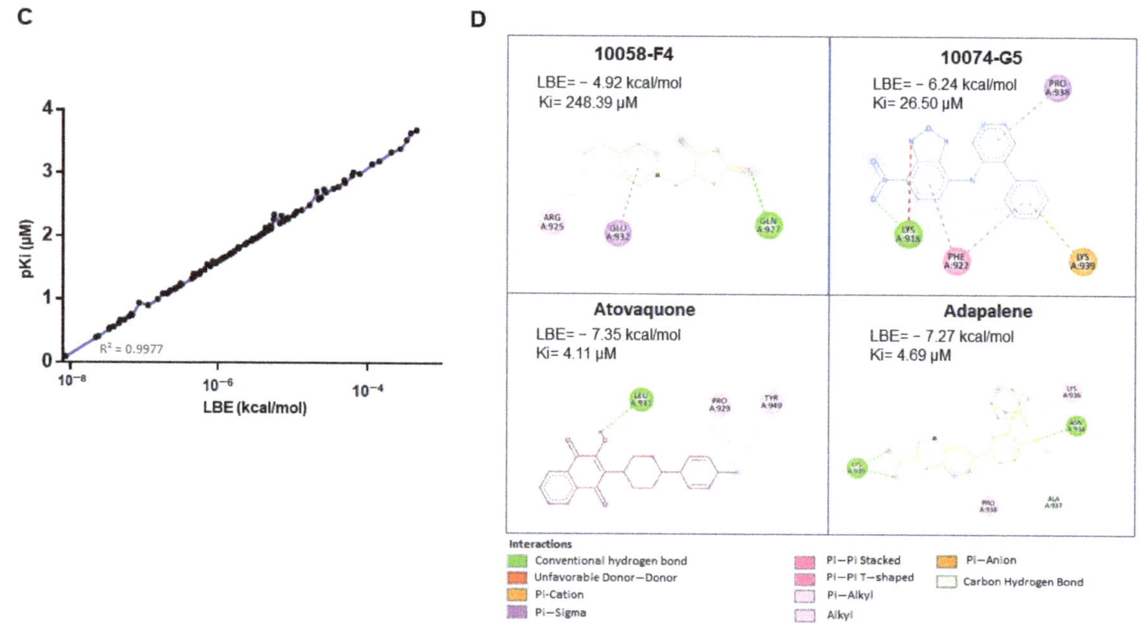

Figure 1. Molecular docking of candidate c-MYC inhibitors. (**A**) Chemical structure of adapalene. (**B**) Pie chart showing the percentage of FDA-approved ligands belonging to a particular lowest binding energy (kcal/mol) range. (**C**) Correlation coefficient representation of predicted inhibition constant (pKi) vs. lowest binding energies (LBE). (**D**) 2D representations of the various interactions between the amino acid residues of c-MYC and the corresponding compounds (10058-F4, 10074-G5, atovaquone, and adapalene) were generated using Discovery Studio Visualizer software (version v.21.1.0.20298). The lowest binding energies (LBE) and the predicted inhibition constant (Ki) of each compound were acquired from AutoDockTools 4.2.6.

2. Materials and Methods

2.1. Virtual Drug Screening and Molecular Docking Analyses

The FDA-approved drug library, consisting of 1577 compounds, was downloaded from the Zinc15 database (https://zinc15.docking.org/, accessed on 25 April 2019) to evaluate the in silico binding strength of those compounds toward c-MYC using PyRx0.9 virtual screening tool and AutoDock 4.2.6 molecular docking.

The 3D structures of the ligands were downloaded as standard data files (sdf). The crystal structure of c-MYC was downloaded from the Protein Data Bank (http://www.rcsb.org/, accessed on 25 April 2019) as a PDB file (PDB ID: 1NKP) [24]. Using AutoDockTool 1.5.6 (The Scripps Research Institute, La Jolla, CA, USA), the protein crystal structure was subsequently improved by removing water molecules and by adding missing hydrogen atoms. Following that, the PDB file was converted to Protein Data Bank Partial Charge and Atom Type (PDBQT) file [25]. Prior to PyRx running, the energy of the FDA-approved ligands was minimized, and the files were converted to PDBQT. The ligands were then sorted according to their lowest binding energy (kcal/mol), which was obtained by the PyRx virtual screening tool.

The top 170 compounds with the lowest binding energy were selected for further molecular docking analysis using AutoDock 4.2.6 (Center for Computational Structural Biology ccsb, La Jolla, CA, USA) [25]. Two known c-MYC inhibitors, 10058-F4 and 10074-G5, were used as positive controls [26,27]. The grid box was set to mask the whole protein with the center of the grid box at x = 65.333, y = 62.507, and z = 42.943 with the number of grid points (npts) of 54 in x, 108 in y, and 70 in z. The calculations were performed using a

Lamarckian algorithm provided by AutoDock with 250 runs and 2,500,000 energy evaluation. The AutoDock RMSD cluster analysis generated the expected results as DLG files. Interacting with amino acids and visualizations was performed with BIOVIA Discovery Studio Visualizer (https://discover.3ds.com/, accessed on 20 May 2019).

2.2. Microscale Thermophoresis

MST was performed to study the in vitro binding of adapalene to recombinant human c-MYC protein (ab169901, Abcam, Cambridge, UK) [28]. Briefly, the Protein Labeling Kit Blue-NHS (L003, NanoTemper Technologies GmbH, Munich, Germany) was used to fluorescently tag the c-MYC protein following the manufacturer's instructions. With a final c-MYC concentration of 200 nM, MST was performed at 50% LED intensity and 40% MST power. Finally, the fit curve and the dissociation constant (K_d) of adapalene were generated with the NanoTemper Analysis Software version 2.2.4.

2.3. MYC Cignal Reporter Assay

The Qiagen cignal MYC reporter assay kit (CCS-012L, Germantown, MD, USA) was used to examine the impact of adapalene on c-MYC activity, as previously described [29]. Briefly stated, HEK293 human embryonic kidney cells were transfected with a c-MYC-luciferase reporter construct and grown in accordance with the instructions provided by the manufacturer. Cells were then exposed to adapalene (5 and 10 μM), DMSO as negative control, or 10058-F4 (127.5 2 μM) as positive control. After 24 h, the Dual-glo® Luciferase Reporter Assay System (E2920, Promega, Madison, WI, USA) was added to each well to quantify the activity of the c-MYC promoter by measuring the luminescence of firefly and renilla luciferases using an Infinite M2000 Pro™ plate reader (Tecan, Crailsheim, Germany).

$$\text{c} - \text{Myc activity} = \frac{\text{firefly luciferase luminescence}}{\text{renilla luciferase luminescence}}$$

$$\text{Relative luciferase} = 100 \times \left(\frac{\text{firefly luciferase luminescence}}{\text{renilla luciferase luminescence}}\right)$$

$$\text{Normalized c} - \text{Myc activity} = \frac{\text{relative luciferase (sample)}}{\text{relative luciferase (DMSO)}}$$

2.4. Cell Lines

Leukemia cells, including the drug-sensitive CCRF-CEM T-cell acute lymphoblastic leukemia (T-ALL) and their multidrug-resistant P-glycoprotein-overexpressing CEM/ADR5000 subline, were provided by Dr. Axel Sauerbrey (Children's Hospital, University of Jena, Jena, Germany). HL60 and U266 were provided by Prof. Markus Munder (University Medical Center of the Johannes Gutenberg University, Mainz, Germany). MM cells, including AMO1, KMS12BM, MolP8, NCI-H929, OPM2, KMS11, L363, and JJN3, were kindly supplied by Dr. Manik Chatterjee (University of Würzburg, Würzburg, Germany). RPMI8226 cells were obtained from the American Type Cell Culture Collection (ATCC® CCL-155™, ATCC, Manassas, VA, USA).

Leukemia cells and MM were maintained in RPMI 1640 (Life Technologies, Darmstadt, Germany), supplemented with 10% FBS (Life Technologies) and 1% penicillin (1000 U/mL)/streptomycin (100 μg/mL) (Life Technologies). Cells were incubated in a 5% CO_2/37 °C incubator.

HEK293 were kindly provided by Prof. Dr. Christina Friedland (Johannes Gutenberg University, Mainz, Germany). Human bone osteosarcoma cells (U2OS) that persistently express an α-tubulin-GFP construct were kindly provided by Dr. Joachim Hehl (Light microscope center, ETH Zurich, Zurich, Switzerland). HEK293 and U2OS were maintained in DMEM (Life Technologies), supplemented with 10% FBS (Life Technologies) and 1% penicillin (1000 U/mL)/streptomycin (100 μg/mL) (Life Technologies). Cells were incubated in a 5% CO_2/37 °C incubator.

Fresh blood samples were obtained from a healthy individual and placed in plastic Monovette EDTA tubes at the Department of Hematology, Oncology, and Pneumology (University Medical Center of the Johannes Gutenberg University, Mainz, Germany).

Histopaque® (Sigma-Aldrich, Taufkirchen, Germany) was used to collect human peripheral blood mononuclear cells (PBMCs). In a few words, 3 mL of fresh blood was cautiously deposited on top of Histopaque® and centrifuged at 400× g/4 °C for 30 min. The buffy coat made up of PBMCs was then isolated, rinsed with PBS, and centrifuged three times at 250 × g, for 10 min each. The resulting cell pellet was cultured in Panserin 413 growth media (PAN-Biotech, Aidenbach, Germany) and supplemented with 2% phytohemagglutinin M (PHA-M, Life Technologies).

2.5. Cell Viability Assessment

The sensitivity of MM cells, leukemia cells, and PBMCs to adapalene was evaluated by the resazurin reduction assay, as previously described [30]. In brief, 10^4 cells were seeded in each well of a flat bottom 96-well plate. Cells were directly treated with 10 different concentrations of adapalene (Activate Scientific, Prien am Chiemsee, Bavaria) which are 3-fold apart from one another, ranging from 100 µM to 0.003 µM for MM and T-ALL cells. However, when 10-fold apart from one another, they ranged from 100 µM to 10^{-7} µM for PBMCs. The plates were incubated for 72 h at 5% CO_2/37 °C and then re-incubated for another 4 h under the same conditions, with 20 µL of resazurin (0.01% w/v; Sigma-Aldrich) added to each well. An Infinite M2000 Pro plate reader (Tecan, Crailsheim, Germany) was used to measure resorufin fluorescence, produced by the reduction of resazurin by live cells, at 544–590 nm (excitation-emission wavelengths). Afterward, cell viability was plotted vs. adapalene concentration, and the IC_{50} values from three separate experiments with six repeats each were calculated with GraphPad Prism 5 software (GraphPad Software, San Diego, CA, USA).

2.6. Cell Cycle Analysis

The cell cycle progression of AMO1 cells incubated with different adapalene concentrations (0.5 × IC_{50}, 1 × IC_{50}, or 2 × IC_{50}) or media for 48 and 72 h was examined by propidium iodide (PI) staining (Thermo Fisher Scientific, Dreieich, Germany). Cells were collected and maintained at −20 °C in 80% ethanol. Following the corresponding incubation time, cells were kept in PI staining solution at 4 °C for 15 min. Later on, the amount of PI staining was assessed with an Accouri C6 flow cytometer (Becton-Dickinson, Heidelberg, Germany). Total DNA content was calculated on FL2-A [31,32].

2.7. Confocal Microscopy of p-H3(Ser10)

AMO1 cells were incubated with adapalene (1 × IC_{50} or 2 × IC_{50}) or DMSO at 5% CO_2/37 °C for 48 h. Afterwards, cells were harvested, washed with PBS, and cytospinned to glass slides (Thermo Fisher Scientific, Dreieich, Germany) for 5 min at 1000 rpm. Cells were then fixed with 4% paraformaldehyde at room temperature for 15 min, washed twice with PBS, and permeabilized with 1% Triton X-100 for 10 min at room temperature. Following permeabilization, cells were again washed twice with PBS. Subsequently, blocking buffer (1% BSA + 10% FBS in PBS) was applied to the cells for 1 h. After blocking, the slides were coated with the primary antibody anti-phospho-histone H3 (Ser10) clone 3H10, FITC Conjugate (Merck, Darmstadt, Germany), at a concentration of 4 µg/mL. The slides had been stored in a humid environment at room temperature. After 1 h of staining, the slides were washed three times with PBS, and the cell nuclei were stained with 1 µg/mL of 4′,6-diamidino-2-phenylindole (DAPI) (Sigma-Aldrich, Darmstadt, Germany) for 5 min. Slides were then washed three times with PBS. Finally, using an AF7000 widefield fluorescent microscope (Leica Microsystems, Wetzlar, Germany), cells were examined after being coated with Fluoromount-G® (SouthernBiotech, Birmingham, AL, USA). FITC was observed at 470/525 nm (excitation/emission wavelengths). DAPI was observed at 470/447 nm (excitation/emission wavelengths) [15].

2.8. Fluorescence Microscopy Imaging of Microtubules Structure

U2OS human osteosarcoma cells persistently expressing α-tubulin-GFP were grown in a μ-Slide 8 Well (30,000 cells/well) (ibidi, Gräfelfing, Germany). Cells were incubated overnight in a 5% CO_2/37 °C incubator. Afterwards, cells were exposed to different adapalene concentrations (1 × IC_{50} or 2 × IC_{50}) or media for 48 h. Cells were then rinsed with PBS and Hoechst 33342 Nuclear Stain (BioVision, Wiesbaden, Germany) was added for 30 min at room temperature in the dark to stain cells nuclei. Later on, excess Hoechst stain was removed with PBS, and the slides were coated with Fluoromount-G®. Living cells were imaged with AF7000 widefield fluorescence microscope (Leica Microsystems, Wetzlar, Germany). GFP was observed at 470/525 nm (excitation/emission wavelengths). Hoechst stain was observed at 470/447 nm (excitation/emission wavelengths). Finally, the software Fiji ImageJ version 1.8.0_322 (National Institutes of Health, Bethesda, MD, USA) was used to analyze images [33].

2.9. Apoptosis Assessment

Apoptosis was examined using fluorescein isothiocyanate (FITC)-conjugated annexin V/propidium iodide (PI) assay kit (eBioscience™ Annexin V; Invitrogen, San Diego, CA, USA). Briefly, 10^6 of AMO1 cells were seeded in each well of a 6-well plate. Cells were directly treated with three different concentrations of adapalene (0.5 × IC_{50}, 1 × IC_{50}, 2 × IC_{50}) or DMSO (used as solvent control), or the positive control bortezomib (1 μM) for 48 and 72 h. Subsequently, cells were collected and washed twice; the first time with cold PBS and the second time with annexin binding buffer (1×). After centrifuging the cells at 1500 rpm, 5 μL of fluorochrome-conjugated annexin V were applied to the cells, and the mixture was then incubated at room temperature for 15 min. PI staining solution (2.5 μL of PI diluted in 400 μL binding buffer (1×)) was used to stain the cells. Apoptosis was assessed using an Accuri C6 flow cytometer (Becton-Dickinson, Heidelberg, Germany). A 530/30 nm band pass filter was used to detect the annexin V-FITC signal after being excited at 488 nm. A 610/20 nm band pass filter was used to detect PI signal after being excited at 561 nm. The F- (forward) and S- (side) scatters gated living cells and the A- (area) and W- (width) scatters gated singlets. 10^4 events/sample were documented from the F- (forward) and S- (side) scatters. Cytograhs were obtained with with FlowJo V10.6.2 software (Becton Dickinson) [34].

2.10. Autophagy Examination

Autophagy was assessed using the autophagy detection kit (ab139484, Abcam, Cambridge, UK). Briefly, 10^6 of AMO1 cells were seeded in each well of a 6-well plate. Cells were directly treated with 3 different concentrations of adapalene (0.5 × IC_{50}, 1 × IC_{50}, 2 × IC_{50}) or DMSO (used as solvent control) for 48 and 72 h. The positive control rapamycin (500 nM) was added 18 h prior to detection. Subsequently, cells were collected, washed with PBS, and suspended in 250 μL of PBS supplemented with 5% FBS. Following that, 250 μL of the diluted green stain solution (1 μL of green detection reagent was diluted in 999 μL of PBS supplemented with 5% FBS) was added to each sample for 30 min at 37 °C in dark. Afterwards, the cells were collected by centrifugation, washed with 1× assay buffer, and resuspended with 500 μL of 1× assay buffer. Autophagy was assessed using an Accouri C6 flow cytometer (Becton Dickinson, Heidelberg, Germany). A 530/30 nm band pass filter was used to detect the green detection reagent after being excited at 488 nm. The F- (forward) and S- (side) scatters gated living cells and the A- (area) and W- (width) scatters gated singlets. 10^4 events/sample were documented from the F- (forward) and S- (side) scatters. Cytographs were obtained with FlowJo V10.6.2 software (Becton-Dickinson, Heidelberg, Germany) [35].

2.11. Western Blot

Aliquots of 10^6 of AMO1 cells were seeded in each well of a 6-well plate and subjected to various concentrations of adapalene (0.5 × IC_{50}, 1 × IC_{50}, or 2 × IC_{50}) or with the negative control DMSO for 48 h at 5% CO_2/37 °C. Cells were then collected and washed twice with PBS. Total protein extraction was accomplished by suspending the cells in M-PER® Mammalian Protein Extraction Reagent supplemented with 1% Halt™ Protease Inhibitor Cocktail (Thermo Scientific, Frankfurt, Germany) and incubated in a 500-rpm shaker at 4 °C for 30 min. Afterwards, the proteins in the supernatant were collected by centrifuging the cells at 1500 rpm at 4 °C for 15 min. A NanoDrop 1000 spectrophotometer (Thermo Scientific, Frankfurt, Germany) was used to determine protein concentration. Following that, 30 µg of proteins were loaded to each loading well of an SDS-PAGE gel (10%). Proteins were transferred onto a polyvinylidene difluoride (PVDF) membrane after being separated by migration in the separating gel. The membrane was then soaked in blocking buffer (5% BSA in TBST) at room temperature for 1 h. Subsequently, membranes were incubated at 4 °C overnight with primary antibodies (1:1000) against c-MYC (#9402), Phospho-Histone H2A.X (Ser139) (20E3) (#9718), GAPDH (D16H11) XP® (#5174), and β-Actin (13E5) (#4970), which were obtained from Cell Signaling Technology (Frankfurt a. M., Germany), and P62 (18420-1-AP), which was obtained from Proteintech (Planegg-Martinsried, Germany). After being washed three times with TBST for 10 min each, membranes were incubated with the proper secondary antibody conjugated with horseradish peroxidase (1:1000) at room temperature for 1 h. Lastly, membranes were photographed using an Alpha Innotech FluorChem Q system (Biozym, Oldendorf, Germany) after being treated with Luminata™ Classico Western HRP substrate (Merck Millipore, Darmstadt, Germany) for 3 min. ImageJ was used to calculate protein expression [36]. Original, uncropped Western blot membranes can be found in Supplementary Figures S1–S5.

2.12. T-ALL Xenograft Zebrafish Model

Adult zebrafish of the wild-type AB strain were ordered from the China Zebrafish Resource Center, Institute of Hydrobiology, China Academy of Science (Wuhan, China) and officially approved by the Association for Assessment and Accreditation of Laboratory Animal Care International (SYXK 2012-0171). 48 h post-fertilization, natural pair-mating procreated zebrafish larvae were grown in an aquaculture space with a photoperiod of 14 h day/10 h night in a row. Zebrafish larvae were nourished with fry flakes (one portion) and live brine shrimps (two portions) every day.

To establish a T-ALL xenograft zebrafish model, CCRF-CEM cells were labelled with red fluorescence CM-Dil at a ratio of 1:1000. After 48 h post-fertilization, CCRF-CEM labelled cells (200 cells/zebrafish) were microinjected into the larvae yolk sac. Following that, 24 h post-tumor growth, the success of the established model was verified with a fluorescent microscope (AZ100, Nikon, Tokyo, Japan). The zebrafish bearing the labelled CCRF-CEM cells were then subjected to different adapalene concentrations, or the positive control cis-platinum for 24 h. The fluorescence intensity (Fi) of the tumor mass was measured in each single zebrafish and the inhibitory rate was determined using the following equation [37]:

$$\% \text{ inhibitory rate} = [1 - (\text{Fi}_{\text{treated group}} / \text{Fi}_{\text{negative control group}})] \times 100\%$$

3. Results

3.1. In Silico Drug Screening

In the field of drug development, virtual screening arose as a potent computational method to swipe vast libraries of small molecules for novel chemical hits with desirable features [38]. In the present study, the FDA-approved Zinc 15 database was screened to assess the in silico binding strength of its compounds toward c-MYC using the PyRx0.9 virtual screening tool. More than 100 compounds with predicted binding affinities of less than −6.10 kcal/mol were identified by PyRx (Supplementary Table S1). Subsequently, molecular docking (blind mode) was performed using AutoDock 4.2.6 to validate the outcomes of the virtual drug screening and to examine the preferential binding site of the ligands. The top 100 ligands with the lowest binding energies (LBEs) are depicted in

Figure 1B (the top 117 ligands with the lowest binding energies (LBEs) are also shown in Supplementary Table S2). Moreover, a significant correlation ($R^2 = 0.9977$) was observed between the LBE (kcal/mol) and the predicted pKi values (µM) (Figure 1C).

Among the top 20 compounds, we focused on atovaquone and adapalene as potential c-MYC inhibitor candidates. The LBE values of atovaquone and adapalene were −7.35 kcal/mol and −7.27 kcal/mol, respectively (Figure 1D). Interestingly, atovaquone and adapalene exerted stronger binding affinities to c-MYC, if compared to the known c-MYC inhibitors, 10058-F4 and 10074-G5 (LBEs of −4.92 kcal/mol and −6.24 kcal/mol, respectively) (Figure 1D). It is noteworthy that atovaquone bound to the same binding cavity as 10058-F4. Moreover, adapalene and 10074-G5 bound to the same binding pocket, and the amino acid residue PRO938 was involved in binding to both substances (Figures 1D and 2).

All compounds had one amino acid involved in H-bonding except for adapalene, which had two amino acids engaged in H-bonding (Figure 1D). The molecular docking further showed that atovaquone and adapalene strongly bound to the bHLHZip domain of c-MYC.

3.2. Effectiveness of Atovaquone and Adapalene against HL60 and U266 Cells

Based on the COSMIC database (https://cancer.sanger.ac.uk/cosmic, accessed on 25 October 2019), HL60 acute myeloid leukemia cells (AML) overexpress c-MYC. On the contrary, Holien et al. (2012) showed that U266 MM cells lack c-MYC expression [39]. To assert these findings, c-MYC protein expression in both cell lines was assessed by us. Our results revealed that HL-60 truly overexpressed c-MYC, while U266 slightly expressed c-MYC. Thus, our U266 findings were contradictory to those of Holien et al. (2012). In our hands, the c-MYC expression is 3× greater in HL-60 than in U266 cells (Figure 3A). In an attempt to examine the specificity of atovaquone and adapalene to c-MYC, we evaluated the cytotoxic effect of atovaquone and adapalene in HL60 and U266 cells, respectively. As expected, HL60 cells overexpressing c-MYC were more susceptible to adapalene and atovaquone than U266 cells that had only a modest c-MYC expression. Moreover, HL60 displayed a greater sensitivity to adapalene ($IC_{50} = 1.19 \pm 0.17$ µM) compared to atovaquone ($IC_{50} = 19.54 \pm 2.26$ µM) (Figure 3B). Therefore, we proceeded with our experiments with adapalene as a potential c-MYC inhibitor candidate.

3.3. Adapalene Strongly Bound to c-MYC

MST is a sensitive approach to confirm the interaction between an unlabeled ligand and a labelled protein [40]. Therefore, we performed MST to verify the in silico predicted binding of adapalene to c-MYC. The fluorescence-labeled recombinant human c-MYC protein was titrated against several adapalene concentrations (Figure 3C). A fit curve was accomplished in accordance with the law of mass action, and adapalene was shown to robustly bind to c-MYC with a K_d value of 3.05 µM. The MST findings were in line with those of the in silico results.

3.4. Adapalene Reduced the Viability of Hematological Cancer Cells

c-MYC plays a crucial role in MM pathophysiology [41]. Given that adapalene might be a novel potential c-MYC inhibitor that has not yet been reported as a therapy for hematological malignancies, we examined the cytotoxic effect of adapalene in MM, T-ALL, and PBMCs using the resazurin cell viability assay. After 72 h of treatment, all evaluated MM cell lines showed substantial sensitivity towards adapalene. The most sensitive cell line, AMO1, had an IC_{50} value of 1.76 ± 0.39 µM, while the least sensitive cell line, JJN3, had an IC_{50} value of 9.10 ± 1.85 µM (Figure 4 and Table 1). Moreover, CCRF-CEM and CEM/ADR5000 cells were sensitive to adapalene to nearly a similar extent ($IC_{50} = 1.83 \pm 0.46$ µM and 2.30 ± 0.09 µM, respectively). Therefore, multidrug-resistant CEM/ADR5000 cells were not cross-resistant to this drug (degree of resistance: 1.26). The concentration of adapalene needed to inhibit the viability of JJN3 cells (the least sensitive cell line) by 50% was lower than the concentration required to inhibit 50% of healthy leucocytes (IC_{50} = 36.72 ± 0.64 μM) (Figure 4 and Table 1), indicating at least some tumor specificity of this compound.

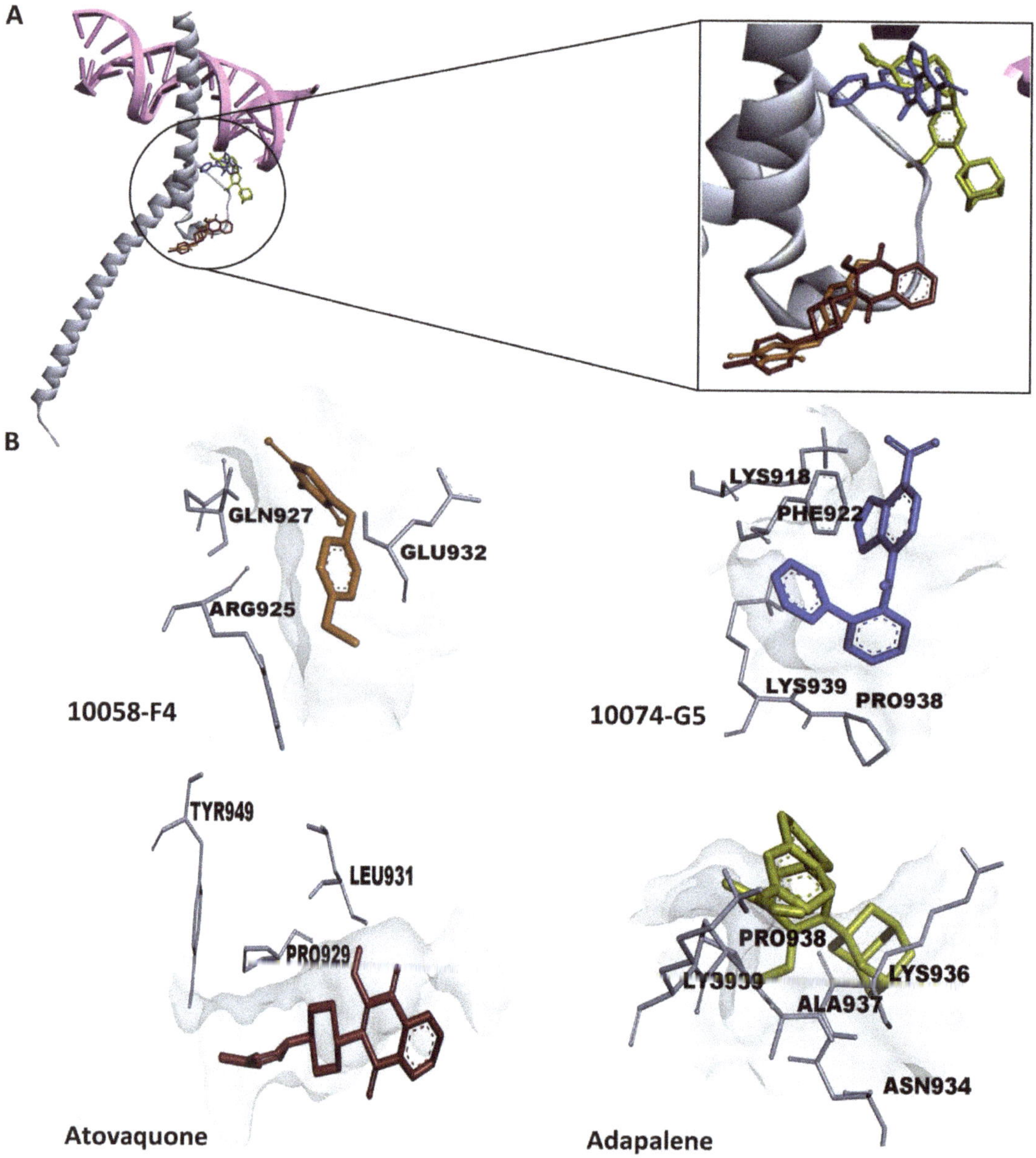

Figure 2. Molecular docking of atovaquone, adapalene, and the known c-MYC:MAX interaction inhibitors: 10058-F4 and 10074-G5. (**A**) Crystal structure of c-MYC (grey) bound to E-Box DNA (pink) (PDB ID: 1NKP). Atovaquone and adapalene shared the same binding cavity as the known inhibitors. (**B**) Amino acids residues expected to be involved in the interaction between c-MYC (grey) and 10058-F4 (orange), 10074-G5 (blue), atovaquone (red), as well as adapalene (yellow), were generated using Discovery Studio Visualizer software (version v.21.1.0.20298).

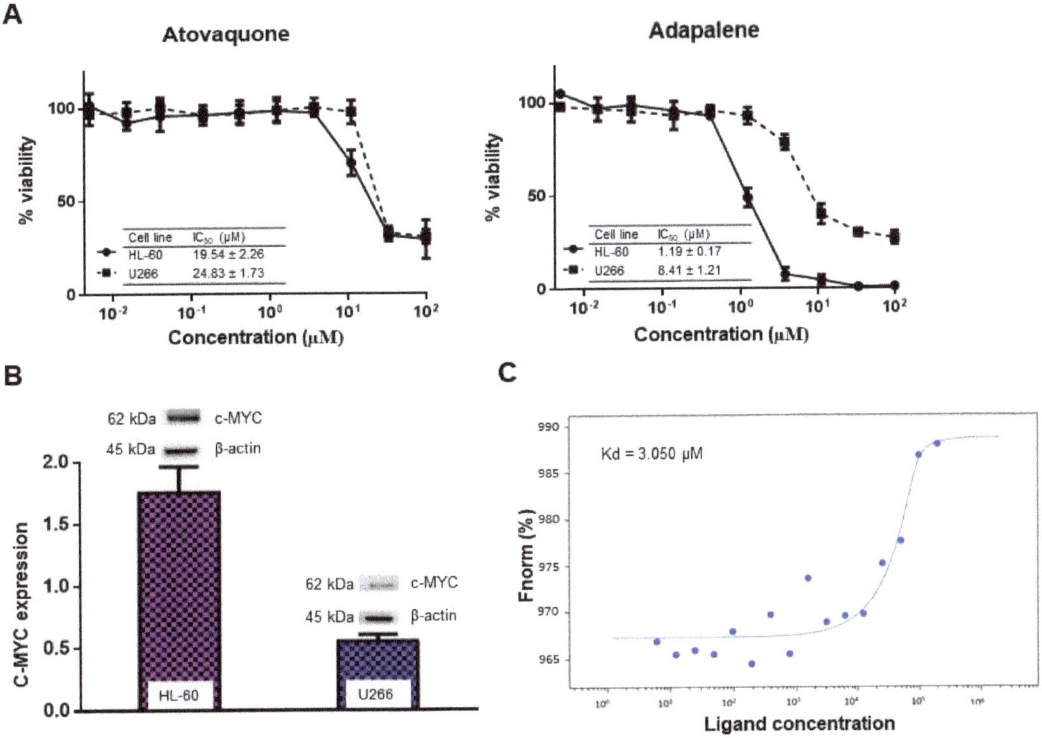

Figure 3. Specificity of atovaquone and adapalene towards c-MYC. (**A**) Assessment of c-MYC protein expression in HL60 and U266 cells by western blot. c-MYC protein expression was three times higher in HL-60 than in U266 cells. The bar diagram was obtained by calculating the mean value ± SD of three independent experiments. (**B**) The cytotoxic effect of atovaquone and adapalene in HL-60 and U266 cells. HL60 cells were more susceptible to adapalene and atovaquone than U266 cells. HL60 cells displayed a greater sensitivity to adapalene than to atovaquone. Adapalene showed higher specificity to c-MYC. (**C**) Binding of adapalene to recombinant human c-MYC as measured by microscale thermophoresis (MST). The fluorescence signal changed depending on the concentration as shown by the binding curve. The law of mass action was used to obtain fitness. MST was conducted with 70% LED power and 10% MST power.

Table 1. Adapalene's IC_{50} values in MM, drug-sensitive T-ALL, and their multidrug-resistant P-glycoprotein-overexpressing leukemia sublines, as well as healthy leukocytes.

Cell Type	Cell Line	IC_{50} (μM)
MM	AMO1	1.76 ± 0.39
	KMS12BM	2.61 ± 0.36
	MOLP8	2.69 ± 0.29
	NCI-H929	4.95 ± 1.21
	RPMI8226	4.97 ± 1.33
	OPM2	5.82 ± 2.07
	KMS11	7.22 ± 1.20
	L363	7.25 ± 0.73
	JJN3	9.10 ± 1.85
Leukemia	CCRF-CEM	1.83 ± 0.46
	CEM/ADR5000	2.30 ± 0.09
Normal leukocytes	PBMCs	36.72 ± 0.64

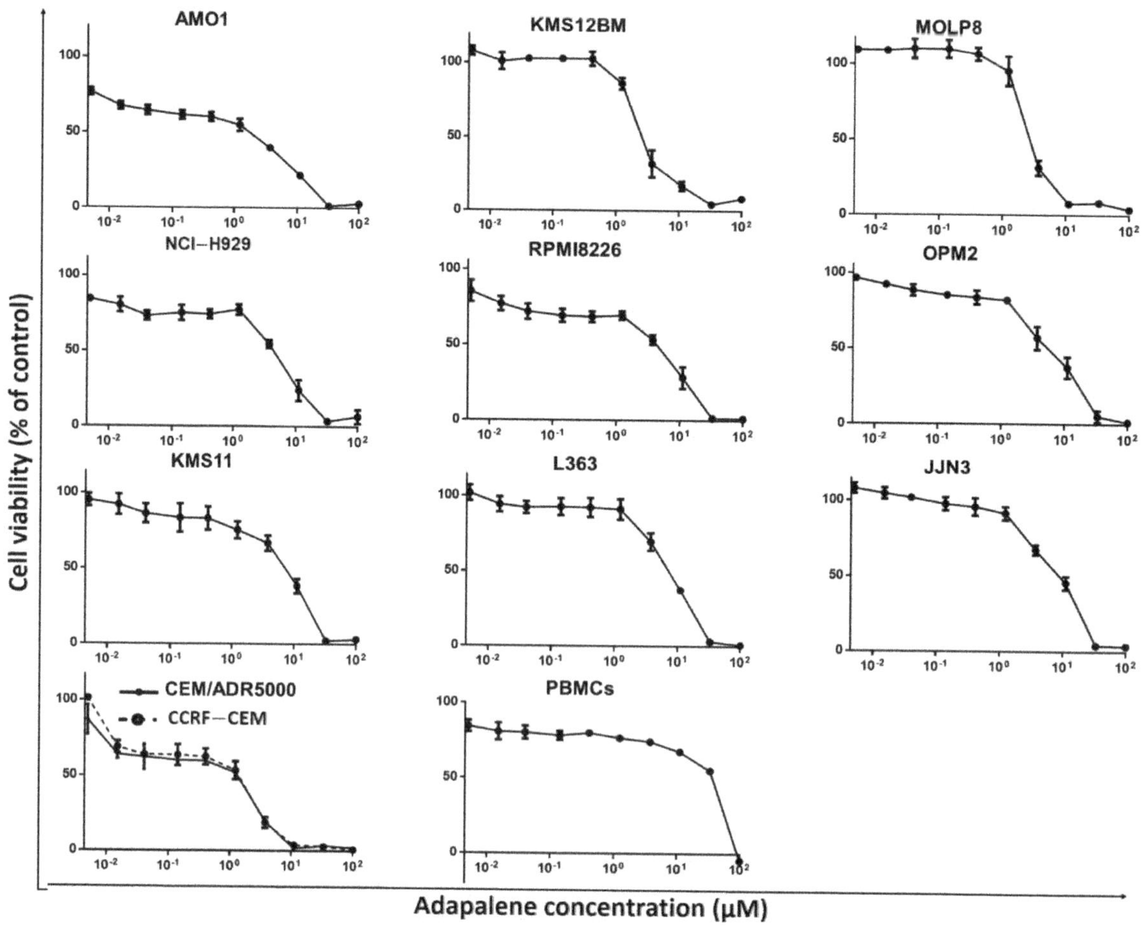

Figure 4. Adapalene's cytotoxic effect in various human MM cell lines (AMO1, KMS12BM, MolP8, NCI-H929, RPMI8226, OPM2, KMS11, L363, and JJN3), in human T-ALL cells (CEM/ADR5000 and CCRF/CEM), and in peripheral blood mononuclear cells (PBMCs). Each value indicates the mean value ± SD of three distinct experiments, each of which had six replicates.

3.5. Adapalene Inhibited c-MYC Expression and Transcriptional Activity In Vitro

Based on the in silico and MST results, we wanted to further confirm the hypothesis that adapalene may be a c-MYC inhibitor. Therefore, we investigated whether adapalene impeded c-MYC expression and transcriptional activity. Adapalene treatment considerably and dose-dependently downregulated c-MYC expression (Figure 5A). In an effort to evaluate whether adapalene's inhibitory effect was not just confined to c-MYC expression but might possibly also involve the inhibition of c-MYC transcriptional activity, a c-MYC reporter luciferase construct was transfected into HEK293 cells. These cells were then subjected to various concentrations of adapalene and 10058-F4, a known c-MYC inhibitor, respectively. Indeed, adapalene dose-dependently suppressed the transcriptional activity of c-MYC. Interestingly, low adapalene concentrations suppressed c-MYC activity more effectively than the established inhibitor 10058-F4, demonstrating the strong c-MYC inhibitory potential of adapalene (Figure 5B).

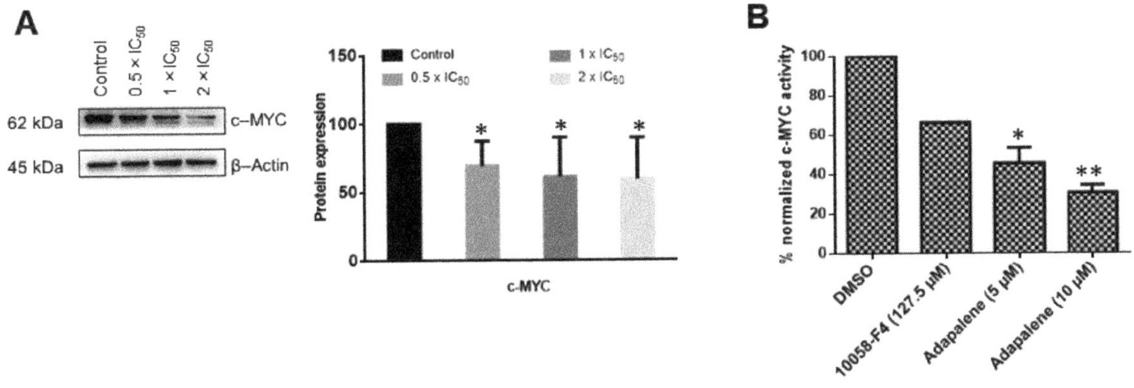

Figure 5. Adapalene affected c-MYC expression and transcriptional activity. (**A**) Effect of adapalene ($0.5 \times IC_{50}$, $1 \times IC_{50}$, and $2 \times IC_{50}$) on c-MYC protein expression in AMO1 cells as displayed by western blot. The bar diagram was created by calculating the mean value ± SD of three independent experiments. The uncropped bolts are shown in Supplementary Materials Figure S2. (**B**) Effect of adapalene and 10058-F4, a known c-MYC inhibitor, on c-MYC transcriptional activity. The bar diagram represents the percentage of normalized c-MYC activity in HEK293 cells transiently expressing a c-MYC-luciferase reporter construct. It was created by calculating the mean value ± SD of two independent experiments. * $p < 0.05$, ** $p < 0.01$, if compared to negative control.

3.6. Cell Cycle Investigations in Adapalene-Treated AMO1 Cells

Many cytotoxic substances exert their anticancer activities by affecting the cell cycle progression of cancer cells [20]. To examine the impact on the cell cycle in AMO1 cells, we incubated the cells for 48 and 72 h with various adapalene concentrations ($0.5 \times IC_{50}$, $1 \times IC_{50}$, and $2 \times IC_{50}$). The percentage of AMO1 cells in the G2/M (indicating mitotic arrest) and sub-G0/G1 phases (indicating cell death) increased in direct proportion with increasing adapalene concentrations (Figure 6).

3.7. Adapalene Induced Mitotic Arrest as Detected by Phospho-Histone-3 (Ser10) Immunofluorescence

Phospho-histone-3 (Ser10) (p-H3(Ser10)) represents a cell cycle marker to assess cells in the late G2/M phase [42]. To confirm whether adapalene induced G2 or M arrest, we examined the effect of adapalene on the expression of p-H3(Ser10), a mitotic hallmark that is crucial in regulating the mitotic catastrophe [43]. Adapalene significantly increased the expression of p-H3(Ser10) in AMO1 cells after treatment for 48 h (Figure 7). Therefore, adapalene indeed induced the accumulation of AMO1 cells in the M-phase.

3.8. Adapalene Mitotic Arrest Involved the Distortion of the Tubulin Network as Detected by Immunofluorescence

Mitotic arrest is most likely caused by the suppression of microtubule polymerization because microtubules are essential for chromosomal separation during mitosis [44]. Considering that adapalene led to G2/M arrest, we examined its impact on the tubulin network. U2OS cells stably transfected with α-tubulin-GFP fusion construct were treated with adapalene ($1 \times IC_{50}$ and $2 \times IC_{50}$) for 48 h, and the tubulin network was visualized by confocal microscopy. Control cells perfectly polymerized the tubulin network. This was demonstrated by the significant amount of tubulin that disseminated throughout the cytoplasm and produced a strong intracellular network. By contrast, the tubulin network appeared in a chaotic shape upon adapalene treatment. Adapalene expanded the tubulin mass surrounding the nucleus while decreasing the growth of microtubules at the borders. Additionally, adapalene-treated cells displayed fragile microtubules at their borders if compared to control cells (Figure 8). Comparing adapalene's effect to positive the control drugs nocodazole (as polymerization inhibitor) and paclitaxel (as depolymerization inhibitor) [45] allowed us to conclude that adapalene prevented the polymerization of the microtubule network in a manner similar to nocodazole.

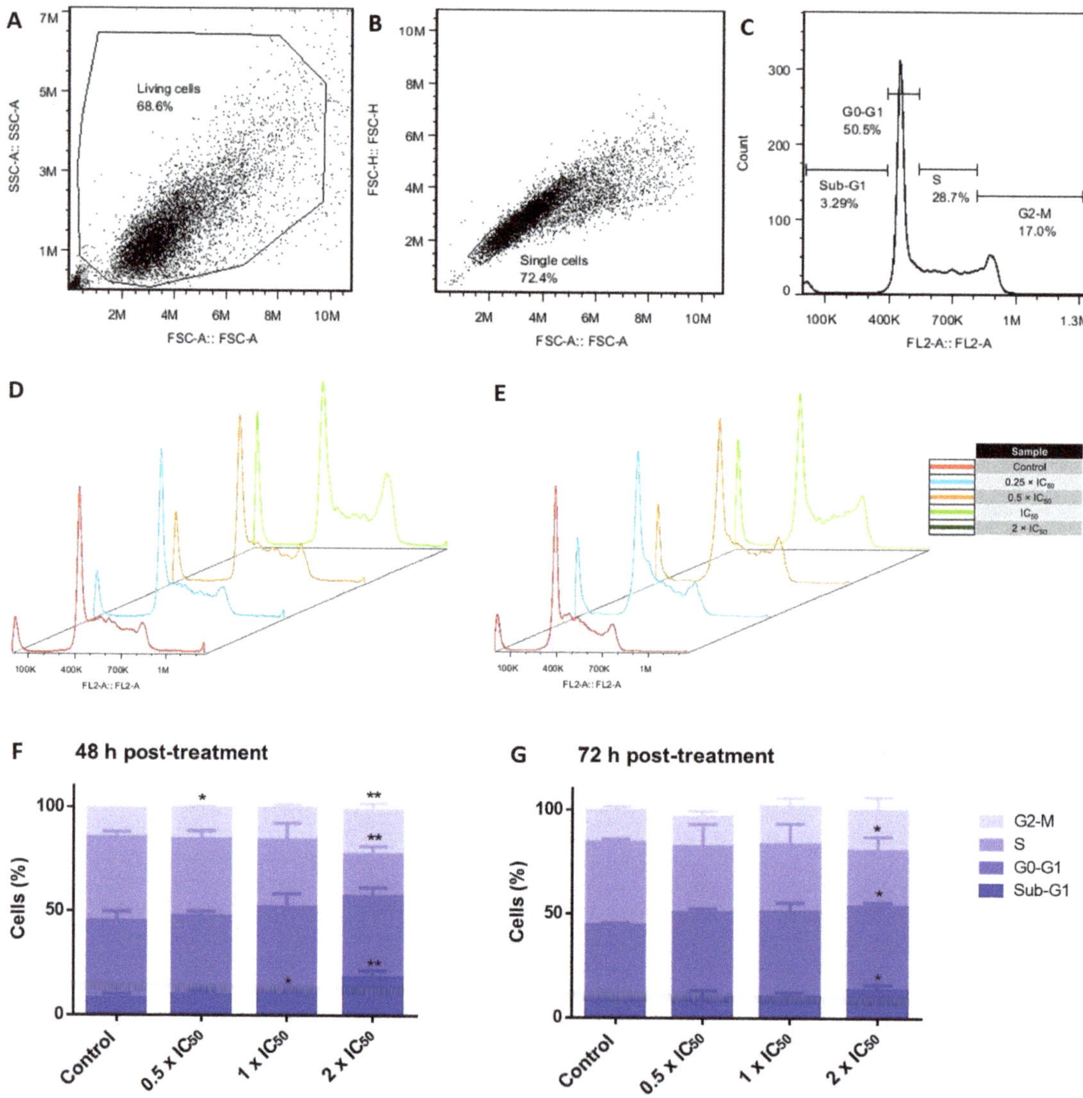

Figure 6. Cell cycle perturbations of AMO1 cells by adapalene. (**A–C**) Gating scheme: (**A**) The first gate (SSC-A vs. FSC-A) intends to get rid of the debris. (**B**) The second gate (FSC-H vs. FSC-A) aims to select only single cells. (**C**) Count vs. FL2-A represents cell cycle histograms. (**D**,**E**) DNA histograms of AMO1 exposed to adapalene (0.5 × IC_{50}, 1 × IC_{50}, and 2 × IC_{50}) for 48 h (**D**) and 72 h (**E**). The histograms were obtained by flow cytometry using an excitation and an emission wavelength of 488 and 530 nm, respectively. (**F**,**G**) The bar diagrams showing the distribution of AMO1 cells treated with adapalene in the distinct phases of the cell cycle after 48 h (**F**) and 72 h (**G**) were created by calculating the mean value ± SD of two independent experiments. * $p < 0.05$, ** $p < 0.01$ if compared to negative control.

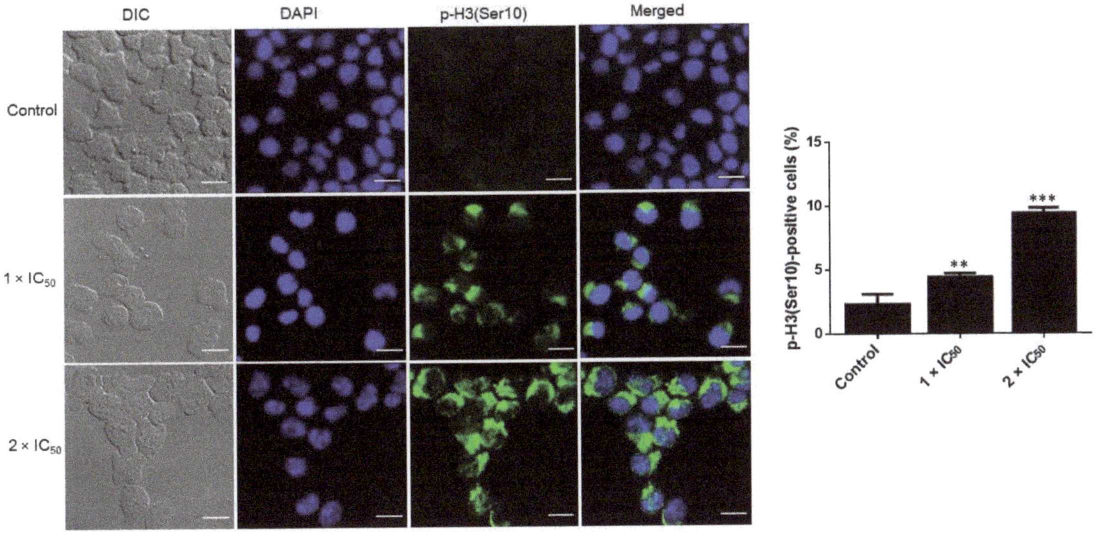

Figure 7. Accumulation of positive p-H3(Ser10) in AMO1 cells treated with adapalene (1 × IC_{50} and 2 × IC_{50}) or DMSO (control) for 48 h. Anti-phospho-histone H3 (Ser10) clone 3H10, FITC-conjugated antibody (green), was used for immunostaining AMO1 cells. DAPI (blue) was used for nuclear staining. An AF7000 widefield fluorescence microscope at 40× magnification (scale bars = 20 μm) was used for imaging. The bar diagram represents the percentage of positive p-H3(Ser10). ** $p < 0.01$, *** $p < 0.001$ if compared to negative control.

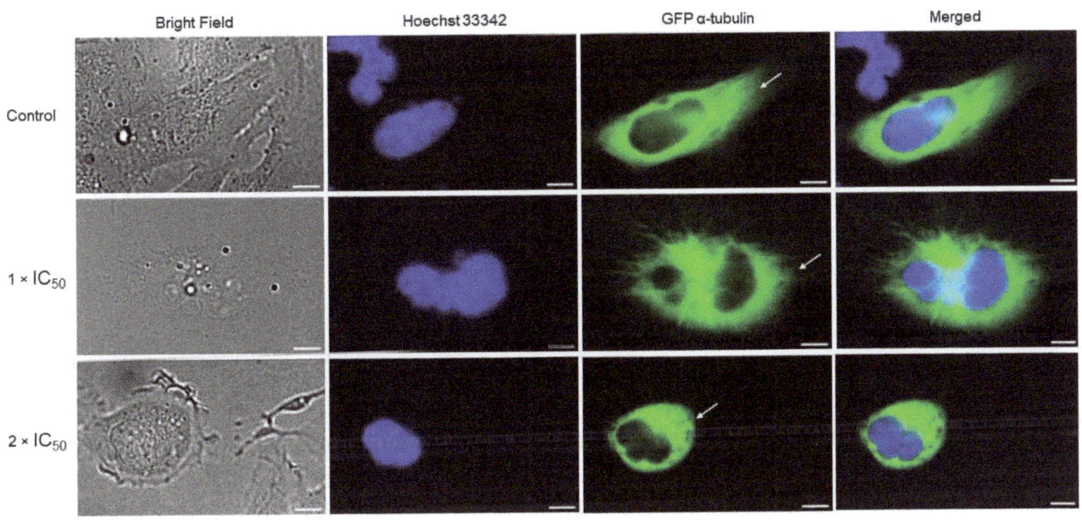

Figure 8. Chaotic microtubule network in U2OS cells stably transfected with GFP-α-tubulin protein upon adapalene treatment (1 × IC_{50} and 2 × IC50) for 48 h. U2OS cells were fixed with 4% paraformaldehyde. Micrographs were snapped 48 h after treatment with DMSO or adapalene treatment (1 × IC_{50} and 2 × IC_{50}). DAPI (blue) was used for nuclear staining. The peripheral tubulin masses are pointed out with white arrows. An AF7000 widefield fluorescence microscope at 40× magnification (scale bars = 7 μm) was used for imaging.

3.9. Adapalene Induced Apoptosis, Autophagy, and DNA Damage in AMO1 Cells

Our cell cycle results showed a dramatical dose-dependent increase in the fraction of cells in the sub-G0/G1 phase, indicating that adapalene promoted cell death. In an effort to determine the cell death mode(s) induced by adapalene, we studied the three main processes of cell death: apoptosis (type I), autophagy (type II), and necrosis (type III) [46]. First, we investigated apoptosis, a form of programmed cell death that most likely takes place in cancer cells treated with cytotoxic drugs. A FITC-conjugated annexin V/PI assay was used to distinguish between living, early apoptotic, late apoptotic, and necrotic cells. Annexin V is usually detected in early and late apoptosis. However, PI is detected in late apoptosis and necrosis. The positive control drug bortezomib effectively induced early and late apoptotic cells after 48 h treatment. Increasing the incubation period to 72 h considerably induced early apoptotic cells without significantly affecting the portion of late apoptotic cells. The number of early and late apoptotic cells significantly increased in a dose-dependent manner upon treatment with adapalene for 48 h. Interestingly, extending the incubation time to 72 h did not considerably change the proportion of apoptotic cells. Moreover, necrotic cells were not detected at all (Figure 9), indicating that adapalene induced apoptosis in a comparable manner after 48 and 72 h.

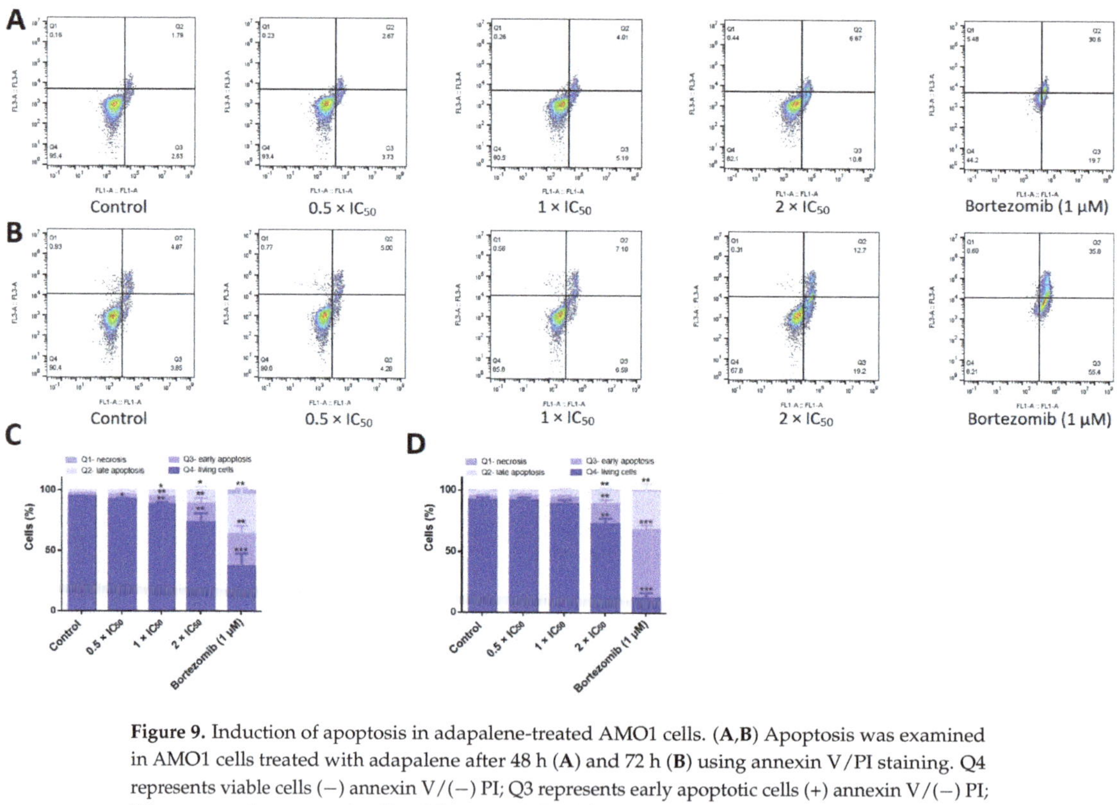

Figure 9. Induction of apoptosis in adapalene-treated AMO1 cells. (**A**,**B**) Apoptosis was examined in AMO1 cells treated with adapalene after 48 h (**A**) and 72 h (**B**) using annexin V/PI staining. Q4 represents viable cells (−) annexin V/(−) PI; Q3 represents early apoptotic cells (+) annexin V/(−) PI; Q2 represents late apoptotic cells exhibit annexin V (+)/PI (+); Q1 represents necrotic cells (−) annexin V/(+) PI. Treatment with adapalene at increasing concentrations greatly enhanced the percentage of early and late apoptotic cells after 48 and 72 h. (**C**,**D**) The bar diagrams showing the distribution of AMO1 cells in the different quadrants after 48 h (**C**) and 72 h (**D**) were created by calculating the mean value ± SD of three trials conducted at distinct times. * $p < 0.05$, ** $p < 0.01$, *** $p < 0.001$ if compared to negative control.

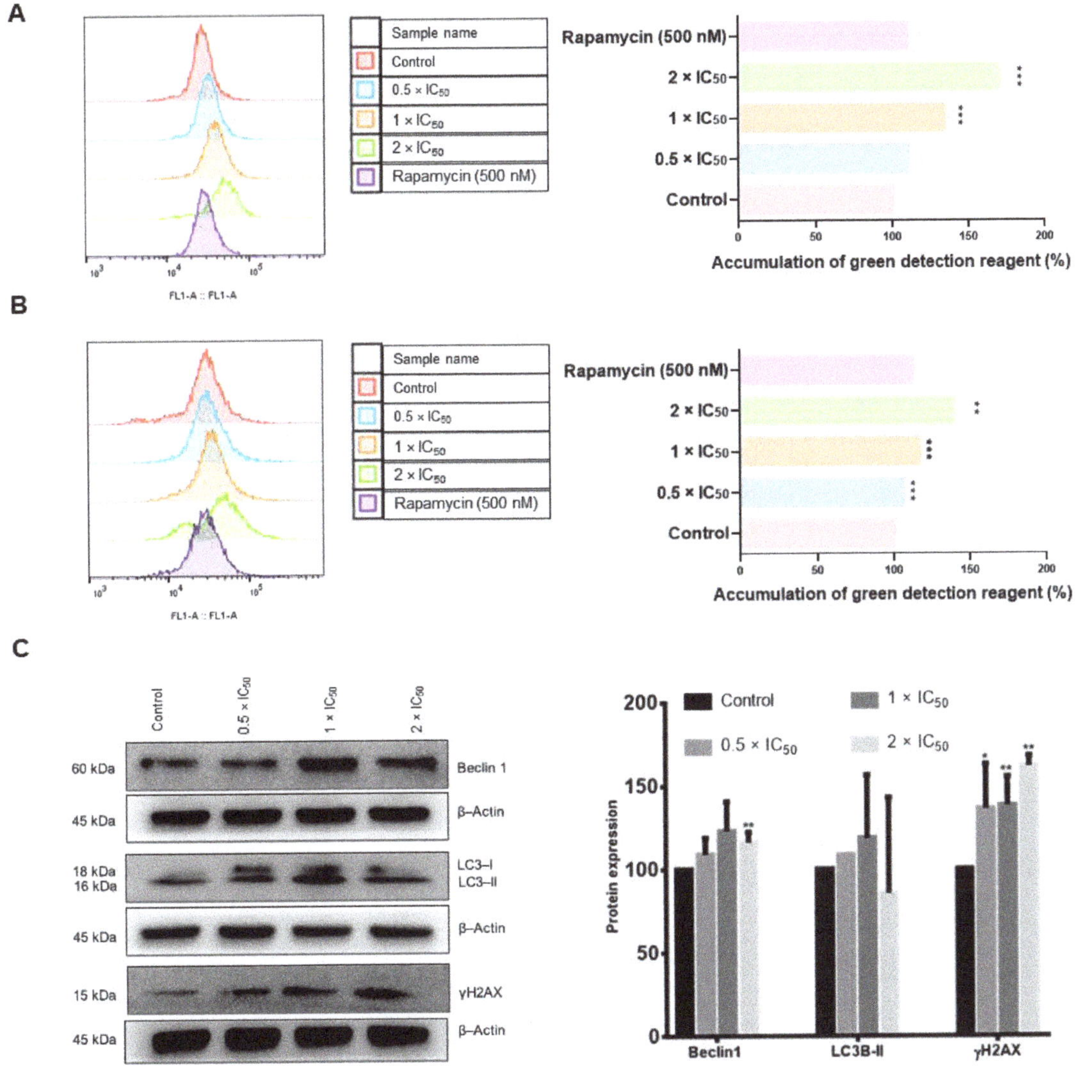

Figure 10. Induction of DNA damage and autophagy in adapalene-treated AMO1 cells. (**A**,**B**) Autophagy was examined in AMO1 cells treated with adapalene after 48 h (**A**) and 72 h (**B**) using green detection reagent. The histograms overlays were obtained by flow cytometry using an excitation and an emission wavelength of 463 and 534 nm, respectively. The bar diagrams were created by calculating the mean value ± SD of three trials conducted at distinct times. (**C**) Effect of adapalene ($0.5 \times IC_{50}$, $1 \times IC_{50}$, and $2 \times IC_{50}$) on the protein expression levels of γH2AX, Beclin 1, and LC3-II in AMO1 cells as detected by western blot. The bar diagram was created by calculating the mean value ± SD of three trials conducted at distinct times. * $p < 0.05$, ** $p < 0.01$, *** $p < 0.001$ if compared to negative control. The uncropped bolts are shown in Supplementary Materials Figures S3–S5.

Next, we examined autophagy as a type II cell death modality. Autophagy detection using flow cytometry revealed that the untreated control cells displayed a weak fluorescence signal. However, the intensity of this signal increased proportionally with increasing adapalene concentrations, reaching an approximately 1.7-fold increase with $2 \times IC_{50}$

after 48 h treatment. Interestingly, adapalene induced autophagy more significantly than rapamycin, a common autophagy inducer (Figure 10A). Adapalene continued to trigger autophagy after 72 h treatment, albeit to a lower extent if compared to 48 h post-treatment (Figure 10B), suggesting a potential switch to another type of cell death. To strengthen our conclusions, we further examined autophagy by detecting the autophagic markers Beclin1 and LC3BII by Western blotting after 48 h treatment. Western blot analyses showed that the protein expression level of Beclin1 and LC3BII increased if AMO1 cells were treated with $0.5 \times IC_{50}$ and $1\times IC_{50}$ of adapalene. However, Beclin1 and LC3BII expression diminished upon treatment with $2 \times IC_{50}$ (Figure 10C), indicating that adapalene prompted autophagy.

It has been known for many years that DNA double-strand breaks and c-MYC dysregulation are tightly related [47]. Given that γH2AX is a marker of DNA double-strand breaks [48], we determined the γH2AX expression 48 h post-adapalene treatment. Western blot analysis revealed that the γH2AX expression effectively increased in a dose-dependent manner in AMO1 cells (Figure 10C), suggesting that adapalene triggered DNA damage.

3.10. Anticancer Activity of Adapalene In Vivo

The anti-tumor efficacy of adapalene has been confirmed in vivo using murine models [20,22]. In this study, a CCRF-CEM xenograft tumor model was established in larvae zebrafish, and the fluorescence intensity was measured to calculate the tumor inhibition rate after 24 h treatment. Comparing the positive control imatinib mesylate with the untreated group revealed that imatinib mesylate significantly reduced the intensity of the fluorescent CCRF-CEM tumors (Figure 11). The same was true for adapalene, which reduced the growth of CCRF-CEM tumors with an inhibitory rate of 38.23% at 3.47 nM. Even though adapalene has been administrated at an extremely low dose, it nonetheless demonstrated a higher inhibitory rate than the positive control drug. Our investigations revealed that adapalene possessed anti-tumor properties in a larvae zebrafish model.

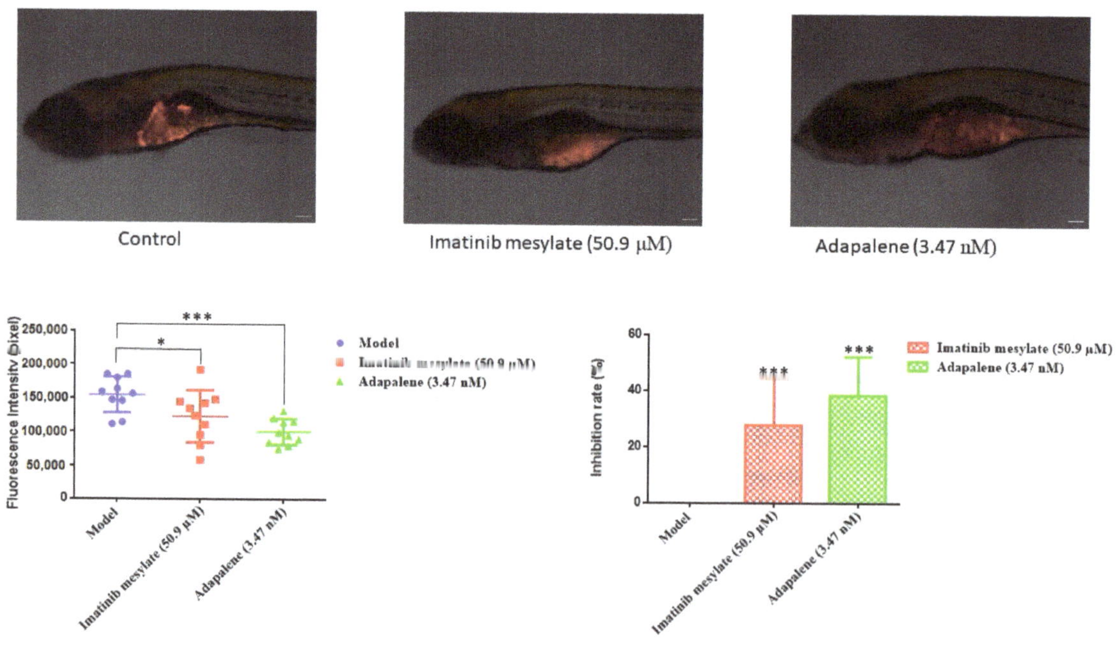

Figure 11. Examination of the acute cytotoxicity (fluorescence intensity and inhibition rate) of CCRF-CEM xenograft tumor zebrafish model ($n = 10$ zebrafish) treated with adapalene. The tumor mass of the CCRF-CEM was highlighted by the red fluorescence. Images were captured at a 60× magnification (scale bars = 100 μm). If compared to the model, * $p < 0.05$, *** $p < 0.001$ are significant.

4. Discussion

Despite substantial improvements in MM treatment, this disease is currently regarded as incurable due to relapse and resistance to chemotherapy, highlighting the need for new treatments with alternative approaches [13]. The proto-oncogene c-MYC is considered as an appealing therapeutic target for MM treatment since its dysregulation is a distinctive genetic feature of MM. Numerous strategies suggested so far focus on c-MYC in MM. However, the pharmacokinetics and efficacy of most of these techniques were unsatisfactory, rendering the direct inhibition of c-MYC very challenging in the context of ligand discovery [13]. This fact urged us to search for novel compounds that directly inhibit c-MYC. Therefore, we performed targeted screening of the FDA-approved drug library using in silico tools (virtual screening and molecular docking). Vitamin A, as well as its natural and synthetic analogues, known as retinoids, are essential for several vital processes such as pattern formation in embryogenesis, bone development, hematopoiesis, differentiation, metabolism, reproduction, and vision [49]. Retinoids have shown a strong antiproliferative effect and have been beneficial in the treatment of a number of human disorders, including cancer [50]. Due to their strong gene regulation capability and receptor-binding affinities, retinoids have been widely claimed to possess anticancer activities [51]. In fact, they have demonstrated promising therapeutic results in clinical studies for solid tumors as prostate cancer, basal cell skin cancer, head and neck cancer, renal cancer, cervical cancer, and breast cancer [52]. Moreover, all-trans-retinoic acid (ATRA)-based differentiation therapy has also been very effective in treating acute promyelocytic leukemia (APL) [53]. In comparison to natural retinoids, synthetic retinoids have demonstrated greater selectivity, stronger efficacy, and reduced toxicity [51]. Adapalene belongs the third generation of retinoids [16]. Although it was originally a topical treatment of acne vulgaris [54], we found that it strongly bound to the c-MYC bHLHZip domain at the same binding pocket as the known inhibitor 10074-G5. This binding pocket represents the MYC/MAX interaction site which is essential for the function of c-MYC. As adapalene shared the same binding pocket with 10074-G5, it is presumed that they exhibit similar modes of action. They inhibit c-Myc/Max heterodimer formation and thus inhibit its transcriptional activity. Interestingly, adapalene showed higher affinity to c-MYC if compared to the positive controls 10058-F4 and 10074-G5. Hence, adapalene might be a novel candidate c-MYC inhibitor, and it may be a third-generation retinoid repurposed for the treatment of MM. To validate this hypothesis, we examined the molecular interaction of adapalene and c-MYC using MST. Indeed, adapalene robustly bound to c-MYC (K_d = 3.05 μM), and these findings were in line with those of the in silico analysis. Next, we investigated the sensitivity of a panel of nine MM cell lines as well as drug-sensitive CCRF-CEM and multidrug-resistant CEM/ADR5000 leukemia cells towards adapalene. All MM cell lines responded to adapalene with different degrees of sensitivity (IC_{50} values from 1.76 ± 0.39 μM to 9.10 ± 1.85 μM). Since AMO1 was the most sensitive cell line (IC_{50} = 1.76 ± 0.39 μM), we investigated the mechanisms of action of adapalene in these cells. It is known that CEM/ADR5000 cells, overexpressing the multidrug-resistance-mediating ABC-transporter P-glycoprotein, extrude chemotherapeutic drugs out of cells resulting in chemotherapy failure [55,56]. According to our findings, CEM/ADR5000 cells and their sensitive counterparts both demonstrated a similar level of sensitivity to adapalene. Furthermore, the resistance ratio was just 1.26, which is far lower than that of doxorubicin, a common chemotherapeutic medication with a cross-resistance ratio much more than 1000 [30]. These findings suggested that adapalene is not involved in the cross-resistance profile conferred by P-glycoprotein. The concentration of adapalene needed to inhibit the proliferation of 50% of human peripheral blood mononuclear cells (PBMCs) was much higher than those of all tested leukemia and MM cell lines. This suggests that the concentration of adapalene required to kill leukemia and MM cells might be also reached in patients without harming healthy hematopoietic cells. To the best of our knowledge, we are the first to demonstrate that the retinoid adapalene inhibited MM cells by suppressing c-MYC, suggesting a novel mode of action of adapalene not as an anti-inflammatory but as a potential anticancer agent.

The oncogene c-MYC is overexpressed in several cancer types, and it is a causative factor of at least 40% of malignancies. On the other hand, c-MYC expression is firmly controlled in healthy cells [57]. c-MYC primarily acts as a transcriptional regulator, modulating the expression of genes that are involved in a variety of cellular activities, including transcription, translation, cell division, metabolism, cell differentiation, DNA repair, apoptosis, autophagy, immune response, and stem cell growth [58]. Its contribution to oncogenesis was initially discovered due to its homology to an avian retrovirus and was highly expressed in Burkitt's lymphoma because of the t(8;14) translocation [59,60]. Moreover, c-MYC deregulation is one of the main features in MM progression. Although targeting c-MYC is challenging, numerous investigations demonstrated the potential significance of c-MYC inhibition for cancer therapy [61]. Currently, no MYC inhibitor has been clinically established, but significant efforts are globally ongoing to realize this possibility for cancer patients [62]. In this context, verifying that adapalene inhibits c-MYC may be a glimmer of hope, especially because it is an FDA-approved drug, and its toxicity profiles, pharmacokinetics, and pharmacodynamics are well established. To further validate adapalene as c-MYC inhibitor, we performed a c-MYC reporter assay. Adapalene significantly reduced the DNA-binding activity of c-MYC. It is interesting to note that this inhibitory impact was substantially stronger than the prominent c-MYC inhibitor 10058-F4. Additionally, adapalene concentrations required to inhibit c-MYC were far lower than that of 10058-F4. Furthermore, adapalene significantly and dose-dependently reduced the expression of c-MYC. Taken together, our in vitro results were in line with those of the in silico data and conclude that adapalene may indeed inhibit c-MYC expression and its transcriptional activity.

c-MYC activates the expression of genes that are essential regulators of the cell cycle, including E2F transcription factors, cyclins, and cyclin-dependent kinases (CDKs). Additionally, c-MYC inhibits Cdk inhibitors such as p21 and p27 by activating SKP2, which is involved in p27 degradation, or by inhibiting CDKN1A, which codes for p21. Furthermore, c-MYC activates CUL1, a component of the E3 ubiquitin ligase complex necessary for the effective ubiquitination and destruction of p27 [63]. Moreover, inhibiting c-MYC caused human myeloid and lymphoid cells arrest the cell cycle [64]. Given the important role of c-MYC for cell cycle control, we examined the cell cycle progression of adapalene-treated AMO1 cells after 48 and 72 h treatment. Adapalene arrested AMO1 cells in the G2/M phase besides an increase in the sub-G0/G1 phase after 48 and 72 h treatment. To investigate the molecular mechanisms underlying the G2/M phase arrest, immunofluorescence microscopy was performed to determine the number of adapalene-treated AMO1 cells that were positive for p-H3(Ser10). Indeed, adapalene treatment caused AMO1 cells to preferentially assemble in the M-phase. Given that Ser10 phosphorylation occurs in early prophase, is maintained during metaphase, is decreased during anaphase, and vanishes entirely during telophase before or at the start of chromosomal decondensation [65], an increase in the number of positive p-H3(Ser10) represents an indication of adapalene's ability to hamper mitotic exit in AMO1 cells. Usually, mitotic catastrophe is the most prevalent outcome of extended mitotic arrest. It is a mechanism that senses mitotic failure and responds by initiating irreparable, anti-proliferative cell death [66]. This may account for the time- and dose-dependent increase of cells in the sub-G0/G1 phase. Our results unexpectedly differed from those of other studies where adapalene induced S-phase arrest in a prostate cancer cell, a triple-negative breast cancer cell, and melanoma cells [22,23], or G1-phase arrest in colorectal cancer cells [19]. It seems that phase-specific cell cycle arrest is tumor cell line-specific.

The accumulation of cells in the G2/M phase may indicate that G2/M mediators are affected by adapalene. Therefore, we studied the impact of adapalene on the microtubule network. Moreover, previous studies demonstrated that c-MYC interacts with α-tubulin and with polymerized microtubules in vitro and in vivo [67]. Microtubules have also been hypothesized to serve as a cytoplasmic repository for c-MYC proteins [68]. Additionally, several drugs that disrupt microtubule dynamics decreased c-MYC expression by reducing the cytoplasmic c-MYC reservoir [69]. Thus, it was fascinating for us to prove whether this reciprocal aspect was true. Microtubules are highly active cytoskeletal structures that are important for many cellular functions such as vesicle transport, cell division, and intracellular organization. Microtubule-targeting agents inhibit the dynamics of microtubules, resulting in a slowdown or blockage of mitosis. This block, which takes place in the G2/M phase, may trigger cell death. Confocal microscopy of adapalene-treated U2OS cells stably expressing α-tubulin-GFP showed an aberrant microtubule arrangement. In fact, adapalene expanded the tubulin mass, surrounding the nucleus while decreasing the growth of microtubules at the borders. Additionally, adapalene-treated cells displayed fragile microtubules at their borders if compared to control cells. To the best of our knowledge, we are the first to decipher that adapalene effectively disrupted the microtubule network, which may account for its cytotoxicity.

Several authors investigated the essential role of c-MYC in DNA damage signaling [70]. Responses to intracellular stress signals as DNA damage resulted in decreased c-MYC levels due to proteasomal degradation [71]. Moreover, DNA damaging agents (e.g., topoisomerase II inhibitors) or ionizing radiation induced DNA damage as well as c-MYC inhibition in MCF-7 breast cancer cells [72,73]. Furthermore, the knockdown of c-MYC in HeLa-630 cells limited their capacity to repair double-strand breaks following ionizing irradiation [74]. Based on the crucial role of c-MYC in DNA damage repair, studies have demonstrated a relationship between c-MYC and γH2AX. Phosphorylated c-MYC displayed a strong co-localization with γH2AX and the phosphorylated DNA-dependent protein kinase, catalytic subunit at the corresponding S2056 cluster. Consequently, the inhibition of c-MYC resulted in double-strand breaks and an increase in γH2AX [74]. Taking into consideration this relationship between c-MYC and γH2AX, we investigated the effect of adapalene on the protein expression level of γH2AX. Intriguingly, adapalene treatment resulted in a dose-dependent increase in γH2AX, suggesting that the ability of adapalene to inhibit MM growth may be due to its capability to induce DNA damage. Our results were in line with other studies, showing that adapalene induced apoptosis through DNA damage in melanoma cells [20]. It also reduced the growth of prostate cancer cells by triggering DNA damage [22].

An eminent function of c-MYC is its ability to sensitize cells to apoptosis. Dysregulated c-MYC expression accompanied by anti-proliferative signals initiates apoptosis [75]. Therefore, we examined whether adapalene-mediated cytotoxicity in AMO1 cells was associated with apoptosis. Our results revealed that adapalene induced both early and late apoptosis. Our findings concurred with those of another study showing that the suppression of c-MYC by CPI-0610, a small-molecule bromodomain and extra-terminal protein inhibitor, induced G0/G1 arrest as well as apoptosis in MM, leading to cancer regression [76]. In addition, adapalene promoted apoptosis in triple-negative breast cancer cells, melanoma cells, colorectal cancer cells, bladder cancer cells, hepatoma cells, prostate cancer cell, and ovarian cancer cell [17,20–23,77,78]. To the best of our knowledge, we are the first to demonstrate that adapalene-mediated c-MYC inhibition induced apoptosis in MM.

Autophagy is a vital catabolic cellular process in which deteriorated organelles, misfolded proteins, and cellular components are digested and recycled by lysosomes. Autophagy is essential for maintaining cellular homeostasis and allowing cells to adjust to harsh conditions. Additionally, it controls both cell survival and death [79]. The microtubule-associated protein light chain 3 (LC3) and Beclin 1 play essential roles in autophagy. Beclin 1 is a member of the phosphatidylinositol 3-kinase complex (PI3K) type III and is necessary for autophagic vesicle formation. LC3 is activated by a ubiquitination-like reaction mediated by Atg3 and Atg7. Initially, LC3 is cleaved into cytosolic LC3-I which is further changed into a membrane-bound form LC3-II. LC3-II is then attracted to autophagosomes. Therefore, it is considered a special autophagy marker [80]. To decipher whether adapalene triggers autophagy in AMO1 cells, we studied the protein expression level of LC3 and Beclin 1. The fact that LC3-II and Beclin 1 were both upregulated upon adapalene treatment approved that the latter induced autophagy in AMO1 cells. Those findings were further confirmed by an autophagy assay. As far as we know, no previous studies reported the ability of adapalene to trigger autophagy. Several groups demonstrated the interplay between c-MYC and the regulation of autophagy. For instance, 4-O-methyl-ascochlorin inhibited c-MYC and triggered autophagy in leukemic cells [81]. The inhibition of c-MYC by 10058-F4 led to the downregulation of miR-150 and restored the miR-150-mediated autophagy defect in NSCLC [82]. Our findings might also indicate that the induction of autophagy could be accredited to c-MYC inhibition. Surprisingly, the expression of Beclin 1 and LC3-II dropped off at high concentrations ($2 \times IC_{50}$). This could be explained by a shift to another cell death as apoptosis. These observations were not detected in the autophagy assay as western blot is more sensitive and detects even minimal changes in protein expression. Numerous reports proved that Beclin 1 is a caspase 3 substrate. Upon caspase 3 activation, Beclin 1 is cleaved and becomes unable to induce autophagy. However, the C-terminal fragment (Beclin 1-C) may relocate to the mitochondria and make cells more susceptible to apoptosis [83]. A reduction of Beclin 1 prompted CED-3/caspase-dependent programmed cell death in *C. elegans* [84]. Moreover, it has been suggested that LC3 can act as a promoter of apoptosis [83].

Several authors verified adapalene's in vivo anti-tumor activity in mice [19,22]. Recently, the zebrafish model proved to be an effective in vivo model for both drug development and toxicity evaluation [85]. In the current investigation, we demonstrated that adapalene inhibited tumor growth in vivo by utilizing a CCRF-CEM xenograft tumor zebrafish model.

One of the study's shortcomings is the inability to examine the impact of adapalene on PBMCs derived from patients with hematological malignancies. In addition, a crucial tool for clinical translation is the analysis of adapalene in murine models of human MM. Therefore, we strive to select the appropriate MM murine model for specific pre-clinical research.

5. Conclusions

In conclusion, the knowledge gained from this work points to the potential of the third-generation retinoid adapalene to significantly suppress tumor growth via autophagic and apoptotic cell death. Furthermore, adapalene possesses a potent cytotoxic activity through c-MYC inhibition, tubulin network suppression, and DNA damage. The discovery of adapalene as a c-MYC inhibitor may significantly lower the drug development costs of new anticancer medications, providing further insights in the future of adapalene-based designs that could result in more effective and targeted innovative therapies for MM.

Supplementary Materials: The following supporting information can be downloaded at: https://www.mdpi.com/article/10.3390/cancers15164136/s1, Figures S1–S5: Original, uncropped Western blot membrane. Table S1. Binding affinities (kcal/mol) of the top 170 FDA compounds as identified by PyRx; Table S2: An overview of the molecular docking results of the top 117 FDA compounds as determined by AutoDock 4.2.6 tools.

Author Contributions: Conceptualization, J.C.B. and T.E.; methodology, J.C.B.; software, J.C.B.; validation, J.C.B. and L.S.; formal analysis, J.C.B.; investigation, J.C.B.; resources, M.C.; data curation, J.C.B.; writing—original draft preparation, J.C.B. and T.E.; writing—review and editing, J.C.B. and T.E.; visualization, J.C.B.; supervision, T.E.; project administration, J.C.B.; funding acquisition, J.C.B. All authors have read and agreed to the published version of the manuscript.

Funding: This research was funded by a private donation of Marc Strobel, Frankfurt, Germany.

Institutional Review Board Statement: The animal study protocol was approved by the Association for Assessment and Accreditation of Laboratory Animal Care International (SYXK 2012-0171).

Informed Consent Statement: Written Informed consent was obtained from all subjects involved in the study.

Data Availability Statement: The data presented in this study are available on request from the corresponding author. The data are not publicly available due to privacy.

Acknowledgments: We gratefully acknowledge the stipend of the Sibylle Kalkhof-Rose-Foundation to J.C.B.

Conflicts of Interest: The authors declare that there is no conflict of interest.

References

1. Banerjee, S.; Parasramka, M.A.; Paruthy, S.B. Garcinol: Preclinical perspective underpinning chemo-and radiosensitization of cancer. In *Role of Nutraceuticals in Cancer Chemosensitization*; Elsevier: Amsterdam, The Netherlands, 2018; pp. 297–324.
2. Pinto, V.; Bergantim, R.; Caires, H.R.; Seca, H.; Guimarães, J.E.; Vasconcelos, M.H. Multiple myeloma: Available therapies and causes of drug resistance. *Cancers* **2020**, *12*, 407. [CrossRef] [PubMed]
3. Van de Donk, N.W.C.J.; Pawlyn, C.; Yong, K.L. Multiple myeloma. *Lancet* **2021**, *397*, 410–427. [CrossRef] [PubMed]
4. Bergsagel, P.L.; Kuehl, W.M. Chromosome translocations in multiple myeloma. *Oncogene* **2001**, *20*, 5611–5622. [CrossRef]
5. Anguiano, A.; Tuchman, S.A.; Acharya, C.; Salter, K.; Gasparetto, C.; Zhan, F.; Dhodapkar, M.; Nevins, J.; Barlogie, B.; Shaughnessy, J.D., Jr. Gene expression profiles of tumor biology provide a novel approach to prognosis and may guide the selection of therapeutic targets in multiple myeloma. *J. Clin. Oncol.* **2009**, *27*, 4197. [CrossRef]
6. Holien, T.; Misund, K.; Olsen, O.E.; Baranowska, K.A.; Buene, G.; Børset, M.; Waage, A.; Sundan, A. Myc amplifications in myeloma cell lines: Correlation with myc-inhibitor efficacy. *Oncotarget* **2015**, *6*, 22698. [CrossRef] [PubMed]
7. Affer, M.; Chesi, M.; Chen, W.D.; Keats, J.J.; Demchenko, Y.N.; Tamizhmani, K.; Garbitt, V.M.; Riggs, D.L.; Brents, L.A.; Roschke, A.V. Promiscuous myc locus rearrangements hijack enhancers but mostly super-enhancers to dysregulate myc expression in multiple myeloma. *Leukemia* **2014**, *28*, 1725–1735. [CrossRef]
8. Chng, W.J.; Huang, G.F.; Chung, T.H.; Ng, S.B.; Gonzalez-Paz, N.; Troska-Price, T.; Mulligan, G.; Chesi, M.; Bergsagel, P.L.; Fonseca, R. Clinical and biological implications of myc activation: A common difference between mgus and newly diagnosed multiple myeloma. *Leukemia* **2011**, *25*, 1026–1035. [CrossRef]
9. Holien, T.; Våtsveen, T.K.; Hella, H.; Rampa, C.; Brede, G.; Grøseth, L.A.G.; Rekvig, M.; Børset, M.; Standal, T.; Waage, A. Bone morphogenetic proteins induce apoptosis in multiple myeloma cells by smad-dependent repression of myc. *Leukemia* **2012**, *26*, 1073–1080. [CrossRef]
10. Kang, B.; Park, H.; Kim, B. Anticancer activity and underlying mechanism of phytochemicals against multiple myeloma. *Int. J. Mol. Sci.* **2019**, *20*, 2302. [CrossRef]
11. Martínez-Martín, S.; Soucek, L. Myc inhibitors in multiple myeloma. *Cancer Drug Resist.* **2021**, *4*, 842. [CrossRef]
12. Wang, C.; Zhang, J.; Yin, J.; Gan, Y.; Xu, S.; Gu, Y.; Huang, W. Alternative approaches to target myc for cancer treatment. *Signal Transduct. Target. Ther.* **2021**, *6*, 117. [CrossRef] [PubMed]
13. Cao, Y.; Shan, H.; Liu, M.; Liu, J.; Zhang, Z.; Xu, X.; Liu, Y.; Xu, H.; Lei, H.; Yu, M. Directly targeting c-myc contributes to the anti-multiple myeloma effect of anlotinib. *Cell Death Dis.* **2021**, *12*, 396. [CrossRef] [PubMed]
14. Pushpakom, S.; Iorio, F.; Eyers, P.A.; Escott, K.J.; Hopper, S.; Wells, A.; Doig, A.; Guilliams, T.; Latimer, J.; McNamee, C. Drug repurposing: Progress, challenges and recommendations. *Nat. Rev. Drug Discov.* **2019**, *18*, 41–58. [CrossRef] [PubMed]
15. Boulos, J.C.; Saeed, M.E.M.; Chatterjee, M.; Bülbül, Y.; Crudo, F.; Marko, D.; Munder, M.; Klauck, S.M.; Efferth, T. Repurposing of the alk inhibitor crizotinib for acute leukemia and multiple myeloma cells. *Pharmaceuticals* **2021**, *14*, 1126. [CrossRef]
16. Tolaymat, L.; Dearborn, H.; Zito, P.M. Adapalene. In *StatPearls*; StatPearls Publishing: St. Petersburg, FL, USA, 2022.
17. Ocker, M.; Herold, C.; Ganslmayer, M.; Zopf, S.; Hahn, E.G.; Schuppan, D. Potentiated anticancer effects on hepatoma cells by the retinoid adapalene. *Cancer Lett.* **2004**, *208*, 51–58. [CrossRef]
18. Rusu, A.; Tanase, C.; Pascu, G.-A.; Todoran, N. Recent advances regarding the therapeutic potential of adapalene. *Pharmaceuticals* **2020**, *13*, 217. [CrossRef]
19. Shi, X.N.; Li, H.; Yao, H.; Liu, X.; Li, L.; Leung, K.S.; Kung, H.F.; Lin, M.C.M. Adapalene inhibits the activity of cyclin-dependent kinase 2 in colorectal carcinoma. *Mol. Med. Rep.* **2015**, *12*, 6501–6508. [CrossRef]
20. Li, H.; Wang, C.; Li, L.; Bu, W.; Zhang, M.; Wei, J.; Tao, L.; Qian, K.; Ma, P. Adapalene suppressed the proliferation of melanoma cells by s-phase arrest and subsequent apoptosis via induction of DNA damage. *Eur. J. Pharmacol.* **2019**, *851*, 174–185. [CrossRef]
21. Wang, Q.; Zhang, Q.; Luan, S.; Yang, K.; Zheng, M.; Li, K.; Chen, L.; Li, H. Adapalene inhibits ovarian cancer es-2 cells growth by targeting glutamic-oxaloacetic transaminase 1. *Bioorg. Chem.* **2019**, *93*, 103315. [CrossRef]
22. Nong, H.-B.; Zhang, Y.-N.; Bai, Y.-G.; Zhang, Q.; Liu, M.-F.; Zhou, Q.; Shi, Z.-H.; Zeng, G.-F.; Zong, S.-H. Adapalene inhibits prostate cancer cell proliferation in vitro and in vivo by inducing DNA damage, s-phase cell cycle arrest, and apoptosis. *Front. Pharmacol.* **2022**, *13*, 801624. [CrossRef]
23. Mehraj, U.; Wani, N.A.; Hamid, A.; Alkhanani, M.; Almilaibary, A.; Mir, M.A. Adapalene inhibits the growth of triple-negative breast cancer cells by s-phase arrest and potentiates the antitumor efficacy of gdc-0941. *Front. Pharmacol.* **2022**, *13*, 958443. [CrossRef] [PubMed]
24. Berman, H.M.; Westbrook, J.; Feng, Z.; Gilliland, G.; Bhat, T.N.; Weissig, H.; Shindyalov, I.N.; Bourne, P.E. The protein data bank. *Nucleic Acids Res.* **2000**, *28*, 235–242. [CrossRef] [PubMed]
25. Morris, G.M.; Huey, R.; Lindstrom, W.; Sanner, M.F.; Belew, R.K.; Goodsell, D.S.; Olson, A.J. Autodock4 and autodocktools4: Automated docking with selective receptor flexibility. *J. Comput. Chem.* **2009**, *30*, 2785–2791. [CrossRef]

26. Clausen, D.M.; Guo, J.; Parise, R.A.; Beumer, J.H.; Egorin, M.J.; Lazo, J.S.; Prochownik, E.V.; Eiseman, J.L. In vitro cytotoxicity and in vivo efficacy, pharmacokinetics, and metabolism of 10074-g5, a novel small-molecule inhibitor of c-myc/max dimerization. *J. Pharmacol. Exp. Ther.* **2010**, *335*, 715–727. [CrossRef] [PubMed]
27. Yap, J.L.; Wang, H.; Hu, A.; Chauhan, J.; Jung, K.-Y.; Gharavi, R.B.; Prochownik, E.V.; Fletcher, S. Pharmacophore identification of c-myc inhibitor 10074-g5. *Bioorg. Med. Chem. Lett.* **2013**, *23*, 370–374. [CrossRef]
28. Elbadawi, M.; Boulos, J.C.; Dawood, M.; Zhou, M.; Gul, W.; ElSohly, M.A.; Klauck, S.M.; Efferth, T. The novel artemisinin dimer isoniazide eli-xxiii-98-2 induces c-myc inhibition, DNA damage, and autophagy in leukemia cells. *Pharmaceutics* **2023**, *15*, 1107. [CrossRef] [PubMed]
29. Boulos, J.C.; Omer, E.A.; Rigano, D.; Formisano, C.; Chatterjee, M.; Leich, E.; Klauck, S.M.; Shan, L.-T.; Efferth, T. Cynaropicrin disrupts tubulin and c-myc-related signaling and induces parthanatos-type cell death in multiple myeloma. *Acta Pharmacol. Sin.* **2023**, 1–17. [CrossRef]
30. Geske, L.; Baier, J.; Boulos, J.C.; Efferth, T.; Opatz, T. Xylochemical synthesis and biological evaluation of the orchidaceous natural products isoarundinin i, bleochrin f, blestanol k, and pleionol. *J. Nat. Prod.* **2022**, *86*, 131–137. [CrossRef]
31. Zhou, M.; Boulos, J.C.; Klauck, S.M.; Efferth, T. The cardiac glycoside zinc253504760 induces parthanatos-type cell death and g2/m arrest via downregulation of mek1/2 phosphorylation in leukemia cells. *Cell Biol. Toxicol.* **2023**, 1–27. [CrossRef]
32. Zhou, M.; Boulos, J.C.; Omer, E.A.; Klauck, S.M.; Efferth, T. Modes of action of a novel c-myc inhibiting 1,2,4-oxadiazole derivative in leukemia and breast cancer cells. *Molecules* **2023**, *28*, 5658. [CrossRef]
33. Khalid, S.A.; Dawood, M.; Boulos, J.C.; Wasfi, M.; Drif, A.; Bahramimehr, F.; Shahhamzehei, N.; Shan, L.; Efferth, T. Identification of gedunin from a phytochemical depository as a novel multidrug resistance-bypassing tubulin inhibitor of cancer cells. *Molecules* **2022**, *27*, 5858. [CrossRef]
34. Saeed, M.E.M.; Boulos, J.C.; Muecklich, S.B.; Leich, E.; Chatterjee, M.; Klauck, S.M.; Efferth, T. Disruption of lipid raft microdomains, regulation of cd38, tp53, and myc signaling, and induction of apoptosis by lomitapide in multiple myeloma cells. *Cancer Genom. Proteom.* **2022**, *19*, 540–555. [CrossRef] [PubMed]
35. Rykowski, S.; Gurda-Woźna, D.; Orlicka-Płocka, M.; Fedoruk-Wyszomirska, A.; Giel-Pietraszuk, M.; Wyszko, E.; Kowalczyk, A.; Stączek, P.; Bak, A.; Kiliszek, A. Design, synthesis, and evaluation of novel 3-carboranyl-1, 8-naphthalimide derivatives as potential anticancer agents. *Int. J. Mol. Sci.* **2021**, *22*, 2772. [CrossRef] [PubMed]
36. Saeed, M.E.M.; Boulos, J.C.; Machel, K.; Andabili, N.; Marouni, T.; Roth, W.; Efferth, T. Expression of the stem cell marker abcb5 in normal and tumor tissues. *In Vivo* **2022**, *36*, 1651–1666. [CrossRef] [PubMed]
37. Lu, X.; Yan, G.; Klauck, S.M.; Fleischer, E.; Klinger, A.; Sugimoto, Y.; Shan, L.; Efferth, T. Cytotoxicity of 4-hydroxy-n-(naphthalen-1-yl)-2-oxo-2h-chromene-3-carboxamide in multidrug-resistant cancer cells through activation of perk/eif2α/atf4 pathway. *Biochem. Pharmacol.* **2021**, *193*, 114788. [CrossRef] [PubMed]
38. Neves, B.J.; Braga, R.C.; Melo-Filho, C.C.; Moreira-Filho, J.T.; Muratov, E.N.; Andrade, C.H. Qsar-based virtual screening: Advances and applications in drug discovery. *Front. Pharmacol.* **2018**, *9*, 1275. [CrossRef]
39. Holien, T.; Våtsveen, T.K.; Hella, H.; Waage, A.; Sundan, A. Addiction to c-myc in multiple myeloma. *Blood J. Am. Soc. Hematol.* **2012**, *120*, 2450–2453. [CrossRef]
40. Wienken, C.J.; Baaske, P.; Rothbauer, U.; Braun, D.; Duhr, S. Protein-binding assays in biological liquids using microscale thermophoresis. *Nat. Commun.* **2010**, *1*, 100. [CrossRef]
41. Delmore, J.E.; Issa, G.C.; Lemieux, M.E.; Rahl, P.B.; Shi, J.; Jacobs, H.M.; Kastritis, E.; Gilpatrick, T.; Paranal, R.M.; Qi, J. Bet bromodomain inhibition as a therapeutic strategy to target c-myc. *Cell* **2011**, *146*, 904–917. [CrossRef]
42. Ozawa, K. Reduction of phosphorylated histone h3 serine 10 and serine 28 cell cycle marker intensities after DNA damage. *Cytom. Part A J. Int. Soc. Anal. Cytol.* **2008**, *73*, 517–527. [CrossRef]
43. Park, C.; Cha, H.-J.; Lee, H.; Hwang-Bo, H.; Ji, S.Y.; Kim, M.Y.; Hong, S.H.; Jeong, J.-W.; Han, M.H.; Choi, S.H. Induction of g2/m cell cycle arrest and apoptosis by genistein in human bladder cancer t24 cells through inhibition of the ros-dependent pi3k/akt signal transduction pathway. *Antioxidants* **2019**, *8*, 327. [CrossRef] [PubMed]
44. Nagai, Y.; Mimura, N.; Rizq, O.; Isshiki, Y.; Oshima, M.; Rizk, M.; Saraya, A.; Koide, S.; Nakajima-Takagi, Y.; Miyota, M. The combination of the tubulin binding small molecule ptc596 and proteasome inhibitors suppresses the growth of myeloma cells. *Sci. Rep.* **2021**, *11*, 2074. [CrossRef]
45. Rashan, L.J.; Özenver, N.; Boulos, J.C.; Dawood, M.; Roos, W.P.; Franke, K.; Papasotiriou, I.; Wessjohann, L.A.; Fiebig, H.-H.; Efferth, T. Molecular modes of action of an aqueous nerium oleander extract in cancer cells in vitro and in vivo. *Molecules* **2023**, *28*, 1871. [CrossRef] [PubMed]
46. Noguchi, M.; Hirata, N.; Tanaka, T.; Suizu, F.; Nakajima, H.; Chiorini, J.A. Autophagy as a modulator of cell death machinery. *Cell Death Dis.* **2020**, *11*, 517. [CrossRef]
47. Li, Z.; Owonikoko, T.K.; Sun, S.-Y.; Ramalingam, S.S.; Doetsch, P.W.; Xiao, Z.-Q.; Khuri, F.R.; Curran, W.J.; Deng, X. C-myc suppression of DNA double-strand break repair. *Neoplasia* **2012**, *14*, 1190–1202, IN32–IN35. [CrossRef]
48. Valdiglesias, V.; Giunta, S.; Fenech, M.; Neri, M.; Bonassi, S. Γh2ax as a marker of DNA double strand breaks and genomic instability in human population studies. *Mutat. Res./Rev. Mutat. Res.* **2013**, *753*, 24–40. [CrossRef] [PubMed]
49. Sacchi, S.; Russo, D.; Avvisati, G.; Dastoli, G.; Lazzarino, M.; Pelicci, P.G.; Bonora, M.R.; Visani, G.; Grassi, C.; Iacona, I. All-trans retinoic acid in hematological malignancies, an update. Ger (gruppo ematologico retinoidi). *Haematologica* **1997**, *82*, 106–121.

50. Chen, S.; Hu, Q.; Tao, X.; Xia, J.; Wu, T.; Cheng, B.; Wang, J. Retinoids in cancer chemoprevention and therapy: Meta-analysis of randomized controlled trials. *Front. Genet.* **2022**, *13*, 1065320. [CrossRef]
51. Jin, Y.; Teh, S.S.; Lau, H.L.N.; Xiao, J.; Mah, S.H. Retinoids as anti-cancer agents and their mechanisms of action. *Am. J. Cancer Res.* **2022**, *12*, 938.
52. Tang, X.-H.; Gudas, L.J. Retinoids, retinoic acid receptors, and cancer. *Annu. Rev. Pathol. Mech. Dis.* **2011**, *6*, 345–364. [CrossRef]
53. Ni, X.; Hu, G.; Cai, X. The success and the challenge of all-trans retinoic acid in the treatment of cancer. *Crit. Rev. Food Sci. Nutr.* **2019**, *59*, S71–S80. [CrossRef] [PubMed]
54. Cunliffe, W.J.; Caputo, R.; Dreno, B.; Förström, L.; Heenen, M.; Orfanos, C.E.; Privat, Y.; Aguilar, A.R.; Poncet, M.; Verschoore, M. Efficacy and safety comparison of adapalene (cd271) gel and tretinoin gel in the topical treatment of acne vulgaris. A european multicentre trial. *J. Dermatol. Treat.* **1997**, *8*, 173–178. [CrossRef]
55. Boulos, J.C.; Idres, M.R.Y.; Efferth, T. Investigation of cancer drug resistance mechanisms by phosphoproteomics. *Pharmacol. Res.* **2020**, *160*, 105091. [CrossRef] [PubMed]
56. Efferth, T.; Konkimalla, V.B.; Wang, Y.-F.; Sauerbrey, A.; Meinhardt, S.; Zintl, F.; Mattern, J.R.; Volm, M. Prediction of broad spectrum resistance of tumors towards anticancer drugs. *Clin. Cancer Res.* **2008**, *14*, 2405–2412. [CrossRef] [PubMed]
57. Miller, D.M.; Thomas, S.D.; Islam, A.; Muench, D.; Sedoris, K. C-myc and cancer metabolism. *Clin. Cancer Res.* **2012**, *18*, 5546–5553. [CrossRef]
58. Dang, C.V. C-myc target genes involved in cell growth, apoptosis, and metabolism. *Mol. Cell. Biol.* **1999**, *19*, 1–11. [CrossRef]
59. Dalla-Favera, R.; Bregni, M.; Erikson, J.; Patterson, D.; Gallo, R.C.; Croce, C.M. Human c-myc onc gene is located on the region of chromosome 8 that is translocated in burkitt lymphoma cells. *Proc. Natl. Acad. Sci. USA* **1982**, *79*, 7824–7827. [CrossRef]
60. Vennstrom, B.; Sheiness, D.; Zabielski, J.; Bishop, J.M. Isolation and characterization of c-myc, a cellular homolog of the oncogene (v-myc) of avian myelocytomatosis virus strain 29. *J. Virol.* **1982**, *42*, 773–779. [CrossRef]
61. Duffy, M.J.; O'Grady, S.; Tang, M.; Crown, J. Myc as a target for cancer treatment. *Cancer Treat. Rev.* **2021**, *94*, 102154. [CrossRef]
62. Whitfield, J.R.; Soucek, L. The long journey to bring a myc inhibitor to the clinic. *J. Cell Biol.* **2021**, *220*, e202103090. [CrossRef]
63. Jovanović, K.K.; Roche-Lestienne, C.; Ghobrial, I.M.; Facon, T.; Quesnel, B.; Manier, S. Targeting myc in multiple myeloma. *Leukemia* **2018**, *32*, 1295–1306. [CrossRef] [PubMed]
64. Bretones, G.; Delgado, M.D.; León, J. Myc and cell cycle control. *Biochim. Biophys. Acta (BBA)-Gene Regul. Mech.* **2015**, *1849*, 506–516. [CrossRef] [PubMed]
65. Boichuk, S.; Galembikova, A.; Zykova, S.; Ramazanov, B.; Khusnutdinov, R.; Dunaev, P.; Khaibullina, S.; Lombardi, V. Ethyl-2-amino-pyrrole-3-carboxylates are novel potent anticancer agents that affect tubulin polymerization, induce g2/m cell-cycle arrest, and effectively inhibit soft tissue cancer cell growth in vitro. *Anti-Cancer Drugs* **2016**, *27*, 620–634. [CrossRef] [PubMed]
66. Mc Gee, M.M. Targeting the mitotic catastrophe signaling pathway in cancer. *Mediat. Inflamm.* **2015**, *2015*, 146282. [CrossRef]
67. Alexandrova, N.; Niklinski, J.; Bliskovsky, V.; Otterson, G.A.; Blake, M.; Kaye, F.J.; Zajac-Kaye, M. The n-terminal domain of c-myc associates with alpha-tubulin and microtubules in vivo and in vitro. *Mol. Cell. Biol.* **1995**, *15*, 5188–5195. [CrossRef] [PubMed]
68. Bressin, C.; Bourgarel-Rey, V.; Carré, M.; Pourroy, B.; Arango, D.; Braguer, D.; Barra, Y. Decrease in c-myc activity enhances cancer cell sensitivity to vinblastine. *Anti-Cancer Drugs* **2006**, *17*, 181–187. [CrossRef]
69. Agut, R.; Falomir, E.; Murga, J.; Martín-Beltrán, C.; Gil-Edo, R.; Pla, A.; Carda, M.; Díaz, J.F.; Josa-Prado, F.; Marco, J.A. Synthesis of n-acyl derivatives of aminocombretastatin a-4 and study of their interaction with tubulin and downregulation of c-myc. *Med. Chem.* **2021**, *17*, 1129–1139. [CrossRef]
70. Jiang, M.-R.; Li, Y.-C.; Yang, Y.; Wu, J.-R. C-myc degradation induced by DNA damage results in apoptosis of cho cells. *Oncogene* **2003**, *22*, 3252–3259. [CrossRef]
71. Popov, N.; Herold, S.; Llamazares, M.; Schülein, C.; Eilers, M. Fbw7 and usp28 regulate myc protein stability in response to DNA damage. *Cell Cycle* **2007**, *6*, 2327–2331. [CrossRef]
72. Watson, N.C.; Di, Y.M.; Orr, M.S.; Fornari, J.K., Jr.; Randolph, K.J.; Magnet, P.T.J.; Gewirtz, D.A. Influence of ionizing radiation on proliferation, c-myc expression and the induction of apoptotic cell death in two breast tumour cell lines differing in p53 status. *Int. J. Radiat. Biol.* **1997**, *72*, 547–559.
73. Lu, H.-R.; Meng, L.-H.; Huang, M.; Zhu, H.; Miao, Z.-H.; Ding, J. DNA damage, c-myc suppression and apoptosis induced by the novel topoisomerase ii inhibitor, salvicine, in human breast cancer mcf-7 cells. *Cancer Chemother. Pharmacol.* **2005**, *55*, 286–294. [CrossRef] [PubMed]
74. Cui, F.; Fan, R.; Chen, Q.; He, Y.; Song, M.; Shang, Z.; Zhang, S.; Zhu, W.; Cao, J.; Guan, H. The involvement of c-myc in the DNA double-strand break repair via regulating radiation-induced phosphorylation of atm and DNA-pkcs activity. *Mol. Cell. Biochem.* **2015**, *406*, 43–51. [CrossRef] [PubMed]
75. Ahmadi, S.E.; Rahimi, S.; Zarandi, B.; Chegeni, R.; Safa, M. Myc: A multipurpose oncogene with prognostic and therapeutic implications in blood malignancies. *J. Hematol. Oncol.* **2021**, *14*, 121. [CrossRef] [PubMed]
76. Siu, K.T.; Ramachandran, J.; Yee, A.J.; Eda, H.; Santo, L.; Panaroni, C.; Mertz, J.A.; Sims Iii, R.J.; Cooper, M.R.; Raje, N. Preclinical activity of cpi-0610, a novel small-molecule bromodomain and extra-terminal protein inhibitor in the therapy of multiple myeloma. *Leukemia* **2017**, *31*, 1760–1769. [CrossRef]
77. Ghosalkar, J.; Iyer, S.; Malhotra, G.; Joshi, K. In vitro and in vivo anticancer potential of adapalene, a third-generation retinoid against bladder cancer. *Cancer Res.* **2018**, *78*, 2316. [CrossRef]

78. Ocker, M.; Herold, C.; Ganslmayer, M.; Hahn, E.G.; Schuppan, D. The synthetic retinoid adapalene inhibits proliferation and induces apoptosis in colorectal cancer cells in vitro. *Int. J. Cancer* **2003**, *107*, 453–459. [CrossRef]
79. Patergnani, S.; Missiroli, S.; Morciano, G.; Perrone, M.; Mantovani, C.M.; Anania, G.; Fiorica, F.; Pinton, P.; Giorgi, C. Understanding the role of autophagy in cancer formation and progression is a real opportunity to treat and cure human cancers. *Cancers* **2021**, *13*, 5622. [CrossRef]
80. Jiang, Z.-F.; Shao, L.-J.; Wang, W.-M.; Yan, X.-B.; Liu, R.-Y. Decreased expression of beclin-1 and lc3 in human lung cancer. *Mol. Biol. Rep.* **2012**, *39*, 259–267. [CrossRef]
81. Hwang, S.-K.; Jeong, Y.-J.; Shin, J.-M.; Magae, J.; Kim, C.-H.; Chang, Y.-C. Mac inhibits c-myc and induces autophagy by downregulation of cip2a in leukemia cells. *Mol. Cell. Toxicol.* **2018**, *14*, 417–424. [CrossRef]
82. Li, H.; Liu, J.; Cao, W.; Xiao, X.; Liang, L.; Liu-Smith, F.; Wang, W.; Liu, H.; Zhou, P.; Ouyang, R. C-myc/mir-150/epg5 axis mediated dysfunction of autophagy promotes development of non-small cell lung cancer. *Theranostics* **2019**, *9*, 5134. [CrossRef]
83. Fan, Y.-J.; Zong, W.-X. The cellular decision between apoptosis and autophagy. *Chin. J. Cancer* **2013**, *32*, 121. [PubMed]
84. Kang, R.; Zeh, H.J.; Lotze, M.T.; Tang, D. The beclin 1 network regulates autophagy and apoptosis. *Cell Death Differ.* **2011**, *18*, 571–580. [CrossRef] [PubMed]
85. Konantz, M.; Balci, T.B.; Hartwig, U.F.; Dellaire, G.; André, M.C.; Berman, J.N.; Lengerke, C. Zebrafish xenografts as a tool for in vivo studies on human cancer. *Ann. N. Y. Acad. Sci.* **2012**, *1266*, 124–137. [CrossRef] [PubMed]

cancers

MDPI

Article

Combining Crocin and Sorafenib Improves Their Tumor-Inhibiting Effects in a Rat Model of Diethylnitrosamine-Induced Cirrhotic-Hepatocellular Carcinoma

Basma Awad [1], Alaaeldin Ahmed Hamza [2,3], Amna Al-Maktoum [1], Suhail Al-Salam [4] and Amr Amin [1,*]

1 Biology Department, College of Science, United Arab Emirates University, Al Ain P.O. Box 15551, United Arab Emirates; basma.a.awad@hotmail.com (B.A.); 202032636@uaeu.ac.ae (A.A.-M.)

2 National Organization for Drug Control and Research, Giza 12611, Egypt; alaa17mm@gmail.com

3 National Committee for Biochemistry and Molecular Biology and Medical Research Council, Academy of Scientific Research, Cairo 11334, Egypt

4 Department of Pathology, College of Medicine and Health Sciences, United Arab Emirates University, Al Ain P.O. Box 15551, United Arab Emirates; suhaila@uaeu.ac.ae

* Correspondence: a.amin@uaeu.ac.ae

Simple Summary: Liver cancer represents one of the most lethal forms of cancer, with hepatocellular carcinoma (HCC) accounting for the majority of its incidences and deaths. Currently, sorafenib is the first-in-line option for treating advanced and unresectable HCC. It is a multi-kinase inhibitor that intervenes with tumor growth and progression. Considering the modest results provided by sorafenib, identifying novel approaches to treating HCC remains a clinical imperative. Based on our previous work, crocin, a constituent of saffron, prevented HCC development. This study aimed to investigate its therapeutic effect in combination with sorafenib against an induced model of hepatocellular carcinoma arising from a cirrhotic milieu in rats. Our results confirmed that combination therapy yielded more effective outcomes compared to crocin and sorafenib monotherapies. It exerted the most pronounced effects in inhibiting inflammation and tumor cell proliferation while activating apoptosis and restoring macroscopic and cellular liver morphology. These results introduce a potential strategy for optimizing the anticancer effects of sorafenib using the bioactive natural compound crocin against HCC.

Abstract: Hepatocellular carcinoma (HCC) is one of the most aggressive malignancies, with continuously increasing cases and fatalities. Diagnosis often occurs in the advanced stages, confining patients to systemic therapies such as sorafenib. Sorafenib (SB), a multi-kinase inhibitor, has not yet demonstrated sufficient efficacy against advanced HCC. There is a strong argument in favor of studying its use in combination with other medications to optimize the therapeutic results. According to our earlier work, crocin (CR), a key bioactive component of saffron, hinders HCC development and liver cancer stemness. In this study, we investigated the therapeutic use of CR or its combination with SB in a cirrhotic rat model of HCC and evaluated how effectively SB and CR inhibited tumor growth in this model. Diethylnitrosamine (DEN) was administered intraperitoneally to rats once a week for 15 weeks, leading to cirrhosis, and then 19 weeks later, leading to multifocal HCC. After 16 weeks of cancer induction, CR (200 mg/kg daily) and SB (10 mg/kg daily) were given orally to rats for three weeks, either separately or in combination. Consistently, the combination treatment considerably decreased the incidence of dyschromatic nodules, nodule multiplicity, and dysplastic nodules when compared to the HCC group of single therapies. Combined therapy also caused the highest degree of apoptosis, along with decreased proliferating and β-catenin levels in the tumor tissues. Additionally, when rats received combined therapy with CR, it showed anti-inflammatory characteristics where nuclear factor kappa B (NF-κB) and cyclooxygenase-2 (Cox-2) were considerably and additively lowered. As a result, CR potentiates the suppressive effects of SB on tumor growth and provides the opportunity to strengthen the therapeutic effects of SB in the treatment of HCC.

Keywords: hepatocellular carcinoma; crocin; sorafenib; inflammation; apoptosis

1. Introduction

Cancer has remained a pervasive health burden despite the advances in its prevention and treatment. It is the second leading cause of death worldwide, with almost 19.3 million cases and 10 million deaths reported in 2020 alone [1]. It has been estimated that cancer might soon potentially surpass heart disease as the leading cause of death [2]. Liver cancer represents the third deadliest cancer worldwide, with a predominance in Asian and African nations [3]. In the UAE, liver cancer ranks as the eighth most lethal cancer [4], with its incidence steadily on the rise [5]. Hepatocellular carcinoma (HCC) is the predominant primary liver cancer, constituting approximately 80% of all liver cancers [6]. Persistent and unresolved chronic inflammation from recurrent injuries to the liver leads to cirrhosis, fibrosis, and ultimately the growth of hepatic tumors [7]. Chronic infections with hepatitis B and C viruses, alcohol abuse, and exposure to environmental carcinogens like aflatoxins and nitrosamines are predisposing factors known to generate hepatic inflammation, ultimately leading to HCC [8–10]. Diethylnitrosamine (DEN), a substance found in tobacco smoke, processed foods, cosmetics, gasoline, and agricultural chemicals, is regarded as an environmental carcinogen to which constant exposure is unavoidable [11–13].

Advanced HCC has an extremely dismal prognosis, with over 50% of all HCC patients being diagnosed at a late stage [14]. Sorafenib (SB) is the primary approach for the treatment of advanced HCC and was approved by the U.S. Food and Drug Administration (FDA) in 2007 [15]. It is an oral multi-kinase inhibitor that targets Raf serine/threonine kinases, c Raf, wild-type, and mutant B Raf signaling to reduce tumor cell growth and promote tumor cell death. It prevents angiogenesis by inhibiting receptor tyrosine kinases, such as platelet-derived growth factor receptor (PDGFR) and vascular endothelial growth factor receptor (VEGFR) 2 and 3 [16,17]. Despite being the first medication to provide a prognostic advantage in advanced HCC, SB's efficacy is very moderate, with a key phase III trial finding that the median overall survival was 10.7 months compared to 7.9 months with a placebo [18]. Additionally, persistent SB use frequently causes tumor cells to lose sensitivity, developing acquired resistance [19]. Combination therapy that targets several signaling pathways may be superior to monotherapy because it may be able to overcome resistance, feedback activation, and compensatory activation of pro-survival pathways [19]. Thus, combining SB with additional anticancer drugs may offer a novel therapeutic approach that could enhance anti-tumor effectiveness and circumvent SB resistance in HCC [15,20].

Historically, nature has provided a dependable and abundant supply of effective anticancer compounds with minimal to nonexistent negative effects [21]. Important anticancer agents such as Vinca alkaloids, podophyllotoxin, taxol, camptothecin, and their derivatives are among the 40% of FDA-approved medicinal chemicals that are of natural origin [21,22]. Many of these compounds are considered to be phytochemicals; therefore, plants have been extensively investigated in the search for potential anticancer agents against HCC [23]. Saffron (stigma of the *Crocus sativus* flower) and its major constituents have been explored for their anti-inflammatory, antioxidant, and anticancer properties [24–26]. For instance, saffron and most of its main components, such as crocin (CR), crocetin, and safranal, have been shown to significantly inhibit the growth of a variety of tumor cell lines, such as prostate, cervical, leukemia, lung, and liver cancer [25–29]. Saffron-derived CR also decreased the incidence of gastric cancer in methyl-3-nitro-1-nitrosoguanidine-induced rodents [30] and HCC in DEN-treated rats [25,26,31–33].

The environmental carcinogen DEN has the ability to generate lesions in rats resembling human benign and malignant tumors [12]. Therefore, it is widely employed to mimic and examine various human benign and malignant tumor types in laboratory settings [34]. Our previous study's initiation-promotion model of cancer development was utilized to simulate the early stages of carcinogenesis [35]. In this investigation, a single dose of DEN, followed by 2-acetylaminofluorene, were intraperitoneally injected into rats to cause HCC. The study examined the therapeutic effects of CR alone or in conjunction with SB in rats during the early phases of hepatocellular tumor promotion. The combination of SB and CR more effectively lowered cell proliferation and carcinogenesis in this liver cancer model by reducing liver damage, oxidative stress, inflammation, and other adverse effects. To date, in vivo testing of SB and CR cotreatment in advanced HCC has yet to take place. In order to determine whether this therapeutic approach could improve the treatment of advanced HCC without causing greater toxicity, we coupled CR and SB in this study. In humans, approximately 80% of advanced HCC develops from cirrhotic livers [36]. Therefore, novel therapeutic approaches ought to be tested in an animal model of HCC occurring on a cirrhotic background. A rat model of DEN-induced liver injury that replicates the evolution of cirrhosis toward HCC was developed for the current study [37]. Multiple smaller doses of DEN are used in this procedure to cause liver cancer in animals. This is implemented to mimic the progression of liver cancer in HCC patients by simulating the inflammatory conditions from which fibrosis and cirrhosis arise before malignant tumors are formed [38]. This animal model with repeated-dose DEN is a useful model regimen for multifocal nodular HCC in the evaluation of novel combination therapy regimens [39]. To investigate the safety and antitumor effectiveness of the combination of SB with CR, we employed the DEN-induced cirrhotic rat model with HCC.

2. Materials and Methods

2.1. Materials

CR, DEN, Folin's reagent, sodium pentobarbital, and bovine albumin were sourced from Sigma Chemical Co. (St. Louis, MO, USA). The alanine transaminase (ALT) (ab105134) and aspartate aminotransferase (AST) (ab105135) kits were purchased from Abcam (Cambridge, CB2 0AX, UK). Rabbit monoclonal antibodies against Bax [E63] (ab32503), β-catenin [E247] (ab32572,) COX2 [EPR12012] (ab179800), Ki67 antibody (ab15580), and NF-κB-p65 (ab16502) were purchased from Abcam (Cambridge, CB2 0AX, UK). Anti-proliferating cell nuclear antigen (PCNA), and anti-caspase-3 were purchased from Cell Signaling Technology Inc. (Danvers, MA, USA). Anti-caspase-9 was sourced from Novus Biologicals (Littleton, CO, USA), and anti-poly ADP-ribose polymerase (PARP), anti-Bcl-2, and anti-Bax for Western Blotting (WB) investigation were purchased from Santa Cruz Biotechnology (Santa Cruz, CA, USA). SB was purchased from Carbosynth Ltd. (Compton, UK).

2.2. Animals

A series of experiments were performed on 40 4-to-5-week-old healthy albino Wistar rats weighing 110–120 g. Upon protocol approval by the Animal Research and Ethics Committee of the College of Medicine and Health Sciences, UAE University (Approval No. A8-15), the rats were sourced from the college's animal research facility. The animals were kept in a controlled environment with 12 h of light/dark cycles and a temperature range from 22 °C to 24 °C. Rats were habituated to the environment with unlimited access to tap water and a typical pellet diet.

2.3. Hepatocarcinogenesis Model

A model of cirrhosis-hepatocellular carcinoma was conducted in adherence to a modified version of the procedure outlined by DePeralta et al. [38] and Schiffer et al. [37]. The rats were separated into two groups at random: the control group and the experimental group. The control group (n = 8) received intraperitoneal injections of phosphate-buffered saline (PBS) once a week for 15 weeks. The experimental group (n = 32) received intraperitoneal injections of DEN at a dose of 50 mg/kg body weight on a weekly basis for 15 weeks, followed by seven days washout period to assess the development of HCC.

2.4. Experimental Design

Rats with established HCC were separated into four groups (n = 8) at the end of the 16-week HCC induction phase (HCC, HCC + SB, HCC + CR, HCC + CR + SB). In the control and HCC groups, 1 mL water containing 0.3% DMSO was administered orally five times each week for three weeks. The HCC-induced groups received treatments of CR and/or SB 5 times a week for 3 weeks. All drugs were administered orally via intragastric tubes. The HCC + SB group received SB dissolved in 0.3% DMSO at a dose of 10 mg/kg b.wt. The HCC + CR group received 200 mg/kg b.wt. of CR after it had been dissolved in 1 mL of water. The last HCC group was treated with both CR and SB. This group received 200 mg/kg b.wt. of CR with the subsequent administration of 10 mg/kg b.wt. of SB. The CR dose utilized in this study was determined based on previous studies assessing its toxicity and anti-inflammatory and anticancer benefits in rats with DEN-induced liver cancer [26,40]. Similarly, rats were given SB at a dose of 10 mg/kg based on findings on its therapeutic effect on the same cirrhotic rat model of hepatocellular carcinoma [19,41]. By the end of the experiment and after a 24 h post-last medication delivery, animals were euthanized by cervical dislocation under 3% sodium pentobarbital (45 mg/kg, i.p.) and dissected under controlled conditions. The experiment's layout is shown in (Figure 1).

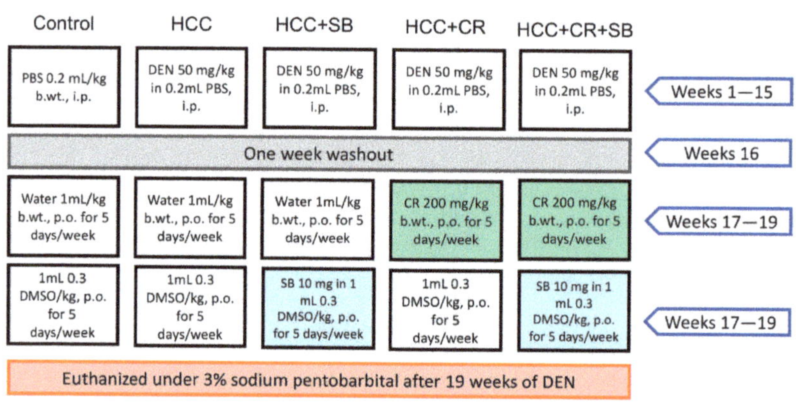

Figure 1. A visual representation of the experimental design. PBS: phosphate-buffered saline, DEN: diethyl nitrosamine, HCC: hepatocellular carcinoma, CR: crocin, SB: sorafenib, DMSO: dimethyl sulfoxide, i.p.: intraperitoneal, p.o.: per. os.

2.5. Sample Preparation

After 19 weeks of treatment with DEN, blood was collected from the retro-orbital plexus of rats under the effect of diethyl ether 24 h post-last treatment. The rats were then euthanized following the administration of 3% sodium pentobarbital (45 mg/kg, i.p.) by a cervical dislocation. The blood samples were centrifuged at 3000 rpm for 20 min (4 °C) for serum separation and collection. Gross livers were dehydrated, rinsed off with an ice-cold saline solution, and then dried out with blotting paper. A portion of the liver was immediately fixed in 10% buffered formalin for histological and immunohistochemical analyses. The remaining parts were flash-frozen in liquid nitrogen and kept at −80 °C for western blotting.

2.6. Liver Gross Appearance and Histopathological Analysis

After liver collection, macroscopic characteristics such as liver color, size, texture, and number of nodules were documented. The dyschromatic nodules were recognizable by their grayish-white color. These surface nodules exceeded 3 mm in size and were counted by two independent investigators. Samples collected from the right, left, and caudate lobes were fixed in 10% buffered formalin for histopathological examination. Fixed tissue samples representing the different groups (control, HCC, HCC + SB, HCC + CR, and HCC

+ CR + SB) were processed simultaneously and embedded in the paraffin block. Tissue blocks were serially cut into 5 μm thick sections, stained with hematoxylin and eosin (H&E), and then examined using an Olympus BX41 microscope (Tokyo, Japan). An experienced pathologist assigned the histopathological ratings. The percentage of the area covered by foci of cytoplasmic vacuolization or hydropic degeneration was used to grade hepatic vacuolization and hydropic degeneration: 0 corresponded to the range of 0–5%, 1 to 33%, 2 to 66%, and 3 to 66% [42]. The degree of inflammation was measured as the number of foci per 200-field: A focus was defined as zero, one to two, two to four, or three to four. The degree of fibrosis was rated as follows: 0 = no fibrosis, 1 = mild fibrosis (collagen fibers extend from the portal triad or central vein to the peripheral region), 2 = moderate fibrosis (collagen fibers create a fibrous septum without compartment development), and 3 = severe fibrosis (thick fibrous septum accompanied by pseudo-lobe formation). Large hepatocytes with hyperchromatic nuclei and dysplastic nodules (DN) were graded according to the proportion of the area they covered: 0 meant no DN, 1 meant 1%–25%, 2 meant 25%–50%, 3 meant 50%–75%, and 4 meant 75%–100% [42].

2.7. Enzyme Markers of Liver Injury

Using a commercially available colorimetric test, the liver enzyme activities of ALT and AST were measured. The Promega GloMax microplate reader was used to measure the concentrations of ALT (ab105134) and AST (ab105135) using the kits that were acquired from Abcam.

2.8. Immunohistochemical Staining

Mounted sections were submerged in sodium citrate buffer (0.1 M, pH 6) and left in a water bath for 15 min to expose antigen epitopes. This was followed by the incubation of the sections with 0.3% H_2O_2 in methanol to prevent any nonspecific binding to endogenous peroxidase. Rabbit anti-rat primary antibodies were added to the sections and incubated overnight at 4 °C. Rabbit monoclonal antibodies against Bax [E63] (ab32503), β-catenin [E247] (ab32572,) COX2 [EPR12012] (ab179800), Ki67 antibody (ab15580), and NF-κB-p65 (ab16502) were purchased from Abcam (Cambridge, CB2 0AX, UK), while anti-PCNA and anti-caspase-3 were purchased from Cell Signaling Technology Inc. (Danvers, MA, USA). Next, the slides were rinsed with PBS and subjected to incubation with the secondary antibody polyvalent biotinylated goat-anti-rabbit for 10 min at room temperature (1:200 dilution). The standard staining protocol was conducted using the Universal LSAB kit and DAB plus substrate kit. Additional counter-staining was carried out using hematoxylin. The slides were examined and photographed under an Olympus DP71 optical microscope. Ten fields were then chosen at random for the quantification of positive cells in individual samples (×400).

2.9. Quantification of Protein Expression in Tissue Sections

The quantitative assessment of different HCC biomarkers expressed in liver tissue sections was achieved by producing digital images using Image-Pro software version 6.0 for Windows. The percentage (%) of positively stained cells was detected by the ImageJ analysis program (NIH, Bethesda, MD, USA). Positively stained cells for Ki-67 and PCNA were counted belonging to five different fields of ten different sections of the different groups. The percentage (%) of the area of immunostaining per image was recorded at a final magnification of ×400. In total, 10 images per probed tissue section were examined corresponding to each group of rats.

2.10. Western Blotting

Cold RIPA buffer containing 2 μL of protease inhibitor and phosphatase inhibitor was utilized to homogenize and lyse the cells of 10 mg liver tissue. The separation of lysates was accomplished by centrifuging the samples at 16,000 rpm for 15 min at 4 °C. Heated samples (20 μg) in Laemmli buffer containing 4% SDS, 10% 2-mercaptoethanol,

20% glycerol, 0.004% bromophenol blue, and 0.125 M Tris HCl were employed to denature proteins in the liver homogenate. The pH was measured and maintained at 6.8. The samples were then heated to 95 degrees for 5 min. The Bradford method (Bio-Rad, Hercules, CA, USA) was used to determine protein concentrations. Protein samples of equal proportions were electrophoresed. Sodium dodecyl sulfate-polyacrylamide gel electrophoresis (SDS-PAGE) was carried out as directed by the manufacturer using a TGX Stain-Free Fast Cast Acrylamide Kit from Bio-Rad Laboratories Inc. (Hercules, CA, USA). Proteins were deposited onto polyvinylidene difluoride membranes (Millipore Bedford, MA) and blocked in bovine serum albumin (BSA, 3%) and Tris buffered saline/tween 20 (TBST) at room temperature for one hour after each sample's protein content was separated on the SDS-PAGE gel. The membranes were treated with primary antibodies for an overnight period at 4 °C following the blocking stage. Anti-PCNA, anti-Caspase-3 (Cell Signaling Technology Inc., (Danvers, MA, USA), anti-caspase-9 (Novus Biologicals, Littleton, CO, USA), anti-poly ADP-ribose polymerase (PARP), anti-Bcl-2, and anti-Bax (Santa Cruz Biotechnology, Santa Cruz, CA, USA) were the main antibodies used for this investigation. After incubating the membranes with primary antibodies overnight, they were thoroughly cleaned with TBST before being re-probed for an hour at room temperature with secondary antibodies such as anti-rabbit IgG and anti-mouse IgG from Cell Signaling Technology, Inc. (Danvers, MA, USA). The signal was then detected and seen using the Bio-Rad ChemiDoc XRS+ System. Protein bands were then recognized using a chemiluminescence solution known as WesternSure PREMIUM. The ImageJ program was used to measure the band's intensity. Considering the upregulation of common housekeeping proteins in HCC, using the amount of total protein was a better alternative for studies of protein expression that require normalization [43,44]. Total protein was utilized as the internal control and was stacked into a single band on a 5% SDS-PAGE stacking gel with no separating gels. SYPRO Ruby protein gel stain was utilized for total protein staining in accordance with the manufacturer's (#170-3125, BIO-RAD, Hercules, CA, USA) protocol [44]. The band intensities were quantified using ImageJ software (National Institutes of Health).

2.11. Statistical Analysis

One-way analysis of variance (ANOVA) of the resulting data was conducted with SPSS statistical program version 25 (SPSS Inc., Chicago, IL, USA). Tukey's post hoc analysis ($p < 0.05$) was carried out to investigate the differences between the means of the treated groups following the detection of significant differences by ANOVA.

3. Results

3.1. CR, SB, and Their Combination Inhibit Nodule Formation and Restore Liver Function of DEN-Induced HCC in Rats

Normal liver morphology and function were almost fully restored following adjuvant therapy with CR and SB in DEN-induced HCC. When observed with the naked eye, gross livers from the untreated HCC group were characterized by having an overall pale color and an ample number of grayish-white nodules (Figure 2A–C). This effect was alleviated to some degree in all the treated groups. SB administration (HCC + SB) markedly improved the macroscopic morphological status of the liver. CR-treated animals (HCC + CR) had a significantly lower number and multiplicity of nodules compared to the livers of animals treated with SB alone (HCC + SB) (Table 1 & Figure 2A,B). The therapeutic administration of both CR and SB (HCC + CR + SB) resulted in the highest level of liver resemblance to the control group. This group presented a glossy dark brown color of the liver and had the lowest nodule multiplicity and incidence (Table 1 & Figure 2A,B). Some rats treated with the combination regimen lacked any macroscopic nodules (Table 1). Biochemical serum markers ALT and AST were measured to assess the severity of liver damage in each of the experimental groups. Hepatic damage caused by DEN administration was indicated by a significant rise in the ALT and AST levels when compared to the control group. Treatment with SB, CR, and CR + SB attenuated the hepatic damage induced by DEN and notably lowered the serum activities of ALT and AST (Figure 2C,D). Co-therapy intensified the effects of SB, leading to a larger reduction in AST and ALT as opposed to the use of SB in isolation (Figure 2D).

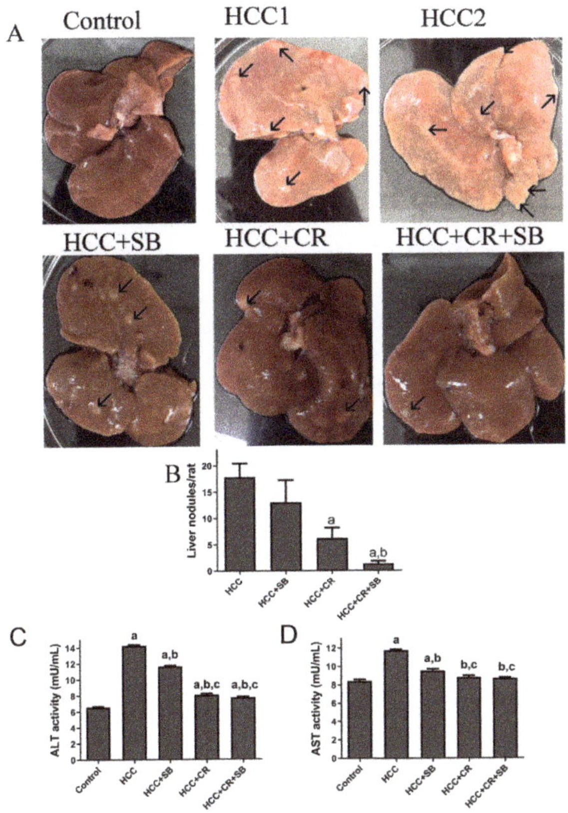

Figure 2. Gross investigations of rat livers: (**A**) Representative macroscopic appearances of livers of DEN-treated male rats administered with CR, SB, and CR + SB, arrows show liver nodules. (**B**) The liver nodule numbers/rat (>3 mm) were calculated. Values represent mean ± SEM of six rats per group. One-way analysis of variance followed by Tukey's post hoc analysis was used to calculate significance values: a $p < 0.05$ vs. HCC group; b $p < 0.05$ vs. HCC + SB. (**C**,**D**) ALT and AST activity is expressed as mU/mL. One-way analysis of variance and a Dunnett's t test were used to determine significance values: a $p < 0.05$ vs. control group; b $p < 0.05$ vs. HCC, c $p < 0.05$ vs. HCC + SB.

Table 1. Effects of CR, SB, and their combination on the incidence of cancer nodules

Groups	Number of Rats with Nodules/Total Number of Rats	Nodule Incidence (%)	Inhibition of Nodule Incidence (%)	Total Number of Nodules	Mean Number of Nodules per Rat [a]	Inhibition of Nodule Multiplicity (%)
HCC	6/6	100%	0%	107	17.83	0%
HCC + SB	6/6	100%	0%	78	13	27.1%
HCC + CR	6/6	100%	0%	37	6.17 [b]	65.40%
HCC + CR + SB	4/6	66.67%	33.33%	8	2 [b,c]	92.52%

[a] Total number of nodules/numbers of animals bearing nodules in each group (multiplicity). [b] $p < 0.05$, as compared to HCC group, [c] $p < 0.05$ as compared to HCC + SB.

3.2. CR, SB, and Their Combination Improve Histological Changes and Decrease Dysplastic Nodule Formation in Livers of HCC-Induced Rats

Histopathological analyses of liver tissue were carried out to inspect the role of CR, SB, and CR + SB in restoring normal cell and tissue morphology. Microscopic examinations of H&E-stained liver sections from the control group displayed proper hepatic architecture. This was characterized by hepatocytes arranged in a polygonal manner, radiating outward from the central vein of each lobule. The lobules had the usual thickness, and the hepatic sinusoids were intact. The hepatocytes possessed 1–2 dark blue nuclei with distinguishable nucleoli (Figure 3A,B). DEN treatment resulted in severe morphological deformations and a collapse of the normal polygonal hepatic architecture. Multi-dysplastic nodules (DN) with proliferating oval cells were observed in the HCC group (Figure 3C). These regions contained irregular dysplastic hepatocytes exhibiting cellular features such as nuclear hyperchromatism, karyomegaly, increased nucleocytoplasmic (N/C) ratios, and multiple nucleoli and nuclei (Figure 3D–F). Additionally, DEN administration generated areas of hydropic degeneration and trabecular HCC. All experimental HCC groups were associated with varying degrees of histological abnormalities. The SB group retained some DEN-induced cellular features associated with foci of hydropic degeneration (HD) (Figure 3G). However, SB clearly improved the histological structure when compared to the HCC group (Figure 3H). Likewise, CR administration demonstrated a decline in the foci of hydropic degeneration (HD) (Figure 3I,J). Cotreatment with CR and SB surpassed the efficacy of either treatment alone in improving the histological conditions and reversing the DEN-induced hepatocyte plate disorganization (Figure 3K,L). The degeneration of foci of hydropic degeneration along with the presence of some hepatocytes with pyknotic nuclei was observed in this group (Figure 3L). As shown in Figure 4, all the treated groups enhanced the histopathological scores for (A) foci of hydropic degeneration, (B) vacuolization, (C) inflammation, (D) fibrosis, and hyperchromatic nuclei with high N/C ratios. However, combined therapy with CR and SB demonstrated the highest impact in improving such scores.

3.3. CR Enhances Antiproliferative Effect of SB and Additively Downregulates β-Catenin Expression in HCC-Induced Rats

Proliferative markers were compared in the liver sections from all the groups. The nuclear proteins Ki-67 and PCNA are established indicators of aberrant cell proliferation that often coincide with tumorigenesis [45]. Liver sections from the HCC group displayed a significantly larger number of Ki-67- and PCNA-positive cells relative to the control group, as detected by IHC staining. After treatment with CR or SB individually, the number of proliferating cells significantly decreased. CR combined with SB exerted an additive effect on hindering cell proliferation and restored Ki-67 and PCNA levels in HCC tissues almost to that of the control group (Figure 5A–C). This effect was further verified by Western blotting, in which PCNA protein levels were markedly lowered in the groups treated with SB, CR, and CR + SB when compared to the HCC group (Figure 5D,E). Combination therapy caused the most dramatic reduction of PCNA, achieving expression levels lower than that of the control group (Figure 5D,E). The overexpression of β-catenin has been shown to be associated with hepatocarcinogenesis [46,47]. This was substantiated through IHC staining of β-catenin in which its expression was considerably higher in the HCC group (Figure 5F–H). The assessment of the number of positively stained cells showed that the HCC group animals had higher levels of cytonuclear expression of β-catenin (Figure 5H). Tissues obtained from the rats treated with SB or CR demonstrated mild β-catenin IHC reactivity. Cotreatment provided the most potent effect, as indicated by β-catenin's intense suppression when compared to the HCC and control groups.

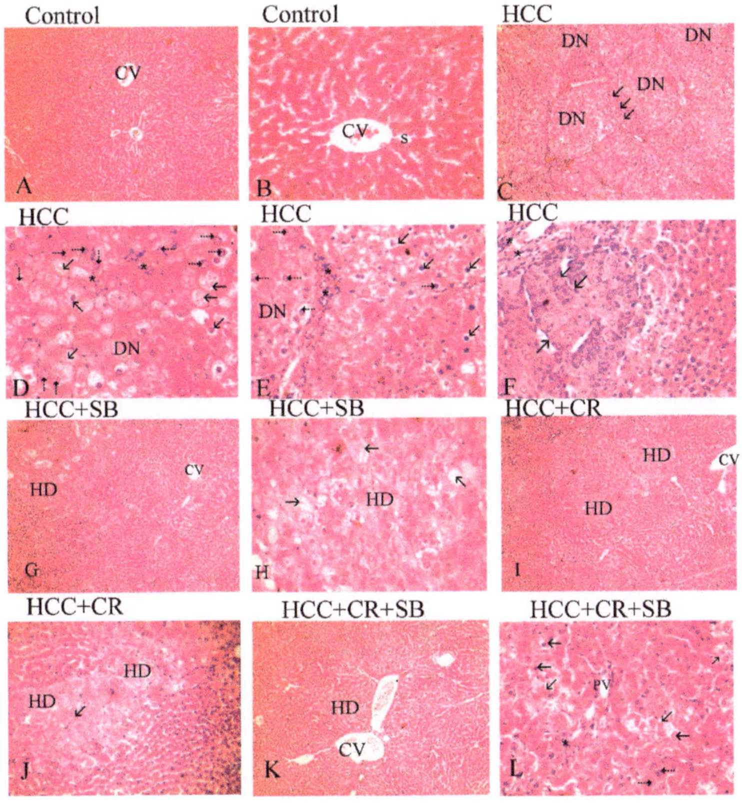

Figure 3. H&E-stained liver sections underwent histopathological analysis, with the control group (**A**,**B**), the HCC group (**C–F**), the HCC + SB group (**G**,**H**), and the HCC + CR + SB group (**K**,**L**). Histopathological investigations of liver sections stained with H&E. (**A**,**B**) control group, (**C–E**) HCC group, (**G**,**H**) HCC + SB group, (**I**,**J**) HCC + CR group, (**K**,**L**) HCC + CR + SB group. (**A**) Demonstrating proper hepatic organization characterized by hepatic lobules and oblique interlobular septa with polygonal hepatocytes extending outward from the central vein (CV) (×100). (**B**) The hepatocytes showed eosinophilic cytoplasm and vesicular nuclei. Flat endothelial cells and Kupffer cells bordered the sinusoidal gaps (S) between the hepatocytes (×400). (**C**) The HCC group displayed a disruption of the hepatic architecture with multi-dysplastic nodules (DN) encircled by proliferating oval cells (↑) (×100). (**D**) Hepatocytes in the HCC group exhibited hydropic degeneration, irregularity, dysplasia, pleomorphic cells with karyomegalic nuclei, conspicuous numerous nucleoli (↑), and other hepatocytes displayed shrunken darkened nuclei and vacuolated cytoplasm (↑). (×400). (**E**) Some hepatocytes showed a high nucleocytoplasmic ratio and hyperchromatic nuclei (↑), whereas others showed vacuolated cytoplasm, shrunken nuclei (↑), and mononuclear cell infiltration (*), (×400). (**F**) Displaying trabecular liver cancer (↑) and inflammation (*). (**G**) A focal hydropic degeneration (HD), (×100), was seen in the HCC + SB group. (**H**) Other samples displayed foci of degeneration with total loss of hepatocytes, a sparse residual population of pyknotic nuclei (↑), and an improvement in the nucleocytoplasmic ratio, (×400). (**I**,**J**) The histological structure of the HCC + CR group showed improvement with a decline foci of hydropic degeneration (HD) (↑). (**K**) Hepatocytes were neatly distributed in cords radiating from the central vein in the HCC + CR + SB group, indicating an improvement in normal liver architecture (CV). (×100). (**L**) Exhibited areas of degeneration with full loss of hepatocytes and a small number of pyknotic nuclei and numerous nucleoli (↑), along with the infiltration of inflammatory cells (*) and an improvement in the nucleocytoplasmic ratio.

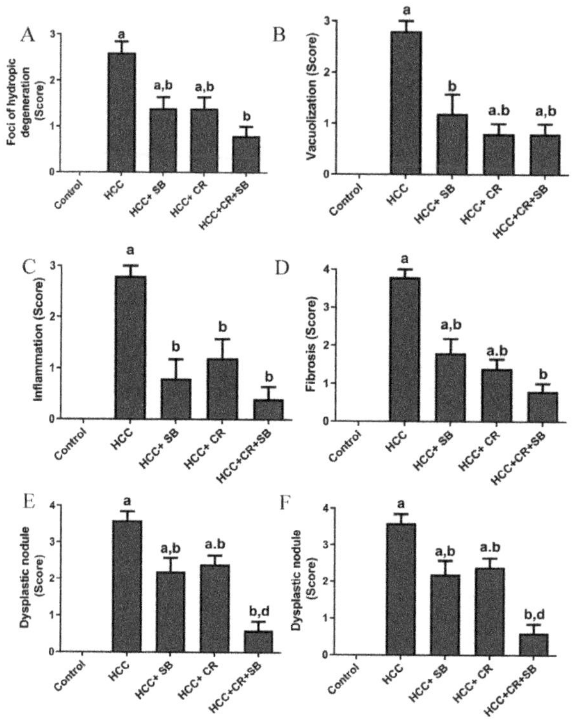

Figure 4. Histopathological scores for (**A**) foci of hydropic degeneration, (**B**) vacuolization, (**C**) inflammation, (**D**) fibrosis, and (**E**) hyperchromatic nuclei with high N/C ration, and (**F**) dysplastic nodules. Values expressed as mean ± SEM for five animals in each group. Significance was determined by one-way analysis of variance followed by Tukey's post hoc analysis: a $p < 0.05$ vs. control group; b $p < 0.05$ vs. HCC group; d $p < 0.05$ vs. HCC + CR group.

3.4. CR Promotes Apoptotic Effect of SB in HCC-Induced Rats

The pro-apoptotic efficacy of CR, SB, and CR + SB against HCC was evident via IHC staining and Western blot analyses measuring the activity of key apoptotic proteins (Figure 6). Pro-apoptotic proteins demonstrated an overall upregulation in all the treated groups when compared to the HCC group. The number of caspase 3- and Bax-positive cells was markedly increased in these groups (Figure 6A–C). However, this elevation was particularly prominent in the group treated with both CR and SB (HCC + CR + SB) (Figure 6A–C). This was corroborated by Western blot results in which the expression of Bax was increased in the SB and CR groups but more significantly in the CR + SB group (Figure 6D,F). This pro-apoptotic pattern was consistent with the downregulation of anti-apoptotic protein Bcl-2 in all the treated groups, especially when CR was combined with SB (Figure 6D,G). Similarly, a considerable reduction of PARP and caspase precursors, pro-caspase 3 and pro-caspase 9, was observed in the CR and SB-treated groups (Figure 6D,E,H,I), indicating the intrinsic activation of apoptosis. The most pronounced reduction was observed in the CR + SB group (Figure 6D,E,H,I). These results reflect CR's role in strengthening the apoptotic capacity of SB against HCC.

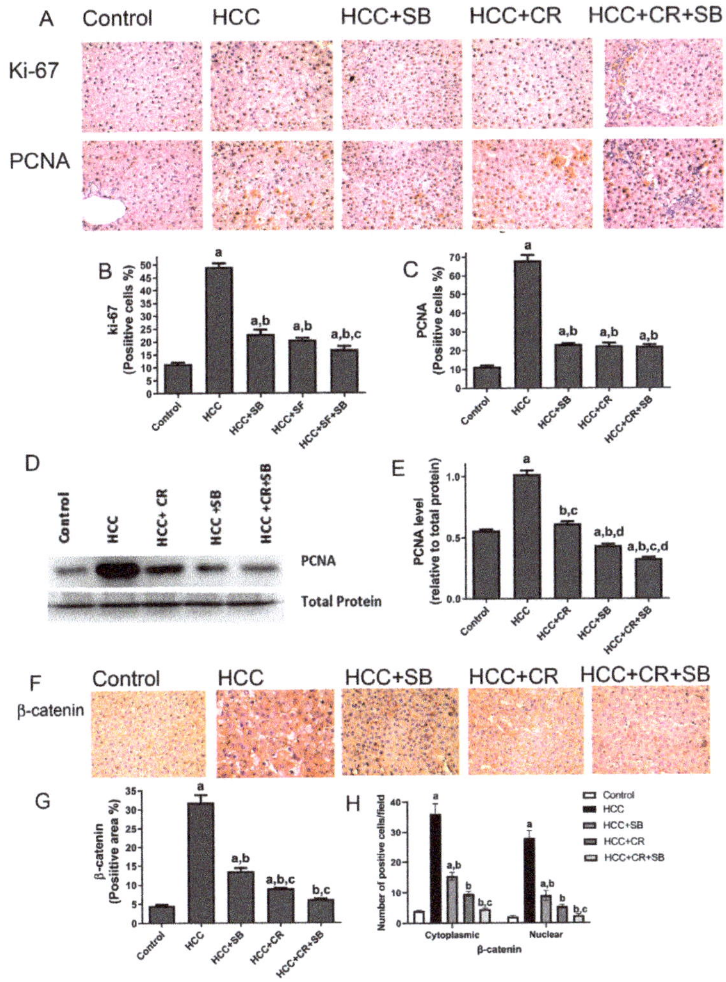

Figure 5. CR potentiates antiproliferative and β-catenin downregulation of SB-induced effects in HCC-induced rats. (**A**) IHC staining of Ki-67 and PCNA in rat liver tissue sections. (**B**,**C**) Graphs reflect the number of cells positively stained for Ki-67 and PCNA, respectively. Positive cell count was determined belonging to five different fields of ten different sections of different groups. (**D**) PCNA concentration in rat tissue lysate of each group quantified by WB. (**E**) Quantification plot illustrating WB signals quantified by ImageJ and normalized relative to the total protein from the liver. (**F**) β-catenin IHC staining in rat liver tissue sections. (**F**) An intense IHC reaction of β-catenin was observed in the HCC group when compared to the control group. Conversely, tissue sections obtained from rats treated with SB, CR, and CR + SB demonstrated a subtle IHC reaction of β-catenin when compared to the control and HCC groups. (**G**) A graphical representation of the IHC staining intensity of β-catenin corresponding to each group. (**H**) Graph showing the number of the positive cells for cytoplasmic and nuclear staining of β-catenin expression in each section by calculating the number in ten fields at ×400 magnifications and then the number of positive cells/fields. Values expressed as mean ± SEM of four animals in each group. The displayed data depicts three independent experiments performed in triplicates and expressed as mean values ± SEM (n = 4). a $p < 0.05$, were significant as compared with normal control rats and b $p < 0.05$ were significant as compared with HCC control group, c $p < 0.05$, were significant as compared with SB group, d $p < 0.05$ vs. HCC + CR group. Original western blots are Presented in Files S1.

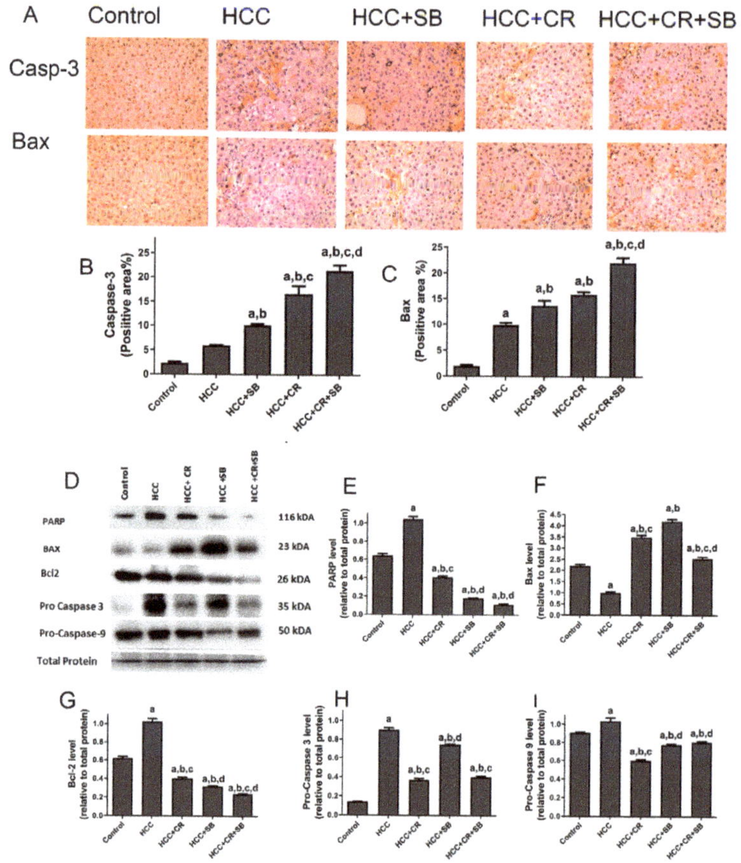

Figure 6. Effects of CR, SB, and CR + SB on apoptotic cell death. (**A**) Representative images exhibiting Bax and caspase 3 IHC staining of liver tissue sections corresponding to all groups (**B**,**C**) show the corresponding IHC-positive staining area graph of Bax and caspase 3-positive area in different experimental groups. The IHC staining of Bax and caspase 3 in each section was calculated by positive area of brown staining in ten fields at ×400 magnifications then the area of positive cells/field. (**D**) Western blot analysis showing the decreased expression of Bcl-2, Pro caspase-3, and Pro caspase-9, and the increased expression of Bax in SB, CR, and CR + SB treated groups. (**E**–**I**) show densitometric analysis representing the expression of PARP, Bax, Bcl-2, Pro caspase-3, and Pro caspase-9 normalized to that of total protein. Values expressed as mean ± SEM for six animals in each group. Significance was determined by one-way analysis of variance followed by Tukey's post hoc analysis: a $p < 0.05$ vs. control group; b $p < 0.05$ vs. HCC group; c $p < 0.05$ vs. HCC + SB group; d $p < 0.05$ vs. HCC + CR group. Original western blots are Presented in Files S1.

3.5. CR Augments the Anti-Inflammatory Capacity of SB in HCC-Induced Rats

Increased expression of the inflammatory proteins COX-2 and NF-κB-p65 was exhibited in the HCC group. These proteins were especially concentrated around the central vein and in the Kupffer cells. There was a substantial decline in NF-κB-p65 and COX-2 immuno-positive cells following treatment with CR, SB, and CR + SB, indicating the inhibition of NF-κB-p65 activation and consequently a downregulation in inflammation. The anti-inflammatory effect of SB was amplified when it was combined with CR, as shown in Figure 7.

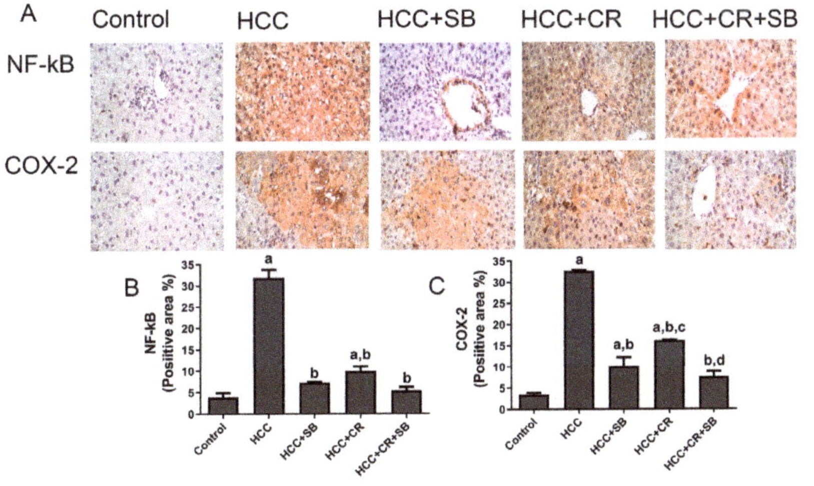

Figure 7. Inhibitory effect of CR, SB, and CR + SB on HCC-induced upregulation in NF-kB-p65 and COX-2 expression in liver. (**A**) Representative images of IHC NF-kB-p65 and COX-2 stained sections in the livers of all groups studied. (**B**,**C**) represent the quantification of COX-2 and NF-kB-p65-positive staining area. Increased NF-kB-p65 and COX-2 immunopositivity staining was observed in livers of the HCC group, as indicated by a brown color, as compared to the control group. The percent of positive staining area was reduced in SB, CR, and CR + SB treated groups. The expression of NF-kB-p65 and COX-2 in each section was determined by calculating the percent of positive area of brown staining in ten fields at ×400 magnifications and then the area of positive cells/field. Values expressed as mean ± SEM of six animals in each group. Significance was determined by one-way analysis of variance followed by Tukey's post hoc analysis: a $p < 0.05$ vs. control group; b $p < 0.05$ vs. HCC group; c $p < 0.05$ vs. HCC + SB group, d $p < 0.05$ vs. HCC + CR group.

4. Discussion

The multi-kinase inhibitor SB targets key hallmark pathways of HCC and has long been the standard therapy for treating advanced HCC as a single agent [15,20]. However, drug resistance, unsatisfactory patient performance, and adverse drug-related side effects continue to impede the success of orally administered SB [18,19]. It has been reported that SB is only effective in about 30% of HCC patients who eventually gain resistance within 6 months [48]. This highlights the urgent need for discovering better therapeutic modalities that tackle SB-related challenges. Employing a combination regimen seems to be a sound strategy for increasing tumor sensitivity to the drug [15,19]. However, increased toxicity is a major drawback associated with this approach. Therefore, identifying well-tolerated and efficient combinations of targeted therapy is necessary for the treatment of HCC patients. In this study, a cirrhotic rat model of HCC was adopted to evaluate the interaction of SB with CR. The progression of HCC from cirrhosis is observed in around 90% of HCC patients, regardless of the etiology of liver disease [49]. This indicates that the animal model utilized in this study accurately reflects the physiopathology of human HCC [38,39]. The amalgamation of SB with CR was shown to offer greater anticancer results against HCC in a synergistic manner when compared to SB and CR monotherapies in rats. Combination therapy caused the most dramatic mitigation of tumor incidence, cell proliferation, and inflammation while promoting apoptosis in DEN-induced HCC.

In the current investigation, dichromatic tumor nodules were significantly more prevalent on the surface of the livers of cirrhotic rats with HCC. The histological study proved that these dichromatic tumor nodules were HCC. DN featured enlarged hyperchromatic nuclei with clear, eosinophilic, or hyper basophilic cytoplasm. These histological characteristics coexisted with other abnormalities such as steatosis, fibrosis, inflammation, hydropic degeneration, and cell necrosis. Under the circumstances of our experiment, administration of CR and SB to DEN-treated rats resulted in a considerable decrease in the number and incidence of dyschromatic nodules as well as a decline in FAH and other histological abnormalities. In terms of the quantity and occurrence of dyschromatic nodules as well as a reduction in FAH with other histological abnormalities, we discovered that the combination of CR and SB outperformed SB and CR monotherapies. These results confirm what was concluded in our recent study on the early stages of carcinogenesis, which proved that the combination of SB and CR increased the effectiveness of SB in lowering cell proliferation and carcinogenesis in this liver cancer model [35].

The status of liver function is often identified by assessing the ALT and AST levels in blood serum. In instances where hepatocytes are subjected to damage, these enzymes leak into circulation and are consequently markers for liver damage. Increased levels of these biochemical parameters often correlate with the incidence of HCC [50]. In this study, the elevated levels of ALT and AST in the HCC group represented the progression of carcinogenesis and showed that liver damage occurred when preneoplastic lesions first appeared. SB or CR monotherapy considerably alleviated the HCC-associated liver injury. These findings align with previous studies on CR's ability in restoring ALT and AST levels in several different hepatotoxic conditions [51–53]. According to the results, the improvement of liver function following SB and CR co-administration was superior to CR or SB monotherapies. These benefits were demonstrated by a notable drop in ALT and AST activity, an indication of diminishing liver damage that may have been attributed to CR's capacity to avoid liver damage and enhance anticancer activity. Our data is consistent with earlier investigations where the combination of anticancer compounds with SB augmented SB's ability in decreasing the ALT and AST levels [54,55].

The characteristic pathways of HCC in cancer cells that promote tumor formation and progression include sustained proliferative signaling and the obstruction of apoptosis [56,57]. In this work, Ki-67 and PCNA were utilized to assess cellular proliferation, as they are exclusively expressed during that process [58]. All HCC animals treated with mono- or combined therapy showed the clear antiproliferative impact of CR and SB, where expressions of Ki-67 and PCNA were markedly downregulated. These results are in line with published research documenting the antiproliferative effects of CR in the liver cancer model induced by DEN [19,26,33,40]. The antiproliferative effects of SB and CR combined exceeded those imposed by CR and SB monotherapies. Increasing the effectiveness of the combination of SB and CR against liver cancer cell proliferation in this model is consistent with the early stages of carcinogenesis in our recent study [35].

Modulation of apoptosis plays a significant role in promoting carcinogenesis and conferring chemoresistance to cancer cells as they evade apoptosis [59,60]. Here, our HCC group demonstrated low Bax levels, whereas Bcl-2, pro-caspase-3, pro-caspase-9, and PARP levels rose, which is consistent with earlier studies by Thomas et al. [61] and Younis et al. [62]. Numerous cancer types have elevated levels of PARP, pro-caspase-3, and pro-caspase-9, and these aberrant expressions indicate that these markers play important roles in the development of oncogenic transformation [63,64]. According to the results presented here, treatment with CR, SB alone, or their combination promoted apoptosis in HCC liver tissue, as shown by the elevated levels of the pro-apoptotic proteins Bax and caspase-3 and the decreased levels of Bcl-2, PARP, pro-caspase-3, and pro-caspase-9 in comparison to the HCC animals. Furthermore, visual examination of the liver samples from various treatment groups confirmed the occurrence of hepatic vacuolation and pyknotic nuclei in cells that may undergo apoptosis, as well as the occurrence of regions displaying cytoplasmic shrinkage and condensation that might be related to apoptotic cell death. Numerous studies have linked CR and SB's ability to inhibit tumor growth in the DEN animal model of cancer to their ability to induce apoptosis by upregulating caspase-3 and Bax and downregulating the anti-apoptotic protein Bcl-2, which in turn encourages apoptosis [33,40,41,62]. Compared to the individual effects, the combined effect was more robust. This is consistent with previous studies that looked at SB combination therapies to reduce SB resistance [65,66]. These combination therapies using natural compounds for HCC increased Bax and caspase-3 and decreased Bcl-2, indicating apoptotic activation to overcome SB resistance.

Treatment with CR, SB, and their combination was highly effective in reducing liver β-catenin overexpression as well as liver tumor and liver proliferation. According to several studies, up to 78% of HCCs have β-catenin activation in their tissue [46,47]. HCC, among other liver cancers, is exacerbated by β-catenin signaling [47,67], which has been linked to an increased β-catenin expression level in DEN-treated rats [68,69]. As a result of β-catenin activation and subsequent trafficking into the nuclei, downstream target genes are stimulated to express themselves, which causes aberrant cell proliferation and ultimately carcinogenesis [67]. Our findings imply that CR, SB, and their combination affected the β-catenin signaling system because they reduced the elevation of β-catenin protein levels in the HCC model. Therefore, by controlling the β-catenin signaling system, treatment with SB and CR reduced HCC cell proliferation and tumorigenicity. The downregulation of the β-catenin effects in the HCC model was shown to be improved by SB and CR combination over CR and SB alone. Here, we demonstrated how CR–SB combination therapy contributed to the additive downregulation of β-catenin tissue expression.

Chronic Inflammation marked by an overexpression of COX-2 has been linked to the development of HCC [70,71]. The rate-limiting enzyme, COX-2, is responsible for mitogenic stimuli and inflammation, which promote the synthesis of prostaglandins in neoplastic tissue and inflamed areas [70,71]. In the current investigation, the rats given DEN had much higher levels of COX-2 than the rats given a control, indicating that this model may be stimulating the inflammatory pathways. Our findings are consistent with previous reports that showed DEN treatment increased COX-2 levels [70,71]. When CR, SB, or both were administered, the inflammatory pathway was markedly suppressed, as evidenced by a substantial drop in the COX-2 levels when compared to rats who had received DEN treatment. In this respect, our findings are consistent with earlier investigations demonstrating the comparable effects of CR and SB on COX-2 [26,40]. The oncogenic transcription factor NF-κB regulates COX-2 in a variety of cancer cell types and mediates cross-talk between inflammation and cancer on a number of different levels [72]. Notably, numerous studies have demonstrated that NF-κB activation encourages the development of cancer. NF-κB promotes angiogenesis, invasion, metastasis, anti-apoptosis, and proliferation [72,73]. The present findings of NF-κB-p65 in the livers of DEN-treated rats imply that inflammation may have taken place as a result of its up-regulation [31]. The up-regulation of NF-κB-p65 in the HCC group was required for the activation of COX-2 and, consequently, inflammation and carcinogenesis, as further corroborated by our findings of NF-κB-p65 in the liver of DEN-induced rats. When comparing HCC-induced rats to those given CR, SB, or both, the level of NF-κB-p65 was dramatically lowered in all the treatments, and the upregulation of NF-κB-p65 levels was additively decreased by the CR–SB combination. In this sense, our findings are consistent with those of prior studies that found CR and SB had comparable effects on NF-κB-p65 levels [26,35,74,75].

5. Conclusions

In conclusion, our findings in the cirrhotic rat model of HCC suggest that CR, when combined with SB, potentiates the anticancer effects of SB. CR promotes apoptosis, and reduces cellular proliferation, making it a viable medication for the treatment of HCC with few side effects. The downregulation of NF-κB-p65, COX-2, and β-catenin is part of the mechanism behind these positive effects (Figure 8). Therefore, both in monotherapy and in combination therapy with already available treatments like SB, this inexpensive agent is a great candidate for pharmacological repurposing as an oncological treatment. These findings point to CR and SB as potential options for further clinical studies in the treatment of HCC. However, it is important to consider the limitations associated with the experimental design presented in this study. Establishing an animal model that reflects the exact etiological complexity and heterogeneity of human HCC is a challenge. It has been reported that DEN may need to be administered for at least a year to effectively induce an HCC model that is equivalent to human HCC [76]. Despite this, DEN-induced HCC in animal models provide reliable insights into the benefits of the presented treatment regimen.

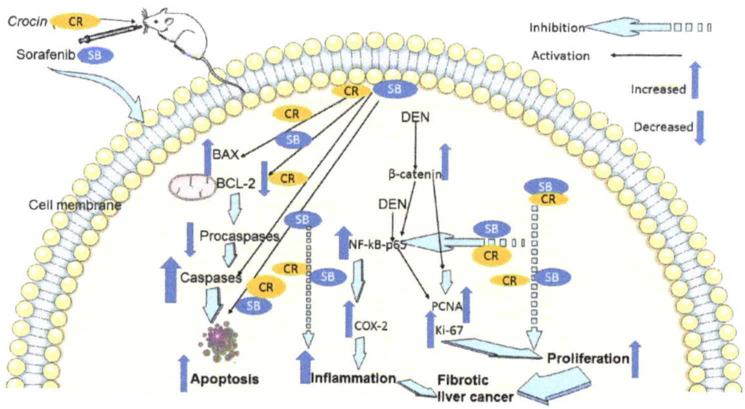

Figure 8. A schematic diagram of the anticancer molecular mechanism of CR and SB in cirrhotic liver cancer model. The pro-apoptotic proteins Bax and caspase-3 are upregulated by combination treatment CR and SB, while Bcl-2, pro-caspase-3, and pro-caspase-9 are downregulated. Thus, caspase-mediated apoptosis is induced. In addition, combination treatment reduces Ki-67 and PCNA proliferative markers. Reducing elevated protein levels of β-catenin and the inflammatory markers NF-κB and COX-2 in the HCC animal model leads to the antiproliferative and anti-inflammatory and apoptotic effects of combination therapy.

Supplementary Materials: The following supporting information can be downloaded at: https://www.mdpi.com/article/10.3390/cancers15164063/s1, File S1: Original western blots.

Author Contributions: A.A. designed the study. B.A., A.A.H. and A.A. performed the experiments and did the statistical analysis. S.A.-S., A.A.-M. and A.A. assisted with methodology and contributed resources. A.A., A.A.H. and A.A.-M. wrote the first draft of the manuscript, and A.A., A.A.H., A.A.-M. and S.A.-S. contributed to the editing of the manuscript. All authors have read and agreed to the published version of the manuscript.

Funding: This research was partially funded by Terry Fox Foundation fund number 21S103 and Zayed Bin Sultan Center for Health Sciences, United Arab Emirates University fund number 12R043.

Institutional Review Board Statement: Animal ethics form has been submitted and approved by the Animal Research Ethics Committee of the College of Medicine and Health Sciences, UAEU (Approval No. A8-15).

Informed Consent Statement: Not applicable.

Data Availability Statement: All data are readily available in the manuscript.

Acknowledgments: Authors are grateful for Chandraprabha Murali for her valuable technical assistance throughout this work and to Aisha Alotaibi for her help reviewing the proof.

Conflicts of Interest: The authors declare no conflict of interest.

References

1. Deo, S.V.S.; Sharma, J.; Kumar, S. GLOBOCAN 2020 Report on Global Cancer Burden: Challenges and Opportunities for Surgical Oncologists. *Ann. Surg. Oncol.* **2022**, *29*, 6497–6500. [CrossRef] [PubMed]
2. ReFaey, K.; Tripathi, S.; Grewal, S.S.; Bhargav, A.G.; Quinones, D.J.; Chaichana, K.L.; Antwi, S.O.; Cooper, L.T.; Meyer, F.B.; Dronca, R.S.; et al. Cancer Mortality Rates Increasing vs. Cardiovascular Disease Mortality Decreasing in the World: Future Implications. *Mayo Clin. Proc. Innov. Qual. Outcomes* **2021**, *5*, 645–653. [CrossRef] [PubMed]

3. Sung, H.; Ferlay, J.; Siegel, R.L.; Laversanne, M.; Soerjomataram, I.; Jemal, A.; Bray, F. Global Cancer Statistics 2020: GLOBOCAN Estimates of Incidence and Mortality Worldwide for 36 Cancers in 185 Countries. *CA Cancer J. Clin.* **2021**, *71*, 209–249. [CrossRef] [PubMed]
4. GLOBOCAN 2020: United Arab. Emirates [Fact. Sheet]; World Health Organization International Agency for Research on Cancer (IARC). 2020. Available online: https://gco.iarc.fr/today/data/factsheets/populations/784-united-arab-emirates-fact-sheets.pdf (accessed on 24 May 2023).
5. Albarrak, J.; Al-Shamsi, H. Current Status of Management of Hepatocellular Carcinoma in The Gulf Region: Challenges and Recommendations. *Cancers* **2023**, *15*, 2001. [CrossRef]
6. Rumgay, H.; Ferlay, J.; de Martel, C.; Georges, D.; Ibrahim, A.S.; Zheng, R.; Wei, W.; Lemmens, V.; Soerjomataram, I. Global, regional and national burden of primary liver cancer by subtype. *Eur. J. Cancer* **2022**, *161*, 108–118. [CrossRef]
7. Crusz, S.M.; Balkwill, F.R. Inflammation and cancer: Advances and new agents. *Nat. Rev. Clin. Oncol.* **2015**, *12*, 584–596. [CrossRef]
8. Plummer, M.; de Martel, C.; Vignat, J.; Ferlay, J.; Bray, F.; Franceschi, S. Global burden of cancers attributable to infections in 2012: A synthetic analysis. *Lancet Glob. Health* **2016**, *4*, e609–e616. [CrossRef]
9. Vogel, A.; Cervantes, A.; Chau, I.; Daniele, B.; Llovet, J.; Meyer, T.; Nault, J.-C.; Neumann, U.; Ricke, J.; Sangro, B. Hepatocellular carcinoma: ESMO Clinical Practice Guidelines for diagnosis, treatment and follow-up. *Ann. Oncol.* **2018**, *29*, iv238–iv255. [CrossRef]
10. Zhou, Y.; Li, Y.; Zhou, T.; Zheng, J.; Li, S.; Li, H.B. Dietary Natural Products for Prevention and Treatment of Liver Cancer. *Nutrients* **2016**, *8*, 156. [CrossRef]
11. Park, D.H.; Shin, J.W.; Park, S.K.; Seo, J.N.; Li, L.; Jang, J.J.; Lee, M.J. Diethylnitrosamine (DEN) induces irreversible hepatocellular carcinogenesis through overexpression of G1/S-phase regulatory proteins in rat. *Toxicol. Lett.* **2009**, *191*, 321–326. [CrossRef]
12. Tolba, R.; Kraus, T.; Liedtke, C.; Schwarz, M.; Weiskirchen, R. Diethylnitrosamine (DEN)-induced carcinogenic liver injury in mice. *Lab. Anim.* **2015**, *49* (Suppl. S1), 59–69. [CrossRef] [PubMed]
13. Santos, N.P.; Colaco, A.A.; Oliveira, P.A. Animal models as a tool in hepatocellular carcinoma research: A Review. *Tumor Biol.* **2017**, *39*, 1010428317695923. [CrossRef] [PubMed]
14. Llovet, J.M.; Zucman-Rossi, J.; Pikarsky, E.; Sangro, B.; Schwartz, M.; Sherman, M.; Gores, G. Hepatocellular carcinoma. *Nat. Rev. Dis. Primers* **2016**, *2*, 16018. [CrossRef] [PubMed]
15. Niu, M.; Yi, M.; Li, N.; Wu, K.; Wu, K. Advances of Targeted Therapy for Hepatocellular Carcinoma. *Front. Oncol.* **2021**, *11*, 719896. [CrossRef] [PubMed]
16. Liu, L.; Cao, Y.; Chen, C.; Zhang, X.; McNabola, A.; Wilkie, D.; Wilhelm, S.; Lynch, M.; Carter, C. Sorafenib blocks the RAF/MEK/ERK pathway, inhibits tumor angiogenesis, and induces tumor cell apoptosis in hepatocellular carcinoma model PLC/PRF. *Cancer Res.* **2006**, *66*, 11851–11858. [CrossRef]
17. Subramaniam, A.; Shanmugam, M.K.; Perumal, E.; Li, F.; Nachiyappan, A.; Dai, X.; Swamy, S.N.; Ahn, K.S.; Kumar, A.P.; Tan, B.K.; et al. Potential role of signal transducer and activator of transcription (STAT)3 signaling pathway in inflammation, survival, proliferation and invasion of hepatocellular carcinoma. *Biochim. Biophys. Acta* **2013**, *1835*, 46–60. [CrossRef] [PubMed]
18. Llovet, J.M.; Ricci, S.; Mazzaferro, V.; Hilgard, P.; Gane, E.; Blanc, J.F.; de Oliveira, A.C.; Santoro, A.; Raoul, J.L.; Forner, A.; et al. Sorafenib in advanced hepatocellular carcinoma. *N. Engl. J. Med.* **2008**, *359*, 378–390. [CrossRef]
19. Jilkova, Z.M.; Kuyucu, A.Z.; Kurma, K.; Ahmad Pour, S.T.; Roth, G.S.; Abbadessa, G.; Yu, Y.; Schwartz, B.; Sturm, N.; Marche, P.N.; et al. Combination of AKT inhibitor ARQ 092 and sorafenib potentiates inhibition of tumor progression in cirrhotic rat model of hepatocellular carcinoma. *Oncotarget* **2018**, *9*, 11145–11158. [CrossRef]
20. Bort, A.; Spinola, E.; Rodriguez-Henche, N.; Diaz-Laviada, I. Capsaicin exerts synergistic antitumor effect with sorafenib in hepatocellular carcinoma cells through AMPK activation. *Oncotarget* **2017**, *8*, 87684–87698. [CrossRef]
21. Changxing, L.; Galani, S.; Hassan, F.U.; Rashid, Z.; Naveed, M.; Fang, D.; Ashraf, A.; Qi, W.; Arif, A.; Saeed, M.; et al. Biotechnological approaches to the production of plant-derived promising anticancer agents: An update and overview. *Biomed. Pharmacother.* **2020**, *132*, 110918. [CrossRef]
22. Man, S.; Luo, C.; Yan, M.; Zhao, G.; Ma, L.; Gao, W. Treatment for liver cancer: From sorafenib to natural products. *Eur. J. Med. Chem.* **2021**, *224*, 113690. [CrossRef] [PubMed]
23. Rodriguez, S.; Skeet, K.; Mehmetoglu-Gurbuz, T.; Goldfarb, M.; Karri, S.; Rocha, J.; Shahinian, M.; Yazadi, A.; Poudel, S.; Subramani, R. Phytochemicals as an Alternative or Integrative Option, in Conjunction with Conventional Treatments for Hepatocellular Carcinoma. *Cancers* **2021**, *13*, 5753. [CrossRef] [PubMed]
24. Das, I.; Das, S.; Saha, T. Saffron suppresses oxidative stress in DMBA-induced skin carcinoma: A histopathological study. *Acta Histochem.* **2010**, *112*, 317–327. [CrossRef] [PubMed]
25. Amin, A.; Hamza, A.A.; Bajbouj, K.; Ashraf, S.S.; Daoud, S. Saffron: A potential candidate for a novel anticancer drug against hepatocellular carcinoma. *Hepatology* **2011**, *54*, 857–867. [CrossRef]
26. Amin, A.; Hamza, A.A.; Daoud, S.; Khazanehdari, K.; Hrout, A.A.; Baig, B.; Chaiboonchoe, A.; Adrian, T.E.; Zaki, N.; Salehi-Ashtiani, K. Saffron-Based Crocin Prevents Early Lesions of Liver Cancer: In vivo, In vitro and Network Analyses. *Recent Pat. Anti-Cancer Drug Discov.* **2016**, *11*, 121–133. [CrossRef]
27. Milajerdi, A.; Djafarian, K.; Hosseini, B. The toxicity of saffron (Crocus sativus L.) and its constituents against normal and cancer cells. *J. Nutr. Intermed. Metab.* **2016**, *3*, 23–32. [CrossRef]

28. Mollaei, H.; Safaralizadeh, R.; Babaei, E.; Abedini, M.R.; Hoshyar, R. The anti-proliferative and apoptotic effects of crocin on chemosensitive and chemoresistant cervical cancer cells. *Biomed. Pharmacother.* **2017**, *94*, 307–316. [CrossRef]
29. Khorasanchi, Z.; Shafiee, M.; Kermanshahi, F.; Khazaei, M.; Ryzhikov, M.; Parizadeh, M.R.; Kermanshahi, B.; Ferns, G.A.; Avan, A.; Hassanian, S.M. Crocus sativus a natural food coloring and flavoring has potent anti-tumor properties. *Phytomedicine* **2018**, *43*, 21–27. [CrossRef]
30. Bathaie, S.Z.; Miri, H.; Mohagheghi, M.A.; Mokhtari-Dizaji, M.; Shahbazfar, A.A.; Hasanzadeh, H. Saffron Aqueous Extract Inhibits the Chemically-induced Gastric Cancer Progression in the Wistar Albino Rat. *Iran. J. Basic Med. Sci.* **2013**, *16*, 27–38.
31. Amin, A. Prevention of Liver Cancer with Safranal-Based Formulations. U.S. Patent 10,912,741, 9 February 2021.
32. Abdalla, Y.; Abdalla, A.; Hamza, A.A.; Amin, A. Safranal Prevents Liver Cancer Through Inhibiting Oxidative Stress and Alleviating Inflammation. *Front. Pharmacol.* **2021**, *12*, 777500. [CrossRef]
33. Amin, A.; Awad, B. Crocin-Sorafenib Combination Therapy for Liver Cancer. U.S. Patent 10,933,076, 2 March 2021.
34. Li, X.; Zhou, X.P.; Guan, Y.S.; Wang, Y.X. Magnetic resonance imaging of hepatocellular carcinoma induced by diethylnitrosamine in Sprague-Dawley rats. *Hepatobiliary Pancreat. Dis. Int.* **2005**, *4*, 427–432. [PubMed]
35. Abdu, S.; Juaid, N.; Amin, A.; Moulay, M.; Miled, N. Therapeutic Effects of Crocin Alone or in Combination with Sorafenib against Hepatocellular Carcinoma: In Vivo & In Vitro Insights. *Antioxidants* **2022**, *11*, 1645.
36. Velasco-Loyden, G.; Perez-Martinez, L.; Vidrio-Gomez, S.; Perez-Carreon, J.I.; Chagoya de Sanchez, V. Cancer chemoprevention by an adenosine derivative in a model of cirrhosis-hepatocellular carcinoma induced by diethylnitrosamine in rats. *Tumor Biol.* **2017**, *39*, 1010428317691190. [CrossRef] [PubMed]
37. Schiffer, E.; Housset, C.; Cacheux, W.; Wendum, D.; Desbois-Mouthon, C.; Rey, C.; Clergue, F.; Poupon, R.; Barbu, V.; Rosmorduc, O. Gefitinib, an EGFR inhibitor, prevents hepatocellular carcinoma development in the rat liver with cirrhosis. *Hepatology* **2005**, *41*, 307–314. [CrossRef] [PubMed]
38. DePeralta, D.K.; Wei, L.; Ghoshal, S.; Schmidt, B.; Lauwers, G.Y.; Lanuti, M.; Chung, R.T.; Tanabe, K.K.; Fuchs, B.C. Metformin prevents hepatocellular carcinoma development by suppressing hepatic progenitor cell activation in a rat model of cirrhosis. *Cancer* **2016**, *122*, 1216–1227. [CrossRef] [PubMed]
39. Gross, C.; Steiger, K.; Sayyed, S.; Heid, I.; Feuchtinger, A.; Walch, A.; Hess, J.; Unger, K.; Zitzelsberger, H.; Settles, M.; et al. Model Matters: Differences in Orthotopic Rat Hepatocellular Carcinoma Physiology Determine Therapy Response to Sorafenib. *Clin. Cancer Res.* **2015**, *21*, 4440–4450. [CrossRef]
40. El-Kharrag, R.; Amin, A.; Hisaindee, S.; Greish, Y.; Karam, S.M. Development of a therapeutic model of precancerous liver using crocin-coated magnetite nanoparticles. *Int. J. Oncol.* **2017**, *50*, 212–222. [CrossRef]
41. El-Ashmawy, N.E.; Khedr, E.G.; El-Bahrawy, H.A.; Abd El-Fattah, E.E. Sorafenib effect on liver neoplastic changes in rats: More than a kinase inhibitor. *Clin. Exp. Med.* **2017**, *17*, 185–191. [CrossRef]
42. Ghufran, H.; Azam, M.; Mehmood, A.; Butt, H.; Riazuddin, S. Standardization of diethylnitrosamine-induced hepatocellular carcinoma rat model with time based molecular assessment. *Exp. Mol. Pathol.* **2021**, *123*, 104715. [CrossRef]
43. Aldridge, G.M.; Podrebarac, D.M.; Greenough, W.T.; Weiler, I.J. The use of total protein stains as loading controls: An alternative to high-abundance single-protein controls in semi-quantitative immunoblotting. *J. Neurosci. Methods* **2008**, *172*, 250–254. [CrossRef]
44. Hu, X.; Du, S.; Yu, J.; Yang, X.; Yang, C.; Zhou, D.; Wang, Q.; Qin, S.; Yan, X.; He, L.; et al. Common housekeeping proteins are upregulated in colorectal adenocarcinoma and hepatocellular carcinoma, making the total protein a better "housekeeper". *Oncotarget* **2016**, *7*, 66679–66688. [CrossRef] [PubMed]
45. Scholzen, T.; Gerdes, J. The Ki-67 protein: From the known and the unknown. *J. Cell Physiol.* **2000**, *182*, 311–322. [CrossRef]
46. Suzuki, T.; Yano, H.; Nakashima, Y.; Nakashima, O.; Kojiro, M. Beta-catenin expression in hepatocellular carcinoma: A possible participation of beta-catenin in the dedifferentiation process. *J. Gastroenterol. Hepatol.* **2002**, *17*, 994–1000. [CrossRef] [PubMed]
47. Tien, L.T.; Ito, M.; Nakao, M.; Niino, D.; Serik, M.; Nakashima, M.; Wen, C.Y.; Yatsuhashi, H.; Ishibashi, H. Expression of beta-catenin in hepatocellular carcinoma. *World J. Gastroenterol.* **2005**, *11*, 2398–2401. [CrossRef] [PubMed]
48. Tang, W.; Chen, Z.; Zhang, W.; Cheng, Y.; Zhang, B.; Wu, F.; Wang, Q.; Wang, S.; Rong, D.; Reiter, F.P.; et al. The mechanisms of sorafenib resistance in hepatocellular carcinoma: Theoretical basis and therapeutic aspects. *Signal Transduct. Target. Ther.* **2020**, *5*, 87. [CrossRef]
49. Llovet, J.M.; Kelley, R.K.; Villanueva, A.; Singal, A.G.; Pikarsky, E.; Roayaie, S.; Lencioni, R.; Koike, K.; Zucman-Rossi, J.; Finn, R.S. Hepatocellular carcinoma. *Nat. Rev. Dis. Primers* **2021**, *7*, 6. [CrossRef]
50. Ishiguro, S.; Inoue, M.; Tanaka, Y.; Mizokami, M.; Iwasaki, M.; Tsugane, S.; Group, J.S. Serum aminotransferase level and the risk of hepatocellular carcinoma: A population-based cohort study in Japan. *Eur. J. Cancer Prev.* **2009**, *18*, 26–32. [CrossRef]
51. Kalantar, M.; Kalantari, H.; Goudarzi, M.; Khorsandi, L.; Bakhit, S.; Kalantar, H. Crocin ameliorates methotrexate-induced liver injury via inhibition of oxidative stress and inflammation in rats. *Pharmacol. Rep.* **2019**, *71*, 746–752. [CrossRef]
52. Gedik, S.; Erdemli, M.E.; Gul, M.; Yigitcan, B.; Gozukara Bag, H.; Aksungur, Z.; Altinoz, E. Hepatoprotective effects of crocin on biochemical and histopathological alterations following acrylamide-induced liver injury in Wistar rats. *Biomed. Pharmacother.* **2017**, *95*, 764–770. [CrossRef]
53. Sokar, S.S.; Alkabbani, M.A.; Akool, E.S.; Abu-Risha, S.E. Hepatoprotective effects of carvedilol and crocin against leflunomide-induced liver injury. *Int. Immunopharmacol.* **2022**, *113 Pt A*, 109297. [CrossRef]

54. Ding, W.; Chen, X.; Yang, L.; Chen, Y.; Song, J.; Bu, W.; Feng, B.; Zhang, M.; Luo, Y.; Jia, X.; et al. Combination of ShuangDan Capsule and Sorafenib Inhibits Tumor Growth and Angiogenesis in Hepatocellular Carcinoma Via PI3K/Akt/mTORC1 Pathway. *Integr. Cancer Ther.* **2022**, *21*, 15347354221078888. [CrossRef] [PubMed]
55. Cheng, Y.; Zheng, H.; Wang, B.; Xu, W.; Xu, J.; Zhu, Y. Sorafenib and fluvastatin synergistically alleviate hepatic fibrosis via inhibiting the TGFbeta1/Smad3 pathway. *Dig. Liver Dis.* **2018**, *50*, 381–388. [CrossRef] [PubMed]
56. Maru, G.B.; Hudlikar, R.R.; Kumar, G.; Gandhi, K.; Mahimkar, M.B. Understanding the molecular mechanisms of cancer prevention by dietary phytochemicals: From experimental models to clinical trials. *World J. Biol. Chem.* **2016**, *7*, 88–99. [CrossRef] [PubMed]
57. Farzaneh, Z.; Vosough, M.; Agarwal, T.; Farzaneh, M. Critical signaling pathways governing hepatocellular carcinoma behavior; small molecule-based approaches. *Cancer Cell Int.* **2021**, *21*, 208. [CrossRef] [PubMed]
58. Bologna-Molina, R.; Mosqueda-Taylor, A.; Molina-Frechero, N.; Mori-Estevez, A.D.; Sanchez-Acuna, G. Comparison of the value of PCNA and Ki-67 as markers of cell proliferation in ameloblastic tumors. *Med. Oral Patol. Oral Cir. Bucal* **2013**, *18*, e174–e179. [CrossRef] [PubMed]
59. Jayakiran, M. Apoptosis-Biochemistry: A Mini Review. *J. Clin. Exp. Pathol.* **2015**, *5*, 205. [CrossRef]
60. Mohammad, R.M.; Muqbil, I.; Lowe, L.; Yedjou, C.; Hsu, H.Y.; Lin, L.T.; Siegelin, M.D.; Fimognari, C.; Kumar, N.B.; Dou, Q.P.; et al. Broad targeting of resistance to apoptosis in cancer. *Semin. Cancer Biol.* **2015**, *35*, S78–S103. [CrossRef]
61. Thomas, N.S.; George, K.; Selvam, A.A.A. Troxerutin subdues hepatic tumorigenesis via disrupting the MDM2-p53 interaction. *Food Funct.* **2018**, *9*, 5336–5349. [CrossRef]
62. Younis, N.S.; Ghanim, A.M.H.; Saber, S. Mebendazole augments sensitivity to sorafenib by targeting MAPK and BCL-2 signalling in n-nitrosodiethylamine-induced murine hepatocellular carcinoma. *Sci. Rep.* **2019**, *9*, 19095. [CrossRef]
63. Li, J.; Dou, D.; Li, P.; Luo, W.; Lv, W.; Zhang, C.; Song, X.; Yang, Y.; Zhang, Y.; Xu, Y.; et al. PARP-1 serves as a novel molecular marker for hepatocellular carcinoma in a Southern Chinese Zhuang population. *Tumor Biol.* **2017**, *39*, 1010428317706914. [CrossRef]
64. Boudreau, M.W.; Peh, J.; Hergenrother, P.J. Procaspase-3 Overexpression in Cancer: A Paradoxical Observation with Therapeutic Potential. *ACS Chem. Biol.* **2019**, *14*, 2335–2348. [CrossRef] [PubMed]
65. Bahman, A.A.; Abaza, M.S.I.; Khoushiash, S.I.; Al-Attiyah, R.J. Sequence-dependent effect of sorafenib in combination with natural phenolic compounds on hepatic cancer cells and the possible mechanism of action. *Int. J. Mol. Med.* **2018**, *42*, 1695–1715. [CrossRef] [PubMed]
66. Dai, N.; Ye, R.; He, Q.; Guo, P.; Chen, H.; Zhang, Q. Capsaicin and sorafenib combination treatment exerts synergistic anti-hepatocellular carcinoma activity by suppressing EGFR and PI3K/Akt/mTOR signaling. *Oncol. Rep.* **2018**, *40*, 3235–3248. [PubMed]
67. He, S.; Tang, S. WNT/beta-catenin signaling in the development of liver cancers. *Biomed. Pharmacother.* **2020**, *132*, 110851. [CrossRef]
68. Tripathy, A.; Thakurela, S.; Sahu, M.K.; Uthanasingh, K.; Behera, M.; Ajay, A.K.; Kumari, R. The molecular connection of histopathological heterogeneity in hepatocellular carcinoma: A role of Wnt and Hedgehog signaling pathways. *PLoS ONE* **2018**, *13*, e0208194. [CrossRef]
69. Yassin, N.Y.S.; AbouZid, S.F.; El-Kalaawy, A.M.; Ali, T.M.; Almehmadi, M.M.; Ahmed, O.M. Silybum marianum total extract, silymarin and silibinin abate hepatocarcinogenesis and hepatocellular carcinoma growth via modulation of the HGF/c-Met, Wnt/beta-catenin, and PI3K/Akt/mTOR signaling pathways. *Biomed. Pharmacother.* **2022**, *145*, 112409. [CrossRef]
70. Kumar, V.; Bhatt, P.C.; Rahman, M.; Al-Abbasi, F.A.; Anwar, F.; Verma, A. Umbelliferon-alpha-d-glucopyranosyl-(2(I)-->1(II))-alpha-Dglucopyranoside ameliorates Diethylnitrosamine induced precancerous lesion development in liver via regulation of inflammation, hyperproliferation and antioxidant at pre-clinical stage. *Biomed. Pharmacother.* **2017**, *94*, 834–842. [CrossRef]
71. Kumar, V.; Al-Abbasi, F.A.; Verma, A.; Mujeeb, M.; Anwar, F. Umbelliferone β-d-galactopyranoside exerts an anti-inflammatory effect by attenuating COX-1 and COX-2. *Toxicol. Res.* **2015**, *4*, 1072–1084. [CrossRef]
72. Maeda, S.; Shibata, W. Nuclear Factor-Kappa B Actions During the Development of Hepatocellular Carcinoma. In *Liver Pathiophysiology*; Academic Press: Cambridge, MA, USA, 2017; pp. 289–293.
73. Xia, Y.; Shen, S.; Verma, I.M. NF-kappaB, an active player in human cancers. *Cancer Immunol. Res.* **2014**, *2*, 823–830. [CrossRef]
74. Chiang, I.T.; Liu, Y.C.; Wang, W.H.; Hsu, F.T.; Chen, H.W.; Lin, W.J.; Chang, W.Y.; Hwang, J.J. Sorafenib inhibits TPA-induced MMP-9 and VEGF expression via suppression of ERK/NF-kappaB pathway in hepatocellular carcinoma cells. *In Vivo* **2012**, *26*, 671–681.
75. Saber, S.; Mahmoud, A.A.A.; Goda, R.; Helal, N.S.; El-Ahwany, E.; Abdelghany, R.H. Perindopril, fosinopril and losartan inhibited the progression of diethylnitrosamine-induced hepatocellular carcinoma in mice via the inactivation of nuclear transcription factor kappa-B. *Toxicol. Lett.* **2018**, *295*, 32–40. [CrossRef] [PubMed]
76. Zhang, H.E.; Henderson, J.M.; Gorrell, M.D. Animal models for hepatocellular carcinoma. *Biochim. Biophys. Acta Mol. Basis Dis.* **2019**, *1865*, 993–1002. [CrossRef] [PubMed]

cancers

MDPI

Review

Cancer Prevention and Treatment with Polyphenols: Type IV Collagenase-Mediated Mechanisms

Wojciech Pawłowski, Miłosz Caban and Urszula Lewandowska *

Department of Biochemistry, Faculty of Medicine, Medical University of Lodz, Mazowiecka 5, 92-215 Lodz, Poland; wojciech.pawlowski1@student.umed.lodz.pl (W.P.); milosz.caban@student.umed.lodz.pl (M.C.)
* Correspondence: urszula.lewandowska@umed.lodz.pl

Simple Summary: Natural polyphenols are well-known dietary supplements that have been used for medical purposes for a long time. Consuming foods and beverages of plant origin, especially those rich in polyphenolic compounds, may have chemopreventive and therapeutic effects on cancer due to the health-promoting properties of these compounds. Polyphenols are characterized by high structural diversity, which contributes to their wide range of therapeutic effects, including anti-oxidant and anti-cancer activities. These compounds can modulate the expression and activity of many proteins, including enzymes, and regulate multiple cell signaling pathways. Among the molecular targets of anti-cancer agents are matrix metalloproteinases, particularly metalloproteinase-2 and metalloproteinase-9, and nuclear factor-kappa B. Matrix metalloproteinases can degrade the protein components of the extracellular matrix and play key roles in physiological processes such as tissue repair and morphogenesis, as well as in carcinogenesis and other pathological processes. The inhibition of their synthesis and activity is closely related to a reduction in the metastasis and invasion of cancer cells. This review discusses the current state of knowledge concerning the anti-invasive and anti-metastatic potential of selected polyphenols, with a focus on in vitro and in vivo evidence.

Abstract: Polyphenols are natural compounds found in many plants and their products. Their high structural diversity bestows upon them a range of anti-inflammatory, anti-oxidant, proapoptotic, anti-angiogenic, and anti-metastatic properties, and a growing body of research indicates that a polyphenol-rich diet can inhibit cancer development in humans. Polyphenolic compounds may modulate the expression, secretion, or activity of compounds that play a significant role in carcinogenesis, including type IV collagenases, such as matrix metalloproteinase-2 (MMP-2) and matrix metalloproteinase-9 (MMP-9), by suppressing cellular signaling pathways such as nuclear factor-kappa B. These enzymes are responsible for the degradation of the extracellular matrix, thus promoting the progression of cancer. This review discusses the current state of knowledge concerning the anti-cancer activity of polyphenols, particularly curcumin, resveratrol, epigallocatechin-3-gallate, genistein, and quercetin, with a specific focus on their anti-invasive and anti-metastatic potential, based on the most recent in vitro and in vivo studies. It appears that polyphenols may be valuable options for the chemoprevention and treatment of cancer via the inhibition of MMP-2 and MMP-9 and the suppression of signaling pathways regulating their expression and activity.

Keywords: polyphenols; anti-cancer; anti-oxidant; chemoprevention; gelatinases; MMP; NF-κB

1. Introduction

Cancer presents significant problems for health care worldwide. The most recent data from GLOBOCAN 2022, prepared by the International Agency for Research on Cancer, indicate that 20 million new cases of cancer occurred globally in 2022, with approximately 10 million cancer-related deaths also being reported [1]. Unfortunately, it is estimated that the incidence of cancer will increase by about 77% by the year 2050 [1]. Unfortunately, many anti-cancer drugs are expensive, and their use is often associated with severe side effects and complications; in addition, resistance to cancer therapy is becoming more prevalent [2,3]. Regrettably, many cancers are diagnosed at an advanced stage of disease, when the efficacy of therapy is limited [4,5]; hence, there is a need for more preventive and therapeutic strategies and to identify new agents that could lower the burden of cancers.

To effectively restrict the development and progression of cancer, any potential chemopreventive agents should be able to inhibit cell viability and migration and demonstrate anti-invasive and anti-metastatic potential. A key step responsible for the invasion and migration of cancer cells is the remodeling of the extracellular matrix (ECM) [6,7]. This tumorigenic process can be divided into three stages: ECM deposition, modification, and degradation. Firstly, cancer-associated fibroblasts deposit collagen and other components, such as fibronectin, laminin, and hyaluronic acid. Then, biochemical modifications of the existing ECM structure take place, consisting of fibrosis, increased ECM stiffness, and the creation of cell migration channels. Finally, matrix metalloproteinases (MMPs) and other enzymes cause the degradation of the ECM structure, which promotes tumor proliferation, migration, invasion, and angiogenesis [7]. Therefore, MMPs play a key role in this process. In particular, the expression and activity of MMP-2 and MMP-9, also known as gelatinases or type IV collagenases, are correlated with the aggressiveness of cancer and a poor prognosis [8,9].

These enzymes degrade ECM components, primarily type IV collagen, enabling cell migration and the formation of pathological blood vessels and metastases [10]. Thus, MMPs are recognized as boosters of tumor growth [11]. Their expression is known to be regulated by certain signaling pathways, mainly nuclear factor-kappa B (NF-κB) or mitogen-activated protein kinases/extracellular-signal-regulated kinases (MAPK/ERK) [12]. Therefore, potential chemopreventive agents should not only reduce the expression and activity of MMP-2 and MMP-9 but also modulate cellular signaling pathway activation.

For centuries, natural compounds of plant origin have been used to treat diseases. Recently, their influence on carcinogenesis has been intensively studied to improve the difficult and challenging process of managing cancer. They are generally characterized by minor side effects and high safety but also, unfortunately, low water solubility and bioavailability. One of the methods to overcome these disadvantages is the use of modern nanodrug delivery systems [7]. Plant-derived compounds, specifically polyphenols—the subject of this review—are suggested to play an important role in preventing cancer progression as MMP, especially MMP-2 and MMP-9, inhibitors [13].

Natural compounds have also been shown to regulate the epithelial–mesenchymal transition (EMT). This term refers to morphological changes in epithelial cells that gain phenotypic characteristics of mesenchymal cells. The EMT includes the deconstruction of epithelial cell-to-cell bonds, the loss of apical–basal polarity, the rebuilding of the actin cytoskeleton, the general prevalence of mesenchymal over epithelial markers, and the increased expression of MMPs. All of these changes occur at the very beginning of cancer development and are responsible for enhanced cell motility, the acquisition of the ability to invade and consequently form distant metastases, and even increased therapeutic resistance [14–16]. Therefore, an attempt to reverse EMT changes, especially those associated with MMPs, could be an attractive way to treat cancer. While studies on synthetic MMP inhibitors, such as marimastat, rebimastat, and tanomastat, failed due to their strong adverse effects, phytochemicals, devoid of such properties, offer an alternative to them [11,15].

This review provides a comprehensive overview of the anti-cancer potential of the most common single polyphenolic compounds, such as curcumin, resveratrol, epigallocatechin-3-gallate (EGCG), quercetin, and genistein (Figure 1), known to modulate the activity and expression of MMP-2 and MMP-9. We selected these polyphenolic compounds due to their various unique pro-health properties and their diverse sources of origin. A brief description of these compounds is provided in Table 1. It also examines the current state of knowledge regarding cellular signaling pathways associated with their expression and activity, particularly the NF-κB pathway, which play roles in the metastasis and invasion of cancers.

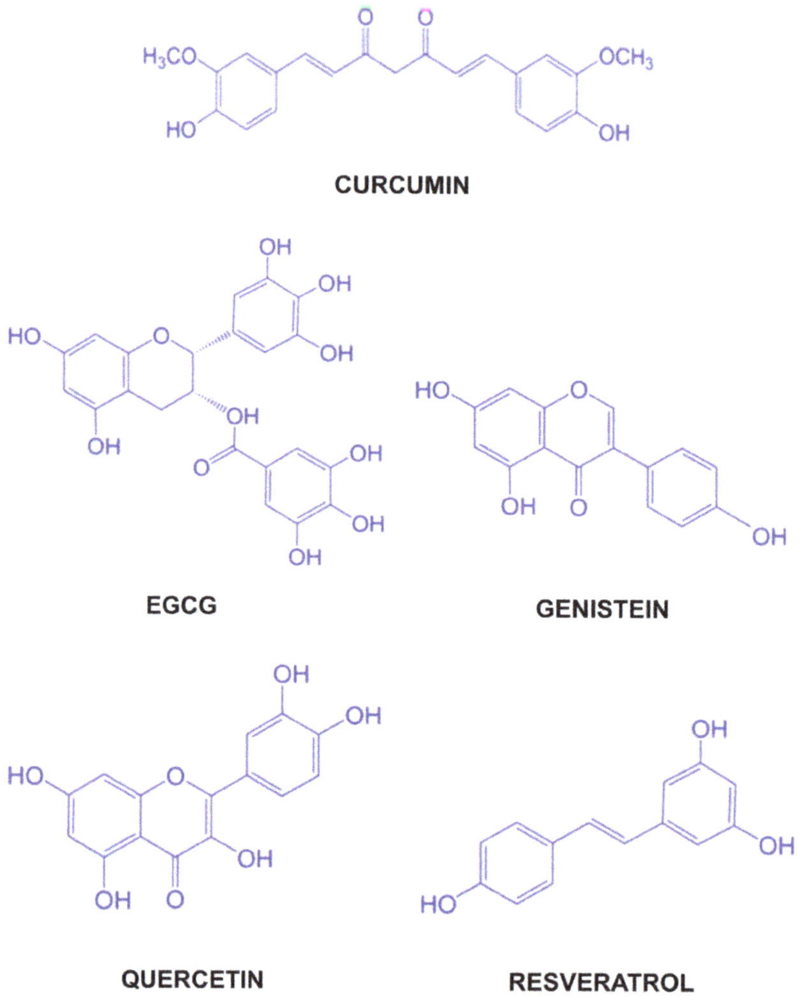

Figure 1. Chemical structures of polyphenolic compounds. Curcumin (1,7-bis(4-hydroxy-3-methoxyphenyl)-1,6-heptadiene-3,5-dione); genistein (4′,5,7-trihydroxyisoflavone); EGCG (2 R,3 R)-3′,4′,5,5′,7-pentahydroxyflavan-3-yl 3,4,5-trihydroxybenzoate); quercetin (3,3′,4′,5,7-pentahydroxyflavone); resveratrol (3,5,4′ trihydroxystilbene).

Numerous review articles describing the potential utility of polyphenols for cancer prevention and therapy have been published [7,10,14–17]. Despite this, there is still a need to identify new compounds that could contribute to the prevention of cancer development as well as enrich current forms of cancer therapies. Polyphenols, as compounds of natural origin, seem to be good candidates and are actually the subject of numerous studies. To confirm their efficacy in chemoprevention and cancer treatment, the constant updating of knowledge is necessary. This is the main reason we created this paper. We focus on five main polyphenols, which we examine after analyzing, in detail, the most recent studies on this topic. Also, we provide the mechanisms of their action.

Table 1. Overview of polyphenols described in this review.

Polyphenol	Class of Compounds	Main Pro-Health Activities	Main Food Sources of Polyphenol
Curcumin (1,7-bis(4-hydroxy-3-methoxyphenyl)-1,6-heptadiene-3,5-dione)	Curcuminoids	Anti-cancer, anti-inflammatory, anti-migratory, anti-metastatic, anti-aging	The rhizome of *Curcuma longa*
EGCG (2 R,3 R)-3′,4′,5,5′,7-pentahydroxyflavan-3-yl 3,4,5-trihydroxybenzoate)	Flavonoids: flavan-3-ols	Anti-oxidative, anti-cancer, anti-inflammatory	Green tea
Genistein (4′,5,7-trihydroxyisoflavone)	Flavonoids: isoflavones	Anti-cancer, anti-oxidant, anti-inflammatory, anti-angiogenic, proapoptotic, neuroprotective	Fermented soya (miso and natto), soy nuts, soy powder, soy milk, tofu
Quercetin (3,3′,4′,5,7-pentahydroxyflavone)	Flavonoids: flavonols	Anti-proliferative, anti-inflammatory, anti-carcinogenic, anti-oxidant, anti-bacterial, anti-viral	Onions, capers, green tea, apples, broccoli, red leaf lettuce, cherries, ginkgo, American elderberry, hypericum
Resveratrol (3,5,4′-trihydroxystilbene)	Stilbenes	Cardioprotective, anti-oxidative, anti-inflammatory, neuroprotective, anti-diabetic, anti-cancer	Grapes, red wine, chocolate, berries, mulberries, peanuts

2. Search Strategy

The PubMed, Google Scholar, Wiley, Springer, Scopus, Embase, and Web of Science databases were systematically and extensively searched to obtain the collected bibliography. The search included all studies published until May 2024 and used the following keywords, alone or in combination: cancer, cancer diseases, curcumin, EGCG, genistein, quercetin, resveratrol, polyphenols, polyphenolic compounds, chemoprevention, MMP-2, MMP-9, gelatinases, type IV collagenases. Clinical trials were searched for using the ClinicalTrials.gov database. The searches were filtered to include only those studies published in English.

3. Polyphenols as Modulators of the Activity and Expression of MMP-2 and MMP-9

Polyphenols are plant secondary metabolites that exhibit strong anti-oxidant properties, thus protecting plants from external stress and danger, for example, insects, as well as UV radiation and drying [18,19]. They are characterized by common structural characteristics, which include at least two phenyl rings and one or more hydroxyl substituents [20]. Polyphenols can be divided into two main groups: flavonoids and non-flavonoids. Flavonoids are, in fact, diphenyl propanes (C6-C3-C6), in which phenolic rings are connected by a heterocyclic ring [20]. According to their structural differences, flavonoids can be further divided into six major subclasses: anthocyanidins, flavanols, flavanones, flavones, flavonols, and isoflavonoids [21]. In turn, nonflavonoids, with a basic structure of only one aromatic ring, consist of many varying subclasses, among which the most important are phenolic acids, stilbenes, and lignans [20,21].

Recent studies indicate that polyphenols can affect various biochemical processes and regulate various intracellular pathways responsible for many pathological conditions, such as inflammation, oxidative stress, angiogenesis, and carcinogenesis [17,22–24]. Polyphenolic compounds may downregulate the expression and activity of MMP-2 and MMP-9 by modulating a number of intracellular signaling pathways, such as the NF-κB, phosphoinositide 3-kinase/protein kinase B (PI3 K/Akt), ERK, and MAPK pathways, among others [10,13,25,26]. Some of the most recent in vitro and in vivo studies investigating the effects of natural and synthetic polyphenols on the expression and activity of MMP-2 and MMP-9 in various cancer models are summarized below.

3.1. Curcumin

Curcumin (1,7-bis(4-hydroxy-3-methoxyphenyl)-1,6-heptadiene-3,5-dione) is the main natural polyphenol present in Curcuma longa (turmeric) and is widely used as a traditional medical herb in Asian cuisine [27]. It is able to modulate many carcinogenesis-related mechanisms and pathways. For instance, type IV collagenase activity has been found to be dysregulated after curcumin treatment [28].

3.1.1. In Vitro Studies

One study evaluated the effect of curcumin treatment on MMP-2 and MMP-9 gene expression in a breast cancer cell line (MDA-MB-231). While low concentrations of curcumin (10 μM) had no effect on MMP gene expression, higher concentrations (20 μM and 40 μM) yielded a significant reduction in MMP expression after 48 and 72 h incubation. This was accompanied by the elevated expression of tissue inhibitors of metalloproteinases (TIMPs), mainly TIMP-1 [29]. TIMPs, in addition to inhibiting MMPs, are also assumed to participate in processes involved in cancer progression and metastasis; in particular, they have been found to inhibit angiogenesis by selectively blocking the action of various growth factors, such as fibroblast growth factor 2 and vascular endothelial growth factor A (VEGF-A) [30]. Lin and co-workers [31] demonstrated that curcumin attenuated the migration and invasion of mouse–rat hybrid retinoblastoma ganglion cells (N18); the authors attribute this to the inhibition of MMP-2 and MMP-9 gene expression and the suppression of various signaling pathways, such as MAPK/ERK and NF-κB. These effects were time- and concentration-dependent. An in vitro study of the anti-tumor activity of curcumin in endometrial adenocarcinoma found that curcumin suppressed cancer cell migration, accompanied by a significant reduction in MMP-2 and MMP-9 protein expression [32].

In a study by Zhao and co-workers [33] on the hepatocellular carcinoma cell lines HepG2 and SK-Hep-1, Western blot analysis showed a significant reduction in MMP-2 and MMP-9 expression, resulting in strong anti-proliferative, anti-metastatic, and anti-invasive effects. Jia et al. [34] demonstrated the anti-cancer properties of curcumin in Wilms' tumor (WT) cells extracted from patients, this being the most common kidney tumor in children. When administered at a concentration of 20 mM, curcumin caused a significant reduction in MMP-2 and MMP-9 at the mRNA and protein levels. It was associated with decreased reversion-inducing cysteine-rich protein with Kazal motifs methylation and reduced proliferative, invasive, and migratory capabilities of the cells in vitro. Another study found curcumin to enhance the anti-cancer activity of metformin, with combined administration yielding stronger effects. However, the curcumin-related reduction in MMP-2 and MMP-9 protein levels was minimal in vitro, which might have resulted from the fact that very small concentrations were used (2.5 or 5 μM). Treatment also downregulated the PI3 K/Akt, NF-κB, and mammalian target of rapamycin (mTOR) signaling pathways, as well as the migration and invasion of hepatocellular carcinoma (HCC) cells [35].

Selected studies investigating the beneficial effects of curcumin in vitro are summarized in Table 2.

Table 2. Overview of in vitro studies related to curcumin.

Polyphenol	Cell Line	Concentration/ Duration	Anti-Cancer Effects	Type IV Collagenase-Mediated Mechanisms	Reference
	N18	7,5, 15 μM for 6, 12, 24, 48 h	↓cell migration ↓cell invasion	↓MMP-2 mRNA, protein ↓MMP-9 protein ↓NF-κB p65 ↓ERK-1/-2	[31]
	MDA-MB-231	10, 20, 40 μM for 24, 48, 72 h	not specified	↓MMP-2, -9 mRNA ↑TIMP-1, -2, -3, -4 mRNA	[29]

Table 2. *Cont.*

Polyphenol	Cell Line	Concentration/ Duration	Anti-Cancer Effects	Type IV Collagenase-Mediated Mechanisms	Reference
Curcumin [1,7-bis(4-hydroxy-3-methoxyphenyl)-1,6-heptadiene-3,5-dione]	Ishikawa Hec-1 B Primary endometrial adenocarcinoma cells	6 µM for 24, 30, 36, 42, 48 h	↓proliferation ↓cell migration	↓MMP-2 protein ↓MMP-9 protein	[32]
	HepG2 PLC/PRF/5	2,5, 5, 10 µM for 12, 24, 48 h with or without 2,5, 5, 10 mM metformin	↓angiogenesis ↓cell migration ↓cell invasion ↓proliferation ↑apoptosis	↓MMP-2, -9 protein, activity ↓PI3 K protein ↓pAkt protein ↓pmTOR protein	[35]
	WT Primary cells WT-1, WT-2, WT-3	10, 20 mM for 6, 12, 18, 24 h	↓cell migration ↓cell invasion ↓proliferation ↑apoptosis	↓MMP-2, -9 mRNA, protein	[34]
	LN229 U87 MG	8, 16, 24 µM for 24, 48, 72 h with or without 0,1, 1, 10 µM of norepinephrine	↓cell migration ↓cell invasion ↓proliferation ↑apoptosis	↓MMP-2, -9 mRNA, protein, activity ↓pERK-1/-2 protein	[36]
	HepG2 SK-Hep-1	20, 40, 60 µM for 24 h	↓cell migration ↓cell invasion ↓proliferation	↓MMP-2, -9 protein	[33]

Legend: ↑ activation or increase; ↓ inhibition or decrease.

3.1.2. In Vivo Studies

Numerous in vivo studies have demonstrated the ability of curcumin to suppress MMPs and subsequently limit the aggressiveness of tumors. Zhu et al. [37] examined the effect of curcumin on acute monocytic leukemia (AML) SHI-1 cells using a subcutaneous xenograft model in female severe combined immunodeficient (SCID) mice. Fifteen-day intraperitoneal therapy with curcumin (15 and 30 mg/kg) in a stand-alone treatment contributed to a significant decrease in tumor volume and weight. In addition, hematoxylin and eosin staining showed signs of intense tumor cell damage. Moreover, curcumin inhibited cell proliferation and enhanced cancer cell apoptosis within the tumor. Most significantly, curcumin suppressed the expression of MMP-2 and MMP-9 at the mRNA and protein levels in a dose-dependent manner, preventing AML metastasis. This decrease in MMP levels was confirmed by immunohistochemical staining. These changes were associated with the downregulation of the NF-κB pathway and the modulation of the MAPK pathway. In endometrial adenocarcinoma, immunohistochemical analysis of xenograft tumor sections in female six-week-old non-obese diabetic SCID (NOD-SCID) mice previously injected with Ishikawa cells demonstrated that curcumin treatment inhibited the expression of MMP-2 and MMP-9 and limited tumor growth observed after 31 days of treatment, which was not associated with any toxic effects, and the mean body weight of the animals remained stable [32].

In a study by Zhao and co-workers [33], hepatoma cells were injected into female Balb/c-nu nude mice to induce subcutaneous tumors, and HepG2 cells were intravenously injected into the caudal vein to create a metastatic tumor model. Curcumin treatment led to a dose-dependent reduction in tumor growth and final volume and a reduction in the number of tumor nodules in the lungs. Reduced MMP-2 and MMP-9 expression was noted in the tumor tissue, inhibiting the invasion and metastasis of neoplastic cells. Wang and co-workers [36] conducted an interesting study evaluating the effect of curcumin on the psychological stress-induced proliferation and invasion of glioma cells. LN229 cells were implanted into female Balb/c nu/nu mice. An adverse stress model was created by placing the animals in a 50 mL multi-well centrifuge without squeezing their bodies. It was found that the MMP-2 and MMP-9 levels in tumor tissue, epinephrine and norepinephrine levels in serum, and the tumor volume were significantly higher in the stressed group than in the non-stressed group. The curcumin treatment reversed these stress-related negative effects and reduced the protein expression of MMPs by half in the non-stressed control group. Due to the ability of curcumin to cross the blood–brain barrier, it may be a promising agent for alleviating the progression of glioma due to psychological stress. Also, in the case of WTs, the mean volume and weight of the tumors in vivo were noticeably lower after 21 days of curcumin treatment [34]. In a model of hepatocellular carcinoma in female Balb/c nu mice, 60 mg/kg curcumin treatment decreased MMP expression by approximately 25% in the xenografts, with the effect being enhanced by the addition of metformin [35].

As curcumin is characterized by low water solubility (hydrophobic), an unstable chemical structure, poor absorption, and rapid metabolism, the oral administration of its pure form does not typically yield significant health-promoting results. Hence, in recent years, studies have evaluated the use of curcumin administered in the form of nanoparticles, liposomes, and micelles. Such methods of delivering the polyphenol directly to target tissues in a living organism have yielded very promising results [38]. Tavakoli and co-workers [39] examined the effects of 12-day administration of pure (15 mg/kg) and nano-encapsulated (30 mg/kg) curcumin in a mouse B16 F10 melanoma tumor model using C57 B16 mice. In both animal groups, the expression of MMP-2 and MMP-9 genes was significantly decreased in tumor tissues, while the TIMP-1 and TIMP-2 genes were overexpressed. Although both forms inhibited tumor growth, the nano-encapsulated curcumin showed a stronger effect. These data confirm that curcumin may impair tumor growth and reduce the metastatic ability of melanoma in vivo by inhibiting MMPs and by stimulating their inhibitors.

Similar results were obtained in another in vivo study by Sesarman et al. [40], who examined the effects of curcumin, alone or combined with doxorubicin, on C26 murine colon carcinoma using male Balb/c mice with subcutaneously injected cancer cells. The animals intravenously received 5 mg/kg curcumin and 2.5 mg/kg doxorubicin in long-circulating liposomes or in free form on days 7 and 10 after tumor cell inoculation. Curcumin in its pure form led to an almost identical reduction in tumor size to that obtained with doxorubicin, i.e., a decrease of approximately 30% compared to controls. Both compounds yielded more significant results in liposomal encapsulation, i.e., about a 70% reduction in the case of curcumin. However, the highest anti-tumor efficacy was achieved when both of them were administered simultaneously, i.e., about 85%. This confirms that curcumin is able to enhance the anti-cancer properties of chemotherapeutics in vivo. The research group identified potential mechanisms. Free curcumin had no significant effect on the activity of either MMP-2 or MMP-9, although MMP-2 activity slightly increased. In turn, liposomal curcumin reduced the activity of MMP-9 by more than half, without any effect on MMP-2. Moreover, curcumin presented an anti-oxidant effect and inhibited the NF-κB pathway and AP-1, reducing the ability of the tumor to metastasize [40].

Selected studies investigating the beneficial effects of curcumin in vivo are summarized in Table 3.

3.2. Epigallocatechin-3-Gallate

Epigallocatechin-3-gallate (2 R,3 R)-3′,4′,5,5′,7-pentahydroxyflavan-3-yl 3,4,5-trihydroxybenzoate) is an important polyphenol occurring in green tea, prepared by brewing leaves from Camellia sinensis. EGCG affects a wide range of processes in humans. It is believed that EGCG may exert anti-oxidative, anti-cancer, and anti-inflammatory activities, as well as decrease blood lipids and glucose, increase insulin sensitivity, or reduce body weight [41,42]. It modulates the activity of genes and various signaling pathways involved in cell proliferation, apoptosis, and the inhibition of cancer, such as pro- and anti-apoptotic proteins (B-cell lymphoma 2 (Bcl-2), Bcl-2-like protein 4 (Bax), B-cell lymphoma-extra large (Bcl-XL)), MAPK/ERK, PI3 K/Akt, and NF-κB, and is involved in the epigenetic downregulation of oncogenes [43]. EGCG was found to have the greatest anti-proliferative effect among 10 representative green tea polyphenols [44] and has long been known to inhibit MMP-2 and MMP-9 expression [45–47].

Table 3. Overview of in vivo studies related to curcumin.

Polyphenol	Animal Model	Dose/ Duration	Anti-Tumor Effects	Type IV Collagenase-Mediated Mechanisms	Reference
Curcumin [1,7-bis(4-hydroxy-3-methoxyphenyl)-1,6-heptadiene-3,5-dione]	NOD-SCID mice injected with Ishikawa	50 mg/kg daily intraperitoneally for 31 days	↓tumor volume	↓MMP-2 protein ↓MMP-9 protein	[32]
	Balb/c mice injected with C26	5 mg/kg curcumin with or without 2.5 mg/kg doxorubicin (in free form or long-circulating liposomes, LCLs) intravenously at days 7 and 10 after inoculation	↓tumor volume	↔MMP-2 activity ↔MMP-9 activity (free curcumin) ↓MMP-9 activity (LCL–curcumin, curcumin with doxorubicin) ↓pNF-κB p65 protein	[40]
	C57 B16 mice injected with B16 F10	15 mg/kg of free curcumin or 30 mg/kg of nano-encapsulated curcumin daily intraperitoneally for 12 days (with or without identical doses of chrysin)	↓tumor volume	↓MMP-2, -9 mRNA ↑TIMP-1, -2 mRNA	[39]
	Balb/c-nu mice injected with HepG2	60 mg/kg daily intraperitoneally for 21 days with or without 150 mg/kg metformin orally	↓tumor volume	↓MMP-2, -9 protein ↓PI3 K protein ↓pAkt protein ↓pmTOR protein	[35]
	Nude mice injected with primary WT-1 and WT-3	20 mg/mL of curcumin in corn oil for 21 days	↓tumor weight ↓tumor volume ↑apoptosis	not specified	[34]
	SCID mice injected with SHI-1	15, 30 mg/kg daily intraperitoneally for 15 days	↓tumor weight ↓tumor volume ↑apoptosis	↓MMP-2, -9 mRNA, protein ↑pp38 protein ↓pERK-1/-2 protein ↓pNF-κB p65 protein	[37]
	Balb/c nu/nu mice injected with LN229	60 mg/kg daily intraperitoneally for 4 weeks, accompanied or not by restraint stress for 8 h per day	↓tumor volume	↓MMP-2, -9 protein	[36]
	Balb/c-nu mice injected with HepG2	0.2 mL of 20, 40, 60 μM curcumin daily intraperitoneally for 10 days	↓tumor volume ↓metastatic incidence in lungs	↓MMP-2, -9 protein	[33]

Legend: ↑ activation or increase; ↓ inhibition or decrease; ↔ no impact.

3.2.1. In Vitro Studies

Multiple studies have demonstrated that EGCG has an inhibitory effect on type IV collagenase expression in cancer cell lines. Roomi and colleagues [48] assessed the role of

EGCG in the regulation of MMP-2 and MMP-9 in human melanoma A-2058 cells using a gelatinase zymography assay and densitometry analysis. The cells were incubated with EGCG alone; EGCG together with phorbol 12-myristate 13-acetate (PMA), a potent tumor promoter; and PMA alone. Melanoma A-2058 is characterized by elevated secretion of both MMP-2 and -9 in comparison to normal cells. Treatment with 100 ng/mL PMA did not affect MMP-2 expression but significantly increased MMP-9 expression. Various concentrations of EGCG (10, 25, 50, 100 μM) inhibited MMP-2 and MMP-9 expression in a concentration-dependent manner, with a 57% reduction noted for MMP-2 and 73% for MMP-9 at the maximum concentration (100 μM).

Similar results were obtained in head and neck squamous carcinoma cells (FaDu) and tongue carcinoma cells (SCC-25). Quantitative densitometry analysis of gelatinase zymography revealed that EGCG (10 μM, 25 μM, 50 μM, 100 μM) decreased both MMP-2 and MMP-9 activity in a concentration-dependent manner [49]. Also, EGCG (10 μM, 25 μM, 50 μM, 100 μM) was found to block the activity of MMP-2 and MMP-9 in pediatric human sarcomata (osteosarcoma U2 OS and rhabdomyosarcoma RD) [50], adult human sarcomata (chondrosarcoma SW-1353, fibrosarcoma HT-1080, liposarcoma SW-872, synovial sarcoma SW-982) [51], the human cervical cancer lines HeLa and DoTc2-4510, the human ovarian cancer line SK-OV-3 [52], and human renal cell carcinoma 786-0 (EGCG in concentrations 10 μM, 50 μM, 100 μM, 200 μM) [53]. Multiple studies indicate that EGCG possesses anti-migratory and anti-cancer properties associated with the downregulation of MMP-2 and MMP-9. In human nasopharyngeal carcinoma cells (NPC-39, HONE-1, NPC-BM), EGCG treatment significantly lowered the expression and activity of MMP-2 and reduced the motility and invasion potential of tumor cells by half. The effect was most evident at a concentration of 50 μM EGCG, at which the activity of MMP-2 was reduced by about 70% in HONE-1 and NPC-BM and 50% in NPC-39. [54]. Likewise, EGCG at concentrations of 20 μM or more was found to inhibit, by about half, the expression and activity of MMP-2 and MMP-9 in human renal carcinoma cells (786-0 and ACHN) and thus reduce their migratory and invasive potential [55].

In cholangiocarcinoma, EGCG treatment decreased the enzymatic activity of MMP-2 and MMP-9 in a concentration-dependent manner, inhibited the invasion and migration capacity, and accelerated the apoptosis of HuCC-T1 cells [56]. In addition, EGCG inhibited the expression of MMP-9 at the mRNA and protein levels and downregulated the NF-κB pathway, as well as suppressed the migration, invasion, and proliferation of SW780 cells and induced their apoptosis. Most importantly, it did not exert any significant cytotoxic activity against normal human bladder epithelial cells [57]. EGCG loaded with poly(lactic-co glycolic acid) (PLGA) nanoparticles suppressed the NF-κB pathway and inhibited the mRNA expression of several downstream molecules, such as MMP-2, cyclooxygenase-2 (COX-2), and tumor necrosis factor α (TNF-α), in the lung cancer cell lines A549 and H1299. PLGA-encapsulated EGCG was far more effective than EGCG in its free form at the same concentration (12.5 μM, 25 μM) [58]. A previous study found that combined therapy with EGCG and a specific NF-κB inhibitor (BAY11-7082) had greater synergistic anti-tumor effects compared to individual drugs. MMP-2 expression was suppressed at the mRNA level in A549 and H1229 cells [59]. In CL1-5 cells, another lung cancer cell line characterized by high invasiveness, EGCG treatment inhibited MMP-2 and MMP-9 at the mRNA and protein levels and reduced enzymatic activity; it also suppressed MMP-2 promoter activity in a concentration-dependent manner and reduced the nuclear translocation of NF-κB and cell invasion and migration [60]. A study by Fang et al. [61] found that EGCG decreased the activity of MMP-2 and MMP-9 in Epstein–Barr virus-negative and -positive nasopharyngeal carcinoma (NPC) cell lines in a concentration-dependent manner, probably by modulating the ERK and NF-κB pathways. MMP-2 expression was also diminished at the mRNA level. As a result, the migration and invasion capabilities of cancer cells were diminished. Finally, EGCG has demonstrated anti-cancer activity in oral squamous cell carcinoma. EGCG decreased the activity of MMP-2 and MMP-9 and the mRNA and protein expression of MMP-2. In addition, TIMP-2 activity and expression were elevated, and the NF-κB and urokinase plasminogen activator (uPA) pathways, known to upregulate MMPs, were suppressed. The cells were found to have reduced motility and invasive and migratory potential, as indicated by the transwell cell invasion and wound-healing migration assays. The authors also noted a decrease in EMT markers [62]. All of these results confirm EGCG's ability to suppress cancer formation, mainly by modulating MMP-2, MMP-9, and associated pathways.

Selected studies investigating the beneficial effects of EGCG in vitro are summarized in Table 4.

Table 4. Overview of in vitro studies related to EGCG.

Polyphenol	Cell Line	Concentration/ Duration	Anti-Cancer Effects	Type IV Collagenase-Mediated Mechanisms	Reference
EGCG [(2 R,3 R)-3′,4′,5,5′,7-pentahydroxy-flavan-3-yl 3,4,5-trihydroxybenzoate]	DU-145	2, 5, 10, 20, 40 μg/mL for 24 h	not specified	↓MMP-2, -9 secretion, activity ↓NF-κB ↓ERK-1/-2 ↓p38	[46]
	786-O	10, 50, 100, 200 μg/mL for 24 h with or without PMA treatment	not specified	↓MMP-2, -9 activity	[53]
	HeLa DoTc2-4510 SK-OV-3	10, 25, 50, 100 μM for 24 h with or without PMA treatment	not specified	↓MMP-2 activity (HeLa, SK-OV-3) ↓MMP-9 activity (HeLa, DoTc2-4510)	[52]
	SCC-9	5, 10, 15, 20 μM for 24 h with or without PMA treatment	↓cell migration ↓cell invasion	↓MMP-2 mRNA, protein, activity ↓MMP-9 activity ↑TIMP-2 mRNA, protein ↓NF-κB protein	[62]
	CL1-5	5, 10, 20, 30, 40, 50 μM for 9, 12, 16, 24 h	↓cell migration ↓cell invasion	↓MMP-2 mRNA, protein, activity, promoter activity ↓MMP-9 mRNA, protein, activity ↓NF-κB nuclear translocation	[60]
	SW-1353, HT-1080, SW-872, SW-982	10, 25, 50, 100 μM for 24 h with or without PMA treatment	not specified	↓MMP-2, -9 activity	[51]
	U2 OS RD	10, 25, 50, 100 μM for 24 h with or without PMA treatment	not specified	↓MMP-2 activity ↓MMP-9 activity	[50]
	TW01 (EBV-negative) NA (EBV-positive, reinfected TW01)	10, 20, 30, 50 μM for 9, 12, 24, 48 h (cells) 1, 2.5, 5, 10, 25 μM for 7 days (spheroid)	↓spheroid formation ↓cell migration ↓cell invasion ↓proliferation	↓MMP-2 mRNA, activity ↓MMP-9 activity ↓pERK-1/-2 protein	[61]
	786-O ACHN	10, 20, 40 μg/mL for 24 h	↓cell migration ↓cell invasion	↓MMP-2, -9 activity, protein	[55]

Table 4. *Cont.*

Polyphenol	Cell Line	Concentration/ Duration	Anti-Cancer Effects	Type IV Collagenase-Mediated Mechanisms	Reference
	HuCC-T1	0.1, 0.5, 1, 5, 10, 20, 50 μg/mL for 24 h	↓cell migration ↓cell invasion ↑apoptosis	↓MMP-2 activity ↓MMP-9 activity	[56]
	SW780	12.5, 25, 50, 100 μM for 24 h	↓cell invasion ↓cell migration ↓proliferation ↑apoptosis	↓MMP-9 mRNA, protein ↓pNF-κB p65 protein ↓NF-κB mRNA	[57]
	A-2058	10, 25, 50, 100 μM for 24 h	not specified	↓MMP-2, -9 activity	[48]
	FaDu SCC-25	10, 25, 50, 100 μM for 24 h with or without PMA treatment	not specified	↓MMP-2, -9 activity	[49]
	NPC-39 HONE-1 NPC-BM	6, 12, 25, 50 μM for 12, 24 h	↓cell migration ↓cell invasion	↓MMP-2 activity, protein	[54]
	A549 H1299	20, 80, 160 μM for 24, 48 h or 20 μM with 0,625, 1.25, 2.5, 5 μM of BAY11-7082 for 24, 48 h	↓proliferation ↑apoptosis ↓cell invasion ↓cell migration	↓MMP-2 mRNA ↓NF-κB, pNF-κB mRNA, protein	[59]
	A549 H1299	12.5, 25 μM for 48 h (free EGCG or PLGA-encapsulated EGCG)	↓proliferation ↑apoptosis	↓MMP-2 mRNA ↓NF-κB, pNF-κB protein	[58]

Legend: ↑ activation or increase; ↓ inhibition or decrease.

3.2.2. In Vivo Studies

The anti-cancer properties of EGCG have been demonstrated in vivo. Shankar and co-workers [63] proved that EGCG was able to inhibit the growth of human pancreatic tumors in an animal model. Briefly, human PANC-1 cells were injected into the pancreas of Balb/c nu/nu mice, and EGCG administration (60, 80, and 100 mg/kg body weight) was begun one week after implantation. The polyphenol inhibited tumor growth in a dose-dependent manner. Interestingly, no visible signs of toxicity were observed, and the mean weight of the mice increased during the treatment. The treatment decreased MMP-2 and MMP-7 mRNA expression, reduced VEGF protein expression, and downregulated the ERK and PI3 K/Akt pathways in the tumor tissue, attenuating the metastatic ability of the cancer cells.

In the in vivo model of cholangiocarcinoma, the tumor xenograft model was established by the subcutaneous implantation of HuCC-T1 cells into the backs of Balb/c male mice. The polyphenol was subcutaneously administered beside the solid tumor at a dose of 20 mg/kg of body weight. The treatment effectively inhibited the expression of MMP-2 and MMP-9 in tumor tissue, assessed by immunohistochemical staining, and significantly decreased the tumor volume, indicating that EGCG has strong anti-cancer activity in vivo [56].

In another study, the polyphenol was used to treat female Balb/c mice injected with SW780 bladder cancer cells. EGCG was intraperitoneally administered at different doses (25, 50, and 100 mg/kg of body weight). The tumor volume and weight decreased dose-dependently. EGCG also inhibited the expression of MMP-9 at the mRNA and protein levels and downregulated the NF-κB pathway in the tumor lysate [57]. Zhang et al. [58] found EGCG loaded with PLGA to possess beneficial properties against human lung cancer in a patient-derived tumor xenograft model. Firstly, small (2–3 mm^3) portions of the patient's resected tumor were injected into male NOD-SCID mice aged eight to ten weeks. Then, when the tumors reached a size of about 1000 mm^3, they were implanted into other Balb/c athymic mice, which were intraperitoneally treated with 10 mg/kg EGCG (free form) or 5 mg/kg (PLGA-encapsulated). The treatment resulted in a reduced tumor volume and weight and lower phospho-NF-κB expression, as indicated by immunoblot analysis. Importantly, encapsulated EGCG clearly suppressed tumor growth more than free EGCG, proving its greater effectiveness in vivo. Interestingly, a combination of EGCG and BAY11-7082 inhibited the growth of lung cancer tumors in vivo more potently than EGCG alone. Hence, supplementing the polyphenol with a specific inhibitor of the NF-κB pathway appears to have stronger effects and can hence reduce potential side effects by allowing lower doses to be used [59].

Moreover, after the injection of CL1-5 cells into Balb/c mice aged six to eight weeks, EGCG treatment reduced cancer invasion and limited tumor metastases in the lungs [60]. In a study by Fang et al. [61], NPC cells were implanted into six-week-old SCID mice that were receiving EGCG at different doses by oral gavage. After eight weeks, all groups treated with the polyphenol developed smaller tumors compared to the control group. The results indicated that EGCG is able to inhibit NPC growth without significant adverse effects. Finally, after subcutaneous implantation of SCC-9 cells into Balb/c nu/nu mice and treatment with 10 mg/kg or 20 mg/kg, EGCG was found to lower tumor weight and volume, indicating its anti-cancer properties in vivo [62].

Selected studies investigating the beneficial effects of EGCG in vivo are summarized in Table 5.

Table 5. Overview of in vivo studies related to EGCG.

Polyphenol	Animal Model	Dose/ Duration	Anti-Tumor Effects	Type IV Collagenase-Mediated Mechanisms	Reference
EGCG [(2 R,3 R)-3′,4′,5,5′,7-pentahydroxy-flavan-3-yl 3,4,5-trihydroxybenzoate]	Balb/c nu/nu mice injected with SCC-9	10, 20 mg/kg daily through oral gavage for 45 days	↓tumor weight ↓tumor volume	not specified	[62]
	Balb/c nude mice injected with CL1-5	50 mg/kg intraperitoneally twice a week for 6 weeks	↓metastatic incidence in lungs	not specified	[60]
	Balb/c nu/nu mice injected with PANC-1	60, 80, 100 mg/kg daily by gavage, 5 days a week for 28 days	↓angiogenesis ↑apoptosis ratio ↓pancreas weight	↓MMP-2 mRNA ↓pAkt protein ↓pPI3 K protein ↓pERK protein	[63]
	SCID mice injected with NA (EBV positive)	30 mg/kg every day or 50 mg/kg every two days, by oral gavage for 8 weeks	↓tumor volume	not specified	[61]
	Balb/c mice injected with HuCC-T1	20 mg/kg once subcutaneously beside tumor when it reached 4–5 mm in diameter	↓tumor volume	↓MMP-2, -9 protein	[56]
	Balb/c mice injected with SW780	25, 50, 100 mg/kg daily intraperitoneally for 3 weeks	↓tumor weight ↓tumor volume	↓MMP-9 mRNA, protein ↓pNF-κB p65 protein ↓NF-κB mRNA	[57]

Table 5. *Cont.*

Polyphenol	Animal Model	Dose/ Duration	Anti-Tumor Effects	Type IV Collagenase-Mediated Mechanisms	Reference
	Balb/c athymic nude mice injected with A549	20 mg/kg with or without 10 mg/kg BAY11-7082, intraperitoneally for 21 days	↓tumor weight ↓tumor volume	↓pNF-κB protein	[59]
	Balb/c athymic nude mice injected with patient-derived lung cancer samples	10 mg/kg (free EGCG) or 5 mg/kg (PLGA-encapsulated EGCG) daily intraperitoneally for a month	↓tumor weight ↓tumor volume	↓pNF-κB protein	[58]

Legend: ↑ activation or increase; ↓ inhibition or decrease.

3.3. *Genistein*

Genistein (4′,5,7-trihydroxyisoflavone) is one of the most commonly known isoflavones. It occurs mainly in soy and soy-based products, which are important elements of Asian cuisine. Its health-promoting properties have been known for a long time, including its anti-cancer, anti-oxidant, anti-inflammatory, anti-angiogenic, and proapoptotic activities [64]. Its activity is believed to be pleiotropic. Genistein has an affinity for estrogen receptors (ERα and ERβ), modifies the expression of various genes and proteins, and modulates various intracellular signaling pathways, including protein tyrosine kinases, NF-κB, PI3 K/Akt, and those associated with apoptosis. However, these beneficial properties depend on the concentration, tissue type, and quantity of ERα. High concentrations of genistein may elicit negative effects in vivo, such as intensified cell proliferation [65,66].

3.3.1. In Vitro Studies

The anti-cancer and anti-metastatic properties of genistein result largely from its ability to inhibit MMP-2 and MMP-9, as proven in many studies on various cancer cell lines. Shafiee et al. [67] examined the effect of genistein on PC3 prostate cancer cells; genistein treatment caused a significant reduction in MMP-2 activity, as measured by gelatinase zymography. At a concentration of 70 μM, MMP-2 activity was reduced by approximately 70%, and the gene expression of p38 MAPK and its active phosphorylated form were downregulated. In addition, the activity of proapoptotic protein caspase-3 was increased. As a consequence, cell viability and metastatic capability were both reduced. Similar effects were observed for colon cancer cells (HT-29). Although the cells demonstrated a slightly more dynamic decrease in MMP-2 activity after genistein treatment than PC3, the two cell lines presented comparable maximal effects at a concentration of 70 μM [68].

Genistein can inhibit the expression of MMP-2 and MMP-9 at both the mRNA and protein levels and can increase the expression of TIMP-1 in HT29 cells. Treatment with 20 μM genistein achieved a 50% decrease in lytic activity by MMP-2 and MMP-9. Also, genistein treatment downregulated the Wnt-1/β-catenin pathway and upregulated E-cadherin expression, exerting strong anti-migratory and anti-invasive effects against colorectal cancer cells [69]. Likewise, genistein treatment inhibited MMP-9 expression and increased the expression of TIMP-1 in HeLa cervical carcinoma cells [70]. In addition, 5 μM genistein inhibited MMP-2 and MMP-9 expression in Mia-PaCa2 pancreatic cancer cells, as assessed by Western blotting, in a time-dependent manner. This effect resulted in a significant deterioration in cell migration [71].

Genistein also induced a concentration-dependent reduction in the secretion and expression of MMP-2 and MMP-9 in melanoma 518 A2 cells, with a stronger effect than two other flavones: chrysin and apigenin. It has also been reported that combining a polyphenol with a metal complex can intensify its biological effect [72]. Indeed, it has been proven that Cu(II)–genistein inhibited the expression and secretion of MMP-2 and MMP-9 several times more effectively, with greater anti-metastatic potential than genistein alone. These results indicate that compounds of polyphenols with metals may mitigate the development of cancer cells more effectively than their native forms [73]. Some studies reported that genistein suppresses the activity of MMP-2, but not MMP-9. Despite this, genistein treatment still reduced the proliferation of A549 non-small-cell lung carcinoma (NSCLC) cells [74] and impaired invasion, metastasis, and the progression of the EMT induced by transforming growth factor β1 (TGF-β1) in Panc-1 human pancreatic cancer cells [75]. Xiao and co-workers [76] found genistein to inhibit mRNA and protein expression of MMP-2 in colorectal cancer cells. Treatment also significantly reduced the migratory and invasive potential of the cells and their viability. Also, in liver cancer cells, genistein diminished cisplatin-induced stimulation of MMP-2 and slowed down cell proliferation [77].

Selected studies investigating the beneficial effects of genistein in vitro are summarized in Table 6.

Table 6. Overview of in vitro studies related to genistein.

Polyphenol	Cell Line	Concentration/ Duration	Anti-Cancer Effects	Type IV Collagenase-Mediated Mechanisms	Reference
Genistein (4′,5,7-trihydroxyisoflavone)	TGF-β1-induced Panc-1	1, 25, 50 μM for 24, 48 h	↓cell migration ↓cell invasion	↓MMP-2 mRNA, activity ↔MMP-9 mRNA, activity ↓uPA mRNA, protein ↓p-p38 MAPK	[75]
	HeLa	5, 25, 100 μM for 6, 24, 48 h	↓cell migration ↑apoptosis	↓MMP-9 mRNA ↑TIMP-1 mRNA	[70]
	A549	25, 50, 75, 100 μM for 24, 48 h	↓proliferation	↓MMP-2 mRNA, activity ↔MMP-9 mRNA, activity	[74]
	HCCLM3	40 μM for 24, 48 h with or without 20 μM of cisplatin	↓proliferation	↓MMP-2 protein	[77]
	518 A2	25, 50 μM for 6, 24, 48 h Free genistein and Cu(II)–genistein complex	↓cell migration ↓cell invasion ↓proliferation	↓MMP-2, -9 secretion, activity	[73]
	HCT116 SW620 HT29	10, 50 μM for 24, 48 h	↓cell migration ↓cell invasion ↓proliferation	↓MMP-2 mRNA, protein	[76]
	HT29	10, 30, 50, 70 μM for 12, 24, 48 h	↓cell migration ↓proliferation ↑apoptosis	↓MMP-2 activity ↓p38 MAPK mRNA ↓p-p38 MAPK	[68]
	Mia-PaCa2	5, 10, 20, 40 μM for 5, 10, 12, 20, 24, 48 h	↓cell migration ↑apoptosis	↓MMP-2, -9 protein	[71]
	HT29	10, 20, 60 μM for 24, 48, 72 h	↓cell migration ↓cell invasion	↓MMP-2, -9 mRNA, protein ↑TIMP-1 mRNA, protein	[69]
	PC3	10, 30, 50, 70 μM for 6, 12, 24 h	↓cell migration ↓proliferation ↑apoptosis	↓MMP-2 activity ↓p38 MAPK mRNA ↓p-p38 MAPK	[67]

Legend: ↑ activation or increase; ↓ inhibition or decrease; ↔ no impact.

3.3.2. In Vivo Studies

Kidani and co-workers [78] assessed the anti-cancer potential of genistein against osteosarcoma. Osteosarcoma LM8 cells were subcutaneously injected into male Balb/cA Jcl-nu nude mice and male C3 H mice. Before implantation, the study group cells had been incubated for three days with 50 μM genistein, whereas the controls had not. The animals were fed with laboratory chow and water and did not receive genistein during the experiment. The results showed that cells pretreated with the polyphenol presented a different phenotype. In the genistein group, the mice generally developed about four-times smaller tumors than controls, with one mouse not developing a tumor at all. Likewise, in the genistein group, the majority of animals did not demonstrate metastatic nodules in the liver and lungs. Immunohistochemical staining revealed significantly lower levels of MMP-2 in primary tumors in the genistein group, indicating that genistein attenuated the metastatic potential of osteosarcoma.

Colorectal cancer cells HCT116-LUC were subcutaneously injected into athymic Balb/c mice aged six to eight weeks. When the tumors developed, they were isolated, cut into small pieces, and transplanted into the cecal wall. This applied model of orthotopic implantation intimately reflects the course of cancer progression in humans, as neoplastic cells have to overcome the intestinal wall, initiate angiogenesis, and form distant metastases. Genistein was orally administered using doses of 25 and 75 mg/kg daily. Significantly fewer metastatic foci were observed in the lungs and livers of the animals treated with genistein compared to the control group. An immunohistochemical assay showed a dose-dependent reduction in MMP-2 expression in tumor sections. Genistein also significantly inhibited angiogenesis in vivo [76].

Chen et al. [77] conducted an interesting study in which they evaluated the effect of genistein on liver cancer recurrence after curative hepatectomy. Hepatocellular cancer cells (HCCLM3) were subcutaneously injected into a single nude Balb/c nu/nu mouse. Subsequently, the developed tumor was removed, divided, and implanted into single lobes of the livers of other mice. After 10 days, the tumor-bearing liver lobes were resected. After hepatectomy, all mice in the control group presented intrahepatic recurrence and lung metastasis. In contrast, the genistein treatment halved the tumor volume and decreased the number of metastases in the lungs. In addition, the treatment also enhanced the inhibitory effect of cisplatin on tumor recurrence and eliminated the cisplatin-induced upregulation of MMP-2. Genistein did not have any clear effect on MMP-2 when applied alone, probably due to the rather low dose used, but halved its mRNA expression in tumor sections when administered together with cisplatin. The treatment also inhibited MMP-2 protein expression, measured by immunochemistry.

Selected studies investigating the beneficial effects of genistein in vivo are summarized in Table 7.

3.4. Quercetin

Quercetin (3,3′,4′,5,7-pentahydroxyflavone) is a flavonol occurring in many fruits, vegetables, leaves, and red wine. It is most commonly found in the form of quercetin glycoside, which is better absorbed by enterocytes. Due to its extremely diverse properties, quercetin has been the subject of extensive research [79]. Quercetin is believed to exert anti-proliferative, anti-inflammatory, anti-carcinogenic, anti-oxidant, anti-bacterial, anti-viral, gastroprotective, radical-scavenging, immune-modulatory, and anti-diabetic activities [80]. In particular, the anti-cancer properties of quercetin result from its ability to promote apoptosis, prevent cell arrest, and suppress metastasis and angiogenesis by modulating various intracellular signaling pathways, such as Wnt/β-catenin, PI3 K/Akt, Janus kinases/signal transducer and activator of transcription proteins (JAK/STAT), MAPK, p53, and NF-κB [81,82].

Table 7. Overview of in vivo studies related to genistein.

Polyphenol	Animal Model	Dose/ Duration	Anti-Tumor Effects	Type IV Collagenase-Mediated Mechanisms	Reference
Genistein (4′,5,7-trihydroxyisoflavone)	Balb/c nu/nu mice injected with HCCLM3; partial hepatectomy 10 days after inoculation	2 mg/kg daily for 4 weeks or 2 mg/kg cisplatin for 7 days or combined therapy of above, intraperitoneally, beginning 3 days after liver lobe resection	↓recurrent tumor volume ↓metastatic incidence in lungs	↓MMP-2 mRNA, protein	[77]
	Balb/cA Jcl-nu and C3 H mice injected with LM8; LM8 previously treated with 50 μM genistein for 3 days	Laboratory chow and water for 25 days (nude) or 36 days (C3 H), no genistein administration	↓tumor weight ↓engraftment rate ↓metastatic incidence in liver ↓metastatic incidence in lungs (by 100%)	↓MMP-2 protein	[78]
	Balb/c athymic mice injected with HCT116-LUC	25, 75 mg/kg daily orally 5 days a week, for 5 weeks	↓tumor weight ↓tumor volume ↓metastatic incidence in liver ↓metastatic incidence in lungs	↓MMP-2 protein	[76]

Legend: ↓ inhibition or decrease.

3.4.1. In Vitro Studies

A number of in vitro studies have found quercetin to suppress MMPs, which act as key pro-angiogenic and pro-metastasis mediators. In lung cancer, which is responsible for the most cancer-related deaths worldwide, quercetin significantly reduced the protein expression of MMP-2 and MMP-9 and increased TIMP-2 expression. The polyphenol was found to deplete the migration and invasive potential of A549 cells by modulating the Akt/MAPK/β-catenin signaling pathway [83]. Quercetin reversed an increase in MMP-9 expression and activity induced by nickel but did not influence MMP-2; treatment also suppressed the NF-κB and Toll-like receptor 4 (TLR4) pathways [84]. Quercetin also yielded promising treatment results in rapidly infiltrating glioblastoma multiforme, another extremely malignant tumor. Liu et al. [85] revealed that quercetin downregulated MMP-2 and MMP-9 protein expression and significantly inhibited migration and invasion in a time- and concentration-dependent manner; however, a noticeable anti-proliferative effect was noted at a concentration of 20 μg/mL. While at a lower concentration of 10 μg/mL, quercetin did not stop cell proliferation, the polyphenol still significantly attenuated cell migration (30%) and invasion and suppressed both MMPs [86].

It is worth emphasizing that quercetin is able to cross the blood–brain barrier [87], making it a potential new agent for the treatment of brain tumors. Quercetin (50 μM) has also been found to reduce the protein levels of MMP-2 and MMP-9 in oral cancers. Treatment lowered cell migration and invasion by regulating the levels of microRNA-16 (miR-16) and homeobox A10, which are involved in tumor progression. Knock-down of miR-16 abrogated the suppressive effect of quercetin on MMP expression in HSC-6 and SCC-9 cells [88].

Interestingly, it has been shown that quercetin can also attenuate the proliferation, invasion, and migration abilities of osteosarcoma by inhibiting parathyroid hormone receptor 1 and by simultaneously downregulating MMP-2 and MMP-9 and upregulating TIMP-1 and TIMP-2 at the mRNA level; this effect is both time- and concentration-dependent (20–100 μM) [89].

The anti-tumor effect of quercetin has also been extensively studied in various gastrointestinal cancers. The administration of quercetin at a concentration of 10 μg/mL decreased the protein expression of MMP-2 and MMP-9, thus inhibiting the migration and invasion of esophageal cancer cells Eca109 [90]. In gastric cancer, quercetin treatment (10 μM for 72 h) also downregulated the expression of MMP-2 and MMP-9, decreasing cell migration and invasion and lowering the protein expression of uPA and the uPA receptor (uPAR). The uPA/uPAR system is considered to play an important role in tumor metastasis. Activated uPA catalyzes the conversion of plasminogen to its active form, plasmin, which, in turn, is responsible for degrading ECM components via the activation of MMPs. In this study, uPA knock-down reduced MMP activity, which was further exacerbated by the quercetin treatment. The authors suggest that quercetin may suppress the uPA/uPAR system by modulating NF-κB, protein kinase C δ, ERK1/2, and 5′-adenosine monophosphate-activated protein kinase α [91].

Quercetin treatment (20 μM, 40 μM, 80 μM) was also found to block MMP-2 and MMP-7 expression in pancreatic cancer [92]. It also suppressed MMPs in metastatic ovarian cancer: treatment (50 μM, 75 μM) inhibited the gene expression, protein expression, and proteolytic activity of MMP-2 and MMP-9, thus attenuating the metastatic potential of ovarian cancer cells [93].

Notably, quercetin may exert bidirectional effects in ER-positive breast cancer. Xu et al. [94] showed that at a low concentration (5 μM), quercetin intensified cell proliferation, reduced apoptosis, and even reversed the anti-proliferative effect of tamoxifen to a certain extent. In contrast, at a high concentration (100 μM), quercetin strongly inhibited cell proliferation and acted synergistically with tamoxifen. This may result from the quercetin treatment modulating the mRNA expression of the many genes involved in tumor progression, including MMPs. High concentrations of quercetin significantly decreased MMP-2 and MMP-9 expression, while low concentrations increased it, which, in turn, enhanced the malignant potential of cancer cells. These dual effects of quercetin resulted from its phytoestrogenic properties and the fact that the polyphenol is able to regulate the relative ratios of different ER subtypes in ER-positive breast cancers. Interestingly, it has been shown that quercetin can act synergistically with chemotherapeutic drugs, such as everolimus, doxorubicin, and lonidamine, enhancing their effects, and inhibit MMP-2 and MMP-9 [95–97].

Tang and co-workers [98] reported that, in breast cancer cells, quercetin significantly inhibited the protein expression of MMP-2 and MMP-9 and increased the TIMP-1 and TIMP-2 levels in a concentration-dependent manner; it also suppressed the activity of MMP-2 and MMP-9 based on gelatin zymography. Furthermore, quercetin decreased the adhesive, invasive, and migratory abilities of breast cancer cells. These findings were confirmed in another study, which also demonstrated reduced levels of MMP-2 and MMP-9 after treatment with quercetin in MDA-MB-231 breast cancer cells [99]. Also, Balakrishnan and co-workers [100] reported the inhibition of MMP-2 and MMP-9 protein expression in MCF-7 and MDA-MB-231 breast carcinoma cells after quercetin treatment. Likewise, the polyphenol downregulated the phosphorylated epidermal growth factor receptor/vascular epithelial growth factor receptor (p-EGFR/VEGFR) pathway and, subsequently, the PI3 K/Akt pathway. The anti-angiogenic properties of quercetin were proven using the tube formation assay. Also, treatment attenuated the invasiveness and migratory potential of the cells and inhibited the EMT. Also, the polyphenol reduced the protein expression of MMP-2 and uPA and limited cell motility via the inhibition of the Snail/Akt pathway in NSCLC cells [101]. In colorectal cancer cells, quercetin lowered MMP-2 and MMP-9 activity, as confirmed by gelatin zymography. Also, MMPs were inhibited at the mRNA level, whereas their inhibitors, TIMP-1 and TIMP-2, were overexpressed, thus yielding an anti-metastatic effect [102]. Likewise, in HCC cells, the protein expression of MMP-2 and MMP-9 was concentration-dependently inhibited by quercetin. The polyphenol suppressed HCC growth by affecting autophagy and the NF-κB pathway [103]. Quercetin was found to exert inhibitory effects against erlotinib-resistant oral squamous cell carcinoma (OSCC). The erlotinib-resistant cell lines ERL-R5 and ERL-R10 were obtained by maintaining HSC-3 human tongue squamous cell carcinoma cells in media with increasing concentrations of erlotinib for six months. At a concentration of 5 μM, treatment caused a reduction in MMP-2 and MMP-9 at the protein level, which was detected in cell lysates from HSC-3, ERL-R5, and ERL-R10 cells. Also, quercetin inhibited cellular invasiveness and migration and induced apoptosis [104].

Selected studies investigating the beneficial effects of quercetin in vitro are summarized in Table 8.

Table 8. Overview of in vitro studies related to quercetin.

Polyphenol	Cell Line	Concentration/ Duration	Anti-Cancer Effects	Type IV Collagenase-Mediated Mechanisms	Reference
Quercetin (3,3′,4′,5,7-pentahydroxyflavone)	A375 A2058 B16 F10	10, 20, 40, 60 μM for 16, 24 h or 60 μM for 3, 6, 12, 24 h or 20, 40, 60, 80 μM for 24 h	↓cell migration ↓cell invasion ↓proliferation ↑apoptosis	↓MMP-2, -9 mRNA, activity ↑pERK, ↑pAkt protein	[105]
	MCF-7 MDA-MB-231	50, 100 μM for 24 h (quercetin or gold-nanoparticle-conjugated quercetin)	↓cell migration ↓cell invasion ↓proliferation ↓angiogenesis	↓MMP-2, -9 protein ↓pPI3 K, ↓Akt, ↓pAkt	[100]
	CT26 MC38 CCD-18 Co	10, 25, 50, 100 μM for 24 h or 50 μM for 3, 6, 9, 12 h or 50 μM for 15, 30, 60 min or 0.1, 1, 10 μM for 24 h	↓cell migration ↓cell invasion ↓proliferation ↑apoptosis	↓MMP-2, -9 mRNA, activity ↑TIMP-1, -2 mRNA ↑pERK, pp38 protein	[102]
	A549 H1975 HCC827	10, 25, 50 μM for 24 h or 50 μM for 10, 30 min, 6, 24 h or 50 μM for 1, 2, 4, 8, 24 h	↓cell migration ↓cell invasion	↓MMP-2 protein ↓pAkt	[101]
	HOS MG63	25, 50, 100 μM for 6, 12, 24 h	↓cell migration ↓cell invasion	↓MMP-2, -9 mRNA, protein	[106]
	U251	10, 20, 30, 40 μg/mL for 24, 48 h	↓cell migration ↓cell invasion ↓proliferation ↑apoptosis	↓MMP-2, -9 protein	[85]
	U251	10 μg/mL for 24, 48 h	↓cell migration ↓cell invasion	↓MMP-2, -9 protein	[86]
	MCF-7	25, 50, 100, 200 μM for 4, 5, 24, 72 h (quercetin) 0.7, 1.4, 2.8, 5.6 mg/mL for 4, 5, 24, 72 h (hyaluronic acid nanohydrogel of quercetin) with or without 1, 10 nM of Everolimus	↓proliferation ↑apoptosis	↓MMP-2, -9 protein	[95]
	IL-6-induced PATU-8988	20, 40, 80 μM for 24, 48 h	↓cell migration ↓cell invasion	↓MMP-2 mRNA, protein	[92]
	MCF-7 MDA-MB-231	20, 30, 40, 60, 80, 100 μM for 6, 24 h	↓cell migration ↓cell invasion	↓MMP-2, -9 protein ↓pAkt protein ↓pmTOR protein	[99]
	BGC823 AGS	10 μM for 72 h	↓cell migration ↓cell invasion ↓proliferation	↓MMP-2, -9 activity ↓pNF-κB p65 protein ↓pERK-1/-2 protein	[91]

Table 8. *Cont.*

Polyphenol	Cell Line	Concentration/ Duration	Anti-Cancer Effects	Type IV Collagenase-Mediated Mechanisms	Reference
	Nickel-induced A549	2, 5 μM for 24 h 2, 5 μM for 4 h before Nickel (1 mM) for 5–10 min or 1, 1.5, 12 h	↓cell migration ↓cell invasion	↓MMP-2 activity ↓MMP-9 activity, protein ↓NF-κB p65 protein ↓IKKβ protein ↓I-κBα protein	[84]
	U2 OS Saos-2	20, 40, 60, 80, 100 μM for 48 h	↓cell migration ↓cell invasion ↓proliferation ↓cell adhesion ↑apoptosis	↓MMP-2, -9 mRNA ↑TIMP-1, -2 mRNA	[89]
	HSC-6 SCC-9	50 μM for 24, 48 h	↓cell migration ↓cell invasion ↓proliferation	↓MMP-2, -9 protein	[88]
	MCF-7	80 μM for 24 h with or without 5 μM of lonidamine	↓proliferation ↑apoptosis	↓MMP-2, -9 mRNA	[97]
	MCF-7	5, 100 μM for 12, 24, 48 h with or without 5 μM of tamoxifen	↑proliferation (5 μM) ↓proliferation (100 μM) ↑cell migration (5 μM) ↓cell migration (100 μM) ↑cell invasion (5 μM) ↓cell invasion (100 μM) ↓apoptosis (5 μM) ↑apoptosis (100 μM)	↑MMP-2 mRNA (5 μM) ↓MMP-2 mRNA (100 μM) ↑MMP-9 mRNA (5 μM) ↓MMP-9 mRNA (100 μM)	[94]
	PA-1	50, 75 μM for 24 h	↓cell migration ↓cell adhesion ↓proliferation	↓MMP-2 mRNA, protein, activity ↓MMP-9 mRNA, protein, activity ↓PI3 K/pPI3 K mRNA, protein ↓Akt/pAkt mRNA, protein ↓mTOR/pmTOR mRNA, protein ↓ERK-1/-2 protein	[93]
	Eca109	5, 10 μg/mL for 8, 12, 24 h	↓cell migration ↓cell invasion ↓proliferation	↓MMP-2, -9 protein	[90]
	MDA-MB-231	50 μM for 24, 48 h with or without 32 nM of doxorubicin	↓cell migration ↓proliferation	↓MMP-2, -9 mRNA	[96]
	A549	20, 40 μM for 24 h	↓proliferation ↓cell migration ↓cell invasion	↓MMP-2, -9 protein ↑TIMP-2 protein ↓pAkt ↓NF-κB	[83]

Table 8. *Cont.*

Polyphenol	Cell Line	Concentration/ Duration	Anti-Cancer Effects	Type IV Collagenase-Mediated Mechanisms	Reference
	H22 HepG2	25, 50, 100 µM for 24, 48, 72 h	↓proliferation ↓cell migration ↓cell invasion ↑autophagy	↓MMP-2, -9 protein ↓pNF-κB p65, ↓pIκBα protein	[103]
	HSC-3 Erlotinib-resistant ERL-R5, ERL-R10	5 µM for 24 h or 5, 10 µM with 5 µM of erlotinib	↓proliferation ↓cell migration ↓cell invasion ↓spheroid formation ↑apoptosis	↓MMP-2, -9 protein	[104]
	ZR-75-1 MCF-7 T47 D MDA-MB-231	2, 5 µM for 2, 10, 12, 24 h	↓proliferation ↓cell migration ↓cell invasion ↓cell adhesion ↑apoptosis	↓MMP-2, -9 protein, activity ↑TIMP-1, -2 protein	[98]

Legend: ↑ activation or increase; ↓ inhibition or decrease.

3.4.2. In Vivo Studies

Pradhan et al. [107] assessed the effect of quercetin on melanoma growth in a mouse model. They subcutaneously implanted B16 F10 melanoma cells into the flanks of four- to six-week-old male C57 BL6 mice. Quercetin at a dose of 15 mg/kg of body weight was injected three times a week into the peripheral parts of the tumors for three weeks. The treatment resulted in the decreased expression of MMP-9 in the tumor sections, as indicated by immunofluorescence analysis, and MMP-9 also demonstrated reduced protein expression and proteolytic activity, as confirmed by Western blot and gelatin zymography assays. As a result, 25% decreases in tumor weight and volume were noted.

In a study by Tang et al. [98], ZR-75-1 and MCF-7 cells were implanted into male Balb/c nude mice, which were then intraperitoneally treated with 20 mg/kg and 40 mg/kg quercetin. The results indicated that quercetin suppressed tumor growth and did not elicit toxic effects in normal tissues. In a similar study, quercetin suppressed tumor growth and inhibited metastasis and glycolysis via the Akt/mTOR pathway [99].

Another study on breast cancer was carried out on female Sprague-Dawley rats. Breast cancer was established using 7,12-dimethylbenz(a)anthracene. After the occurrence of tumors, the rats were treated with intratumoral injections of quercetin (25 mg/kg) or gold-nanoparticle-conjugated quercetin (25 mg/kg) for eight days. In the tumor-bearing animals, both the simple polyphenol and encapsulated polyphenol successfully suppressed tumor growth and restored the mammary epithelial tissue architecture. The anti-angiogenic properties of quercetin were proven using a chick embryo angiogenesis assay [100]. Chang et al. [101] examined the effect of quercetin on NSCLC cells in an orthotopic xenograft model. A549 cells were injected into the left lateral thorax of female SCID mice. The animals were intraperitoneally treated with quercetin (500 mg/kg of body weight). The treatment yielded an anti-metastatic effect in vivo, inhibited tumor growth, and prolonged survival time. Also, quercetin has been found to prevent metastasis formation in colorectal cancer in vivo. An experimental lung metastasis model was established by injecting mouse colon carcinoma CT26 cells into the lateral tail veins of five-week-old Balb/c female mice. The animals treated with quercetin developed fewer tumor nodules in the lungs [102]. Similar results indicating the inhibition of cancer metastasis development in the lungs via the suppression of MMPs have also been confirmed in osteosarcoma and melanoma [105,106]. In another study, H22 human hepatocellular carcinoma cells were subcutaneously injected into four-week-old male Balb/c mice to create a xenograft model.

Quercetin was administered through gavage at different doses (25, 50, and 100 mg/kg of body weight). The tumor weight and volume were significantly decreased in animals treated with the polyphenol [103].

Finally, quercetin was found to have beneficial properties in an animal model of erlotinib-resistant OSCC. A tumor model was developed by subcutaneously injecting four-week-old male nude mice with ERL-R5 cells, and the mice were intraperitoneally treated with quercetin (2 or 10 mg/kg) for 18 days. The results showed a dose-dependent depletion in tumor weight and volume after the treatment [104].

Selected studies investigating the beneficial effects of quercetin in vivo are summarized in Table 9.

Table 9. Overview of in vivo studies related to quercetin.

Polyphenol	Animal Model	Dose/ Duration	Anti-Tumor Effects	Type IV Collagenase-Mediated Mechanisms	Reference
Quercetin (3,3′,4′,5,7-pentahydroxyflavone)	C57 BL6 mice injected with B16 F10	15 mg/kg daily thrice a week into the peripheral sites of tumors for 3 weeks or 7.5 mg/kg quercetin with 1.75 mg/kg sulforaphane or 15 mg/kg quercetin with 3.5 mg/kg sulforaphane, the same way	↓tumor weight ↓tumor volume	↓MMP-9 protein, activity	[107]
	Balb/c nu/nu mice injected with A375 (xenograft) C57 BL/6 mice injected with B16 F10 (metastasis model)	100 mg/kg daily intragastrically for 21 days (xenograft) 100 mg/kg daily intragastrically, 1 day before cell injection and for next 24 days (metastatic model)	↓tumor weight ↓tumor volume ↓metastatic incidence in lungs	not specified	[105]
	Sprague-Dawley rats stimulated by DMBA	25 mg/kg free quercetin or 25 mg/kg gold-nanoparticle-conjugated quercetin by daily intratumoral injections for 8 days	↓tumor weight ↓tumor volume ↑normal breast tissue architecture	not specified	[100]
	Balb/c mice injected with CT26	10, 50 mg/kg intraperitoneally 2 h prior to cell injection and then once every 2 days for 14 days	↓lung weight ↓metastatic incidence in lungs	not specified	[102]
	SCID mice injected with A549 pretreated with quercetin for 24 h (metastatic model) or not (xenograft)	500 mg/kg daily intraperitoneally for 5 weeks (xenograft model)	↑survival time ↓metastatic incidence in distant organs (xenograft) ↓metastatic incidence in bones ↓metastatic incidence in lungs (metastatic model)	not specified	[101]
	Balb/c nu/nu mice injected with stably transfected HOS	25, 50, 100 mg/kg intraperitoneally, twice daily for a month	↓metastatic incidence in lungs	not specified	[106]
	Balb/c nude mice injected with MCF-7	50 mg/kg, intraperitoneally, twice daily for 25 days	↓tumor volume	↓pAkt protein	[99]
	Balb/c mice injected with H22	25, 50, 100 mg/kg, by gavage, once a day for 21 days	↓tumor weight ↓tumor volume	not specified	[103]
	Nude mice injected with erlotinib-resistant HSC-3, ERL-R5	2, 10 mg/kg, intraperitoneally, daily for 18 days	↓tumor weight ↓tumor volume	not specified	[104]
	Balb/c nude mice injected with ZR-75-1 and MCF-7	20, 40 mg/kg daily, intraperitoneally for 28 days	↓tumor weight ↓tumor volume	not specified	[98]

Legend: ↑ activation or increase; ↓ inhibition or decrease.

3.5. Resveratrol

Resveratrol (3,5,4′-trihydroxystilbene) occurs naturally in many plants, including peanuts, pistachios, and berries; it is also present in grapes and, thus, red wine. Interest continues to grow in resveratrol as its broad biological properties are being discovered; it is currently recognized as having cardioprotective, anti-oxidative, anti-inflammatory, neuroprotective, anti-diabetic, and anti-tumor properties [108,109]. Various studies have shown that resveratrol affects many stages of carcinogenesis. It plays a role in initiation by reactive oxygen species scavenging, protecting DNA from damage and anti-mutagenic activity; it influences promotion through its proapoptotic and anti-inflammatory properties and by inhibiting cell proliferation via interference with the PI3 K/Akt, mTOR, MAPK, Wnt/β-catenin, and NF-κB signaling pathways; and it also inhibits progression and metastasis via the suppression of MMPs and its anti-angiogenic and anti-migratory properties [110,111]. Hence, resveratrol appears to be a very promising agent in the inhibition of cancer development. In particular, many scientific works indicate that resveratrol slows carcinogenesis by inhibiting MMP-2 and MMP-9.

3.5.1. In Vitro Studies

In glioblastoma, the most common and lethal malignant tumor of the central nervous system, resveratrol treatment (40 μM) suppressed the protein expression and enzymatic activity of MMP-2 and significantly inhibited the migration and invasion of cancer cells in vitro [112]. Resveratrol has been found to suppress MMPs in various OSCC cell lines, most likely through the inhibition of the MAPK/ERK pathway [113,114]. OSCC is characterized by relatively high resistance to chemotherapy. It has been proven that resveratrol can act synergistically with conventional drugs, e.g., cisplatin and cetuximab, and even overcome drug resistance [115]. In a cisplatin-resistant OSCC cell line, non-toxic concentrations (50 μM) of resveratrol depleted the migration and invasive capabilities of cancer cells by reducing the mRNA and protein expression of MMP-2 and MMP-9 [114].

In lung cancer cells (A549), resveratrol (10 μM, 30 μM) decreased MMP-9 mRNA expression and activity and its promoter activity, without any significant impact on MMP-2. This effect resulted from the suppression of NF-κB and activator protein 1, which are directly involved in MMP-9 transcription [116]. Resveratrol treatment has been found to influence similar processes when administered with gold nanoparticles in breast cancer cells: treatment (10 μM) inhibited MMP-9 at the mRNA and protein levels and reduced its activity by downregulating the NF-κB, PI3 K/Akt, and MAPK/ERK pathways. These effects were accompanied by slightly increased protein expression of TIMP-1 and TIMP-2. Consequently, the migratory capacity and invasive ability of the cells were significantly suppressed [117]. Resveratrol at a concentration of up to 50 μM also inhibited both MMP-2 and MMP-9 in other breast cancer cell lines. Interestingly, in addition to blocking MMPs, it was found to attenuate the metastasis and migration of breast cancer cells by reversing the EMT and interfering with tumor–stromal cross-talk [118,119].

Resveratrol (20 μM, 40 μM) also suppressed the migratory and invasive abilities of cervical cancer cells by reducing MMP-2 and MMP-9 protein expression [120]. Interestingly, another stilbene, pterostilbene, was found to exert stronger effects and demonstrate greater bioavailability than resveratrol at the same concentration; it is structurally similar to the latter but with two methoxy groups instead of two hydroxyl groups. However, further research is still needed to better verify its therapeutic potential [120].

In colorectal cancer, resveratrol (5 μM) reduced the MMP-9 protein level by modulating the cellular response to TNF-β and downregulating the NF-κB pathway. It is also able to re-chemosensitize cancer cells to 5-fluorouracil and prevent the expression of EMT markers [121,122]. Also, it was proven that resveratrol (12.5 μM, 25 μM, 50 μM) impaired the expression of EMT-related genes, including MMP-2 and MMP-9, in pancreatic cancer; such inhibition via the suppression of the NF-κB, PI3 K/Akt and uPA pathways reduced cell proliferation, invasion, and metastasis in a concentration-dependent manner [123,124].

In HCC, resveratrol (10 μg/mL) limited the expression of MMP-2 and MMP-9 at the mRNA and protein levels and increased TIMP-1 and TIMP-2. Together with the modulation of multiple signaling pathways, this effect lessened cell viability and stimulated apoptosis [125]. Furthermore, resveratrol could enhance the anti-cancer activity of paclitaxel and gemcitabine in HCC and pancreatic cancer [125,126]. Also, resveratrol treatment (25 μM, 50 μM, 100 μM) limited the proliferation, migration, and invasion of neoplastic cells in renal cancer by inhibiting MMP-2 and MMP-9 and stimulating TIMP-1 by modulating the MAPK/ERK and PI3 K/Akt pathways [127]. However, it must be emphasized that these effects may result from the polyphenol regulating histone acetylation in renal carcinoma [128]. Additionally, resveratrol used at different concentrations, detailed in Table 6, has been found to mitigate the adhesive, migratory, and invasive properties of cancer cells by simultaneously downregulating MMP-2 and MMP-9 and upregulating TIMP-1 and TIMP-2 in bladder cancer [129], prostate cancer [130], and thyroid carcinoma [131]. Resveratrol treatment has also demonstrated similar effects in several mesenchymal cancers, e.g., osteosarcoma [132] and chondrosarcoma [133]. In contrast, resveratrol significantly increased MMP-9 activity and expression and improved cell motility in fibrosarcoma, promoting disease progression [134].

Resveratrol's anti-metastatic properties were confirmed in mouse breast cancer 4 T1 cells, where it reduced the activity and expression of MMP-9 in a concentration-dependent manner and mitigated cell adhesion, motility, and invasion [135]. Similar effects were demonstrated in SKBR3/paclitaxel-resistant (SKBR3/PR) breast cancer cells. Free resveratrol and resveratrol–solid lipid nanoparticles, with or without D-α-tocopheryl polyethylene glycol 1000 succinate, were found to inhibit the protein expression of MMP-2 and MMP-9 and to modulate EMT markers, thus attenuating cell migration and invasion [136]. In a model of oral cancer, resveratrol suppressed the metastasis and invasion of H-357 cells by inhibiting the activity of MMP-2 and MMP-9 and numerous inflammation mediators, e.g., NF-κB, COX-2, inducible nitric oxide synthase (iNOS), TLR4, TNF-α, interleukin-1 β (IL-1 β), and interleukin-6 (IL-6). Additionally, resveratrol administration suppressed angiogenesis in the cancer cells, as indicated by the Chick Chorioallantoic Membrane assay [137]. An investigation by Yang et al. [138] found resveratrol to have anti-cancer effects on gastric cancer. In SGC-7901 and HSC-39 cells, the polyphenol reversed IL-6-induced overexpression of MMP-2 and MMP-9. Resveratrol inhibited TGF-β1-induced expression of MMP-2 and MMP-9 in LoVo cells [139]. Wang and co-workers [140] assessed the impact of resveratrol on malignant C6 rat glioma cells. Treatment downregulated multiple signaling pathways and mediators, such as NF-κB, PI3 K/Akt, mTOR, COX-2, EGFR, and VEGF, in a concentration-dependent manner. Immunohistochemical staining confirmed the diminished expression of MMP-9 and NF-κB. A similar experiment, but on glioblastoma-initiating cells (GICs), revealed reduced MMP-2 activity and protein expression, probably due to the downregulation of the NF-κB and PI3 K/Akt/mTOR pathways [141]. Finally, Yang and co-workers [142] evaluated the anti-cancer effect of resveratrol against human osteosarcoma. The treatment of HOS cells caused the concentration-dependent suppression of MMP-2 mRNA and protein expression, enzymatic activity, or promoter activity. Additionally, resveratrol inhibited MMP-2 transcriptional activity by blocking the DNA-binding activity of cAMP response-element binding, a form of transcription factor. Interestingly, TIMP-2 expression was not affected by resveratrol. In addition, resveratrol also modulated some cellular signaling pathways, such as Akt or c-Jun N-terminal kinases; this could be responsible for suppressing MMP-2 and weakening cancer cell motility, adhesion, and invasion.

Selected studies investigating the beneficial effects of resveratrol in vitro are summarized in Table 10.

Table 10. Overview of in vitro studies related to resveratrol.

Polyphenol	Cell Line	Concentration/ Duration	Anti-Cancer Effects	Type IV Collagenase-Mediated Mechanisms	Reference
Resveratrol (3,5,4′-trihydroxystilbene)	PMA-induced A549 HeLa	10, 30 μM for 24 h	↓proliferation ↓cell migration ↓cell invasion	↔MMP-2 mRNA, activity ↓MMP-9 mRNA, activity ↓NF-κB activity	[116]
	4 T1	10, 20, 30 μM for 12, 16, 24, 48 h	↓cell adhesion ↓cell migration ↓cell invasion	↓MMP-9 mRNA, activity	[135]
	HT1080	50 μM for 10, 30 min, 1, 3, 6, 12, 24 h or 10, 20, 30, 40, 50 μM for 24 h or 20, 30, 50 μM for 24, 48 h	↓proliferation ↑cell migration	↑MMP-9 protein, activity ↓pp38 ↓pAkt	[134]
	BxPC-3 Panc-1	12.5, 25, 50 μM for 24, 48 h	↓proliferation ↓cell migration ↓cell invasion	↓MMP-2, -9 mRNA, protein ↓pNF-κB protein ↓pAkt protein	[123]
	HTB94	50 μM for 10, 30 min, 1, 3, 6, 12, 24 h or 10, 20, 30, 40, 50 μM for 24 h	↓proliferation	↓MMP-2, -9 protein, activity ↑pp38	[133]
	TGF-β1-induced LoVo	6, 12 μM for 24, 48 h	↓proliferation ↓cell migration ↓cell invasion	↓MMP-2, -9 protein	[139]
	Glioblastoma-initiating cells (GICs) derived from patients	5, 10, 20 μM for 24, 48 h	↓proliferation ↓cell adhesion ↓cell migration ↓cell invasion	↓MMP-2 protein, activity ↓NF-κB p65 nuclear translocation ↑I-κBα, ↓pI-κBα protein ↑IKKα/β, ↓pIKKα/β protein ↓pAkt, ↓pmTOR protein	[141]
	TPA-induced SCC-9	25, 50, 75, 100 μM for 24 h	↓proliferation ↓cell migration ↓cell invasion	↔MMP-2 activity ↓MMP-9 mRNA, protein, activity ↓pERK protein	[113]
	C6	50, 100, 150 μM for 24, 48 h	↓proliferation ↑apoptosis	↓MMP-9 protein ↓PI3 K, pAkt, mTOR, STAT3 protein ↓NF-κB protein	[140]
	HOS MNNG/HOS 143 B	25, 50, 75, 100 μM for 12, 24, 48 h or 100 μM for 2, 4 h	↓proliferation ↓cell adhesion ↓cell migration ↓cell invasion	↓MMP-2 mRNA, protein, activity, promoter activity ↔TIMP-2 protein ↓pp38, pAkt protein ↑pERK protein	[142]
	SW579	10 μg/mL for 24 h with 100, 200 μg/mL of lentinan	↓proliferation ↑apoptosis	↓MMP-2, -9 mRNA ↑TIMP-1, -2 mRNA ↓NF-κB mRNA ↑I-κBα mRNA	[131]
	Hypoxia-induced BxPC-3 Panc-1	12.5, 25, 50 μM for 24, 48 h	↓proliferation ↓cell migration ↓cell invasion	↓MMP-2 mRNA, protein	[124]

Table 10. *Cont.*

Polyphenol	Cell Line	Concentration/ Duration	Anti-Cancer Effects	Type IV Collagenase-Mediated Mechanisms	Reference
	TPA-stimulated MCF-7	10 µM for 1, 24 h (resveratrol) 1, 5, 10 µM for 1, 4, 12, 24 h (gold-conjugated resveratrol nanoparticles)	↓proliferation ↓cell migration ↓cell invasion	↓MMP-2 protein ↓MMP-9 mRNA, protein, activity, secretion ↑TIMP-1, -2 protein ↓NF-κB p65/pNF-κB p65 protein ↓pAkt, pERK protein	[117]
	U87 MG T98 G U251	40 µM for 24, 48 h	↓proliferation ↓cell migration ↓cell invasion	↓MMP-2 protein, activity	[112]
	T24	10, 25, 50 µM for 6, 12, 24 h	↓cell migration ↓cell invasion	↓MMP-2, -9 protein ↓pERK-1/-2 protein	[129]
	SW480 HCT116	5 µM for 12, 24 h or 10, 28 days	↓proliferation ↓cell invasion (in alginate culture) ↑apoptosis	↓MMP-9 protein ↓pNF-κB p65 protein ↓pNF-κB p50 protein	[121]
	HepG2	10 µg/mL for 24 h with 5, 10 µg/mL of paclitaxel	↑apoptosis	↓MMP-2, -9 mRNA, protein ↑TIMP-1, -2 mRNA, protein ↓NF-κB mRNA, protein ↑I-κBα mRNA, protein	[125]
	U2 OS	6, 12 µg/mL for 24, 48 h	↓proliferation ↓cell migration ↓cell invasion ↑apoptosis	↓MMP-2, -9 protein	[132]
	HCT116 5-Fluorouracil-resistant HCT116 R	5 µM for 24, 72 h or 10 days	↓proliferation ↓cell invasion (in alginate culture) ↑apoptosis	↓MMP-9 protein ↓pNF-κB p65 protein	[122]
	Cancer-associated fibroblasts (CAF)-induced MCF-7 MDA-MB-231	50 µM for 24, 36, 48 h	↓proliferation ↓cell migration ↓cell invasion	↓MMP-2, -9 mRNA ↓pAkt	[119]
	IL 6 induced SGC-7901 HSC-39	10, 20 µM for 48 h	↓proliferation ↓cell invasion	↓MMP-2, -9 activity ↓pERK protein	[138]
	ACHN A498	25, 50, 100 µM for 24, 48 h	↓proliferation ↓cell migration ↓cell invasion	↓MMP-2, -9 protein ↑TIMP-1 protein ↓pAkt, ERK-1/-2, pERK-1/-2	[127]
	TGF-1 β-induced MDA-MB-231 MDA-MB-436 MDA-MB-453 BT549	12.5, 25, 50 µM for 24 h	↓proliferation ↓cell migration ↓cell invasion	↓MMP-2 protein, secretion (MDA-MB-231) ↓MMP-9 protein, secretion (MDA-MB-231) ↓pAkt, pPI3 K	[118]

Table 10. *Cont.*

Polyphenol	Cell Line	Concentration/ Duration	Anti-Cancer Effects	Type IV Collagenase-Mediated Mechanisms	Reference
	HeLa Cancer Stem Cells (CSCs)	10, 20, 40 μM for 24, 48 h	↓proliferation ↑cell migration (slightly, after 24 h) ↓cell migration (after 48 h) ↓cell invasion ↑apoptosis	↓MMP-2, -9 protein	[120]
	PC3 DU145 LNCap	150 μM for 12, 24, 48 h	↓cell migration ↓cell invasion	↓MMP-2, -9 protein ↑TIMP-2, -3 protein ↓TIMP-2, -3 methylation level	[130]
	Cisplatin-resistant CAL27	25, 50, 75 μM for 6, 12, 18, 24 h	↓proliferation ↓cell migration ↓cell invasion	↓MMP-2, -9 protein ↓pERK, pp38 protein	[114]
	H-357	1, 3.5, 5 μM for 48 h (resveratrol nanoparticles)	↓angiogenesis ↓proliferation ↓cell invasion	↓MMP-2, -9 activity ↓NF-κB, IKKα protein ↓Akt, MAPK protein	[137]
	Paclitaxel-resistant SKBR3/PR	30 μM for 24, 48 h (free resveratrol) or equivalent dose (resveratrol–solid lipid nanoparticles with or without TPGS)	↓proliferation ↓cell migration ↓cell invasion ↑apoptosis	↓MMP-2, -9 protein	[136]

Legend: ↑ activation or increase; ↓ inhibition or decrease; ↔ no impact.

3.5.2. In Vivo Studies

The anti-cancer properties of resveratrol were demonstrated in an in vivo model of HCC. HCC was chemically induced in male Sprague-Dawley rats using diethylnitrosamine and carbon tetrachloride. The following experimental variants were used: alone in low (300 mg/kg) and high (450 mg/kg) doses for 9 months, pretreated for 4 weeks before the administration of carcinogenic compounds and for 9 months after it, or without the pretreatment for 9 months. The tumor-bearing animals treated with the polyphenol demonstrated significantly lower MMP-2 and MMP-9 serum concentrations compared to the untreated group. Interestingly, the post-treated group presented a more noticeable effect than the pretreated. Also, resveratrol reduced the serum concentrations of sirtuin 1 and VEGF, as well as those of heparanase and elastase, two other enzymes known to degrade the ECM. The histopathological assessment demonstrated that resveratrol partially reversed the morphological changes in the liver induced by carcinogens, indicating the anti-proliferative, anti-metastatic, and anti-angiogenic properties of resveratrol [143].

A study performed by Ganapathy et al. [144] found resveratrol to have anti-tumor properties against prostate cancer. A xenograft model was established by injecting PC-3 cells into the right flank of athymic Balb/c nu/nu nude mice. The oral application of resveratrol (30 mg/kg) caused the significant inhibition of MMP-2 and MMP-9 expression, as detected by immunohistochemistry and Western blotting. Also, the growth of tumors and the expression of pro-angiogenic VEGF were limited, confirming the anti-metastatic and anti-angiogenic effects.

To evaluate the effects of resveratrol on metastasis formation in vivo, breast cancer cells were intravenously injected into the tail veins of five-week-old female Balb/c mice. The polyphenol was orally administered at different doses (100 and 200 mg/kg of body weight).

The cancer foci were significantly smaller in the resveratrol groups, possibly due to the decreased activity of MMP-9 in plasma, as confirmed using gelatin zymography [135]. In a study by Wang et al. [136], SKBR3/PR cells were implanted into the right flank of female Balb/c nude mice, which were then intraperitoneally treated with resveratrol (20 mg/kg) five times a day for 21 days. The treatment limited tumor growth and decreased its volume. In a xenograft model of oral cancer, created by injecting H-357 cells into Balb/c mice, resveratrol treatment caused a reduction in tumor volume [137].

In a study by Yang et al. [138], resveratrol attenuated the formation of metastases in the lungs of male NOD-SCID mice with HSC-39 cells injected into the tail vein. The results demonstrate the potential of resveratrol to inhibit IL-6-related cancer progression and metastasis. Another study assessed the effect of resveratrol against LoVo colorectal cancer. Briefly, female Balb/c nude mice aged four to six weeks were subjected to orthotopic implantation and tail injection with the cancer cells. Fragments of a tumor developed in one mouse were transplanted into the appendixes of other animals. The mice treated with a three-week intragastric administration of resveratrol at increasing doses (50, 100, and 150 mg/kg) resulted in fewer metastases in the lungs and suppressed local invasion and tumor growth. These effects were dose-dependent [139].

In a study by Wang and co-workers [140], C6 cells were stereotactically implanted into the right caudate nucleus of Wistar rats. The oral application of resveratrol prolonged survival time. Interestingly, only small amounts of cancer cells were visible in histopathological examination. Moreover, reduced MMP-9 expression was confirmed in tumor sections by immunohistochemistry. In a similar study, GICs acquired from patients were stereotactically injected into the right corpus striatum of six-week-old male NOD-SCID mice. Resveratrol (10 mg/kg) administered intraperitoneally once a day for four weeks suppressed cancer invasion. Tumors in the resveratrol-treated group were characterized by smoother borders and infiltrated the gray and white matter less clearly than in the control group [141]. In an orthotopic graft model using SCID mice with MNNG/HOS cells injected into the proximal tibia, the oral application of resveratrol resulted in less metastatic foci in the lungs and smaller origin tumors. Immunohistochemical staining also revealed decreased MMP-2 expression in tumor tissue [142].

Selected studies investigating the beneficial effects of resveratrol in vivo are summarized in Table 11.

Table 11. Overview of in vivo studies related to resveratrol.

Polyphenol	Animal Model	Dose/ Duration	Anti-Tumor Effects	Type IV Collagenase-Mediated Mechanisms	Reference
Resveratrol (3,5,4′-trihydroxystilbene)	Balb c nu/nu mice injected with PC-3	30 mg/kg through gavage thrice a week, with or without 15 mg/kg TRAIL intravenously on days 1, 7, 14, 21	↓angiogenesis ↓tumor volume	↓MMP-2, -9 protein	[144]
	Balb/c mice injected with 4 T1	100, 200 mg/kg orally, daily, for 21 days	↓metastatic incidence in lungs	↓MMP-9 activity (in plasma)	[135]
	Sprague-Dawley rats stimulated by DENA and CCl4	diet containing resveratrol 300, 450 mg/kg for 9 months; 300, 450 mg/kg for 4 weeks as pretreatment and for 9 months as post-treatment	↑normal hepatic tissue architecture (post-treatment group)	↓MMP-2, -9 serum concentration	[143]

Table 11. *Cont.*

Polyphenol	Animal Model	Dose/ Duration	Anti-Tumor Effects	Type IV Collagenase-Mediated Mechanisms	Reference
	Balb/c nude mice injected with LoVo	50, 100, 150 mg/kg via intragastric administration daily for 3 weeks	↓metastatic incidence in lungs (metastatic model and xenograft) ↓metastatic incidence in liver (xenograft) ↓tumor weight (xenograft)	not specified	[139]
	NOD-SCID mice injected with glioblastoma-initiating cells (GICs) derived from patients	10 mg/kg daily intraperitoneally for 28 days	↓mean depth of tumor invasion	not specified	[141]
	Wistar rats injected with C6	8 mg/kg daily orally for different lengths of time, depending on the animals' lifespan, minimum 13 days, maximum 90 days	↑survival time ↑apoptosis ↓tumor growth	↓MMP-9 protein ↓NF-κB protein	[140]
	SCID mice injected with MNNG/HOS	40, 100 mg/kg five times a week by oral gavage for 24 days	↓tumor volume ↓metastatic incidence in lungs	↓MMP-2 protein	[142]
	NOD-SCID mice injected with HSC-39	10, 20 μM for 3 weeks	↓metastatic incidence in lungs	not specified	[138]
	Balb/c mice injected with H-357	40 mg/kg daily orally for 55 days (resveratrol–nanoparticles)	↓tumor volume	not specified	[137]
	Balb/c nude mice injected with SKBR3/PR	20 mg/kg (free resveratrol) or equivalent dose (resveratrol–solid lipid nanoparticles with or without TPGS), intraperitoneally, 5 times a day for 21 days	↓tumor weight ↓tumor volume	not specified	[136]

Legend: ↑ activation or increase; ↓ inhibition or decreaset.

3.6. Human Studies

Clinical studies assessing the effectiveness and utility of polyphenols in cancer diseases by suppressing MMP expression are ongoing, and their number is limited. We searched for studies using the ClinicalTrials.gov platform. There are many studies that are in the phase of recruiting or have been completed without available results. Nonetheless, most of them focus on the beneficial effects of curcumin on cancer. In a study with patients with advanced pancreatic cancer, a phase II trial (NCT00094445) determined the effect of oral curcumin (8 mg per day for 8 weeks) on six-month survival and response rate and assessed the biological activity in tumor and blood mononuclear cells by examining signaling and apoptotic pathways. However, detailed results were not published. Another study (NCT00113841) was performed to assess clinical tolerance and response to curcumin alone and in combination with Bioperine in subjects with multiple myeloma (MM). Also, the evaluation of the biological effects of curcumin on the expression of NF-κB and related genes in MM was a primary objective. Two grams of the polyphenol was orally used in two divided doses. The percent change in NF-κB protein expression in peripheral blood mononuclear cells was assessed at baseline and after four weeks of treatment. The particular results were not presented. In turn, a phase I/II pilot study conducted on 13 patients with metastatic colorectal cancer analyzed the association between adding genistein to the regimens of FOLFOX or FOLFOX-Avastin and therapy tolerability, progression-free survival, and response rate measured by radiologic RECIST criteria (NCT01985763). Oral genistein at a dose of 60 mg per day for seven days every two weeks was applied. The therapy contributed to a significant percent regression in tumor size, as well as being associated with a good radiological response. Also, genistein may be useful in prostate cancer. A randomized phase II trial (NCT01126879) determined whether treatment with genistein could reduce the number of circulating prostate cancer cells and tumor growth via the downregulation of the expression of factors promoting tumor growth, including MMP-2, in prostate tissue. In this study, genistein was generally applied once daily for three months beginning at least one month prior to radical prostatectomy. Unfortunately, the trial was closed due to low accrual. There are some clinical trials assessing the efficacy of polyphenols for cancer prevention, as well as for improving the safety and effectiveness of chemotherapy (NCT01538316, NCT01496521, NCT06080841, NCT06398405, NCT06015022, NCT02891538, NCT01912820, NCT00027495, NCT01490996); however, their detailed status is unknown, patients are still being recruited, or detailed results have not been posted yet. The number of human studies confirming the safety and utility of polyphenols is insufficient. Moreover, outcomes from existing studies are not always positive. This results from several factors, such as the higher doses of the compounds used in animal studies compared to those applied in humans, among other factors. Large-scale, well-controlled human clinical trials are needed to confirm the health-promoting effects of consuming polyphenols.

4. The Mechanisms of MMP-2 and MMP-9 Regulation via Polyphenols

Many signaling pathways are responsible for the modulation of type IV collagenase expression and activity, which can affect cell growth, survival, migration, invasiveness, or even metastasis formation. The enhanced expression and activity of MMP-2 and MMP-9 are associated with the increased activity of various cellular signaling pathways, such as NF-κB, MAPK, or Akt. Also, it has been found that by suppressing these pathways, polyphenols may inhibit MMP activity [10]. The PI3 K/Akt cellular signaling pathway has a significant role in cell growth and survival, determining the development of potential cell malignancy and invasiveness. Several studies indicate that polyphenols have anti-cancer potential that is realized through the inhibition of MMPs by suppressing the PI3 K/AKT pathway. Resveratrol was found to suppress the activity of the PI3 K/Akt pathway, thus limiting the EMT, cell migration, and metastasis [118]. In addition, EGCG and curcumin appear to restrict the proliferation of bladder cancer and colon cancer, as well as limiting tumor growth and progression, by inhibiting the PI3 K/Akt pathway [145,146].

The activation of the MAPK and NF-κB pathways enhances the expression of MMP-2 and MMP-9, thus promoting cell invasion and migration and cancer disease progression [147,148]. However, curcumin treatment inhibited the proliferation and invasion of glioma cells by downregulating the ERK/MAPK pathway [36]. In turn, curcumin suppressed the growth and invasion of human monocytic leukemia cells by reducing MMP-2 and MMP-9 mRNA transcription and protein expression by downregulating the ERK and NF-κB signaling pathways [36]. Also, curcumin is able to reduce the resistance of lung cancer cells to therapy by suppressing NF-κB [149]. Furthermore, other polyphenols described in our article were demonstrated as compounds having the ability to suppress intracellular pathways. Quercetin was found to exert anti-cancer effects, cause cell cycle arrest, leading to cancer cell death, and limit the progression of the disease by downregulating the PI3 K/Akt, MAPK/ERK, JNK, p38, and NF-κB pathways [150,151]. In turn, genistein inactivates MAPK, Akt, NF-κB, and ERK1/2, which cause downstream MMP expression, and, consequently, exerts anti-cancer and anti-angiogenic effects [64].

The mechanisms by which polyphenols suppress type IV collagenases via cellular signaling pathways are summarized in Figure 2.

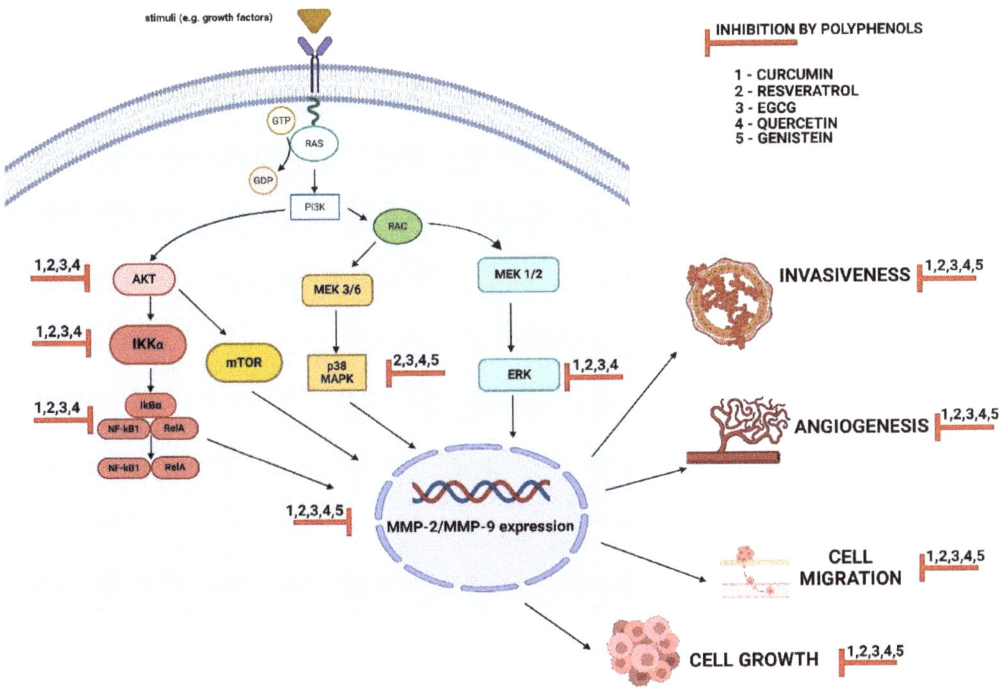

Figure 2. A schematic representation of the PI3 K/AKT, MAPK, and NF-κB pathways involved in the inhibition of expression and activity of MMP-2/9 by polyphenols (created by BioRender). AKT—protein kinase B; ERK—extracellular-signal-regulated kinase; IKK—I kappa B kinase; IKKα—catalytic subunit of IKK; IκBα—inhibitor alpha of nuclear factor-kappa B; GTP—guanosine-5′-triphosphate; MEK—mitogen-activated protein kinase; MMP-2/9—matrix metalloproteinase-2/9 (type IV collagenases); mTOR—mammalian target of rapamycin; NF-κB—nuclear factor-kappa B; PI3 K—phosphatidylinositol 3-kinase; p38 MAPK—p38 mitogen-activated protein kinase; RAS—rat sarcoma, subfamily of small GTPases; RelA—subunit of NF-κB; EGCG—epigallocatechin-3-gallate.

5. Summary and Conclusions

A considerable body of research has accumulated regarding the effects of individual polyphenols, such as curcumin, resveratrol, EGCG, genistein, and quercetin, as treatments for cancer. They are believed to exert their anti-invasive and anti-metastatic activities by downregulating the expression and activity of type IV collagenases and by suppressing cellular signaling pathways, particularly NF-κB and MAPK. Pre-clinical studies employing both in vitro and animal models suggest that they mostly act by inhibiting MMP-2 and MMP-9 or their related pathways, indicating that polyphenolic compounds have considerable potential against the development and progression of cancers.

The preventive and therapeutic efficacy of polyphenols as modulators of gelatinases in cancers remains controversial due to some limitations in the research described. Most of the studies described herein focus on the use of natural polyphenolic compounds in pre-clinical studies. These findings show that polyphenols are able to prevent cancer development by inhibiting MMP-2/MMP-9 and suppressing various signaling pathways. Unfortunately, the number of human studies is small, and those available were restricted to small participant groups, short-term administration, and usually one dose without a placebo group. The results of this review hint at the potential benefits associated with polyphenolic compounds, but more studies on patients are necessary to establish the efficacy and safety of polyphenols as inhibitors of MMP-2 and MMP-9. The large variation in the bioavailability of ingested compounds and incomplete information in food composition databases are only some of the main challenges related to their use. The effects of single polyphenolic compounds applied in pharmacological doses in epidemiological studies and animal models may, however, not be transferable to polyphenol levels achievable with normal human diets.

The most recent data show that polyphenols are characterized by unsatisfactory bioavailability and bioaccessibility, which may significantly limit the efficacy of their oral administration [152]. Therefore, there is a need to create new formulations or delivery systems with greater bioavailability. Nevertheless, taking into account their properties and metabolism, polyphenols offer promise as chemopreventive agents rather than as therapeutic ones. Further studies, primarily involving human participants in clinical trials, are necessary to confirm the anti-cancer properties of polyphenols as agents with chemopreventive activity.

Author Contributions: Conceptualization, U.L. and W.P.; methodology, W.P., M.C. and U.L.; investigation, writing—original draft preparation, W.P. and M.C.; writing—review and editing, U.L. visualization, M.C.; supervision, U.L. All authors have read and agreed to the published version of the manuscript.

Funding: The study was supported by grant No. 503/1-156-04/503-11-001 from the Medical University of Lodz, Poland.

Conflicts of Interest: The authors declare no conflicts of interest.

References

1. Laversanne, M.; Sung, H.; Ferlay, J.; Siegel, R.L.; Soerjomataram, I.; Jemal, A. Global Cancer Statistics 2020: GLOBOCAN Estimates of Incidence and Mortality Worldwide for 36 Cancers in 185 Countries. *CA Cancer J. Clin.* **2024**, *74*, 229–263.
2. Schirrmacher, V. From chemotherapy to biological therapy: A review of novel concepts to reduce the side effects of systemic cancer treatment. *Int. J. Oncol.* **2019**, *54*, 407–419. [CrossRef] [PubMed]
3. Zhang, C.; Liu, X.; Jin, S.; Chen, Y.; Guo, R. Ferroptosis in cancer therapy: A novel approach to reversing drug resistance. *Mol. Cancer* **2022**, *21*, 47. [CrossRef] [PubMed]
4. Dekker, E.; Tanis, P.J.; Vleugels, J.L.A.; Kasi, P.M.; Wallace, M.B. Colorectal cancer. *Lancet* **2019**, *394*, 1467–1480. [CrossRef] [PubMed]
5. Miller, M.; Hanna, N. Advances in systemic therapy for non-small cell lung cancer. *BMJ* **2021**, *375*, n2363. [CrossRef]
6. Chojnacka, K.; Owczarek, K.; Caban, M.; Sosnowska, D.; Kajszczak, D.; Lewandowska, U. Chemopreventive effects of Japanese quince (*Chaenomeles japonica* L.) phenol leaf extract on colon cancer cells through the modulation of extracellular signal-regulated kinases/Akt signaling pathway. *J. Physiol. Pharmacol.* **2022**, *73*, 41–52.
7. Liang, D.; Liu, L.; Zhao, Y.; Luo, Z.; He, Y.; Li, Y.; Tang, S.; Tang, J.; Chen, N. Targeting extracellular matrix through phytochemicals: A promising approach of multi-step actions on the treatment and prevention of cancer. *Front. Pharmacol.* **2023**, *14*, 1186712. [CrossRef]
8. Li, H.; Qiu, Z.; Li, F.; Wang, C. The relationship between MMP-2 and MMP-9 expression levels with breast cancer incidence and prognosis. *Oncol. Lett.* **2017**, *14*, 5865–5870. [CrossRef]
9. Zhou, W.; Yu, X.; Sun, S.; Zhang, X.; Yang, W.; Zhang, J.; Zhang, X.; Jiang, Z. Increased expression of MMP-2 and MMP-9 indicates poor prognosis in glioma recurrence. *Biomed. Pharmacother.* **2019**, *118*, 109369. [CrossRef]
10. Chojnacka, K.; Lewandowska, U. Chemopreventive effects of polyphenol-rich extracts against cancer invasiveness and metastasis by inhibition of type IV collagenases expression and activity. *J. Funct. Foods* **2018**, *46*, 295–311. [CrossRef]
11. Alaseem, A.; Alhazzani, K.; Dondapati, P.; Alobid, S.; Bishayee, A.; Rathinavelu, A. Matrix Metalloproteinases: A challenging paradigm of cancer management. *Semin. Cancer Biol.* **2019**, *56*, 100–115. [CrossRef] [PubMed]
12. Caban, M.; Owczarek, K.; Lewandowska, U. The Role of Metalloproteinases and Their Tissue Inhibitors on Ocular Diseases: Focusing on Potential Mechanisms. *Int. J. Mol. Sci.* **2022**, *23*, 4256. [CrossRef] [PubMed]
13. Anuar, N.N.M.; Zulkafali, N.I.N.; Ugusman, A. Modulation of Matrix Metalloproteinases by Plant-derived Products. *Curr. Cancer Drug Targets* **2021**, *21*, 91–106. [CrossRef] [PubMed]
14. Ang, H.L.; Mohan, C.D.; Shanmugam, M.K.; Leong, H.C.; Makvandi, P.; Rangappa, K.S.; Bishayee, A.; Kumar, A.P.; Sethi, G. Mechanism of epithelial-mesenchymal transition in cancer and its regulation by natural compounds. *Med. Res. Rev.* **2023**, *43*, 1141–1200. [CrossRef] [PubMed]

15. Das, B.; Sarkar, N.; Bishayee, A.; Sinha, D. Dietary phytochemicals in the regulation of epithelial to mesenchymal transition and associated enzymes: A promising anticancer therapeutic approach. *Semin. Cancer Biol.* **2019**, *56*, 196–218. [CrossRef] [PubMed]
16. Proença, C.; Freitas, M.; Ribeiro, D.; Rufino, A.T.; Fernandes, E.; Ferreira de Oliveira, J.M.P. The role of flavonoids in the regulation of epithelial-mesenchymal transition in cancer: A review on targeting signaling pathways and metastasis. *Med. Res. Rev.* **2023**, *43*, 1878–1945. [CrossRef] [PubMed]
17. Niedzwiecki, A.; Roomi, M.W.; Kalinovsky, T.; Rath, M. Anticancer Efficacy of Polyphenols and Their Combinations. *Nutrients* **2016**, *8*, 552. [CrossRef]
18. Lang, Y.; Gao, N.; Zang, Z.; Meng, X.; Lin, Y.; Yang, S.; Yang, Y.; Jin, Z.; Li, B. Classification and antioxidant assays of polyphenols: A review. *J. Future Foods* **2024**, *4*, 193–204. [CrossRef]
19. Zhang, L.; Han, Z.; Granato, D. Polyphenols in foods: Classification, methods of identification, and nutritional aspects in human health. *Adv. Food Nutr. Res.* **2021**, *98*, 1–33.
20. Singla, R.K.; Dubey, A.K.; Garg, A.; Sharma, R.K.; Fiorino, M.; Ameen, S.M.; Haddad, M.A.; Al-Hiary, M. Natural Polyphenols: Chemical Classification, Definition of Classes, Subcategories, and Structures. *J. AOAC Int.* **2019**, *102*, 1397–1400. [CrossRef]
21. Burcher, J.T.; DeLiberto, L.K.; Allen, A.M.; Kilpatrick, K.L.; Bishayee, A. Bioactive phytocompounds for oral cancer prevention and treatment: A comprehensive and critical evaluation. *Med. Res. Rev.* **2023**, *43*, 2025–2085. [CrossRef] [PubMed]
22. Fraga, C.G.; Croft, K.D.; Kennedy, D.O.; Tomás-Barberán, F.A. The effects of polyphenols and other bioactives on human health. *Food Funct.* **2019**, *10*, 514–528. [CrossRef] [PubMed]
23. Leri, M.; Scuto, M.; Ontario, M.L.; Calabrese, V.; Calabrese, E.J.; Bucciantini, M.; Stefani, M. Healthy Effects of Plant Polyphenols: Molecular Mechanisms. *Int. J. Mol. Sci.* **2020**, *21*, 1250. [CrossRef] [PubMed]
24. Caban, M.; Lewandowska, U. Polyphenols and the potential mechanisms of their therapeutic benefits against inflammatory bowel diseases. *J. Funct. Foods* **2022**, *95*, 105181. [CrossRef]
25. Caban, M.; Owczarek, K.; Chojnacka, K.; Podsędek, A.; Sosnowska, D.; Lewandowska, U. Chemopreventive properties of spent hops (*Humulus lupulus* L.) extract against angiogenesis, invasion and migration of colorectal cancer cells. *J. Physiol. Pharmacol.* **2022**, *73*, 431–442.
26. Caban, M.; Owczarek, K.; Podsędek, A.; Sosnowska, D.; Lewandowska, U. Spent hops extract (*Humulus lupulus* L.) attenuates inflammation and angiogenesis of the retina via the nuclear factor-kappaB and protein kinase B/extracellular signal-regulated kinase pathways. *J. Physiol. Pharmacol.* **2023**, *74*, 537–549.
27. Pulido-Moran, M.; Moreno-Fernandez, J.; Ramirez-Tortosa, C.; Ramirez-Tortosa, M. Curcumin and Health. *Molecules* **2016**, *21*, 264. [CrossRef]
28. Bhatia, M.; Bhalerao, M.; Cruz-Martins, N.; Kumar, D. Curcumin and cancer biology: Focusing regulatory effects in different signalling pathways. *Phytother. Res.* **2021**, *35*, 4913–4929. [CrossRef]
29. Hassan, Z.K.; Daghestani, M.H. Curcumin effect on MMPs and TIMPs genes in a breast cancer cell line. *Asian Pac. J. Cancer Prev.* **2012**, *13*, 3259–3264. [CrossRef]
30. Sun, J. Matrix metalloproteinases and tissue inhibitor of metalloproteinases are essential for the inflammatory response in cancer cells. *J. Signal Transduct.* **2010**, *2010*, 985132. [CrossRef]
31. Lin, H.J.; Su, C.C.; Lu, H.F.; Yang, J.S.; Hsu, S.C.; Ip, S.W.; Wu, J.J.; Li, Y.C.; Ho, C.C.; Wu, C.C.; et al. Curcumin blocks migration and invasion of mouse-rat hybrid retina ganglion cells (N18) through the inhibition of MMP-2, -9, FAK, Rho A and Rock-1 gene expression. *Oncol. Rep.* **2010**, *23*, 665–670. [PubMed]
32. Sirohi, V.K.; Popli, P.; Sankhwar, P.; Kaushal, J.B.; Gupta, K.; Manohar, M.; Dwivedi, A. Curcumin exhibits anti-tumor effect and attenuates cellular migration via Slit-2 mediated down-regulation of SDF-1 and CXCR4 in endometrial adenocarcinoma cells. *J. Nutr. Biochem.* **2017**, *44*, 60–70. [CrossRef] [PubMed]
33. Zhao, Z.; Su, J.; Zhao, J.; Chen, J.; Cui, X.; Sun, M.; Zhang, X. Curcumin inhibits invasion and metastasis of human hepatoma cells through Bclaf1-mediated Wnt/β-catenin signalling. *Food Agric. Immunol.* **2022**, *33*, 664–676. [CrossRef]
34. Jia, W.; Deng, F.; Fu, W.; Hu, J.; Chen, G.; Gao, X.; Tan, X.; Li, G.; Liu, G.; Zhu, S. Curcumin suppresses wilms' tumor metastasis by inhibiting RECK methylation. *Biomed. Pharmacother.* **2019**, *111*, 1204–1212. [CrossRef]
35. Zhang, H.H.; Zhang, Y.; Cheng, Y.N.; Gong, F.L.; Cao, Z.Q.; Yu, L.G.; Guo, X.L. Metformin incombination with curcumin inhibits the growth, metastasis, and angiogenesis of hepatocellular carcinoma in vitro and in vivo. *Mol. Carcinog.* **2018**, *57*, 44–56. [CrossRef]
36. Wang, P.; Hao, X.; Li, X.; Yan, Y.; Tian, W.; Xiao, L.; Wang, Z.; Dong, J. Curcumin inhibits adverse psychological stress-induced proliferation and invasion of glioma cells via down-regulating the ERK/MAPK pathway. *J. Cell. Mol. Med.* **2021**, *25*, 7190–7203. [CrossRef]
37. Zhu, G.; Shen, Q.; Jiang, H.; Ji, O.; Zhu, L.; Zhang, L. Curcumin inhibited the growth and invasion of human monocytic leukaemia SHI-1 cells in vivo by altering MAPK and MMP signalling. *Pharm. Biol.* **2020**, *58*, 25–34. [CrossRef]
38. Chopra, H.; Dey, P.S.; Das, D.; Bhattacharya, T.; Shah, M.; Mubin, S.; Maishu, S.P.; Akter, R.; Rahman, M.H.; Karthika, C.; et al. Curcumin Nanoparticles as Promising Therapeutic Agents for Drug Targets. *Molecules* **2021**, *26*, 4998. [CrossRef]
39. Tavakoli, F.; Jahanban-Esfahlan, R.; Seidi, K.; Jabbari, M.; Behzadi, R.; Pilehvar-Soltanahmadi, Y.; Zarghami, N. Effects of nano-encapsulated curcumin-chrysin on telomerase, MMPs and TIMPs gene expression in mouse B16F10 melanoma tumour model. *Artif. Cells Nanomed. Biotechnol.* **2018**, *46*, 75–86. [CrossRef]
40. Sesarman, A.; Tefas, L.; Sylvester, B.; Licarete, E.; Rauca, V.; Luput, L.; Patras, L.; Porav, S.; Banciu, M.; Porfire, A. Co-delivery of curcumin and doxorubicin in PEGylated liposomes favored the antineoplastic C26 murine colon carcinoma microenvironment. *Drug Deliv. Transl. Res.* **2019**, *9*, 260–272. [CrossRef]

41. Gan, R.Y.; Li, H.B.; Sui, Z.Q.; Corke, H. Absorption, metabolism, anti-cancer effect and molecular targets of epigallocatechin gallate (EGCG): An updated review. *Crit. Rev. Food Sci. Nutr.* **2018**, *58*, 924–941. [CrossRef] [PubMed]
42. Li, F.; Gao, C.; Yan, P.; Zhang, M.; Wang, Y.; Hu, Y.; Wu, X.; Wang, X.; Sheng, J. EGCG Reduces Obesity and White Adipose Tissue Gain Partly Through AMPK Activation in Mice. *Front. Pharmacol.* **2018**, *9*, 1366. [CrossRef] [PubMed]
43. Negri, A.; Naponelli, V.; Rizzi, F.; Bettuzzi, S. Molecular Targets of Epigallocatechin-Gallate (EGCG): A Special Focus on Signal Transduction and Cancer. *Nutrients* **2018**, *10*, 1936. [CrossRef] [PubMed]
44. Du, G.J.; Zhang, Z.; Wen, X.D.; Yu, C.; Calway, T.; Yuan, C.S.; Wang, C.Z. Epigallocatechin Gallate (EGCG) Is the Most Effective Cancer Chemopreventive Polyphenol in Green Tea. *Nutrients* **2012**, *4*, 1679–1691. [CrossRef] [PubMed]
45. Benelli, R.; Venè, R.; Bisacchi, D.; Garbisa, S.; Albini, A. Anti-invasive effects of green tea polyphenol epigallocatechin-3-gallate (EGCG), a natural inhibitor of metallo and serine proteases. *Biol Chem.* **2002**, *383*, 101–105. [CrossRef]
46. Vayalil, P.K.; Katiyar, S.K. Treatment of epigallocatechin-3-gallate inhibits matrix metalloproteinases-2 and -9 via inhibition of activation of mitogen-activated protein kinases, c-jun and NF-kappaB in human prostate carcinoma DU-145 cells. *Prostate* **2004**, *59*, 33–42. [CrossRef]
47. Huang, Y.J.; Wang, K.L.; Chen, H.Y.; Chiang, Y.F.; Hsia, S.M. Protective Effects of Epigallocatechin Gallate (EGCG) on Endometrial, Breast, and Ovarian Cancers. *Biomolecules* **2020**, *10*, 1481. [CrossRef]
48. Roomi, M.W.; Kalinovsky, T.; Niedzwiecki, A.; Rath, M. Modulation of MMP-2 and -9 secretion by cytokines, inducers and inhibitors in human melanoma A-2058 cells. *Oncol. Rep.* **2017**, *37*, 3681–3687. [CrossRef]
49. Roomi, M.W.; Bhanap, B.; Niedzwiecki, A.; Rath, M. In vitro modulation of MMP-2 and MMP-9 secretion by cytokines, inducers, and inhibitors in head and neck squamous carcinoma cells (FaDu) and tongue carcinoma cells (SCC-25). *J. Otolaryngol. Rhinol.* **2017**, *3*, 29. [CrossRef]
50. Roomi, M.W.; Kalinovsky, T.; Rath, M.; Niedzwiecki, A. In vitro modulation of MMP-2 and MMP-9 in pediatric human sarcoma cell lines by cytokines, inducers and inhibitors. *Int. J. Oncol.* **2014**, *44*, 27–34. [CrossRef]
51. Roomi, M.W.; Kalinovsky, T.; Monterrey, J.; Rath, M.; Niedzwiecki, A. In vitro modulation of MMP-2 and MMP-9 in adult human sarcoma cell lines by cytokines, inducers and inhibitors. *Int. J. Oncol.* **2013**, *43*, 1787–1798. [CrossRef] [PubMed]
52. Roomi, M.W.; Monterrey, J.C.; Kalinovsky, T.; Rath, M.; Niedzwiecki, A. In vitro modulation of MMP-2 and MMP-9 in human cervical and ovarian cancer cell lines by cytokines, inducers and inhibitors. *Oncol. Rep.* **2010**, *23*, 605–614. [PubMed]
53. Roomi, M.W.; Ivanov, V.; Kalinovsky, T.; Niedzwiecki, A.; Rath, M. Modulation of human renal cell carcinoma 786-0 MMP-2 and MMP-9 activity by inhibitors and inducers in vitro. *Med. Oncol.* **2006**, *23*, 245–250. [CrossRef] [PubMed]
54. Ho, H.C.; Huang, C.C.; Lu, Y.T.; Yeh, C.M.; Ho, Y.T.; Yang, S.F.; Hsin, C.H.; Lin, C.W. Epigallocatechin-3-gallate inhibits migration of human nasopharyngeal carcinoma cells by repressing MMP-2 expression. *J. Cell. Physiol.* **2019**, *234*, 20915–20924. [CrossRef]
55. Chen, S.J.; Yao, X.D.; Peng, B.O.; Xu, Y.F.; Wang, G.C.; Huang, J.; Liu, M.; Zheng, J.H. Epigallocatechin-3-gallate inhibits migration and invasion of human renal carcinoma cells by downregulating matrix metalloproteinase-2 and matrix metalloproteinase-9. *Exp. Ther. Med.* **2016**, *11*, 1243–1248. [CrossRef]
56. Kwak, T.W.; Park, S.B.; Kim, H.J.; Jeong, Y.I.; Kang, D.H. Anticancer activities of epigallocatechin-3-gallate against cholangiocarcinoma cells. *Onco Targets Ther.* **2016**, *10*, 137–144. [CrossRef]
57. Luo, K.W.; Chen, W.; Lung, W.Y.; Wei, X.Y.; Cheng, B.H.; Cai, Z.M.; Huang, W.R. EGCG inhibited bladder cancer SW780 cell proliferation and migration both in vitro and in vivo via down-regulation of NF-κB and MMP-9. *J. Nutr. Biochem.* **2017**, *41*, 56–64. [CrossRef]
58. Zhang, L.; Chen, W.; Tu, G.; Chen, X.; Lu, Y.; Wu, L.; Zheng, D. Enhanced Chemotherapeutic Efficacy of PLGA-Encapsulated Epigallocatechin Gallate (EGCG) Against Human Lung Cancer. *Int. J. Nanomed.* **2020**, *15*, 4417–4429. [CrossRef]
59. Zhang, L.; Xie, J.; Gan, R.; Wu, Z.; Luo, H.; Chen, X.; Lu, Y.; Wu, L.; Zheng, D. Synergistic inhibition of lung cancer cells by EGCG and NF-κB inhibitor BAY11-7082. *J. Cancer* **2019**, *10*, 6543–6556. [CrossRef]
60. Deng, Y.T.; Lin, J.K. EGCG inhibits the invasion of highly invasive CL1-5 lung cancer cells through suppressing MMP-2 expression via JNK signaling and induces G2/M arrest. *J. Agric. Food Chem.* **2011**, *59*, 13318–13327. [CrossRef]
61. Fang, C.Y.; Wu, C.C.; Hsu, H.Y.; Chuang, H.Y.; Huang, S.Y.; Tsai, C.H.; Chang, Y.; Tsao, G.S.; Chen, C.L.; Chen, J.Y. EGCG inhibits proliferation, invasiveness and tumor growth by up-regulation of adhesion molecules, suppression of gelatinases activity, and induction of apoptosis in nasopharyngeal carcinoma cells. *Int. J. Mol. Sci.* **2015**, *16*, 2530–2558. [CrossRef] [PubMed]
62. Chen, P.N.; Chu, S.C.; Kuo, W.H.; Chou, M.Y.; Lin, J.K.; Hsieh, Y.S. Epigallocatechin-3 gallate inhibits invasion, epithelial-mesenchymal transition, and tumor growth in oral cancer cells. *J. Agric. Food Chem.* **2011**, *59*, 3836–3844. [CrossRef] [PubMed]
63. Shankar, S.; Marsh, L.; Srivastava, R.K. EGCG inhibits growth of human pancreatic tumors orthotopically implanted in Balb C nude mice through modulation of FKHRL1/FOXO3a and neuropilin. *Mol. Cell. Biochem.* **2013**, *372*, 83–94. [CrossRef]
64. Tuli, H.S.; Tuorkey, M.J.; Thakral, F.; Sak, K.; Kumar, M.; Sharma, A.K.; Sharma, U.; Jain, A.; Aggarwal, V.; Bishayee, A. Molecular Mechanisms of Action of Genistein in Cancer: Recent Advances. *Front. Pharmacol.* **2019**, *10*, 1336. [CrossRef] [PubMed]
65. Russo, M.; Russo, G.L.; Daglia, M.; Kasi, P.D.; Ravi, S.; Nabavi, S.F.; Nabavi, S.M. Understanding genistein in cancer: The "good" and the "bad" effects: A review. *Food Chem.* **2016**, *196*, 589–600. [CrossRef]
66. Mukund, V.; Mukund, D.; Sharma, V.; Mannarapu, M.; Alam, A. Genistein: Its role in metabolic diseases and cancer. *Crit. Rev. Oncol. Hematol.* **2017**, *119*, 13–22. [CrossRef]
67. Shafiee, G.; Saidijam, M.; Tayebinia, H.; Khodadadi, I. Beneficial effects of genistein in suppression of proliferation, inhibition of metastasis, and induction of apoptosis in PC3 prostate cancer cells. *Arch. Physiol. Biochem.* **2022**, *128*, 694–702. [CrossRef]

68. Shafiee, G.; Saidijam, M.; Tavilani, H.; Ghasemkhani, N.; Khodadadi, I. Genistein Induces Apoptosis and Inhibits Proliferation of HT29 Colon Cancer Cells. *Int. J. Mol. Cell. Med.* **2016**, *5*, 178–191.
69. Zhu, J.; Ren, J.; Tang, L. Genistein inhibits invasion and migration of colon cancer cells by recovering WIF1 expression. *Mol. Med. Rep.* **2018**, *17*, 7265–7273. [CrossRef]
70. Hussain, A.; Harish, G.; Prabhu, S.A.; Mohsin, J.; Khan, M.A.; Rizvi, T.A.; Sharma, C. Inhibitory effect of genistein on the invasive potential of human cervical cancer cells via modulation of matrix metalloproteinase-9 and tissue inhibitors of matrix metalloproteinase-1 expression. *Cancer Epidemiol.* **2012**, *36*, e387–e393. [CrossRef]
71. Bi, Y.L.; Min, M.; Shen, W.; Liu, Y. Genistein induced anticancer effects on pancreatic cancer cell lines involves mitochondrial apoptosis, G0/G1cell cycle arrest and regulation of STAT3 signalling pathway. *Phytomedicine* **2018**, *39*, 10–16. [CrossRef] [PubMed]
72. Dowling, S.; Regan, F.; Hughes, H. The characterisation of structural and antioxidant properties of isoflavone metal chelates. *J. Inorg. Biochem.* **2010**, *104*, 1091–1098. [CrossRef] [PubMed]
73. Spoerlein, C.; Mahal, K.; Schmidt, H.; Schobert, R. Effects of chrysin, apigenin, genistein and their homoleptic copper(II) complexes on the growth and metastatic potential of cancer cells. *J. Inorg. Biochem.* **2013**, *127*, 107–115. [CrossRef]
74. Noori, D.M.; Saffari, M.; Saydi, D.O.; Rahmani, B.; Noori, D.A.; Salehi, A.; Ghazarian, A. Study of antimetastatic effect of genistein through inhibition of expression of matrix metalloproteinase in A-549 cell line. *J. Sci. Islam. Repub. Iran* **2012**, *23*, 115–122.
75. Han, L.; Zhang, H.W.; Zhou, W.P.; Chen, G.M.; Guo, K.J. The effects of genistein on transforming growth factor-β1-induced invasion and metastasis in human pancreatic cancer cell line Panc-1 in vitro. *Chin. Med. J.* **2012**, *125*, 2032–2040.
76. Xiao, X.; Liu, Z.; Wang, R.; Wang, J.; Zhang, S.; Cai, X.; Wu, K.; Bergan, R.C.; Xu, L.; Fan, D. Genistein suppresses FLT4 and inhibits human colorectal cancer metastasis. *Oncotarget* **2015**, *6*, 3225–3239. [CrossRef]
77. Chen, P.; Hu, M.D.; Deng, X.F.; Li, B. Genistein reinforces the inhibitory effect of Cisplatin on liver cancer recurrence and metastasis after curative hepatectomy. *Asian Pac. J. Cancer Prev.* **2013**, *14*, 759–764. [CrossRef]
78. Kidani, T.; Nakamura, A.; Kamei, S.; Norimatsu, Y.; Miura, H.; Masuno, H. Overexpression of cytoplasmic β-catenin inhibits the metastasis of the murine osteosarcoma cell line LM8. *Cancer Cell Int.* **2014**, *14*, 31. [CrossRef]
79. Aghababaei, F.; Hadidi, M. Recent Advances in Potential Health Benefits of Quercetin. *Pharmaceuticals* **2023**, *16*, 1020. [CrossRef]
80. Kim, J.K.; Park, S.U. Quercetin and its role in biological functions: An updated review. *EXCLI J.* **2018**, *17*, 856–863.
81. Tang, S.M.; Deng, X.T.; Zhou, J.; Li, Q.P.; Ge, X.X.; Miao, L. Pharmacological basis and new insights of quercetin action in respect to its anti-cancer effects. *Biomed. Pharmacother.* **2020**, *121*, 109604. [CrossRef] [PubMed]
82. Asgharian, P.; Tazekand, A.P.; Hosseini, K.; Forouhandeh, H.; Ghasemnejad, T.; Ranjbar, M.; Hasan, M.; Kumar, M.; Beirami, S.M.; Tarhriz, V.; et al. Potential mechanisms of quercetin in cancer prevention: Focus on cellular and molecular targets. *Cancer Cell Int.* **2022**, *22*, 257. [CrossRef] [PubMed]
83. Elumalai, P.; Ezhilarasan, D.; Raghunandhakumar, S. Quercetin Inhibits the Epithelial to Mesenchymal Transition through Suppressing Akt Mediated Nuclear Translocation of β-Catenin in Lung Cancer Cell Line. *Nutr Cancer* **2022**, *74*, 1894–1906. [CrossRef] [PubMed]
84. Wu, T.C.; Chan, S.T.; Chang, C.N.; Yu, P.S.; Chuang, C.H.; Yeh, S.L. Quercetin and chrysin inhibit nickel-induced invasion and migration by downregulation of TLR4/NF-κB signaling in A549 cells. *Chem. Biol. Interact.* **2018**, *292*, 101–109. [CrossRef]
85. Liu, Y.; Tang, Z.G.; Lin, Y.; Qu, X.G.; Lv, W.; Wang, G.B.; Li, C.L. Effects of quercetin on proliferation and migration of human glioblastoma U251 cells. *Biomed. Pharmacother.* **2017**, *92*, 33–38. [CrossRef]
86. Liu, Y.; Tang, Z.G.; Yang, J.Q.; Zhou, Y.; Meng, L.H.; Wang, H.; Li, C.L. Low concentration of quercetin antagonizes the invasion and angiogenesis of human glioblastoma U251 cells. *Onco. Targets Ther.* **2017**, *10*, 4023–4028. [CrossRef]
87. Faria, A.; Pestana, D.; Teixeira, D.; Azevedo, J.; De Freitas, V.; Mateus, N.; Calhau, C. Flavonoid transport across RBE4 cells: A blood-brain barrier model. *Cell Mol Biol Lett.* **2010**, *15*, 234–241. [CrossRef]
88. Zhao, J.; Fang, Z.; Zha, Z.; Sun, Q.; Wang, H.; Sun, M.; Qiao, B. Quercetin inhibits cell viability, migration and invasion by regulating miR-16/HOXA10 axis in oral cancer. *Eur. J. Pharmacol.* **2019**, *847*, 11–18. [CrossRef]
89. Li, S.; Pei, Y.; Wang, W.; Liu, F.; Zheng, K.; Zhang, X. Quercetin suppresses the proliferation and metastasis of metastatic osteosarcoma cells by inhibiting parathyroid hormone receptor 1. *Biomed. Pharmacother.* **2019**, *114*, 108839. [CrossRef]
90. Liu, Y.; Li, C.L.; Xu, Q.Q.; Cheng, D.; Liu, K.D.; Sun, Z.Q. Quercetin inhibits invasion and angiogenesis of esophageal cancer cells. *Pathol. Res. Pract.* **2021**, *222*, 153455. [CrossRef]
91. Li, H.; Chen, C. Quercetin Has Antimetastatic Effects on Gastric Cancer Cells via the Interruption of uPA/uPAR Function by Modulating NF-κb, PKC-δ, ERK1/2, and AMPKα. *Integr. Cancer Ther.* **2018**, *17*, 511–523. [CrossRef]
92. Yu, D.; Ye, T.; Xiang, Y.; Shi, Z.; Zhang, J.; Lou, B.; Zhang, F.; Chen, B.; Zhou, M. Quercetin inhibits epithelial-mesenchymal transition, decreases invasiveness and metastasis, and reverses IL-6 induced epithelial-mesenchymal transition, expression of MMP by inhibiting STAT3 signaling in pancreatic cancer cells. *Onco Targets Ther.* **2017**, *10*, 4719–4729. [CrossRef] [PubMed]
93. Dhanaraj, T.; Mohan, M.; Arunakaran, J. Quercetin attenuates metastatic ability of human metastatic ovarian cancer cells via modulating multiple signaling molecules involved in cell survival, proliferation, migration and adhesion. *Arch. Biochem. Biophys.* **2021**, *701*, 108795. [CrossRef] [PubMed]
94. Xu, Z.; Zhao, D.; Zheng, X.; Huang, B.; Xia, X.; Pan, X. Quercetin exerts bidirectional regulation effects on the efficacy of tamoxifen in estrogen receptor-positive breast cancer therapy: An in vitro study. *Environ. Toxicol.* **2020**, *35*, 1179–1193. [CrossRef] [PubMed]

95. Quagliariello, V.; Iaffaioli, R.V.; Armenia, E.; Clemente, O.; Barbarisi, M.; Nasti, G.; Berretta, M.; Ottaiano, A.; Barbarisi, A. Hyaluronic Acid Nanohydrogel Loaded With Quercetin Alone or in Combination to a Macrolide Derivative of Rapamycin RAD001 (Everolimus) as a New Treatment for Hormone-Responsive Human Breast Cancer. *J. Cell. Physiol.* **2017**, *232*, 2063–2074. [CrossRef]
96. Roshanazadeh, M.; Babaahmadi Rezaei, H.; Rashidi, M. Quercetin Enhances the Suppressive Effects of Doxorubicin on the Migration of MDA-MB-231 Breast Cancer Cell Line. *Int. J. Cancer Manag.* **2021**, *14*, e119049. [CrossRef]
97. Ozkan, E.; Bakar-Ates, F. Potentiation of the Effect of Lonidamine by Quercetin in MCF-7 human breast cancer cells through downregulation of MMP-2/9 mRNA Expression. *An. Acad. Bras. Cienc.* **2020**, *92*, e20200548. [CrossRef]
98. Tang, H.; Kuang, Y.; Wu, W.; Peng, B.; Fu, Q. Quercetin inhibits the metabolism of arachidonic acid by inhibiting the activity of CYP3A4, thereby inhibiting the progression of breast cancer. *Mol Med.* **2023**, *29*, 127. [CrossRef]
99. Jia, L.; Huang, S.; Yin, X.; Zan, Y.; Guo, Y.; Han, L. Quercetin suppresses the mobility of breast cancer by suppressing glycolysis through Akt-mTOR pathway mediated autophagy induction. *Life Sci.* **2018**, *208*, 123–130. [CrossRef]
100. Balakrishnan, S.; Bhat, F.A.; Raja Singh, P.; Mukherjee, S.; Elumalai, P.; Das, S.; Patra, C.R.; Arunakaran, J. Gold nanoparticle-conjugated quercetin inhibits epithelial-mesenchymal transition, angiogenesis and invasiveness via EGFR/VEGFR-2-mediated pathway in breast cancer. *Cell Prolif.* **2016**, *49*, 678–697. [CrossRef]
101. Chang, J.H.; Lai, S.L.; Chen, W.S.; Hung, W.Y.; Chow, J.M.; Hsiao, M.; Lee, W.J.; Chien, M.H. Quercetin suppresses the metastatic ability of lung cancer through inhibiting Snail-dependent Akt activation and Snail-independent ADAM9 expression pathways. *Biochim. Biophys. Acta Mol. Cell Res.* **2017**, *1864*, 1746–1758. [CrossRef] [PubMed]
102. Kee, J.Y.; Han, Y.H.; Kim, D.S.; Mun, J.G.; Park, J.; Jeong, M.Y.; Um, J.Y.; Hong, S.H. Inhibitory effect of quercetin on colorectal lung metastasis through inducing apoptosis, and suppression of metastatic ability. *Phytomedicine* **2016**, *23*, 1680–1690. [CrossRef] [PubMed]
103. Wu, R.; Zhou, T.; Xiong, J.; Zhang, Z.; Tian, S.; Wang, Y.; Chen, J.; Tian, X. Quercetin, the Ingredient of Xihuang Pills, Inhibits Hepatocellular Carcinoma by Regulating Autophagy and Macrophage Polarization. *Front. Biosci. (Landmark Ed.)* **2022**, *27*, 323. [CrossRef] [PubMed]
104. Chan, C.Y.; Hong, S.C.; Chang, C.M.; Chen, Y.H.; Liao, P.C.; Huang, C.Y. Oral Squamous Cell Carcinoma Cells with Acquired Resistance to Erlotinib Are Sensitive to Anti-Cancer Effect of Quercetin via Pyruvate Kinase M2 (PKM2). *Cells* **2023**, *12*, 179. [CrossRef] [PubMed]
105. Cao, H.H.; Tse, A.K.; Kwan, H.Y.; Yu, H.; Cheng, C.Y.; Su, T.; Fong, W.F.; Yu, Z.L. Quercetin exerts anti-melanoma activities and inhibits STAT3 signaling. *Biochem. Pharmacol.* **2014**, *87*, 424–434. [CrossRef]
106. Lan, H.; Hong, W.; Fan, P.; Qian, D.; Zhu, J.; Bai, B. Quercetin Inhibits Cell Migration and Invasion in Human Osteosarcoma Cells. *Cell. Physiol. Biochem.* **2017**, *43*, 553–567. [CrossRef]
107. Pradhan, S.J.; Mishra, R.; Sharma, P.; Kundu, G.C. Quercetin and sulforaphane in combination suppress the progression of melanoma through the down-regulation of matrix metalloproteinase-9. *Exp. Ther. Med.* **2010**, *1*, 915–920. [CrossRef]
108. Vervandier-Fasseur, D.; Latruffe, N. The Potential Use of Resveratrol for Cancer Prevention. *Molecules* **2019**, *24*, 4506. [CrossRef]
109. Ren, B.; Kwah, M.X.; Liu, C.; Ma, Z.; Shanmugam, M.K.; Ding, L.; Xiang, X.; Ho, P.C.; Wang, L.; Ong, P.S.; et al. Resveratrol for cancer therapy: Challenges and future perspectives. *Cancer Lett.* **2021**, *515*, 63–72. [CrossRef]
110. Ko, J.H.; Sethi, G.; Um, J.Y.; Shanmugam, M.K.; Arfuso, F.; Kumar, A.P.; Bishayee, A.; Ahn, K.S. The Role of Resveratrol in Cancer Therapy. *Int. J. Mol. Sci.* **2017**, *18*, 2589. [CrossRef]
111. Najafiyan, B.; Bokaii Hosseini, Z.; Esmaelian, S.; Firuzpour, F.; Rahimipour Anaraki, S.; Kalantari, L.; Hheidari, A.; Mesgari, H.; Nabi-Afjadi, M. Unveiling the potential effects of resveratrol in lung cancer treatment: Mechanisms and nanoparticle-based drug delivery strategies. *Biomed. Pharmacother.* **2024**, *172*, 116207. [CrossRef]
112. Xiong, W.; Yin, A.; Mao, X.; Zhang, W.; Huang, H.; Zhang, X. Resveratrol suppresses human glioblastoma cell migration and invasion via activation of RhoA/ROCK signaling pathway. *Oncol. Lett.* **2016**, *11*, 484–490. [CrossRef] [PubMed]
113. Lin, F.Y.; Hsieh, Y.H.; Yang, S.F.; Chen, C.T.; Tang, C.H.; Chou, M.Y.; Chuang, Y.T.; Lin, C.W.; Chen, M.K. Resveratrol suppresses TPA-induced matrix metalloproteinase-9 expression through the inhibition of MAPK pathways in oral cancer cells. *J. Oral Pathol. Med.* **2015**, *44*, 699–706. [CrossRef] [PubMed]
114. Chang, W.S.; Tsai, C.W.; Yang, J.S.; Hsu, Y.M.; Shih, L.C.; Chiu, H.Y.; Bau, D.T.; Tsai, F.J. Resveratrol inhibited the metastatic behaviors of cisplatin-resistant human oral cancer cells via phosphorylation of ERK/p-38 and suppression of MMP-2/9. *J. Food Biochem.* **2021**, *45*, e13666. [CrossRef] [PubMed]
115. Angellotti, G.; Di Prima, G.; Belfiore, E.; Campisi, G.; De Caro, V. Chemopreventive and Anticancer Role of Resveratrol against Oral Squamous Cell Carcinoma. *Pharmaceutics* **2023**, *15*, 275. [CrossRef] [PubMed]
116. Kim, Y.S.; Sull, J.W.; Sung, H.J. Suppressing effect of resveratrol on the migration and invasion of human metastatic lung and cervical cancer cells. *Mol. Biol. Rep.* **2012**, *39*, 8709–8716. [CrossRef]
117. Park, S.Y.; Chae, S.Y.; Park, J.O.; Lee, K.J.; Park, G. Gold-conjugated resveratrol nanoparticles attenuate the invasion and MMP-9 and COX-2 expression in breast cancer cells. *Oncol. Rep.* **2016**, *35*, 3248–3256. [CrossRef] [PubMed]
118. Sun, Y.; Zhou, Q.M.; Lu, Y.Y.; Zhang, H.; Chen, Q.L.; Zhao, M.; Su, S.B. Resveratrol Inhibits the Migration and Metastasis of MDA-MB-231 Human Breast Cancer by Reversing TGF-β1-Induced Epithelial-Mesenchymal Transition. *Molecules* **2019**, *24*, 1131. [CrossRef]
119. Suh, J.; Kim, D.H.; Surh, Y.J. Resveratrol suppresses migration, invasion and stemness of human breast cancer cells by interfering with tumor-stromal cross-talk. *Arch. Biochem. Biophys.* **2018**, *643*, 62–71. [CrossRef]
120. Shin, H.J.; Han, J.M.; Choi, Y.S.; Jung, H.J. Pterostilbene Suppresses both Cancer Cells and Cancer Stem-Like Cells in Cervical Cancer with Superior Bioavailability to Resveratrol. *Molecules* **2020**, *25*, 228. [CrossRef]

121. Buhrmann, C.; Shayan, P.; Goel, A.; Shakibaei, M. Resveratrol Regulates Colorectal Cancer Cell Invasion by Modulation of Focal Adhesion Molecules. *Nutrients* **2017**, *9*, 1073. [CrossRef] [PubMed]
122. Buhrmann, C.; Yazdi, M.; Popper, B.; Shayan, P.; Goel, A.; Aggarwal, B.B.; Shakibaei, M. Resveratrol Chemosensitizes TNF-β-Induced Survival of 5-FU-Treated Colorectal Cancer Cells. *Nutrients* **2018**, *10*, 888. [CrossRef] [PubMed]
123. Li, W.; Ma, J.; Ma, Q.; Li, B.; Han, L.; Liu, J.; Xu, Q.; Duan, W.; Yu, S.; Wang, F.; et al. Resveratrol inhibits the epithelial-mesenchymal transition of pancreatic cancer cells via suppression of the PI-3K/Akt/NF-κB pathway. *Curr. Med. Chem.* **2013**, *20*, 4185–4194. [CrossRef] [PubMed]
124. Li, W.; Cao, L.; Chen, X.; Lei, J.; Ma, Q. Resveratrol inhibits hypoxia-driven ROS-induced invasive and migratory ability of pancreatic cancer cells via suppression of the Hedgehog signaling pathway. *Oncol. Rep.* **2016**, *35*, 1718–1726. [CrossRef] [PubMed]
125. Jiang, Q.; Yang, M.; Qu, Z.; Zhou, J.; Zhang, Q. Resveratrol enhances anticancer effects of paclitaxel in HepG2 human liver cancer cells. *BMC Complement. Altern. Med.* **2017**, *17*, 477. [CrossRef]
126. Harikumar, K.B.; Kunnumakkara, A.B.; Sethi, G.; Diagaradjane, P.; Anand, P.; Pandey, M.K.; Gelovani, J.; Krishnan, S.; Guha, S.; Aggarwal, B.B. Resveratrol, a multitargeted agent, can enhance antitumor activity of gemcitabine in vitro and in orthotopic mouse model of human pancreatic cancer. *Int. J. Cancer* **2010**, *127*, 257–268. [CrossRef]
127. Zhao, Y.; Tang, H.; Zeng, X.; Ye, D.; Liu, J. Resveratrol inhibits proliferation, migration and invasion via Akt and ERK1/2 signaling pathways in renal cell carcinoma cells. *Biomed. Pharmacother.* **2018**, *98*, 36–44. [CrossRef]
128. Dai, L.; Chen, L.; Wang, W.; Lin, P. Resveratrol inhibits ACHN cells via regulation of histone acetylation. *Pharm. Biol.* **2020**, *58*, 231–238. [CrossRef]
129. Bai, Y.; Yang, H.; Zhang, G.; Hu, L.; Lei, Y.; Qin, Y.; Yang, Y.; Wang, Q.; Li, R.; Mao, Q. Inhibitory effects of resveratrol on the adhesion, migration and invasion of human bladder cancer cells. *Mol. Med. Rep.* **2017**, *15*, 885–889. [CrossRef]
130. Wang, K.; Chen, Z.; Shi, J.; Feng, Y.; Yu, M.; Sun, Y.; Zhuang, Q.; Liang, B.; Luo, G.; Xu, X.; et al. Resveratrol inhibits the tumor migration and invasion by upregulating TET1 and reducing TIMP2/3 methylation in prostate carcinoma cells. *Prostate* **2020**, *80*, 977–985. [CrossRef]
131. Chen, H.; Zhu, M.; Luo, T.; Huang, H. Resveratrol raises in vitro anticancer effects of lentinan in SW579 human thyroid squamous cell carcinoma. *Int. J. Clin. Exp. Med.* **2016**, *9*, 20777–20789.
132. Xie, D.; Zheng, G.Z.; Xie, P.; Zhang, Q.H.; Lin, F.X.; Chang, B.; Hu, Q.X.; Du, S.X.; Li, X.D. Antitumor activity of resveratrol against human osteosarcoma cells: A key role of Cx43 and Wnt/β-catenin signaling pathway. *Oncotarget* **2017**, *8*, 111419–111432. [CrossRef] [PubMed]
133. Gweon, E.J.; Kim, S.J. Resveratrol attenuates matrix metalloproteinase-9 and -2-regulated differentiation of HTB94 chondrosarcoma cells through the p38 kinase and JNK pathways. *Oncol. Rep.* **2014**, *32*, 71–78. [CrossRef] [PubMed]
134. Gweon, E.J.; Kim, S.J. Resveratrol induces MMP-9 and cell migration via the p38 kinase and PI-3K pathways in HT1080 human fibrosarcoma cells. *Oncol Rep.* **2013**, *29*, 826–834. [CrossRef]
135. Lee, H.S.; Ha, A.W.; Kim, W.K. Effect of resveratrol on the metastasis of 4T1 mouse breast cancer cells in vitro and in vivo. *Nutr. Res. Pract.* **2012**, *6*, 294–300. [CrossRef]
136. Wang, W.; Zhou, M.; Xu, Y.; Peng, W.; Zhang, S.; Li, R.; Zhang, H.; Zhang, H.; Cheng, S.; Wang, Y.; et al. Resveratrol-Loaded TPGS-Resveratrol-Solid Lipid Nanoparticles for Multidrug-Resistant Therapy of Breast Cancer: In Vivo and In Vitro Study. *Front. Bioeng. Biotechnol.* **2021**, *9*, 762489. [CrossRef]
137. Pradhan, R.; Chatterjee, S.; Hembram, K.C.; Sethy, C.; Mandal, M.; Kundu, C.N. Nano formulated Resveratrol inhibits metastasis and angiogenesis by reducing inflammatory cytokines in oral cancer cells by targeting tumor associated macrophages. *J. Nutr. Biochem.* **2021**, *92*, 108624. [CrossRef]
138. Yang, T.; Zhang, J.; Zhou, J.; Zhu, M.; Wang, L.; Yan, L. Resveratrol inhibits Interleukin-6 induced invasion of human gastric cancer cells. *Biomed. Pharmacother.* **2018**, *99*, 766–773. [CrossRef]
139. Ji, Q.; Liu, X.; Han, Z.; Zhou, L.; Sui, H.; Yan, L.; Jiang, H.; Ren, J.; Cai, J.; Li, Q. Resveratrol suppresses epithelial-to-mesenchymal transition in colorectal cancer through TGF-β1/S expression. *BMC Cancer* **2015**, *15*, 97. [CrossRef]
140. Wang, G.; Dai, F.; Yu, K.; Jia, Z.; Zhang, A.; Huang, Q.; Kang, C.; Jiang, H.; Pu, P. Resveratrol inhibits glioma cell growth via targeting oncogenic microRNAs and multiple signaling pathways. *Int. J. Oncol.* **2015**, *46*, 1739–1747. [CrossRef]
141. Jiao, Y.; Li, H.; Liu, Y.; Guo, A.; Xu, X.; Qu, X.; Wang, S.; Zhao, J.; Li, Y.; Cao, Y. Resveratrol Inhibits the Invasion of Glioblastoma-Initiating Cells via Down-Regulation of the PI3K/Akt/NF-κB Signaling Pathway. *Nutrients* **2015**, *7*, 4383–4402. [CrossRef] [PubMed]
142. Yang, S.F.; Lee, W.J.; Tan, P.; Tang, C.H.; Hsiao, M.; Hsieh, F.K.; Chien, M.H. Upregulation of miR-328 and inhibition of CREB-DNA-binding activity are critical for resveratrol-mediated suppression of matrix metalloproteinase-2 and subsequent metastatic ability in human osteosarcomas. *Oncotarget* **2015**, *6*, 2736–2753. [CrossRef] [PubMed]
143. Abdel-Halim, A.H.; Fyia, A.A.; Ali, M.M.; Soliman, S.M. Anticancer properties of resveratrol on chemically induced hepatocellular carcinoma in rats: Inhibition of metastasis and angiogenesis. *J. Chem. Pharm. Res.* **2015**, *7*, 913–921.
144. Ganapathy, S.; Chen, Q.; Singh, K.P.; Shankar, S.; Srivastava, R.K. Resveratrol enhances antitumor activity of TRAIL in prostate cancer xenografts through activation of FOXO transcription factor. *PLoS ONE* **2010**, *5*, 15627. [CrossRef] [PubMed]
145. Luo, K.W.; Lung, W.Y.; Luo, X.L.; Huang, W.R. EGCG inhibited bladder cancer T24 and 5637 cell proliferation and migration via PI3K/AKT pathway. *Oncotarget* **2018**, *9*, 12261–12272. [CrossRef]
146. He, Q.; Liu, C.; Wang, X.; Rong, K.; Zhu, M.; Duan, L.; Zheng, P.; Mi, Y. Exploring the mechanism of curcumin in the treatment of colon cancer based on network pharmacology and molecular docking. *Front. Pharmacol.* **2023**, *14*, 1102581. [CrossRef]

147. Wu, Z.; He, D.; Zhao, S.; Wang, H. IL-17A/IL-17RA promotes invasion and activates MMP-2 and MMP-9 expression via p38 MAPK signaling pathway in non-small cell lung cancer. *Mol. Cell. Biochem.* **2019**, *455*, 195–206. [CrossRef]
148. Lee, G.H.; Jin, S.W.; Kim, S.J.; Pham, T.H.; Choi, J.H.; Jeong, H.G. Tetrabromobisphenol A Induces MMP-9 Expression via NADPH Oxidase and the activation of ROS, MAPK, and Akt Pathways in Human Breast Cancer MCF-7 Cells. *Toxicol. Res.* **2019**, *35*, 93–101. [CrossRef]
149. Rasheduzzaman, M.; Jeong, J.K.; Park, S.Y. Resveratrol sensitizes lung cancer cell to TRAIL by p53 independent and suppression of Akt/NF-κB signaling. *Life Sci.* **2018**, *208*, 208–220. [CrossRef]
150. Biswas, P.; Dey, D.; Biswas, P.K.; Rahaman, T.I.; Saha, S.; Parvez, A.; Khan, D.A.; Lily, N.J.; Saha, K.; Sohel, M.; et al. A Comprehensive Analysis and Anti-Cancer Activities of Quercetin in ROS-Mediated Cancer and Cancer Stem Cells. *Int. J. Mol. Sci.* **2022**, *23*, 11746. [CrossRef]
151. Neamtu, A.A.; Maghiar, T.A.; Alaya, A.; Olah, N.K.; Turcus, V.; Pelea, D.; Totolici, B.D.; Neamtu, C.; Maghiar, A.M.; Mathe, E. A Comprehensive View on the Quercetin Impact on Colorectal Cancer. *Molecules* **2022**, *27*, 1873. [CrossRef] [PubMed]
152. Caban, M.; Lewandowska, U. Encapsulation of Polyphenolic Compounds Based on Hemicelluloses to Enhance Treatment of Inflammatory Bowel Diseases and Colorectal Cancer. *Molecules* **2023**, *28*, 4189. [CrossRef] [PubMed]

cancers

MDPI

Review

Nature's Green Potential: Anticancer Properties of Plants of the Euphorbiaceae Family

Víctor Jiménez-González [1,*], Tomasz Kowalczyk [2,*], Janusz Piekarski [3], Janusz Szemraj [4], Patricia Rijo [5,6] and Przemysław Sitarek [7]

1 Department of Pharmacology, Faculty of Pharmacy, University of Seville, 41012 Seville, Spain
2 Department of Molecular Biotechnology and Genetics, Faculty of Biology and Environmental Protection, University of Lodz, Banacha 12/16, 90-237 Lodz, Poland
3 Department of Surgical Oncology, Medical University in Lodz, 93-513 Lodz, Poland; janusz.piekarski@umed.lodz.pl
4 Department of Medical Biochemistry, Medical University of Lodz, 92-215 Lodz, Poland; janusz.szemraj@umed.lodz.pl
5 CBIOS-Lusófona University's Research Center for Biosciences and Health Technologies, 1749-024 Lisbon, Portugal; p1609@ulusofona.pt
6 Instituto de Investigação do Medicamento (iMed.ULisboa), Faculdade de Farmácia, Universidade de Lisboa, 1649-003 Lisbon, Portugal
7 Department of Medical Biology, Medical University of Lodz, 90-151 Lodz, Poland; przemyslaw.sitarek@umed.lodz.pl
* Correspondence: vjimenez3@us.es (V.J.-G.); tomasz.kowalczyk@biol.uni.lodz.pl (T.K.)

Simple Summary: Euphorbiaceae is a large family of flowering plants that includes a wide spectrum of useful plants, from edible plants to toxic and medicinal plants. They are cosmopolitan plants that have very different shapes, from little herbaceous plants to big trees and cactus-like forms. This review article focuses on the potential anticancer activity of extracts, isolated compounds, and nanoparticles generated from the plants of the Euphobiaceae family based on in vitro and in vivo experiments. Possible mechanisms of action are also discussed.

Abstract: The number of cancer cases will reach 24 million in 2040, according to the International Agency for Research on Cancer. Current treatments for cancer are not effective and selective for most patients; for this reason, new anticancer drugs need to be developed and researched enough. There are potentially useful drugs for cancer isolated from plants that are being used in the clinic. Available information about phytochemistry, traditional uses, in vitro and in vivo experiments with plants, and pure compounds isolated from the Euphorbiaceae family indicates that this family of plants has the potential to develop anticancer drugs. This review examines selected species from the Euphorbiaceae family and their bioactive compounds that could have potential against different types of cancer cells. It reviews the activity of crude extracts, isolated compounds, and nanoparticles and the potential underlying mechanisms of action.

Keywords: Euphorbiaceae family; in vitro; in vivo; anticancer; extracts; pure compounds; nanoparticles

1. Introduction

Nowadays, cancer is a serious health problem that represents a great cost to national health systems around the world. Usually cells live, repair errors, divide, and die, and new cells replace the old ones. But sometimes, a mutation in the DNA of a cell that can not repair itself through reparation mechanisms leads to multiple abnormal divisions. These multiple divisions could activate oncogenes (inducing cell growth) or/and deactivate tumor suppressor genes (repressing cell growth), leading to an uncontrolled cell cycle. All these fast divisions, without control, accumulate different mutations that could imply fast growth and cancer cell death evasion. These mutations could also favor the loss of adhesion of tumor cells, which would facilitate their movement to other areas of the body through epithelial-mesenchymal transition, promoting tumor invasion and metastasis. In addition, it has been established that tumors release some angiogenic cytokines that affect vessel formation, tumor development, invasion, and metastasis. The most important angiogenic cytokines are vascular endothelial growth factor (VEGF) and basic fibroblast growth factor (bFGF), which are also poor markers of the prognostic and aggressiveness of the illness in patients [1,2].

More than 19 million new cases of cancer and 10 million deaths from cancer were reported in 2020 [3]. The most frequently diagnosed cancer was breast cancer (11.7%), lung cancer (11.6%), colorectal cancer (10%), and prostate cancer (7.3%). Furthermore, estimates made by experts expect that in 2040 there will be 24.8 million cases of cancer (47% more than in 2020) [4]. With this future perspective, new treatments and the development of new drugs will be difficult to achieve if governments do not increase the share devoted to cancer, and this lack of financing may be a problem in receiving quality care [5]. New therapies for cancer are usually directed toward developing more effective drugs and trying to avoid the side effects of the actual anticancer drugs. But all these strategies are usually very complex or hard and expensive to achieve, using new molecular targets, nanomedicine, and bioengineering [6]. However, the plant kingdom is still being unexplored; nonetheless, several very useful anticancer drugs are of plant origin, such as Paclitaxel, Vincristine, Vinblastine, Irinotecan, Topotecan, and Etoposide [7–9].

The Euphorbiaceae family of plants is a group of plants that has gained the interest of the scientific community due to their traditional uses in ethnomedicine, their high diversity of compounds, the potential toxicity of these compounds, and their easy access to these cosmopolitan plants [10]. Different plants from the genus of the family, such as Euphorbia, Croton, Jatropha, and Cnidoscolus, have been tested in vitro for their anticancer activity with excellent results [11–13]. This gives us an opportunity to continue delving deeper into the compounds present in these plants and their mechanisms of action as potential anticancer drugs. Several secondary metabolites have been described in the Euphorbiaceae family; for example, there is a high diversity of terpenoids with different types of original skeleton configurations [14–16]. Some common flavonoids, like quercetin and apigenin, have been isolated from this plant family [17–20]. Additionally, it has been documented that these plants contain certain tryptamine-derived alkaloids [21].

The main purpose of this review is to bring together all the information available about the anticancer effect in vitro or in vivo of plant extracts or pure compounds isolated from the Euphorbiaceae family published in the last ten years.

2. Criteria for the Selection of Experimental Papers

This review is based on primary literature published between 2012 and 2023 (to date). The papers were selected from different electronic databases: PubMed, Google Scholar, Scopus, and Web of Science. The following terms were used to achieve the search: Euphorbiaceae with: family, anticancer, antiproliferative, cytotoxic, plant extract, pure compound, in vitro, in vivo, and nanoparticles. The articles reporting extracts or pure compounds from the Euphorbiaceae family with some anticancer, antiproliferative, or cytotoxic activity in vitro or in vivo were included. Other articles reporting different types of reviews, articles in different languages than English, articles without full text access, lacking specific plant names, without reports of clear objectives and methodology, published more than ten years ago, using plant species other than Euphorbiaceae, were excluded. Duplicate articles from different database searching results were also excluded. All the inclusion/exclusion criteria were checked again after the removal of these articles. Each selected research paper was examined, and the following data were selected and presented in the tables: scientific plant name, parts of the plants used for extract preparation or pure compound isolation, type of extract, class of compounds or different compounds identified in the extract, cancer cell lines used or animal model/cell line inoculated with cancer-inducing compounds, activity or mechanism of action, and reference. Articles explaining the mechanisms of action of Euphorbiaceae plant extracts or isolated compounds were discussed before the tables in the main text.

3. The Euphorbiaceae Family of Plants

The Euphorbiaceae family of plants has about 228 plant genera accepted according to Plants of the World Online by Royal Botanic Garden Kew [22] and more than 7000 species of plants according to the Global Biodiversity Information Facility [23]. This family of green plants has a very different overall shape. There are habits from herbaceous plants (for example, *Euphorbia peplus* L.) to shrubs (like *Ricinus communis* L.) or woody trees (*Hevea brasiliensis* (Willd. ex A.Juss.) Müll.Arg.) and cactus-like shapes (*Euphorbia ingens* (E.Mey. ex Boiss.)). These plants can be annuals or perennials, monoics or dioics, and usually present some type of latex. The leaves are oppositive (sometimes alternatives) and have stipules that could be transformed into spines or glands. The flowers gather in an inflorescence called cyathium, and sometimes they are inconspicuous flowers that lack a corolla. Sometimes the cyathium contains several masculine flowers and only one feminine flower. Androecium with one or numerous stamens, and gynoecium with two or three styles and carpels. The fruits are usually contained in capsules, and they separate easily from each other [24–26]. Among the best-known genera of this family, we find *Euphorbia*, *Jatropha*, *Croton*, *Acalypha*, *Cnidoscolus*, and *Ricinus* (Figure 1) [22]. Some plants in the family are very important for humans; for example, *Mannihot sculenta* L. is an edible plant that is cultivated in many countries and is considered a basic food. This crop is easy to grow in a variety of environments, is undemanding, and has very good nutritional properties [27,28]. *Mannihot sculenta* L. was grown as a crop on more than one million hectares in countries such as Ghana, Angola, Cote d'Ivoire, Brazil, Thailand, the Democratic Republic of the Congo, and Nigeria in 2021, according to the Food and Agriculture Organization of the United Nations [29]. Other plants are considered toxic to be consumed but still useful; for example, in the proper dosage, *Ricinus communis* L., commonly known as Castor oil, has been used in the past as a purgative [30] and is approved by the US Food and Drug Administration as an antisticking additive agent to produce hard candy [31]. Many other uses of castor's oil have been reported, including uterine contraction [32], antiviral [33], antibacterial [34], and antinflammatory [30]. In addition, the oils extracted from the seeds are very useful for industrial applications [31,35].

Plants of the most numerous genera, *Euphorbia*, have been used traditionally around the world for different purposes, for example, to feed animals, as additives in food, as fuels, or for environmental uses, but the two main purposes have been to poison different animals and as folk medicines [10]. These two main purposes take advantage of the toxicological properties of the diverse phytochemistry present in these plants. For example, it is well known that different species of Euphorbiaceae, for example, *Euphorbia tirucalli* L., have been used in Africa to poison fish. This is a very common way of fishing with the help of plant metabolites that spread through water and poison animals [36]. On the other hand, when used as folk medicines, they are known to be used mainly for digestive disorders, skin or subcutaneous tissue disorders, infections, inflammation, or respiratory disorders [10]. For example, for digestive disorders, decoctions of *Euhprobia hirta* L. are recorded to be used in distant places such as Burundi, the Philippines, and China as antidiarrheal [37–39]. *Euphorbia lathyris* L. is recorded as being used as a purgative in different countries in Europe. For skin disorders, *Euphorbia maculata* L. is well known to be used in folk medicine against warts [40]. To treat infections, for example, *Euphorbia hirta* L. had been used in the past for gonorrhoea in Africa [41]. The same plant has been reported to be used in Australia for bronchitis (inflammation) [42]. For respiratory disorders, it is used in Nepal for the treatment of asthma [43].

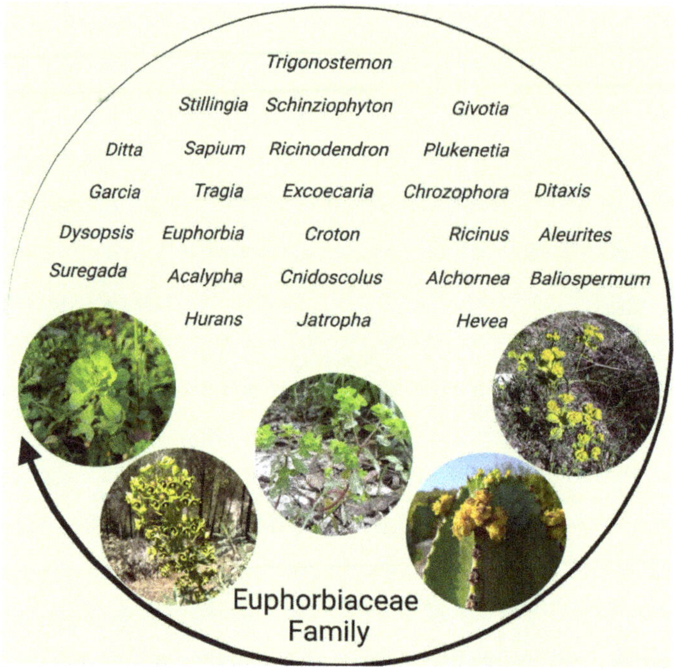

Figure 1. The Euphorbiaceae family of green plants. (created by BioRender).

3.1. Phytochemistry of the Euphorbiaceae Family

This family of plants is very diverse and rich in secondary metabolites. Different compounds have been isolated, for example, terpenoids and flavonoids. The first class of compounds in Euphorbiaceae are terpenoids, classified into diterpenoids, triterpenoids, and sesquiterpenoids. These metabolites have been studied in this family for a long time for their different biological activities. The diterpenoids are cyclized from the precursor geranyl-geranyl-phosphate to the corresponding diterpenoid skeleton. In the Euphorbiaceae family, compounds have been isolated with different types of diterpenoid skeletons [44–46].

For example, in the genus *Euphorbia*, different types of diterpenoids have been described, such as labdane, abietane, atisane, kaurane, isopimarane, rosane, dolabrane, casbane, cembrane, rharnnofolane, gaditanone, ingenane, ingol, jatrophane, jatropholane, lathyrane, cyclomyrsinol, myrsinol, premyrsinol, paraliane, pepluane, presegetane, segetane, tigliane, cyclojatrophane, and expoxyjatropholane [44,45]. Due to the high diversity of plants and metabolites in this genus, every year new diterpenoids are discovered. Zhu et al. [47] using the roots *Euphorbia fischeriana* L. described two new *ent*-abietane diterpenoids, euphonoids H and I. Zhang et al. [48] using the same plant species have reported for the first time the presence of a new *ent*-rosane diterpene, named ebracteolatas D. On the other hand, in the *Croton* genus, labdanes, clerodanes, trachylobane, kaurene, cembrane, and isopimarane diterpenoids have been identified [46]. Wang et al. [49] reported the isolation of a new *ent*-abietane diterpenoid (7b,13a,15-tri-hydroxy-*ent*-abieta-8(14)-en-3-one) from the leaves of *Croton lachnocarpus* Benth. In the genus *Jatropha*, different diterpenoids' skeletons have also been described, such as tigliane, casbene, daphnane, lathyrane, jatrophane, podocarpane, and rhamnofolane [50]. For example, the team led by Yuan et al. [51] isolated jatropodagins A, a new lathyrane-type diterpenoid.

Triterpenoids are also very common and diverse in the family. In the genus *Euphorbia*, different types of skeletons have been described, for example, tirucallane, euphane, lanostane, cycloartanes, lupane, oleanane, taraxarane, friedoursane, friedelane, and ursane [52].

And still, nowadays, new compounds are being discovered. A new cycloartane-type triterpene (23 R/S-3b-hydroxycycloart-24-ene-23-methyl ether) was isolated from the aerial parts of *Euphorbia dendroides* L [53]. In the genus *Croton*, several triterpenoids have been described [46]. For example, lupeol has been isolated from different parts of the species *Croton sylvaticus* Hochst. and *Croton zambezicus* Müll. Arg. [54,55]. β-Sitosterol has been isolated from *Croton zambezicus* Müll. Arg. and *Croton steenkampianus* Gerstner [15,56]. Betulinic acid, betulin, and lupenone have been isolated from the fruits of *Croton zambezicus* [57]. Jatrogrossidione, a triterpenoid isolated from the branches and leaves of *Jatropha gossypiifolia* L., was isolated by Zhan et al. [58].

Also, a few sesquiterpenoids have been reported from *Euphorbia, Croton, Jatropha*, etc. [46,59,60]. Aryanin, a new sesquiterpene lactone, was isolated from the aerial parts of *Euphorbia microsphaera* Boiss by Azizi et al. [61]. Another sesquiterpene, caryophyllene, was reported to be present in *Croton* species as a volatile constituent [46].

The presence of flavonoids in this family is widespread. These compounds could have an impact on health, for example, as potential anticancer agents that have been previously reported [62]. For example, quercitrin has been isolated from *Euphorbia hirta* L. [63], and apigenin has been isolated from *Croton betulaster* Mull, *Jatropha gossypiifolia* L., and *Macaranga gigantifolia* Merr. [17,20,64].

Some alkaloids have been isolated from this family also, from latex, roots, or other parts of the plants. Alkaloids are important chemicals; some of them have been isolated or developed for cancer treatment, such as the alkaloids of vinca [65]. For example, Novello et al. [66] have isolated, from *Croton echioides* Baill, a new alkaloid (*N-trans*-feruloyl-3,5-dihydroxyindolin-2-one) as a mixture with other already known alkaloids (*N-trans-p*-coumaroyl-tryptamine, *N-trans-p*-coumaroyl-5-hydroxytryptamine, *N-trans*-4-methoxy-cinnamoyl-5-hydroxytryptamine, and *N-trans*-feruloyl-5-hydroxytryptamine.

3.2. *Cytotoxic and Anticancer Effects of* Euphorbiaceae *Extracts In Vitro Studies*

Testing plant extracts is one of the first steps in the search for new compounds with potential biological properties, including an anticancer effect. Many articles confirm the preliminary cytotoxic properties of extracts from many medicinal plant families, which can induce apoptosis in many cancer lines. The Euphorbiaceae family is a source of many interesting compounds with broad medicinal applications. The first step of our analysis was to analyze the effect of plant extracts on cytotoxic effects in in vitro studies. Mesas et al. [67] showed that an ethanolic extract of *Euphorbia lathyris* seeds rich in polyphenols such as esculetin, euphorbetin, gaultherin, and kaempferol-3-rutinoside had an antiproliferative effect against colon cancer cell lines (T84 and HCT-15) and glioblastoma multiforme. The authors demonstrated that the induction of apoptosis is associated with overexpression of caspase-9 (casp-9), caspase-3 (casp-3), and caspase-8 (casp-8) and activation of autophagy. In another study, Sultana et al. [68] showed that an aqueous leaf extract of *Excoecaria agallocha* (L.), where the head compound was bergenin, effectively reduced the proliferation of SiHa cervical cancer cells by inducing autophagy and apoptosis in a coordinated manner, with simultaneous stimulation of mitophagy and cell cycle arrest in the G2/M phase. In contrast, Kwan et al. [69] showed that a methanolic extract of *Euphorbia hirta* exhibited significant inhibition of MCF-7 breast cancer cell survival through induction of apoptosis via a casp-3-independent pathway, activation of caspase-2, caspase-6, casp-8, and casp-9, accumulation of cells in the S and G2/M phases, and DNA fragmentation. Similarly, Mfotie Njoya et al. [70] showed that *Croton gratissimus* leaf extract exhibited cytotoxic effects on various cancer lines (A549, Caco-2, HeLa, MCF-7) and inhibited cancer cell growth through induction of caspase-3 (casp-3)/caspase-7 (casp-7) activation, with the highest induction (1.83-fold change) obtained on HeLa cells. Vargas-Madriz et al. [71] presented that *Cnidoscolus aconitifolius* and *Porophyllum ruderale*, rich in polyphenols, reduced the metabolic activity of human SW480 colon adenocarcinoma cells. In addition, both extracts increased the total number of apoptotic cells and arrested the cell cycle in the G0/G1 phases. Other studies are presented in Table 1.

Table 1. Cytotoxic properties of selected extracts from the Euphorbiaceae family against cancer cells.

Name of the Species	Part of the Plant	Type of Extract	Class of Compounds/Compounds Identified in Extract	Cell Lines	IC_{50}	Activity/ Mechanism/ Effect	Ref.
Acalypha fruticosa Forssk.	Aerial parts	Methanol	-	MCF-7, HCT-116, and HepG-2	12.2 ± 0.6 µg/mL, 4.81 ± 0.4 µg/mL, and 5.21 ± 0.7 µg/mL, respectively.	Cytotoxic	[72]
Acalypha indica L.	Leaves	Hexane	-	MCF-7	50 µg/mL	Cytotoxic	[73]
Acalypha monostachya Cav.	Aerial parts	Distilled water, absolute methanol, and *n*-hexane	Phenols, coumarins, lactones, flavonoids, saponins, aromatic compounds, carbohydrates, and carbonyl groups. Methanol and hexane: steroids and terpenoids. Aqueous: alkaloids.	HeLa and MDA-MB-231	-	Cytotoxic	[74]
Baliospermum montanum (Willd.) Müll.Arg.	Leaves	Methanol	-	Jurkat	298 µg/mL	Cytotoxic	[75]
Baliospermum montanum (Willd.) Müll.Arg.	Roots	Ethanol	Propiophenones	HepG2 and KKU M156	HepG2 (0.06 ± 0.02 µg/mL) and KKU M157 (0.16 ± 0.02 µg/mL)	Cytotoxic	[76]
Blumeodendron toxbrai (Blume.)	Stem Bark	Hexane, Dichloromethane, and Methanolic	-	MCF-7	Hexane extract 121.24 ± 0.15 µg/mL, Dichloromethane extract 55 ± 0.48 µg/mL, and methanolic extract 70.71 ± 0.15 µg/mL	Cytotoxic	[77]
Croton sylvaticus Hochst.	Leaves	Acetone and ethanol	-	A549, Caco-2, HeLa, and MCF-7	Acetone extract: A549 (32.78 ± 2.55 µg/mL), Caco-2 (150.63 ± 8.79 µg/mL), HeLa (169.09 ± 13.0 µg/mL), MCF-7 (13.13 ± 2.76 µg/mL). Ethanol extract: A549 (1.75 ± 0.62 µg/mL), Caco-2 (103.73 ± 1.47 µg/mL), HeLa (106.52 ± 4.50 µg/mL), MCF-7 (6.02 ± 1.60 µg/mL).	Cytotoxic. casp-3/casp7 pathway.	[70]

Table 1. *Cont.*

Name of the Species	Part of the Plant	Type of Extract	Class of Compounds/Compounds Identified in Extract	Cell Lines	IC_{50}	Activity/ Mechanism/ Effect	Ref.
Chrozophora oblongifolia (Delile) Spreng.	Root Bark	Aqueous methanol, fractions with *n*-hexane, methylene chloride, and ethyl acetate	Carbohydrates and/or glycosides, sterols and/or triterpenes, tannins, alkaloids, and saponins	MCF-7 and Huh-7	Cytotoxic activity (%) of the methanolic extracts MCF-7 (15.82 ± 0.66) and Huh-7 (31.28 ± 0.68). *n*-hexane MCF-7 (59.55 ± 0.76) and Huh-7 (54.17 ± 0.46). Methylene chloride, MCF-7 (83.83 ± 0.37) and Huh-7 (82.79 ± 0.55). Ethyl acetate MCF-7 (22.25 ± 0.13) and Huh-7 (72.52 ± 0.23).	Cytotoxic	[78]
Chrozophora plicata (Vahl) A.Juss. ex Spreng.	Leaves	Petroleum ether, chloroform, hexane, ethyl acetate, methanol, and water	flavonoids, alkaloids, glycosides, and lignans.	DAL	25–50 µg/mL	Cytotoxic	[79]
Cnidoscolus aconitifolius (Mill.) I.M. Johnst.	Leaves	Methanol	Saponins, tannins, terpenes, and flavonoids	MCF-7 and NCI-H460	4.50 ± 0.58 µg/mL and 3.29 ± 4.57 µg/mL, respectively.	Cytotoxic	[80]
Cnidoscolus chayamansa McVaugh.	Leaves	Ethanolic	-	HT-29	CTC50 (µg/mL) ≥ 1000 ± 0.00	Cytotoxic	[81]
Cnidoscolus multilobus (Pax) I.M. Johnst	Leaves	Ethanol-water (70:30)		HeLa	130–160 µg/mL	Cytotoxic	[82]
Cnidoscolus quercifolius Pohl	Bark root	Methanol, chloroform fraction	Faveline, Faveline methyl ether, Deoxofaveline, and Neofavelanone	OVCAR-8, HCT-116, and HL-60	OVCAR-8 15.23 ± 2.0 µg/mL, HCT-116 7.07 ± 0.59 µg/mL, and HL-60 4.95 ± 0.19 µg/mL	Cytotoxic	[83]
Croton acutifolius Esser	Twigs and leaves	Hexane, ethyl acetate, and methanol	Retusin	KKU-M213, FaDu, HT-29, MDA-M, B-231, SH-SY5Y, A 549 and MMNK-2	Ethyl acetate extract against KKU-M213, MDA-MB-231, A-549, and MMNK-1 with the ED50 at 3.31 µg/mL, 0.58 µg/mL, 0.58 µg/mL, and 0.65 µg/mL, respectively.	Cytotoxic	[84]

Table 1. *Cont.*

Name of the Species	Part of the Plant	Type of Extract	Class of Compounds/Compounds Identified in Extract	Cell Lines	IC_{50}	Activity/ Mechanism/ Effect	Ref.
Croton bonplandianus Baill.	Leaves	Acetone	-	A549	15.68 ± 0.006 µg/mL	Cytotoxic, apoptosis, and G2M phase arrest	[85]
Croton caudatus Geiseler	Leaves	Chloroform, ethanol and aqueous	-	HeLa	80 µg/mL	Cytotoxic, increased DNA damage	[86]
Croton caudatus Geiseler	Leaves	Chloroform, ethanol, and aqueous	Alkaloids, saponins, tannins, and cardiac glycosides.	Dalton's lymphoma (DL)	28.36 µg/mL	Cytotoxic	[87]
Croton caudatus Geiseler	Leaves	Methanol		HeLa	59.70 µg/mL	Cytotoxic	[88]
Croton fluviatilis Esser	Stems	Hexane, ethyl acetate, and methanol	β-amyrin (1), stigmasterol, and β-sitosterol	KKU-M213, FaDu, HT-29, MDA-M, B-231, SH-SY5Y, A-549, and MMNK-1	Hexane extract cytotoxicity against KKU-M213, MDA-MB-231, and A-549 at the ED50 values of 1.70 µg/mL, 2.62 µg/mL, and 0.60 µg/mL, respectively	Cytotoxic	[84]
Croton heliotropiifolius Kunth	Leaves	Methanol	Gallic acid	NCI-H292, MCF-7, Hep-2, and HL-60	% inhibitor activity in NCI-H292 (46.5 ± 2.6), MCF-7 (21.7 ± 3.7), Hep-2 (26.7 ± 7.1), and HL-60 (59.5 ± 2.9)	Inhibitory activity	[89, 90]

Table 1. *Cont.*

Name of the Species	Part of the Plant	Type of Extract	Class of Compounds/Compounds Identified in Extract	Cell Lines	IC_{50}	Activity/ Mechanism/ Effect	Ref.
Croton membranaceus Müll. Arg.	Roots	Hydroethanolic	5-Hydroxypipecolic acid, Phenol, 3, 5-bis(1, 1-dimethylethyl)-, 2-Octenoic acid, 5, 5, 7-trihyroxy, 9, 10-Secocholeasta-5,7,10(19)-tiene-1,3-diol, 25-[(trimethylsilyl)oxy]-, Phenol, 4-(3-hydroxy-1-propenyl)-2-methoxy, *n*-Hexadecanoic acid, Benzene, 1,2,4,5-tetrakis(1-methylethyl)-, Prednisolone acetate, 1H, 4H-Pyrazolo[3,4-b]pyran-5-carbonitrile, 6-amino-4-(2, 4, 5-trimethoxyphenyl)-3-methyl and Astaxanthin	22Rv1	3.809 µg/mL	Cytotoxic, inhibit colony-forming and migration abilities	[91]
Croton sphaerogynus Baill.	Leaves	Hexane, dichloromethane, and methanol	Abieta-8,11-diene-3-one, Podocarp-7-ene,13-methyl-13-vinyl-3-one, Abieta-8,11,13-trien12-ol, Podocarp-7-ene-3-ol, 13-methyl-13-vinyl, 13-Hydroxy-abieta8,11-dien-7-one, and Crotonin derivative	786-0, HT-29, K562, NCI-ADR/RES, NCI-H460, MCF-7, PC-3, OVCAR-3, U251, and UACC-62.	Hexane and dichloromethane against NCI-H460 (GI50 0.26 µg/mL and 0.33 µg/mL, respectively) and K562 (GI50 0.60 µg/mL and <0.25 µg/mL, respectively).	Antiproliferative	[92]
Croton thorelii Gagnep.	Stems	Hexane, ethyl acetate, and methanol	5-hydroxy-7,4′-dimethoxyflavone	KKU-M213, FaDu, HT-29, MDA-M, B-231, SH-SY5Y, A-549, and MMNK-3	KKU-M213, MDA-MB-231, and A-549 had ED50 values of 0.55 µg/mL, 0.72 µg/mL, and 1.75 µg/mL, respectively.	Cytotoxic	[84]

Table 1. *Cont.*

Name of the Species	Part of the Plant	Type of Extract	Class of Compounds/Compounds Identified in Extract	Cell Lines	IC_{50}	Activity/ Mechanism/ Effect	Ref.
Croton tiglium L.	Seeds	Ethylether and methanol	Isoguanosine, 12-O-Acetylphorbol-13-tigliate, and 13-O-Acetylphorbol-20-linoleate	A549	-	Apoptosis via apoptosis regulator or bcl-2-like protein 4/B-cell lymphoma 2 protein (Bax/Bcl-2) Pathways	[13]
Croton urucurana Baill	-	Hydroalcoholic	-	U937 and THP1	402.2 μg/mL and 360.3 μg/mL, respectively.	Cytotoxic and Apoptosis	[93]
Drypetes sepiaria (Wight & Arn.) Pax & K.Hoffm.	Leaves	Methanol	Phenolics and flavonoids	SiHa	10 μg/mL	Cytotoxic, apoptosis, or necrosis. casp-3 activation.	[94]
Euphorbia cactus Ehrenb. ex Boiss.		Methanol	Phenols, flavonoids, diterpenes, sesquiterpenoids, terpenoids, anthocyanins, tannins, steroids, cerebrosides, anthraquinones, phloracetophenones, glycerols, alkaloids, and carbohydrates	A549, LoVo, and MCF-7	A549 (20.1 ± 0.5 μg/mL), LoVo (53.2 ± 0.4 μg/mL), and MCF-7 (58.80 ± 1.83 μg/mL)	Cytotoxic, in A549, G2M cell cycle arrest. changes in the level of gene expression of Bax, Bcl-2, and casp-3	[95]

Table 1. *Cont.*

Name of the Species	Part of the Plant	Type of Extract	Class of Compounds/Compounds Identified in Extract	Cell Lines	IC_{50}	Activity/ Mechanism/ Effect	Ref.
Euphorbia caducifolia Haines	Aerial parts	Ethanol and fractions: aqueous, ethyl acetate, and petroleum ether.	Friedooleanane-3- ol, (3α)-, 1,2-Benzendicarboxylic acid, mono (2-ethylhexyl) ester, Docosanoic acid, methyl ester; methyl behenate, Hexadecanoic acid methyl ester, methyl palmitate, 9, 12-Octadecadienoic Acid (Z,Z)-, methyl ester; methyl Linoleate (Z,Z)-isomer 9-Octadecenoic acid (z)-, methyl ester; methyl oleate	MCF-7, NCI-H460, PC-3, and HeLa	MCF-7 (61 ± 1.0 μg/mL), NCI-H460 (19 ± 6.3 μg/mL), PC-3 (135 ± 3 μg/mL), and HeLa (80 ± 2 μg/mL)	Cytotoxic	[96]
Euphorbia davidii Subils	Whole plant	*n*-Hexane and chloroform	kaempferol 3-O-rhamnoside, myricetin 3-O-rhamnoside, and quercetin 3-O-rhamnoside.	HeLa, MCF7, A2781, and A431	GI %: *n*-Hexane extract against HeLa (22.44 ± 2.66), MCF7 (45.88 ± 1.58), A2780 (26.72 ± 0.91) and A431 (25.65 ± 2.99) and chloroform extract against HeLa (22.28 ± 2.74), MCF7 (52.63 ± 0.88), A2781 (47.10 ± 0.68) and A431 (21.64 ± 0.37)	Cytotoxic	[97]

Table 1. *Cont.*

Name of the Species	Part of the Plant	Type of Extract	Class of Compounds/Compounds Identified in Extract	Cell Lines	IC_{50}	Activity/ Mechanism/ Effect	Ref.
Euphorbia dendroides L	Aerial parts	Ethanol	Ellagic acid, pyrogallol, e-vanillic acid, benzoic acid, catechin, epi-catechin, alpha-coumaric acid, and salicylic acid	HepG2, HCT116 and MCF	HepG2 (9.5 mg/mL), HCT-116 (13.6 mg/mL), and MCF-7 (20.9 mg/mL).	Antiproliferative	[98]
Euphorbia graminea Jacq.	Leaves	Aqueous Methanol, fractions with *n*-hexane, ethyl acetate, chloroform, and water	Tannins, flavonoids, saponins, cardiac glycosides, and terpenes	MCF7 and NCI-H460	At 250 µg/mL, the extract recorded −3.1 and +75% cytotoxic and growth inhibitory effects on MCF-7 and NCI-H460 cell lines, respectively. While the cytotoxic effect became more pronounced on MCF-7 cell lines as −2.19 and −9.6% cytotoxicities were recorded by the chloroform fraction at 75 and 100 µg/mL, the ethyl acetate fraction recorded +58.72 and +89.33% inhibitory effects at similar concentrations.	Cytotoxic	[99]
Euphorbia grandicornis Blanc	Aerial parts	Dichloromethane	Methyl 2,5-dihydroxybenzoate, *n*-octylbenzoate, Friedelanol, Germanicol, β-glutinol, β-amyrin, Stigmasterol, β-Sitosterol, (24R)-tirucalla-8,25-diene-3β, 24-diol, Euphorbol, Hexyl (E)-3-(4-hydroxy-3-methoxyphenyl)-2 propenoate	HeLa	83.84 ± 2.94 µg/mL	-	[100]

Table 1. *Cont.*

Name of the Species	Part of the Plant	Type of Extract	Class of Compounds/Compounds Identified in Extract	Cell Lines	IC_{50}	Activity/ Mechanism/ Effect	Ref.
Euphorbia grandicornis Blanc	Roots and aerial parts	Dichloromethane	β-glutinol, β-amyrin, 24-methylenetirucalla-8-en-3β-ol, (−)-tirucalla-8, 25-diene-3β-24R-diol, Stigmasterol, Sitosterol, Hexyl (E)-3-(4-hydroxy-3-methoxyphenyl)-2-propenoate	MCF-7 and HCC70	For roots, extract MCF-7 (0.83 ± 1.14 μg/mL) and HCC70 (0.83 ± 1.14 μg/mL), and for aerial parts, extract MCF-7 (1.03 ± 1.15 μg/mL), and HCC70 (0.31 ± 1.06 μg/mL)	Cytotoxic	[101]
Euphorbia grantii Oliv.	Aerial parts	Methanol and dichloromethane fraction	Friedelin, 3-b-firedelinol, epifriedelanol, euphol, cycloartenol, cycloartenyl acetate, epifriedelinyl acetate, and euphylbenzoate	MCF-7 and MCF-7ADR	Methanol extracts MCF-7 (16.47 μg/mL) and MCF-7ADR (19.55 μg/mL)Dichloromethane fraction, MCF-7 (10.31 μg/mL) and MCF-7ADR (10.41 μg/mL)	Cytotoxic	[102]
Euphorbia granulata Forssk.	Whole plant	Methanol	t-cinnamic acid, *p*-hydroxybenzoic acid, vanillic acid, 3,4-dihydroxybenzoic acid, syringic acid, *p*-coumaric acid, gallic acid, ferulic acid, caffeic acid, and sinapic acid	MCF-7, A2780 and HT-29	MCF-7 (16.23 ± 4.50 μg/mL), A2780 (22.80 ± 1.55 μg/mL), and HT-29 (41.89 ± 0.07 μg/mL)	Cytotoxic	[103]
Euphorbia helioscopia L.	Powdered	Hexane, acetone, methanol, and water		DLD-1	140.83 ± 0.31 μg/mL	Cytotoxic	[104],
Euphorbia helioscopia L.	Whole plant	Ethanol	-	Hep-2, T-47D, HT-29, and PC-3	%GI Hep-2 (27), T-47D (7), HT-29 (0), and PC-3 (11)	Cytotoxic	[12]
Euphorbia heterophylla Desf.	-	Methanol		HepG2	-	cell cycle arrest	[105]
Euphorbia hierosolymitana Boiss.	Whole plant	Methanol		MCF-7, HepG-2, HCT-116, PC-3	HCT-116 (4.22 ppm)	Cytotoxic. Changed the cell cycle and affected the gene expression of her2, Bax, and Bcl-2.	[106]

Table 1. *Cont.*

Name of the Species	Part of the Plant	Type of Extract	Class of Compounds/Compounds Identified in Extract	Cell Lines	IC_{50}	Activity/ Mechanism/ Effect	Ref.
Euphorbia hierosolymitana Boiss.	Aerial parts	Ethyl acetate and *n*-butanol fraction	2-Myristynoyl acid pantethene, Palmitic acid, methyl ester, Pyrrolidine,1-bicyclo 3,2,1Oct-2-En-3-Yl, Desulphosinigrin	MCF-7, PC3, A549 and Caco-2.	MCF-7 (93 µg/mL), PC3 (100 µg/mL), A549 (103 µg/mL), and Caco-2 (170 µg/mL). For the *n*-butanol fraction, for MCF-7, PC3, and A549 (>500 µg/mL), and for Caco-2 (152 µg/mL).	Cytostatic	[107]
Euphorbia hirta L.	Leaves	Ethanol	Anthroquinone, terpenoids, alkaloids, phenolic compounds, tannins, flavonoids, steroids, coumarins, and saponins	DLA and EAC	DLA (560.83 µg/mL) and EAC (384.7 µg/mL)	Cytotoxic	[108]
Euphorbia hirta L.	Roots	Ethanolic	-	MCF-7	From 10 µg/mL (61.57 ± 0.16 µg/mL) to 100 µg/mL (48.08 ± 0.30 µg/mL)	Cytotoxic	[109]
Euphorbia hirta L.	Whole plant	Ethanol	9,12,15-Octadecatrien-1-ol, Pentadecylic acid, Ethyl palmitate, Methyl linoleate, 5-Hydroxymethyl-2-furancarboxaldehyde, Ethyl linoleolate	HL-60	50–100 µg/mL	Anticancer	[110]
Euphorbia hirta L.	Whole plant	Petroleum Ether and Chloroform	-	HepG2	Petroleum ether 200 µg/mL and Chloroform 150 µg/mL	Cytotoxic	[111]
Euphorbia hirta L.	Whole plant	Methanol and distilled water	-	HCT-15	510.66 µg/mL	Cytotoxic	[112]
Euphorbia hyssopifolia L.	Aerial parts	Ethanol	Mono and sesquiterpenes, triterpenes, steroids, flavonoids, cynnamic derivatives, hydrolysable tannins, and saponnins	HepG2	-	Cytotoxic and genotoxic	[113]

Table 1. *Cont.*

Name of the Species	Part of the Plant	Type of Extract	Class of Compounds/Compounds Identified in Extract	Cell Lines	IC_{50}	Activity/ Mechanism/ Effect	Ref.
Euphorbia inarticulata Schweinf.	-	Ethanolic	Catechol, syringic acid, cinnamic acid, caffeic acid, gallic acid, ellagic acid, and benzoic acid	Huh-7 and HeLa	Huh-7 104.52 ± 2.74 µg/mL and HeLa 145.11 ± 6.21 µg/mL	Cytotoxic	[114]
Euphorbia ingens E.Mey. ex Boiss.	Root	Dichlorometh-ane:methanol (36.25%) and ethyl acetate fraction	Mayor constituents: 6-pentylidene-4,5-secoandrostane-4,17 beta-diol, 2-bornanol, 1-octadecene, 1-tridecene, and 1-dodecene	DU-145	9.71 ± 0.40 µg/mL	Cytotoxic, Regulation of the Phospho-inositide 3-kinases/Protein kinase B (PI3K/Akt), MAPK, and tumor protein p53 (p53) signalling pathways	[115]
Euphorbia lactea Haw.	Stems	Hydroalcoholic	-	HN22	250–500 µg/mL	Cytotoxic and anti-migratory activity	[116]
Euphorbia macroclada Boiss.	Leaves, flower and body	Acetone	-	MCF-7 and L-929	Leaves (8.91 ± 0.10 µg/mL)	Cytotoxic	[117]
Euphorbia milii Des Moul.	Aerial parts	Methanol	-	HepG-2	HepG-2 (87.1 ± 9.4 µg/mL)	Cytotoxic	[118]
Euphorbia nivulia Buch.-Ham	Aerial parts	Aqueous ethanol	Phenols, flavonoids, terpenoids, glycosides, alkaloids, saponins, steroids, and tannins	HeLa cells	-	Cytotoxic	[119]

Table 1. *Cont.*

Name of the Species	Part of the Plant	Type of Extract	Class of Compounds/Compounds Identified in Extract	Cell Lines	IC_{50}	Activity/ Mechanism/ Effect	Ref.
Euphorbia paralias L.	Aerial parts	Methanol, fractions with dichloromethane, and ethyl acetate	Gallic acid, ellagic acid, Kaempferol-3-O-(600-O-galloyl-b-D-glucopyranoside), Quercetin-3-O-b-D-glucopyranoside, and Quercetin-3-O-b-D-arabinopyranoside	HepG2	HepG2 (26.4 ± 1.2 mg/mL)	Cytotoxic	[120]
Euphorbia platyphyllos L.	Whole plant	Diethyl ether, petroleum ether, ethyl acetate, methanol, water infusion, and water decoction	-	MCF-7	>300 µg/mL, 98.07 ± 0.58 µg/mL, 46.24 ± 0.57 µg/mL, 97.16 ± 0.51 µg/mL, 38.29 ± 0.57 µg/mL and 27.79 ± 0.58 µg/mL respectively.	Cytotoxic, Apoptosis	[121]
Euphorbia pulcherrima Willd. ex Klotzsch	-	Methanol		HepG2	-	cell cycle arrest	[105]
Euphorbia rigida M.Bieb.	Aerial parts	Methanol	-	Hep3B and HepG2	-	Cytotoxic	[122]
Euphorbia royleana Boiss.	Aerial parts	Methanol	-	HepG-2, HCT-116 and MCF-7	HepG-2 (0.42 ± 0.7), and HCT-116 (285.1 ± 19.2)	Cytotoxic	[118]
Euphorbia tirucalli L.	Aerial parts	Ethanol and fractions with ethanol, hexane, dichloromethane, ethyl acetate, and aqueous fractions AGS	Aqueous and ethyl acetate fractions (ellagic acid, 1-o-Galloyl-β-d-glucose, sucrose or isomers, Quercitrin, 2,3-hexahydroxydiphenoyl-d-glucose or isomers, rutin, corilagin or isomers, and pedunculagin/casuariin)	AGS	AGS fractions: ethanol (11.73 ± 0.31 µg/mL), hexane (10.33 ± 2.01 µg/mL), dichloromethane (85.00 ± 9.5 µg/mL), ethyl acetate (120.9 ± 2.21 µg/mL), and aqueous (13.08 ± 0.99 µg/mL)	Cytotoxic	[123]

Table 1. *Cont.*

Name of the Species	Part of the Plant	Type of Extract	Class of Compounds/Compounds Identified in Extract	Cell Lines	IC_{50}	Activity/ Mechanism/ Effect	Ref.
Euphorbia tirucalli L.	Aerial parts	Hexanic and hydroalcoholic	-	HCT-116	25.26 ± 0.18 µg/mL	Cytotoxic, Increase in the expression of casp-3 and p53	[124]
Euphorbia triaculeata Forssk.	Whole plant	Methanol	-	MCF-7, PC-3, HEPG2 and MCF-10A	0–50 µg/mL	Cytotoxicity and genotoxicity	[125]
Euphorbia turcomanica Boiss.	Aerial parts	Heptane, ethyl acetate, dichloromethane, acetone, methanol, and methanol-water (70–30)	Flavonoid, alkaloid, anthraquinone, and tannin.	Hela and HT-29	Methanol-water (50 µg/mL), acetone (90 µg/mL), dichloromethane (230 µg/mL), methanol (420 µg/mL), and heptane (450 µg/mL) in HeLa cells. Methanol-water (43 µg/mL), acetone (115 µg/mL), dichloromethane (125 µg/mL), methanol (250 µg/mL), and heptane (390 µg/mL) in HT-29 cells.	Cytotoxic	[126]
Euphorbia umbellata (Pax) Bruyns	Fresh stems and leaves	Methanol	-	U-251, MCF-7, 786-0, NCI-H460	Stems extract (GI50 between 8.1 and 30.3 mg/mL) Leaf extract (GI50 between 35.6 and >250 mg/mL). Acetone fraction (GI50, between 0.37 and 2.9 mg/mL)	Antiproliferative	[127]
Euphorbia umbellata (Pax) Bruyns	Bark	Ethanol:water (70:30), chloroform fraction	Euphol, sitosterol, lanosterol, lupeol, cycloartenol, friedelin-3b-ol, friedelin	Jurkat clone E6-1	29.00 ± 1.49 µg/mL, 10.06 ± 1.48 µg/mL and 4.83 ± 2.25 µg/mL for 24, 48 and 72 h	Cytotoxic, apoptosis and cell cycle arrest	[128]

Table 1. *Cont.*

Name of the Species	Part of the Plant	Type of Extract	Class of Compounds/Compounds Identified in Extract	Cell Lines	IC_{50}	Activity/ Mechanism/ Effect	Ref.
Euphorbia umbellata (Pax) Bruyns	Green branches and leaves	Water, methanol, ethanol, and chloroform	Flavonoids, phenols and tannins, terpenoids, steroids, carbohdraates, alkaloids and saponins.	A549	Water (90.15 ± 2.50 μg/mL), ethanol (125.27 ± 2.00 μg/mL), chloroform (197.66 ± 2.40 μg/mL), and methanol (4.30 ± 0.44 μg/mL)	Cytotoxic	[129]
Excoecaria agallocha L.	Leaves	Methanol and Chloroform	-	Hep 2	Methanol extract range between 125–200 μg/mL and chloroform extract, 15–30 μg/mL	Cytotoxic	[130]
Excoecaria agallocha L.	Leaves	Methanol	-	M14, SKMEL5, SKMEL2, SKMEL28, MALME3M, UACC62, UACC257, U251, SNB19, MDA-MB-231, MCF-7, T47D, BT549, Ovcar3, Ovcar5, HCC2998, Colo205, HCT15, KM12, HeLa, SIHA and C33A	M14 (47.5 ± 4.12 μg/mL), SKMEL5 (89.2 ± 4.62 μg/mL), SKMEL2 (30.0 ± 2.12 μg/mL), SKMEL28 (29.8 ± 2.46 μg/mL), MALME3M (35.0 ± 3.12 μg/mL), UACC62 (34.0 ± 2.90 μg/mL), UACC257 (26.0 ± 3.12 μg/mL), U251 (19.44 ± 1.14 μg/mL), SNB19 (19.84 ± 1.60 μg/mL), MDA-MB-231 (15.56 ± 1.14 μg/mL), MCF-7 (20.24 ± 1.16 μg/mL), T47D (19.20 ± 0.15 μg/mL), BT549 (63.42 ± 5.12 μg/mL), Ovcar3 (39.44 ± 1.14 μg/mL), Ovcar5 (19.84 ± 0.60 μg/mL), HCC2998 (20.28 ± 0.56 μg/mL), Colo205 (12.0 ± 2.12 μg/mL), HCT15 (39.0 ± 3.82 μg/mL), KM12 (20.0 ± 1.70 μg/mL) HeLa (18.60 ± 2.20 μg/mL), SIHA (23.42 ± 1.90 μg/mL) and C33A (39.9 ± 3.10 μg/mL)	Cytotoxic	[131]

Table 1. *Cont.*

Name of the Species	Part of the Plant	Type of Extract	Class of Compounds/Compounds Identified in Extract	Cell Lines	IC_{50}	Activity/ Mechanism/ Effect	Ref.
Flueggea leucopyrus Willd.	Leaves and bark	Ethyl acetate and methanol.	Bergenin and bergenin isomers	A2780	Methanol extract of bark 12.58 ± 1.02 µg/mL, Ethyl acetate extract of leaves 36.35 ± 0.17 µg/mL	Cytotoxic and antiprolifera-tive effect	[132]
Hura crepitans L.	Leaves	Methanol and *n*-butanol	-	HepG2	-	Cytotoxic	[133]
Jatropha curcas L.	Leaves	Methanol	Hexadecanoic acid, hexadecanoic acid methyl ester, anethole, estragol, oleic acid, phytol, and carvacrol, octadecanoic acid methyl ester, and thymol	HepG2	47.2 ± 2.48 µg/mL	Cytotoxic	[11]
Jatropha curcas L.	Leaves	Ethanol	-	T-47D, SiHa, and OVCAR-7	%GI T-47D (0), SiHa (47), and OVCAR-7 (30)	Cytotoxic	[12]
Jatropha dioica Sesse ex Cerv.	Roots	Aqueous	Alkaloids, flavonoids, saponins, phenols, tannins, and carbohydrates		-		
Jatropha gossypifolia L.	Leaves	Methanol	-	HepG2	15.3 ± 0.95 µg/mL	Cytotoxic	[11]
Jatropha multifida L.	Leaves	Methanol	-	HepG2	29.6 ± 1.27 µg/mL	Cytotoxic	[11]
Jatropha podagrica Hook.	Leaves	Methanol and distilled water (80:20)	-	A549 and PC12	GI > 80% at 100 µg/mL	Antiproliferative	[11]
Jatropha zeyheri Sond.	Roots	Ethyl acetate	Mayor contents: Hexadecanoic acid, Octadecanoic acid, (Z)-9-Octadecenamide, 11-*n*-Decylheneicosane, Octacosane, 9-Hexacosene, Ethyl vallesiachotamate, Cyclooctacosane, Cyclotetracosane, and Tricosane	Caco-2, A547 and MCF-7	8.83 ± 0.00 µg/mL, 224.48 ± 0.01 µg/mL, and 102.88 ± 2.17 µg/mL respectively	Cytotoxic	[134]

Table 1. *Cont.*

Name of the Species	Part of the Plant	Type of Extract	Class of Compounds/Compounds Identified in Extract	Cell Lines	IC_{50}	Activity/ Mechanism/ Effect	Ref.
Mallotus cumingii Müll.Arg.	Leaves	Methanol, fractions with hexane and ethyl acetate	Phenolic compounds, flavonoids, terpenoids, cardiac glicosides and saponins.	HCT-116	Methanol (31.51 µg/mL), hexane fraction (17.49 µg/mL) and ethyl acetate fraction (7.75 µg/mL)	Cytotoxic	[135]
Mallotus phillippensis (Lam.) Müll.Arg.	Leaves	Methanol	alkaloids, flavonoids, tannins, diterpenes, steroids, and phenolic compounds	MCF-7	190 g/mL	Cytotoxic and apoptosis through the intrinsic pathway	[136]
Manihot esculenta Crantz	Aerial parts	Ether and chloroform fraction	-	A-549	Inhibition ratio % (69.71 ± 1.18) at 50 µg/mL	Cytotoxic	[137]
Mercurialis annua L.	Aerial parts	Ethanolic	Kaempferol, Isorhamnetin, Quercetin, and Rutin	K562, MCF-7, Hela, and A562	%GI 100 µM K562 (28.52 ± 0.57), MCF-7 (20.74 ± 6.96), Hela (14.44 ± 2.16), and A562 (10.33 ± 2.75)	Antiproliferative	[138]
Plukenetia volubilis L.	Leaves	Methanol, ethanol, chloroform, hexane, and water	terpenoids, saponins, and flavonoids	HeLa, and A549	Inhibition of 40–50% rate.	Antiproliferative effect	[139]
Ricinus communis L	Leaves	Aqueous	-	A375	48 µg/mL.	Cytotoxic	[140]
Ricinus communis L	Stems and seeds	Ethanol	-	A549, HT-29, SW-20, SiHa, Hep-2, T-47D, OVCAR-5 and PC-3	Seed extract activity was 41%, 11%, 12%, and 14% against A549, OVCAR-5, PC-5 respectively. Stem extract activity was 9%, 31% and 40% activity against Hep-2, HT-29, and SiHa cell lines (100 µg/mL).	Cytotoxic	[141]

Table 1. *Cont.*

Name of the Species	Part of the Plant	Type of Extract	Class of Compounds/Compounds Identified in Extract	Cell Lines	IC_{50}	Activity/ Mechanism/ Effect	Ref.
Ricinus communis L.	Stems	Ethanol	-	Hep-2, HT-29, SiHa, and OVCAR-6	%GI Hep-2 (9), HT-29 (31), SiHa (47), and OVCAR-6 (30).	Cytotoxic	[12]
Ricinus communis L.	Seeds	Ethanol	-	502713, A549, OVCAR-5, and PC-6	%GI 502713 (41), A549 (11), OVCAR-5 (12) and PC-5 (14).	Cytotoxic	[12]
Ricinus communis L.	Different part of the seeds (testa, tegmen, embryo, endosperm, etc)	Methanol	Phorbol esters	THP-1	testa extract in THP-1 (109.9 μg/mL)	Cytotoxic	[142]
Schinziophyton rautanenii (Schinz) Radcl.-Sm.	Root and bark	Aqueous and methanolic	Alkaloids, flavonoids, anthraquinones, coumarins and triterpenenes	TK10, MCF-7, and UACC-62	Aqueous (100–150 μg/mL) and methanolic (70–120 μg/mL) for both cell lines.	Cytotoxic	[143]
Tragia involucrata L.	Whole plant	Ethanol	Clionasterol, Squalene, 2-Ethylhexyl phthalate, Phytol, neophytadiene, ethyl palmitate, ethyl linolate, linolenic acid, viminalol, etc	YAC-1	-	Cytotoxic	[144]

Data not reported are represented by "-".

3.3. Cytotoxic and Anticancer Effects of Euphorbiaceae Pure Compounds In Vitro Studies

Many studies have focused on investigating the induction of apoptosis through various signaling pathways in cancer cells as a result of isolated plant compounds. In their study, Wisniewski et al. [145] showed that, of the compounds derived from Euphorbia sp., latilagascene B is an effective *P*-glycoprotein inhibitor capable of increasing doxorubicin accumulation in resistant cells (human colon carcinoma LoVo cells). In contrast, Li et al. [146] showed that Trigothysoid N, a natural diterpenoid isolated from *Trigonostemon thyrsoideus*, revealed a strong ability to inhibit the proliferation of A549 lung cancer cells through cell cycle arrest. In addition, the compound can inhibit tumor proliferation and migration by targeting mitochondria, regulating the signal transducer and activator of transcription 3/focal adhesion quinase) signaling pathway (STAT3/FAK), and inhibiting angiogenesis. In another study, Lin et al. [147] showed that Euphorbia L2, a lathyrane diterpenoid isolated from the seeds of *Euphorbia lathyris* L., possessed potent cytotoxicity against A549 lung cancer cells and induced apoptosis through the mitochondrial pathway via an increase in reactive oxygen species (ROS), loss of mitochondrial potential, release of cytochrome c, activation of casp-9 and casp-3, and cleavage of poly(ADP-ribose) polymerase. In turn, Fan et al. [148] showed that the 8,9-seco-*ent*-kaurane diterpenoid isolated from *Croton kongensis* induced apoptosis, autophagy, and metastasis suppression in triple-negative breast cancer (TNBC) cells by inhibiting Akt. Additionally, in in vivo studies, it significantly inhibited TNBC tumor growth without causing side effects. Wongprayoon et al. [149] noted that *Euphorbia lactea* triterpenoid friedelan-3β-ol was cytotoxic to several cancer cell lines, including HN22, HepG2, HCT116, and HeLa. Furthermore, the authors showed that the compound induced S-phase cell cycle arrest in HN22 cells without inducing apoptosis at the same concentration and exposure time. Studies about isolated compounds are presented in Table 2 below.

Table 2. Cytotoxic properties of isolated compounds from the Euphorbiaceae family of plants against cancer cells.

Name of the Species	Part of the Plant	Type of Extract	Class of Compounds/ Compounds Identified in Extract	Cell Lines	IC50	Activity/ Mechanism/Effect	Ref.
Croton crassifolius Geiseler	Roots	Ethanol	Crotonpyrone A	HeLa and NCI-446	HeLa (10.21 μg/mL) and NCI-446 (6.59 μg/mL)	Cytotoxic	[150]
Croton crassifolius Geiseler	Roots	Ethanol	Crotonpyrone B	HeLa and NCI-446	HeLa (9.54 μg/mL) and NCI-446 (6.52 μg/mL)	Cytotoxic	[150]
Croton damayeshu Y.T.Chang	Twigs and leaves	Ethanol	Crodamoid H	A549	A549 (0.9 ± 0.6 μM)	Cytotoxic	[151]
Croton damayeshu Y.T.Chang	Twigs and leaves	Ethanol	Crodamoid I	A549 and HL-60	A549 (1.3 ± 0.2 μM) and HL-60 (2.4 ± 1.0 μM)	Cytotoxic	[151]
Croton damayeshu Y.T.Chang	Twigs and leaves	Ethanol	4α-deoxyphorbol-12-tiglate-13-isobutyrate	A549 and HL-60	A549 (1.9 ± 0.1 μM) and HL-60 (1.8 ± 0.8 μM)	Cytotoxic	[151]
Croton echioides Baill.	Stem bark	EtOH/H_2O	*N-trans*-4-Methoxy-cinnamoyl-5-hydroxytryptamine	HCT-116	HCT-116 (86.8 μmol L^{-1})	Cytotoxic	[21]
Croton floribundus SPRENG.	Root bark	Hexane	*ent*-kaur-16-en-6a,19-diol	HCT-116, HL60, MDA-MB-435, and HCT-8	HCT-116 (12.1 μg/mL), MDA-MB-435 (14.3 μg/mL), and HCT-9 (13.5 μg/mL)	Cytotoxic	[152]
Croton lachnocarpus Benth.	Leaves	Ethanol	7b,15-dihydroxy-*ent*-abieta-8,11,13-trien-3-one	A549, BGC-823, HepG2, HL-60, MCF-7,	A549 (56.3 μM), BGC-823 (68.7 μM), HepG2 (66.9 μM), HL-60 (52.3 μM), MCF-7 (56.2 μM), W480 (59.4 μM)	Cytotoxic	[49]
Croton lachnocarpus Benth.	Leaves	Ethanol	2b,15-dihydroxy-*ent*-abieta-8,11,13-triene	A549, BGC-823, HepG2, HL-60, MCF-7, W480	A549 (52.3 μM), BGC-823 (52.2 μM), HepG2 (59.7 μM), HL-60 (49.4 μM), MCF-7 (60.1 μM), W480 (57.6 μM)	Cytotoxic	[49]
Croton lachnocarpus Benth.	Leaves	Ethanol	7b,13a,15-tri-hydroxy-*ent*-abieta-8(14)-en-3-one	A549, BGC-823, HepG2, HL-60, MCF-7, W480	A549 (28.7 μM), BGC-823 (26.6 μM), HepG2 (25.3 μM), HL-60 (31.7 μM), MCF-7 (27.1 μM), W480 (24.9 μM)	Cytotoxic	[49]
Croton laui Merr. & F.P.Metcalf			crotonolide A	HL-60 and P-388	HL-60 (9.42 μM) and P-388 (7.45 μM)	Cytotoxic	[153]

Table 2. *Cont.*

Name of the Species	Part of the Plant	Type of Extract	Class of Compounds/ Compounds Identified in Extract	Cell Lines	IC50	Activity/ Mechanism/Effect	Ref.
Croton tiglium L.	Seeds	Ethanol	4-deoxy-20-oxophorbol 12-tiglyl 13-acetate	K562, A549, and Huh-7	K562 (0.03 μM), A549 (6.88 μM), and Huh-7 (3.85 μM)	Cytotoxic	[154]
Croton tiglium L.	Seeds	Ethanol	7-oxo-5-ene-phorbol-13-(2-methylbutyrate	K562, A549, and Huh-7	K562 (0.03 μM), A549 (6.33 μM), and Huh-7 (20.9 μM)	Cytotoxic	[154]
Croton tiglium L.	Seeds	Ethanol	crotignoid C	K562, A549, and Huh-7	K562 (0.07 μM), A549 (8.86 μM), and Huh-7 (11.6 μM)	Cytotoxic	[154]
Croton tiglium L.	Seeds	Ethanol	13-O-(2-metyl)butyryl-phorbol	K562, A549, and Huh-7	K562 (0.05 μM), A549 (43.5 μM), and Huh-7 (34.2 μM)	Cytotoxic	[154]
Croton tiglium L.	Seeds	Ethanol	12-O-tiglylphorbol-13-acetate	K562, A549, and Huh-7	K562 (0.07 μM), A549 (8.50 μM), and Huh-7 (3.36 μM)	Cytotoxic	[154]
Croton tiglium L.	Seeds	Ethanol	crotignoid F	K562, A549, and Huh-7	K562 (0.05 μM), A549 (3.11 μM), and Huh-7 (4.41 μM)	Cytotoxic	[154]
Croton tiglium L.	Seeds	Ethanol	phorbol	K562, A549, and Huh-7	K562 (0.10 μM), A549 (15.3 μM), and Huh-7 (5.93 μM)	Cytotoxic	[154]
Croton tiglium L.	Seeds	Methanol	13-O-acetylphorbol-20-oleate.	SNUB387	SNUB387 (1.2 ± 0.1 μM)	Cytotoxic	[155]
Croton tiglium L.	Seeds	Methanol	13-O-acetyl-4-deoxy-4α-phorbol-20-linoleate.	SNUB387	SNUB387 (8.1 ± 1.3 μM)	Cytotoxic	[155]
Croton tiglium L.	Seeds	Methanol	13-O-acetyl-4-deoxy-4α-phorbol-20-oleate.	SNUB387	SNUB387 (6.6 ± 0.9 μM)	Cytotoxic	[155]
Croton tiglium L.	Branches and leaves	Ethanol	12-O-acetylphorbol-13-isobutyrate	K562, MOLT-4, U937, MCF-7, Hela, DU145, A549, SGC-7091, H1975, HL60	K562 (4.0 μM), MOLT-4 (2.4 μM), U937 (6.8 μM), MCF-7 (13 μM), Hela (3.9 μM), DU145 (7.2 μM), A549 (5.8 μM) SGC-7091 (13 μM), H1975 (10 μM), HL60 (12 μM)	Cytotoxic	[156]

Table 2. *Cont.*

Name of the Species	Part of the Plant	Type of Extract	Class of Compounds/ Compounds Identified in Extract	Cell Lines	IC50	Activity/ Mechanism/Effect	Ref.
Croton tiglium L.	Branches and leaves	Ethanol	12-O-benzoylphorbol-13-(2-methyl)butyrate	K562, MOLT-4, U937, MCF-7, Hela, DU145, A549, SGC-7091, H1975, HL60	K562 (15 µM), MOLT-4 (12 µM), U937 (17 µM), MCF-7 (20 µM), Hela (4.6 µM), DU145 (4.3 µM), A549 (6.9 µM), SGC-7091 (10 µM), H1975 (3.3 µM), HL60 (6.8 µM)	Cytotoxic	[156]
Croton tiglium L.	Branches and leaves	Ethanol	12-O-tiglyl-7-oxo-5-ene-phorbol-13-(2-methylbutyrate)	K562, MOLT-4, U937, MCF-7, Hela, DU145, A549, SGC-7091, H1975, HL60	K562 (17 µM), MOLT-4 (4.8 µM), U937 (21 µM), MCF-7 (20 µM), Hela (5.0 µM), DU145 (10 µM), A549 (19 µM), SGC-7091 (23 µM), H1975 (10 µM), HL60 (10 µM)	Cytotoxic	[156]
Croton tiglium L.	Branches and leaves	Ethanol	13-O-(2-metyl)butyryl-4-deoxy-4a-phorbol.	K562, MOLT-4, U937, MCF-7, Hela, DU145, A549, SGC-7091, H1975, HL60	K562 (8 µM), MOLT-4 (9.9 µM), U937 (18 µM), MCF-7 (24 µM), Hela (10 µM), DU145 (10 µM), A549 (4.5 µM), SGC-7091 (5.4 µM), H1975 (3.3 µM), HL60 (9.8 µM)	Cytotoxic	[156]
Croton tiglium L.	Branches and leaves	Ethanol	12-O-tiglylporbol-13-propionate	K562, MOLT-4, U937, MCF-7, Hela, DU145, A549, SGC-7091, H1975, HL60	K562 (4.4 µM), MOLT-4 (1.1 µM), U937 (5.5 µM), MCF-7 (>50 µM), Hela (9.2 µM), DU145 (1.1 µM), A549 (32 µM), SGC-7091 (43 µM), H1975 (10 µM), HL60 (1.2 µM)	Cytotoxic	[156]
Croton tiglium L.	Branches and leaves	Ethanol	12-O-tiglylphor-bol-13-isobutyrate	K562, MOLT-4, U937, MCF-7, Hela, DU145, A549, SGC-7091, H1975, HL60	K562 (2.2 µM), MOLT-4 (1.0 µM), U937 (2.6 µM), Hela (10 µM), DU145 (5.0 µM), H1975 (10 µM), HL60 (1.2 µM)	Cytotoxic	[156]
Croton tiglium L.	Branches and leaves	Ethanol	12-O-tiglylphorbol-13-(2-methyl)butyrate	K562, MOLT-4, U937, MCF-7, Hela, DU145, A549, SGC-7091, H1975, HL60	K562 (7.2 µM), MOLT-4 (10 µM), U937 (14 µM), MCF-7 (>50 µM), Hela (10 µM), DU145 (11 µM), A549 (>50 µM), SGC-7091 (>50 µM), H1975 (10 µM), HL60 (9.9 µM)	Cytotoxic	[156]

Table 2. *Cont.*

Name of the Species	Part of the Plant	Type of Extract	Class of Compounds/ Compounds Identified in Extract	Cell Lines	IC50	Activity/ Mechanism/Effect	Ref.
Croton tiglium L.	Branches and leaves	Ethanol	tiglin A	K562, MOLT-4, U937, MCF-7, Hela, DU145, A549, SGC-7091, H1975, HL60	K562 (15 µM), MOLT-4 (12 µM), U937 (17 µM), MCF-7 (20 µM), Hela (4.6 µM), DU145 (4.3 µM), A549 (6.9 µM), SGC-7091 (10 µM), H1975 (3.3 µM), HL60 (6.8 µM)	Cytotoxic	[156]
Croton tiglium L.	Seeds	Acetone	7-Keto-12-O-tiglylphorbol-13-acetate	HL60 and A549	HL60 (6.22 ± 3.24 µg/mL) and A549 (18.0 ± 9.48 µg/mL)	Cytotoxic	[157]
Croton tiglium L.	Seeds	Acetone	Phorbol-12-isobutyrate	HL60 and A549	HL60 (0.22 ± 0.15 µg/mL) and A549 (0.74 ± 0.48 µg/mL)	Cytotoxic	[157]
Croton tiglium L.	Seeds	Acetone	12-O-Tiglylphorbol-13-acetate	HL60 and A549	HL60 (0.02 ± 0.01 µg/mL) and A549 (0.10 ± 0.03 µg/mL)	Cytotoxic	[157]
Croton tiglium L.	Seeds	Acetone	12-O-(2-methyl)-butyrylphorbol-13-aetate	HL60 and A549	HL60 (<0.01µg/mL) and A549 (0.01 ± 0.00 µg/mL)	Cytotoxic	[157]
Croton tiglium L.	Seeds	Acetone	12-O-tiglyl-phorbol-13-isobutyrate	HL60 and A549	HL60 (<0.01 µg/mL) and A549 (<0.01 µg/mL)	Cytotoxic	[157]
Croton tiglium L.	Seeds	Acetone	phorbol-12-tigliate	HL60 and A549	HL60 (83.1 ± 2.89 µg/mL) and A549 (38.6 ± 30.1 µg/mL)	Cytotoxic	[157]
Croton tiglium L.	Seeds	Acetone	phorbol-12-tetradecanoate	HL60 and A549	HL60 (3.14 ± 2.17 µg/mL) and A549 (4.71 ± 1.92 µg/mL)	Cytotoxic	[157]
Croton tiglium L.	Seeds	Acetone	phorbol-13-aetate	HL60 and A549	HL60 (80.9 ± 11.6 µg/mL)	Cytotoxic	[157]
Croton tiglium L.	Seeds	Acetone	phorbol-13-decanoate	HL60 and A549	HL60 (0.02 ± 0.02 µg/mL) and A549 (0.94 ± 0.01 µg/mL)	Cytotoxic	[157]
Croton tiglium L.	Seeds	Acetone	4-deoxy-4α-phorbol-13-acetate	HL60 and A549	HL60 (89.0 ± 0.76 µg/mL)	Cytotoxic	[157]
Croton urucurana Baill.	Bark	Ethanol	Orbitide [1−9-NαC]-crourorb A1	786-O, HT29, MCF7, ADR-RES, Hep-G2, and PC-03	786-O (18.69 ± 0.82 µg/mL), HT29 (37.28 ± 0.57 µg/mL), MCF7 (35.49 ± 2.59 µg/mL), ADR-RES (3.98 ± 0.20 µg/mL), Hep-G2 (41.31 ± 2.70 µg/mL) and PC-03 (29.80 ± 0.34 µg/mL)	Cytotoxic	[158]

Table 2. *Cont.*

Name of the Species	Part of the Plant	Type of Extract	Class of Compounds/ Compounds Identified in Extract	Cell Lines	IC50	Activity/ Mechanism/Effect	Ref.
Croton velutinus Baill.	Roots	Methanol	(E)-1-(7,8-epoxypropen) phenyl benzoate	B16F10, HL-60, HCT116, MCF-7, and HepG2	B16F10 (14.4 ± 0.5 µM), HL-60 (9.8 ± 2.6 µM), HCT116 (12.9 ± 1.8 µM), MCF-7 (6.8 ± 1.59 µM) and HepG2 (16.7 ± 0.7 µM)	Cytotoxic	[159]
Croton velutinus Baill.	Roots	Methanol	sellovicine B	B16F10, HL-60, HCT116, MCF-7, and HepG2	B16F10 (13.8 ± 01 µM), HL-60 (11.4 ± 3.6 µM), HCT116 (13.2 ± 1.0 µM), MCF-7 (11.1 ± 1.4 µM) and HepG2 (18.3 ± 1.8 µM)	Cytotoxic	[159]
Drypetes hainanensis Merr.	Leaves and stems	Ethanol	4β-hydroxy-23-nor-friedel-3-one	BEL-7402, A549, HL60	GI rates: BEL-7402 (3.0%), A549 (9.7%), HL60 (4.1%)	Cytotoxic	[160]
Drypetes hainanensis Merr.	Leaves and stems	Ethanol	friedelin	BEL-7402, A549, HL60	HL60 (1.3%)	Cytotoxic	[160]
Drypetes hainanensis Merr.	Leaves and stems	Ethanol	friedelane-3,7-dione	BEL-7402, A549, HL60	BEL-7402 (4.6%), A549 (21.1%), HL60 (43.1%)	Cytotoxic	[160]
Euphorbia ammak Schweinf.	Leaves	Ethanol	euphol	HeLa	HeLa (9.25 mg/mL)	Cytotoxic	[161]
Euphorbia ammak Schweinf.	Leaves	Ethanol	α-glutinol	HeLa	HeLa (7.6 mg/mL)	Cytotoxic	[161]
Euphorbia ammak Schweinf.	Leaves	Ethanol	stigmasterol	HeLa	HeLa (10 mg/mL)	Cytotoxic	[161]
Euphorbia balsamifera Aiton	Aerial parts	Ethanol	Kampferol-3,40-dimethyl ether	HCT-116, HePG2, and MCF7	HCT116 (111.46 mM), HePG2 (42.67 mM) and MCF7 (44.90 mM)	Cytotoxic	[162]
Euphorbia connata Boiss.	Aerial flowering parts	Dichlorom-ethane/Acetone	3,7,14,15-tetraacetyl-5-propanoyl-13(17)-epoxy-8,10(18)-myrsinadiene	MDA-MB-231 and MCF-7	MDA-MB-231 (24.53 ± 3.39 µM) and MCF-7 (37.73 ± 3.41 µM)	Cytotoxic	[163]

Table 2. *Cont.*

Name of the Species	Part of the Plant	Type of Extract	Class of Compounds/ Compounds Identified in Extract	Cell Lines	IC50	Activity/ Mechanism/Effect	Ref.
Euphorbia connata Boiss.	Aerial flowering parts	Dichloro-methane/Acetone	3,7,10,14,15-pentaacetyl-5-butanoyl-13,17-epoxy-8-myrsinene	MDA-MB-231 and MCF-7	MDA-MB-231 (26.67 ± 1.41 μM) and MCF-7 (34.57 ± 2.12 μM)	Cytotoxic	[163]
Euphorbia dendroides L.	Aerial parts	Methanol	23 R/S-3b-hydroxycycloart-24-ene23-methyl ether	HepG2, Huh-7, KLM-1, 1321N1, HeLa	HepG2 (20.67 ± 0.72 μM), Huh-7 (16.24 ± 0.53 μM), KLM-1 (22.59 ± 0.94 μM), 1321N1 (25.99 ± 0.31 μM), HeLa (40.50 ± 3.14 μM)	Cytotoxic	[164]
Euphorbia dendroides L.	Aerial parts	Methanol	24-methylene cycloartan-3b-ol	HepG2, Huh-7, KLM-1, 1321N1, HeLa	HepG2 (10.93 ± 0.21 μM), Huh-7 (7.42 ± 0.16 μM), KLM-1 (21.48 ± 0.60 μM), 1321N1 (12.32 ± 0.58 μM), HeLa (13.68 ± 0.16 μM)	Cytotoxic	[164]
Euphorbia dendroides L.	Aerial parts	Methanol	cycloart-23-ene-3b,25-diol monoacetate	HepG2, Huh-7, KLM-1, 1321N1, HeLa	HepG2 (12.81 ± 0.73 μM), Huh-7 (<0.47 μM), KLM-1 (22.48 ± 0.64 μM), 1321N1 (25.17 ± 0.32 μM), HeLa (54.05 ± 1.11 μM)	Cytotoxic	[164]
Euphorbia dendroides L.	Aerial parts	Methanol	3b-hydroxy-cycloart-23-ene-25 methyl ether	HepG2, Huh-7, KLM-1, 1321N1, HeLa	HepG2 (12.72 ± 2.38 μM), Huh-7 (<0.44 μM), KLM-(<0.44 μM), 1321N1 (0.63 ± 0.15 μM), HeLa (3.7 ± 0.39 μM)	Cytotoxic	[164]
Euphorbia dendroides L.	Aerial parts	Methanol	24 R/S-3b-hydroxy-25-methylene Figure 1. Chemical structures of compounds 1–11, isolated from Euphorbia dendroides L. aerial parts. 830 A. R. HASSAN ET AL. cycloartan-24-ol	HepG2, Huh-7, KLM-1, 1321N1, HeLa	HepG2 (15.54 ± 1.95), Huh-7 (16.33 ± 1.22), KLM-1 (22.38 ± 1.29), 1321N1 (13.53 ± 0.33), HeLa (>4.52)	Cytotoxic	[164]
Euphorbia denticulata Lam	-	Acetone	taraxast-12-ene-3β,20,21(α)-triol	DU-145	DU-145 (12.2 ± 2.9 μM)	Cytotoxic	[165]

Table 2. *Cont.*

Name of the Species	Part of the Plant	Type of Extract	Class of Compounds/ Compounds Identified in Extract	Cell Lines	IC50	Activity/ Mechanism/Effect	Ref.
Euphorbia denticulata Lam	-	Acetone	cycloartane-3β,25-diol	DU-145	DU-145 (27.5 ± 4.9 μM)	Cytotoxic	[165]
Euphorbia denticulata Lam	-	Acetone	cycloartane-3β,24,25-triol	DU-145	DU-145 (18.3 ± 1.4 μM)	Cytotoxic	[165]
Euphorbia ebracteolata Hayata	Roots	Ethanol	Ebracteolata A	HL60, A549, SMMC-7721, MCF-7, and SW480	HL60 (17.5 μM), A549 (11.0 μM), SMMC-7721 (16.8 μM), MCF-7 (17.5 μM), and SW480 (18.0 μM)	Cytotoxic	[166]
Euphorbia ebracteolata Hayata	Roots	Ethanol	Yuexiandajisu F	HL60, A549, SMMC-7721, MCF-7, and SW480	HL60 (16.8 μM), A549 (19.7 μM), SMMC-7721 (18.4 μM), MCF-7 (15.3 μM), and SW480 (15.3 μM)	Cytotoxic	[166]
Euphorbia ebracteolata Hayata	Roots	Ethanol	jolkinol B	HL60, A549, SMMC-7721, MCF-7, and SW480	HL60 (5.0 μM), A549 (11.5 μM), SMMC-7721 (3.5 μM), MCF-7 (15.8 μM), and SW480 (9.5 μM)	Cytotoxic	[166]
Euphorbia fischeriana Steud	Roots	Ethanol	ebracteolatas D	HCT116, A549, HeLa, SW620, MCF-7, HepG-2	HCT116 (>40 μM), A549 (22.03 μM), HeLa (>40 μM), SW620 (>40 μM), MCF-7 (>40 μM), HepG-2 (>40 μM)	Cytotoxic	[48]
Euphorbia fischeriana Steud	Roots	Ethanol	ebractenoid Q	HCT116, A549, HeLa, SW620, MCF-7, HepG-2	HCT116 (33.18 μM), A549 (2.81 μM), HeLa (>40 μM), SW620 (>40 μM), MCF-7 (>40 μM), HepG-2 (27.24 μM)	Cytotoxic	[48]
Euphorbia fischeriana Steud	Roots	Ethanol	Euphonoid H	MDA-MB-231, HCT-15, RKO, C4-2B, C4-2B/ENZR	MDA-MB-231 (21.80 ± 2.35 μM), HCT-15 (28.57 ± 1.16 μM), RKO (20.46 ± 1.43 μM), C4-2B (5.52 ± 0.65 μM), C4-2B/ENZR (4.16 ± 0.42 μM)	Cytotoxic	[47]
Euphorbia fischeriana Steud	Roots	Ethanol	Euphonoid I	MDA-MB-231, HCT-15, RKO, C4-2B, C4-2B/ENZR	MDA-MB-231 (7.95 ± 0.82 μM), HCT-15 (12.45 ± 3.24 μM), RKO (8.78 ± 2.45 μM), C4-2B (4.49 ± 0.78 μM), C4-2B/ENZR (5.74 ± 0.45 μM)	Cytotoxic	[47]

Table 2. *Cont.*

Name of the Species	Part of the Plant	Type of Extract	Class of Compounds/ Compounds Identified in Extract	Cell Lines	IC50	Activity/ Mechanism/Effect	Ref.
Euphorbia fischeriana Steud	Roots	EtOH	17-Hydroxyljolkinolide B	MCF-10A, MCF-7, ZR-75-1 and MDA-MB-231	MCF-10A (3.4 ± 0.1 μg/mL), MCF-7 (4.7 ± 0.2 μg/mL), ZR-75-1 (2.2 ± 0.1 μg/mL) and MDA-MB-231 (1.1 ± 0.1 μg/mL)	Cytotoxic	[167]
Euphorbia fischeriana Steud	Roots	EtOH	17-Acetyljolkinolide B	MCF-10A, MCF-7, ZR-75-1 and MDA-MB-231	MCF-10A (4.3 ± 0.1 μg/mL), MCF-7 (3.4 ± 0.1 μg/mL), ZR-75-1 (1.2 ± 0.1 μg/mL) and MDA-MB-231 (1.7 ± 0.1 μg/mL)	Cytotoxic	[167]
Euphorbia fischeriana Steud	Roots	Ethanol	Euphorfiatnoid B	HepG2, H460, and MCF-7	H460 (9.97 μM)	Cytotoxic	[168]
Euphorbia fischeriana Steud	Roots	Ethanol	Euphorfiatnoid A	HepG2, H460, and MCF-7	HepG2 (11.64 μM), H460 (28.54 ± 1.20 μM), and MCF-7 (40.02 ± 0.47 μM)	Cytotoxic	[168]
Euphorbia fischeriana Steud	Roots	Ethanol	Euphorfiatnoid C	HepG2, H460, and MCF-7	HepG2 (13.10 ± 0.35 μM), H460 (14.88 ± 0.57 μM), and MCF-7 (32.95 ± 0.40 μM)	Cytotoxic	[168]
Euphorbia fischeriana Steud.	Roots	Ethanol	Euphorfischerin A	HeLa, N460 and Namalwa	HeLa (4.6 ± 0.11 μM), N460 (11.5 ± 0.04 μM) and Namalwa (16.4 ± 0.07 μM)	Cytotoxic	[169]
Euphorbia fischeriana Steud.	Roots	Ethanol	Euphorfischerin B	HeLa, N460 and Namalwa	HeLa (9.5 ± 0.16 μM), N460 (17.4 ± 0.34 μM) and Namalwa (13.3 ± 0.19 μM)	Cytotoxic	[169]
Euphorbia fischeriana Steud.	Aerial parts	Methanol	3α-acetoxy-14-hydroxy-*ent*-abieta-8(9),13(15)-dien-16,12-olide	HL-60, SMMC-7721 and SGC-7901	HL-60 (15.3 μM), SMMC-7721 (23.2 μM) and SGC-7901 (29.0 μM)	Cytotoxic	[170]
Euphorbia helioscopia L.	Aerial parts	Ethanol aqueous	Euphoheliphane A	OS-RC-2, Ketr-3, 769-P, G401, GRC-1 and ACHN	OS-RC-2 (47 μM), Ketr-3 (45 μM), 769-P (43 μM), G401 (38 μM), GRC-1 (41 μM) and ACHN (40 μM)	Cytotoxic	[171]
Euphorbia helioscopia L.	Aerial parts	Ethanol aqueous	Euphoheliphane B	OS-RC-2, Ketr-3, 769-P, G401, GRC-1 and ACHN	OS-RC-2 (31 μM), Ketr-3 (32 μM), 769-P (30 μM), G401 (34 μM), GRC-1 (33 μM) and ACHN (35 μM)	Cytotoxic	[171]

Table 2. *Cont.*

Name of the Species	Part of the Plant	Type of Extract	Class of Compounds/ Compounds Identified in Extract	Cell Lines	IC50	Activity/ Mechanism/Effect	Ref.
Euphorbia helioscopia L.	Aerial parts	Ethanol aqueous	Euphoheliphane C	OS-RC-2, Ketr-3, 769-P, G401, GRC-1 and ACHN	OS-RC-2 (35 µM), Ketr-3 (41 µM), 769-P (39 µM), G401 (32 µM), GRC-1 (38 µM) and ACHN (36 µM)	Cytotoxic	[171]
Euphorbia heliosocpia L	Whole plant	Methanol	Euphohelinoid A	HepG2, Hela, HL-60, SMMC-7721	HepG2 (24.3 ± 1.5 µM), Hela (28.4 ± 1.8 µM), HL-60 (18.6 ± 1.1 µM), SMMC-7721 (29.6 ± 1.5 µM)	Cytotoxic	[172]
Euphorbia heliosocpia L	Whole plant	Methanol	Euphohelinoid B	HepG2, Hela, HL-60, SMMC-7721	HepG2 (10.2 ± 1.4 µM), Hela (9.3 ± 1.2 µM), HL-60 (8.1 ± 0.7 µM), SMMC-7721 (9.8 ± 1.3 µM)	Cytotoxic	[172]
Euphorbia heliosocpia L	Whole plant	Methanol	Euphohelinoid C	HepG2, Hela, HL-60, SMMC-7721	HepG2 (>50 µM), Hela (>50 µM), HL-60 (>50 µM), SMMC-7721 (>50 µM)	Cytotoxic	[172]
Euphorbia heliosocpia L	Whole plant	Methanol	Euphohelinoid D	HepG2, Hela, HL-60, SMMC-7721	HepG2 (>50 µM), Hela (34.5 ± 2.3 µM), HL-60 (34.1 ± 1.6 µM), SMMC-7721 (30.1 ± 1.9 µM)	Cytotoxic	[172]
Euphorbia heliosocpia L	Whole plant	Methanol	Euphohelinoid F	HepG2, Hela, HL-60, SMMC-7721	HepG2 (12.5 ± 1.6 µM), Hela (14.1 ± 0.8 µM), HL-60 (13.3 ± 1.2 µM), SMMC-7721 (11.1 ± 1.7 µM)	Cytotoxic	[172]
Euphorbia heliosocpia L	Whole plant	Methanol	euphornin L	HepG2, Hela, HL-60, SMMC-7721	HepG2 (22.8 ± 1.7 µM), Hela (25.7 ± 2.2 µM), HL-60 (13.1 ± 1.8 µM), SMMC-7721 (14.3 ± 2.2 µM)	Cytotoxic	[172]
Euphorbia heliosocpia L	Whole plant	Methanol	helioscopianoid O	HepG2, Hela, HL-60, SMMC-7721	HepG2 (>50 µM), Hela (26.2 ± 1.4 µM), HL-60 (18.2 ± 1.9 µM), SMMC-7721 (19.5 ± 1.2 µM)	Cytotoxic	[172]

Table 2. *Cont.*

Name of the Species	Part of the Plant	Type of Extract	Class of Compounds/ Compounds Identified in Extract	Cell Lines	IC50	Activity/ Mechanism/Effect	Ref.
Euphorbia helioscopia L	Whole plant	Methanol	euphoscopin I	HepG2, Hela, HL-60, SMMC-7721	HepG2 (24.1 ± 1.2 μM), Hela (29.7 ± 2.1 μM), HL-60 (14.3 ± 1.1 μM), SMMC-7721 (18.7 ± 1.1 μM)	Cytotoxic	[172]
Euphorbia helioscopia L	Whole plant	Methanol	euphoscopin J	HepG2, Hela, HL-60, SMMC-7721	HepG2 (14.9 ± 1.3 μM), Hela (13.7 ± 1.4 μM), HL-60 (12.4 ± 1.2 μM), SMMC-7721 (15.0 ± 1.7 μM)	Cytotoxic	[172]
Euphorbia helioscopia L	Whole plant	Methanol	euphoscopin B	HepG2, Hela, HL-60, SMMC-7721	HepG2 (23.3 ± 1.3 μM), Hela (29.2 ± 1.6 μM), HL-60 (20.2 ± 1.5 μM), SMMC-7721 (27.1 ± 1.4 μM)	Cytotoxic	[172]
Euphorbia heterophylla L.	Roots	*n*-hexane, DCM and MeOH	13-epicupressic acid	EJ-138, HepG2, A549, MCF-7 and PC3	EJ-138 (>200 μg/mL), HepG2 (>200 μg/mL), A549 (157.4 ± 3.24 μg/mL), MCF-7 (139.1 ± 2.14 μg/mL) and PC3 (>200 μg/mL)	Cytotoxic	[173]
Euphorbia heterophylla L.	Roots	*n*-hexane, DCM and MeOH	imbricatholic acid	EJ-138, HepG2, A549, MCF-7, and PC3	EJ-138 (>200 μg/mL), HepG2 (>200 μg/mL), A549 (>200 μg/mL), MCF-7 (173.5 ± 4.34 μg/mL) and PC3 (>200 μg/mL)	Cytotoxic	[173]
Euphorbia heterophylla L.	Roots	*n*-hexane, DCM and MeOH	α-hydroxy sandaracopimaric acid	EJ-138, HepG2, A549, MCF-7, and PC3	EJ-138 (173.3 ± 2.37 μg/mL), HepG2 (>200 μg/mL), A549 (>200 μg/mL), MCF-7 (>250 μg/mL) and PC3 (>250 μg/mL)	Cytotoxic	[173]
Euphorbia heterophylla L.	Roots	*n*-hexane, DCM and MeOH	13-epicupressic acid	EJ-138, HepG2, A549, MCF-7, and PC3	EJ-138 (182.2 ± 1.18 μg/mL), HepG2 (>200 μg/mL), A549 (>200 μg/mL), MCF-7 (>200 μg/mL) and PC3 (>250 μg/mL)	Cytotoxic	[173]

Table 2. *Cont.*

Name of the Species	Part of the Plant	Type of Extract	Class of Compounds/ Compounds Identified in Extract	Cell Lines	IC50	Activity/ Mechanism/Effect	Ref.
Euphorbia heterophylla L.	Roots	*n*-hexane, DCM and MeOH	β-hydroxy sandaracopimaric acid 13-epicupressic acid	EJ-138, HepG2, A549, MCF-7, and PC3	EJ-138 (>200 µg/mL), HepG2 (>200 µg/mL), A549 (67.4 ± 2.45 µg/mL), MCF-7 (111.7 ± 3.75 µg/mL) and PC3 (>200 µg/mL)	Cytotoxic	[173]
Euphorbia heterophylla L.	Roots	*n*-hexane, DCM and MeOH	5,7,3′,4′-pentahydroxyflavone	EJ-138, HepG2, A549, MCF-7, and PC3	EJ-138 (>200 µg/mL), HepG2 (>200 µg/mL), A549 (135.8 ± 7.41 µg/mL), MCF-7 (117.4 ± 3.71 µg/mL) and PC3 (>200 µg/mL)	Cytotoxic	[173]
Euphorbia heterophylla L.	Roots	*n*-hexane, DCM and MeOH	quercitrin	EJ-138, HepG2, A549, MCF-7, and PC3	EJ-138 (>250 µg/mL), HepG2 (>200 µg/mL), A549 (138.1 ± 4.62 µg/mL), MCF-7 (105.3 ± 6.19 µg/mL), and PC3 (>200 µg/mL)	Cytotoxic	[173]
Euphorbia hypericifolia L	Whole herb	Ethanol	euphypenoid A	HCT-116	HCT-116 (12.8 ± 1.6 µM)	Cytotoxic	[174]
Euphorbia hypericifolia L	Whole herb	Ethanol	20(S),24(R)-20,24-epoxy-24-methyldammaran-3β-ol	HCT-116	HCT-116 (26.8 ± 4.6 µM)	Cytotoxic	[174]
Euphorbia hypericifolia L	Whole herb	Ethanol	3β-hydroxycycloart-24-one	HCT-116	HCT-116 (7.4 ± 0.2 µM)	Cytotoxic	[174]
Euphorbia hypericifolia L	Whole herb	Ethanol	isomotiol	HCT-116	HCT-116 (10.6 ± 1.2 µM)	Cytotoxic	[174]
Euphorbia kansui S.L.Liou ex S.B.Ho	Roots	Ethanol	Euphorikanin A	HeLa and NCI-446	HeLa (28.85 ± 1.41 µM) and NCI-446 (20.89 ± 1.67 µM)	Cytotoxic	[175]
Euphorbia lactea Haw.	Aerial parts	Ethanol, *n*-hexane fraction	friedelin	HN22, HepG2, and HCT116	-	Cytotoxic	[149]
Euphorbia lactea Haw.	Aerial parts	Ethanol, *n*-hexane fraction	taraxerol	HN22, HepG2, and HCT116	-	Cytotoxic	[149]

Table 2. *Cont.*

Name of the Species	Part of the Plant	Type of Extract	Class of Compounds/ Compounds Identified in Extract	Cell Lines	IC50	Activity/ Mechanism/Effect	Ref.
Euphorbia lactea Haw.	Aerial parts	Ethanol, *n*-hexane fraction	friedelan-3α-ol	HN22, HepG2, and HCT116	-	Cytotoxic	[149]
Euphorbia lagascae Spreng.	Seeds	Methanol	Esculetin	LoVo and LoVo/Dx	LoVo (56.81 ± 5.42%) and LoVo/Dx (68.42 ± 7.56%)	Cytotoxic	[145]
Euphorbia microsphaera Boiss	Aerial parts	Hexane, chloroform and methanol	Aryanin (3aR,4S,4aS,5R,7aS,9aS)-5-hydroxy-5,8-dimethyl-3-methylene-2-oxo2,3,3a,4,4a,5,6,7,7a, 9a decahydroazuleno [6,5-b] furan-4-yl acetate)	MCF-7	MCF-7 (13.81 μg/mL)	Cytotoxic	[61]
Euphorbia nematocypha Hand.-Mazz.	Roots	Ethanol	16-O-caffeoyl-16-hydroxyldodecanoic acid	MCF-7 and HeLa	MCF-7 (20.22 ± 1.2 μmol/L) and HeLa (27.8 ± 1.4 μmol/L)	Cytotoxic	[176]
Euphorbia nematocypha Hand.-Mazz.	Aerial parts	Methylene chloride	*trans*, *trans*-2′,4′-hexadienedioicacid-1′-β-amyrin ester	MCF7 and HeLa	MCF7 (29.5 ± 3.4 μmol /L) and HeLa (23.2± 4.2 μmol /L)	Cytotoxic	[177]
Euphorbia nematocypha Hand.-Mazz.	Roots	Ethanol	Nematocynine	HCC1806, ST486, CT26, HeLa, and A549	HCC1806 (16.96 ± 0.16 μM), ST486 (60.94 ± 0.74 μM), CT26 (52.04 ± 1.96 μM), and HeLa (52.70 ± 0.52 μM)	Cytotoxic	[178]
Euphorbia neriifolia Linn.	Aerial parts	Ethanol	Phonerilin B	A549 and HL60	A549 (8.6 ± 1.7 μM) and HL60 (9.1 ± 0.02 μM)	Cytotoxic	[179]
Euphorbia neriifolia Linn.	Aerial parts	Ethanol	Phonerilin E	A549 and HL60	A549 (4.9 ± 0.06 μM) and HL60 (9.2 ± 0.09 μM)	Cytotoxic	[179]
Euphorbia neriifolia Linn.	Aerial parts	Ethanol	Phonerilin F	A549 and HL60	A549 (3.8 ± 0.2 μM) and HL60 (4.5 ± 0.7 μM)	Cytotoxic	[179]
Euphorbia neriifolia Linn.	Aerial parts	Ethanol	Phonerilin H	A549 and HL60	A549 (7.5 ± 0.8 μM) and HL60 (5.7 ± 1.0 μM)	Cytotoxic	[179]
Euphorbia neriifolia Linn.	Aerial parts	Ethanol	20-O-diacetyl-ingenol	A549 and HL60	HL60 (3.1 ± 0.2 μM)	Cytotoxic	[179]

Table 2. *Cont.*

Name of the Species	Part of the Plant	Type of Extract	Class of Compounds/ Compounds Identified in Extract	Cell Lines	IC50	Activity/ Mechanism/Effect	Ref.
Euphorbia neriifolia Linn.	Aerial parts	Ethanol	7,12-O-diacetyl-8-O-tigloylingol	A549 and HL60	A549 (6.4 ± 0.2 μM) and HL60 (9.5 ± 0.04 μM)	Cytotoxic	[179]
Euphorbia osyridea Bioss.	Aerial flowering parts	Dichloromethane/Acetone	2,7,9,14-tetraacetyl-3-benzoyl-8-butanoyl-5,15-dihydroxy-6(17),11(E)-jatrophadiene	Caov-4, and OVCAR	Caov-4 (46.27 ± 3.86 μM) and OVCAR (38.81 ± 3.30 μM)	Cytotoxic	[180]
Euphorbia osyridea Bioss.	Aerial flowering parts	Dichloromethane/Acetone	2,7,9,14-tetraacetyl-3-benzoyl-propionyl ester-5,15-dihydroxy-6(17),11(E)-jatrophadiene	Caov-4, and OVCAR	Caov-4 (36.48 ± 3.18), and OVCAR (42.59 ± 4.50 μM)	Cytotoxic	[180]
Euphorbia pekinensis Rupr.	Roots	Ethanol	Pekinenin G (11a,12b-epoxy-18-hydroxy-1bH, 2aH-casba-3E and 7E-dien-5-one)	BGC823, A549, HT-29, and MCF-7	BGC823 (42.7 μM), A549 (40.8 μM), HT-29 (47.8 μM), and MCF-7 (48.5 μM)	Cytotoxic	[181]
Euphorbia pekinensis Rupr.	Roots	Ethanol	Pekinenin G (11a,12b-epoxy-18-hydroxy-1bH, 2aH-casba-3E and 7E-dien-5-one) 2	BGC823, A549, HT-29, and MCF-8	BGC823 (53.9 μM), A549 (88.8 μM), HT-29 (70.1 μM), and MCF-7 (70.5 μM)	Cytotoxic	[181]
Euphorbia pekinensis Rupr.	Roots	Ethanol	Pekinenin G (11a,12b-epoxy-18-hydroxy-1bH, 2aH-casba-3E and 7E-dien-5-one) 3	BGC823, A549, HT-29, and MCF-9	BGC823 (15.6 μM), A549 (21.9 μM), HT-29 (25.1 μM), and MCF-7 (22.3 μM)	Cytotoxic	[181]
Euphorbia pekinensis Rupr.	Roots	Ethanol	Pekinenin G (11a,12b-epoxy-18-hydroxy-1bH, 2aH-casba-3E and 7E-dien-5-one) 4	BGC823, A549, HT-29, and MCF-10	BGC823 (25.1 μM), A549 (35.1 μM), HT-29 (30.2 μM), and MCF-7 (32.3 μM)	Cytotoxic	[181]
Euphorbia pekinensis Rupr.	Roots	Ethanol	Pekinenin G (11a,12b-epoxy-18-hydroxy-1bH, 2aH-casba-3E and 7E-dien-5-one) 5	BGC823, A549, HT-29, and MCF-11	BGC823 (54.8 μM), A549 (90.2 μM), HT-29 (110.7 μM), and MCF-7 (87.9 μM)	Cytotoxic	[181]

Table 2. *Cont.*

Name of the Species	Part of the Plant	Type of Extract	Class of Compounds/ Compounds Identified in Extract	Cell Lines	IC50	Activity/ Mechanism/Effect	Ref.
Euphorbia pekinensis Rupr.	Roots	Ethanol	Pekinenin G (11a,12b-epoxy-18-hydroxy-1bH, 2aH-casba-3E and 7E-dien-5-one) 6	BGC823, A549, HT-29, and MCF-12	BGC823 (12.1 µM), A549 (15.6 µM), HT-29 (11.3 µM), and MCF-7 (21.2 µM)	Cytotoxic	[181]
Euphorbia pekinensis Rupr.	Roots	Ethanol	(−)-(1S)-15-hydroxy-18-carboxycembrene	Hela, PC-3, HT1080, A375-S2, and MDA23	Hela (35.3 ± 3.6 µM), PC-3 (53.9 ± 6.2 µM), HT1080 (37.3 ± 2.0 µM), A375-S2 (28.7 ± 3.8 µM), and MDA24 (43.5 ± 5.1 µM)	Cytotoxic	[182]
Euphorbia pekinensis Rupr.	Roots	Ethanol	Jolkinol B	U-937 and LOVO	U-937 (3.60 ± 0.02 µM) and LOVO (8.44 ± 0.03 µM)	Cytotoxic	[183]
Euphorbia pekinensis Rupr.	Roots	Ethanol	Euphodane A	U-937	U-937 (5.92 ± 0.38 µM)	Cytotoxic	[183]
Euphorbia pekinensis Rupr.	Roots	Ethanol	Isopimara-7,15-dien-3β-ol	K-562	K-562 (0.87 ± 0.02 µM)	Cytotoxic	[183]
Euphorbia pseudocactus A.Berger	Aerial parts	Methanol	Gallic acid	LS-174T	LS-174T (18.27 µg/mL)	Cytotoxic	[184]
Euphorbia pseudocactus A.Berger	Aerial parts	Methanol	Ethyl gallate	LS-174T	LS-174T (25.42 µg/mL)	Cytotoxic	[184]
Euphorbia royleana Boiss.	Whole plant	Ethanol	(3b,23Z)-9,19-cyclolanost-23-ene-3,25-diol	A549	A549 (4.84 ± 0.56 µM)	Cytotoxic	[185]
Euphorbia royleana Boiss.	Whole plant	Ethanol	taraxerol	A549	A549 (7.11 ± 1.65 µM)	Cytotoxic	[185]
Euphorbia sanctae-catharinae Fayed	Aerial parts	Dichloromethane/Methanol (1:1)	4,12,20-trideoxyphorbol-13-(2,3-dimethyl) butyrate	A549 and Caco-2	A549 (3.3 (0.996) µM) and Caco-2 (29.4 (0.972) µM)	Cytotoxic	[175]
Euphorbia schimperi C.Presl	Aerial parts	MeOH/H_2O (70:30 *V*/*V*)	Cycloschimperol A	MCF-7, HepG2, and HCT-116	MCF-7 (55.4 ± 3 µM), HepG2 (19.7 ± 3 µM), and HCT-116 (20.25 ± 5 µM)	Cytotoxic	[186]

Table 2. *Cont.*

Name of the Species	Part of the Plant	Type of Extract	Class of Compounds/ Compounds Identified in Extract	Cell Lines	IC50	Activity/ Mechanism/Effect	Ref.
Euphorbia schimperi C.Presl	Aerial parts	MeOH/H_2O (70:30 *V/V*)	Cycloschimperol B	MCF-7, HepG2, and HCT-116	MCF-7 (2.1 ± 0.01 µM), HepG2 (1.4 ± 0.1 µM), and HCT-116 (1.8 ± 0.1 µM)	Cytotoxic	[186]
Euphorbia schimperi C.Presl	Aerial parts	MeOH/H_2O (70:30 *V/V*)	Cycloart-25-en-3-one	MCF-7, HepG2, and HCT-116	MCF-7 (4.7 ± 0.1 µM), HepG2 (2.3 ± 0.2 µM), and HCT-116 (1.9 ± 0.4 µM)	Cytotoxic	[186]
Euphorbia schimperiana Scheele	Aerial parts	Ethanol	3,30-di-O-methylellagic acid	PC3	PC3 (5.5 mg/mL)	Cytotoxic	[187]
Euphorbia sogdiana Popov	Aerial parts	Acetone/Dichloromethane (1:2)	Tigliane diterpene	EJ-138 and Jurkat T	EJ-138 (12.1 µM) and Jurkat T (16.1 µM)	Cytotoxic	[188]
Euphorbia stracheyi Boiss	Whole plant	Methanol	3-O-benzoyl-20-deoxymgenol	HL-60, A-549, SMMC-7721, MCF-7, and SW480	HL-60 (0.5 ± 0.18 µM), A-549 (21.47 ± 0.17 µM), SMMC-7721 (18.36 ± 1.17 µM), MCF-7 (18.82 ± 0.84 µM), and SW481 (16.25 ± 0.71 µM)	Cytotoxic	[189]
Euphorbia stracheyi Boiss.	Roots	Methanol	Euphstrachenol A	MV4-11	MV4-11 (12.29 µM)	Cytotoxic	[190]
Euphorbia stracheyi Boiss.	Roots	Methanol	Euphstrachenol B	MV4-11	MV4-11 (14.80 µM)	Cytotoxic	[190]
Euphorbia stracheyi Boiss.	Roots	Methanol	Euphstrachenol C	MV4-11	MV4-11 (5.92 µM)	Cytotoxic	[190]
Euphorbia taurinensis All.	Whole plant	MeOH	Ingenane diterpene	L5178Y mouse T-lymphoma cells parent and MDR L5178Y	L5178Y mouse T-lymphoma cells parent (82.47 µM) and MDR L5178Y (62.81 µM)	Cytotoxic	[191]
Euphorbia tirucalli L.	Sap	Hexane	euphol	73 human cancer lines from 15 tumor types	Range from 1.41 to 38.89 µM	Cytotoxic	[192]

Table 2. *Cont.*

Name of the Species	Part of the Plant	Type of Extract	Class of Compounds/ Compounds Identified in Extract	Cell Lines	IC50	Activity/ Mechanism/Effect	Ref.
Euphorbia tithymaloides L.	Stems	Methanol	friedelane-3β-ol, 3-oxo-friedelane, euphane-7, 24-diene, 3β-ol (butyrospermol), and euphane -7, 25-diene, 3, 24-β-diols in addition to the diterpene derivative 1 α, 13 β, 14 α-trihydroxy-3 β, 7 β-dibenzenzoyloxy-9 β, 15 β-diacetoxyjatropha-5, 11-E-diene and the phytosterol β-sitosterol	HepG2, HCT-116, MCF-7 and PC-3	Only for compound: 1 α, 13 β, 14 α-trihydroxy-3 β, 7 β-dibenzenzoyloxy-9 β, 15 β-diacetoxyjatropha-5, 11-E-diene, HepG2 (12.99 ± 0.9 μM), HCT-116 (18.63 ± 1.4 μM), MCF-7 (24.40 ± 1.9 μM), and PC-3 (37.12 ± 2.3 μM)	Cytotoxic	[164]
Euphorbia umbellata (Pax) Bruyns	Stems and leaves	Methanol	3,4,12,13-tetraacetylphorbol-20-phenylacetate	U251, MCF-7, NCI-ADR/RES, 786-0, NCI-H460, HT29, and K562	U251 (25.2 mg/mL), MCF-7 (>250 mg/mL), NCI-ADR/RES (>250 mg/mL), 786-0 (24.1 mg/mL), NCI-H460 (31.1 mg/mL), HT29 (>250 mg/mL), and K563 (65.3 mg/mL)	Cytotoxic	[127]
Excoecaria agallocha L.	Leaves and twigs	Ethanol	excagallonoid A	RKO	RKO (8.7 ± 1.98 μM)	Cytotoxic	[193]
Excoecaria agallocha L.	Leaves and twigs	Ethanol	2-hydroxy-atis-1,16-diene-3,14-dione	RKO	RKO (2.6 ± 2.81 μM)	Cytotoxic	[193]
Jatropha gossypifolia L.	Stem bark	-	Jatrophone	HepG2, WiDr, HeLa, and AGS	HepG2 (3.2 μM), WiDr (8.97 μM), HeLa (5.13), and AGS (2.5 μM)	Cytotoxic	[194]
Jatropha gossypiifolia L.	Branches and leaves	Ethanol	Jatrogrossidione	RKO	2.6 μM	Cytotoxicity Apoptosis associated with G2/M-phase cell cycle arrest.	[58]

Table 2. *Cont.*

Name of the Species	Part of the Plant	Type of Extract	Class of Compounds/ Compounds Identified in Extract	Cell Lines	IC50	Activity/ Mechanism/Effect	Ref.
Jatropha tanjorensis J.L.Ellis & Saroja	Leaves	Hexane, chloroform and methanol	R (+) 4-hydroxy-2-pyrrolidinone	HEP-2, B16F10, A549, and NRK 49F	HEP-2 (42.26 ± 0.03 μg/mL), B16F10 (44.56 ± 0.02 μg/mL), A549 (48.26 ± 0.03 μg/mL), and NRK 49F (47.28 ± 0.03 μg/mL).	Cytotoxic	[195]
Macaranga barteri Müll.Arg.	Leaves	*N*-hexane, dichloromethane and methanol	macabartebenes A	MCF7, HeLa, A549, and PC3	MCF7 (0.68 ± 0.01 μM), HeLa (0.60 ± 0.01 μM), A549 (0.79 ± 0.01 μM), and PC3 (0.66 ± 0.01 μM)	Cytotoxic	[196]
Macaranga barteri Müll.Arg.	Leaves	*N*-hexane, dichloromethane and methanol	macabartebenes B	MCF7, HeLa, A549, and PC3	MCF7 (0.71 ± 0.02 μM), HeLa (0.72 ± 0.01 μM), A549 (0.74 ± 0.01 μM), and PC3 (0.69 ± 0.01 μM)	Cytotoxic	[196]
Macaranga barteri Müll.Arg.	Leaves	*N*-hexane, dichloromethane and methanol	macabartebenes C	MCF7, HeLa, A549, and PC3	MCF7 (1.73 ± 0.01 μM), HeLa (1.67 ± 0.01 μM), A549 (1.81 ± 0.00 μM), and PC3 (1.61 ± 0.01 μM)	Cytotoxic	[196]
Macaranga barteri Müll.Arg.	Leaves	*N*-hexane, dichloromethane and methanol	vedelianin	MCF7, HeLa, A549, and PC3	MCF7 (0.32 ± 0.03 μM), HeLa (0.51 ± 0.01 μM), A549 (0.54 ± 0.02 μM), and PC3 (0.39 ± 0.01 μM)	Cytotoxic	[196]
Macaranga barteri Müll.Arg.	Leaves	*N*-hexane, dichloromethane and methanol	schweinfurthin G	MCF7, HeLa, A549, and PC3	MCF7 (0.95 ± 0.02 μM), HeLa (1.18 ± 0.01 μM), A549 (1.10 ± 0.09 μM), and PC3 (0.91 ± 0.01 μM)	Cytotoxic	[196]
Macaranga barteri Müll.Arg.	Leaves	*N*-hexane, dichloromethane and methanol	8-prenylkaempferol	MCF7, HeLa, A549, and PC3	MCF7 (6.22 ± 0.13 μM), HeLa (6.88 ± 0.16 μM), A549 (6.61 ± 0.21 μM), and PC3 (6.53 ± 0.11 μM)	Cytotoxic	[196]
Macaranga barteri Müll.Arg.	Leaves	*N*-hexane, dichloromethane and methanol	mappain	MCF7, HeLa, A549, and PC3	MCF7 (0.71 ± 0.02 μM), HeLa (0.71 ± 0.01 μM), A549 (0.81 ± 0.02 μM), and PC3 (0.77 ± 0.01 μM)	Cytotoxic	[196]

Table 2. *Cont.*

Name of the Species	Part of the Plant	Type of Extract	Class of Compounds/ Compounds Identified in Extract	Cell Lines	IC50	Activity/ Mechanism/Effect	Ref.
Macaranga barteri Müll.Arg.	Leaves	N-hexane, dichloromethane and methanol	broussoflavonol F	MCF7, HeLa, A549, and PC3	MCF7 (4.13 ± 0.00 µM), HeLa (4.10 ± 0.01 µM), A549 (3.83 ± 0.01 µM), and PC3 (3.99 ± 0.01 µM)	Cytotoxic	[196]
Macaranga barteri Müll.Arg.	Leaves	N-hexane, dichloromethane and methanol	isomacarangin	MCF7, HeLa, A549, and PC3	MCF7 (8.43 ± 0.26 µM), HeLa (8.49 ± 0.21 µM), A549 (8.72 ± 0.21 µM), and PC3 (8.5 ± 0.31 µM)	Cytotoxic	[196]
Macaranga gigantea (Rchb.f. & Zoll.) Müll.Arg.	Leaves	Methanol	Glyasperin	P-388	P-388 (3.44 µg/mL)	Cytotoxic	[197]
Macaranga gigantea (Rchb.f. & Zoll.) Müll.Arg.	Leaves	Methanol	Meliternatin	P-388	P-388 (30.04 µg/mL)	Cytotoxic	[197]
Macaranga gigantifolia Merr.	Leaves	Methanol, ethyl acetate fraction	Apigenin	P-388	P-388 (14.13 µg/mL)	Cytotoxic	[64]
Macaranga hispida (Blume) Mull.Arg	Leaves	Methanol	5,7,3′,4′-tetrahydroxy-6-geranyl flavonol	P388	P388 (0.22 µg/mL)	Cytotoxic	[19]
Macaranga hispida (Blume) Mull.Arg	Leaves	Methanol	kaemferol 7–O-β-glucoside	P388	P388 (101.5 µg/mL)	Cytotoxic	[19]
Macaranga kurzii (Kuntze) Pax & K.Hoffm.	Twigs	Ethanol	kurzphenol A	HepG2	HepG2 (30.14 µg/mL)	Cytotoxic	[198]
Macaranga kurzii (Kuntze) Pax & K.Hoffm.	Twigs	Ethanol	kurzphenol C	A549	A549 (17.11 µg/mL)	Cytotoxic	[198]
Macaranga kurzii (Kuntze) Pax & K.Hoffm.	Twigs	Ethanol	8-prenylnaringenin	A549	A549 (9.76 µg/mL)	Cytotoxic	[198]

Table 2. *Cont.*

Name of the Species	Part of the Plant	Type of Extract	Class of Compounds/ Compounds Identified in Extract	Cell Lines	IC50	Activity/ Mechanism/Effect	Ref.
Macaranga kurzii (Kuntze) Pax & K.Hoffm.	Twigs	Ethanol	glepidotin B	A549	A549 (15.32 µg/mL)	Cytotoxic	[198]
Macaranga kurzii (Kuntze) Pax & K.Hoffm.	Twigs	Ethanol	acetylatractylodinol	A549	A549 (18.22 µg/mL)	Cytotoxic	[198]
Macaranga kurzii (Kuntze) Pax & K.Hoffm.	Twigs	Ethanol	blumenol A	A549	A549 (18.23 µg/mL)	Cytotoxic	[198]
Macaranga kurzii (Kuntze) Pax & K.Hoffm.	Twigs	Ethanol	alicylic acid	A549	A549 (12.01 µg/mL)	Cytotoxic	[198]
Macaranga recurvata Gage	Leaves	Methanol	Macarecurvatin A	MCF7 and MCF7/TAMR	MCF7 (5.26 µM) and MCF7/TAMR (5.66 µM)	Cytotoxic	[199]
Macaranga recurvata Gage	Leaves	Methanol	Macarecurvatin B	MCF7 and MCF7/TAMR	MCF7 (0.96 µM) and MCF7/TAMR (1.25 µM)	Cytotoxic	[199]
Macaranga recurvata Gage	Leaves	Methanol	6,8-diisoprenylaromadendrin	MCF7 and MCF7/TAMR	MCF7 (5.03 µM) and MCF7/TAMR (5.83 µM)	Cytotoxic	[199]
Mallotus conspurcatus Croizat	Aerial parts	Methanol	6-Prenylnaringenin	HeLa and A549	HeLa (30.12 ± 1.21 µM) and A549 (70.25 ± 0.89 µM)	Cytotoxic	[200]
Mallotus conspurcatus Croizat	Aerial parts	Methanol	8-Prenylnaringenin	HeLa and A549	HeLa (60.16 ± 0.91 µM) and A549 (99.36 ± 1.94 µM)	Cytotoxic	[200]
Mallotus conspurcatus Croizat	Aerial parts	Methanol	7-O-Methyl-8-prenylnaringenin	HeLa and A549	HeLa (45.03 ± 0.82 µM) and A549 (89.16 ± 0.61 µM)	Cytotoxic	[200]
Mallotus conspurcatus Croizat	Aerial parts	Methanol	7-O-Methyl-6-prenylnaringenin	HeLa and A549	HeLa (19.69 ± 0.65 µM) and A549 (55.26 ± 1.87 µM)	Cytotoxic	[200]
Mallotus conspurcatus Croizat	Aerial parts	Methanol	4′-O-Methyl-6-prenylnaringenin	HeLa and A549	HeLa (10.08 ± 1.06 µM) and A549 (47.26 ± 0.82 µM)	Cytotoxic	[200]
Manniophyton fulvum Müll.Arg.	Twigs	Methanol	Betulinic acid	HeLa	4% at 62.5 µg/mL	Cytotoxic	[201]

Table 2. *Cont.*

Name of the Species	Part of the Plant	Type of Extract	Class of Compounds/ Compounds Identified in Extract	Cell Lines	IC50	Activity/ Mechanism/Effect	Ref.
Mareya micrantha Müll. Arg.	Leaves	Ethanol/Water	29-nor-2β,15α,20β-trihydroxy-16α-acetyl-3,1,22-trioxo-cucurbita-4,23-diene	Hep3B	Hep3B (0.12 ± 0.05 μM)	Cytotoxic	[202]
Mareya micrantha Müll. Arg.	Leaves	Ethanol/Water	29-nor-2β,15α,20β-trihydroxy-16α-acetyl-3,1,22-trioxo-cucurbita-4,23-diene 29-nor-1,2,3,4,5,10-dehydro-3,15α,20β-trihydroxy-16α-acetyl-11,22-dioxo-cucurbita-23-ene 2-O-β-D-glucopyranoside	Hep3B	Hep3B (43.8 ± 5.7 μM)	Cytotoxic	[202]
Mareya micrantha Müll. Arg.	Leaves	Ethanol/Water	29-nor-2β,15α,20β-trihydroxy-16α-acetyl-3,11,22 trioxo-cucurbita-4,23-diene 2-O-β-D glucopyranoside	Hep3B	Hep3B (>50 μM)	Cytotoxic	[202]
Mareya micrantha Müll. Arg.	Leaves	Ethanol/Water	dihydro-epi-isocucurbitacin D	Hep3B	Hep3B (18.2 ± 2.8 μM)	Cytotoxic	[202]
Mareya micrantha Müll. Arg.	Leaves	Ethanol/Water	tetrahydro-cucurbitacin I	Hep3B	Hep3B (14.9 ± 3.3 μM)	Cytotoxic	[202]
Mareya micrantha Müll. Arg.	Leaves	Ethanol/Water	cucurbitacin L	Hep3B	Hep3B (11.3 ± 6.2 μM)	Cytotoxic	[202]
Margaritaria discoidea (Baill.) G. L. Webste	Stem bark	Dichloromethane and methanol (1:1).	Securinine	OVCAR-8, A2780, and A2780cis	OVCAR-8 (16.2 ± 0.5 μM), A2780 (2.7 ± 0.7 μM), and A2780cis (6.5 ± 0.4 μM)	Cytotoxic	[203]
Margaritaria discoidea (Baill.) G. L. Webste	Stem bark	Dichloromethane and methanol (1:1).	Gallic acid	OVCAR-8, A2780, and A2780cis	OVCAR-8 (5.2 ± 0.1 μM), A2780 (6.2 ± 0.3 μM), and A2780cis (5.4 ± 0.3 μM)	Cytotoxic	[203]

Table 2. *Cont.*

Name of the Species	Part of the Plant	Type of Extract	Class of Compounds/ Compounds Identified in Extract	Cell Lines	IC50	Activity/ Mechanism/Effect	Ref.
Ricinodendron heudelotii (Baill.) Heckel	Leaves	Ethanol	Corilagin	HL-60, SMMC-7721, A-549, MCF-7, and SW-480	HL-60 (25.81 ± 0.67 μg/mL), MCF-7 (33.18 ± 0.76 μg/mL), and SW-480 (37.04 ± 1.06 μg/mL)	Cytotoxic	[204]
Suregada zanzibariensis Baill.	Stem bark	Dichloromethane/Methanol (1:1)	Mangiolide	TK10, UACC62, and MCF7	TK10 (0.02 μg/mL), UACC62 (0.03 μg/mL), and MCF7 (0.05 μg/mL)	Cytotoxic	[205]
Suregada zanzibariensis Baill.	Stem bark	Dichloromethane/Methanol (1:1)	Jolkinolide B	TK10, UACC62, and MCF8	TK10 (3.31 μg/mL), UACC62 (0.94 μg/mL), and MCF7 (2.99 μg/mL)	Cytotoxic	[205]
Trewia nudiflora L.	Fruits	Ethanol	*N*-methyltreflorine	HeLa, MV-4–11, MCF-7, and MCF-7/ADR	HeLa (0.54 nM), MV-4–11 (3.6 nM), MCF-7 (8.6 nM), and MCF-7/ADR (13 nM)	Cytotoxic and inhibited tubulin polymerization in vitro	[206]
Trewia nudiflora L.	Fruits	Ethanol	Methyltrewiasine	HeLa, MV-4–11, MCF-7, and MCF-7/ADR	HeLa (1.6 nM), MV-4–11 (3.1 nM), and MCF-7 (10 nM)	Cytotoxic and inhibited tubulin polymerization in vitro	[206]
Trewia nudiflora L.	Fruits	Ethanol	Treflorine	HeLa, MV-4–11, MCF-7, and MCF-7/ADR	HeLa (0.74 nM), MV-4–11 (0.12 nM), and MCF-7 (5.5 nM)	Cytotoxic	[206]
Trewia nudiflora L.	Fruits	Ethanol	Trenudine	HeLa, MV-4–11, MCF-7, and MCF-7/ADR	HeLa (0.41 nM), MV-4–11 (4.8 nM), MCF-7 (11 nM), and MCF-7/ADR (28)	Cytotoxic	[206]
Trewia nudiflora L.	Fruits	Ethanol	Colubrinol	HeLa, MV-4–11, MCF-7, and MCF-7/ADR	HeLa (0.28 nM), MV-4–11 (0.21 nM), and MCF-7 (3.2 nM)	Cytotoxic	[206]

Table 2. *Cont.*

Name of the Species	Part of the Plant	Type of Extract	Class of Compounds/ Compounds Identified in Extract	Cell Lines	IC50	Activity/ Mechanism/Effect	Ref.
Trigonostemon heterophyllus Merr.	Stems and leaves	Ethanol	Trigoheterophines A	HL60, SMMC-7721, A-549, MCF-7, and SW480	HL60 (0.58 ± 0.06 μM), SMMC-7721 (1.42 ± 0.07 μM), A-549 (3.18 ± 0.11 μM), MCF-7 (0.28 ± 0.02 μM), and SW480 (0.93 ± 0.05 μM)	Antiproliferative	[207]
Trigonostemon heterophyllus Merr.	Stems and leaves	Ethanol	Trigoheterophines B	HL60, SMMC-7721, A-549, MCF-7, and SW480	HL60 (0.66 ± 0.04 μM), SMMC-7721 (1.98 ± 0.08 μM), A-549 (0.52 ± 0.03 μM), MCF-7 (0.75 ± 0.05 μM), and SW480 (2.08 ± 0.11 μM)	Antiproliferative	[207]
Trigonostemon heterophyllus Merr.	Stems and leaves	Ethanol	(Z, Z, E, E)-1, 4-epoxy-16-hydroxyheneicos-1, 3, 12, 14-tetraene	HL60, SMMC-7721, A-549, MCF-7, and SW480	HL60 (2.12 ± 0.10 μM), SMMC-7721 (3.26 ± 0.09 μM), A-549 (2.20 ± 0.07 μM), MCF-7 (1.68 ± 0.06 μM), and SW480 (2.72 ± 0.08 μM)	Antiproliferative	[207]
Trigonostemon heterophyllus Merr.	Stems and leaves	Ethanol	(Z, Z, E, E, E)-1, 4-epoxy-16-hydroxyheneicos-1, 3, 12, 14, 18-pentaene	HL60, SMMC-7721, A-549, MCF-7, and SW480	HL60 (3.98 ± 0.12 μM), SMMC-7721 (1.42 ± 0.07 μM), A-549 (3.18 ± 0.11 μM), MCF-7 (0.45 ± 0.05 μM), and SW480 (2.23 ± 0.10 μM)	Antiproliferative	[207]
Trigonostemon heterophyllus Merr.	Stems and leaves	Ethanol	2-(hexadecyl)furan	HL60, SMMC-7721, A-549, MCF-7, and SW480	HL60 (2.07 ± 0.06 μM), SMMC-7721 (1.83 ± 0.03 μM), A-549 (4.86 ± 0.10 μM), MCF-7 (1.78 ± 0.06 μM), and SW480 (4.28 ± 0.09 μM)	Antiproliferative	[207]
Trigonostemon heterophyllus Merr.	Stems and leaves	Ethanol	2-(octadecyl)furan	HL60, SMMC-7721, A-549, MCF-7, and SW480	HL60 (1.05 ± 0.06 μM), SMMC-7721 (2.97 ± 0.13 μM), A-549 (6.32 ± 0.15 μM), MCF-7 (3.02 ± 0.07 μM), and SW480 (12.06 ± 0.11 μM)	Antiproliferative	[207]

Table 2. *Cont.*

Name of the Species	Part of the Plant	Type of Extract	Class of Compounds/ Compounds Identified in Extract	Cell Lines	IC50	Activity/ Mechanism/Effect	Ref.
Trigonostemon xyphophylloides (Croizat) L.K.Dai & T.L.Wu	Twigs	Ethanol	Trigoxyphin P	SPC-A-1, BEL-7402, SGC-7901, and K-562	SPC-A-1 (1.70 µM) and K-562 (2.24 µM)	Cytotoxic	[208]
Trigonostemon xyphophylloides (Croizat) L.K.Dai & T.L.Wu	Twigs	Ethanol	Trigoxyphin Q	SPC-A-1, BEL-7402, SGC-7901, and K-562	SPC-A-1 (1.42 µM), SGC-7901 (2.88 µM), and K-562 (0.37 µM)	Cytotoxic	[208]
Trigonostemon xyphophylloides (Croizat) L.K.Dai & T.L.Wu	Twigs	Ethanol	Trigoxyphin R	SPC-A-1, BEL-7402, SGC-7901, and K-562	SPC-A-1 (12.42 µM) and K-562 (17.18 µM)	Cytotoxic	[208]
Trigonostemon xyphophylloides (Croizat) L.K.Dai & T.L.Wu	Twigs	Ethanol	Trigoxyphin T	SPC-A-1, BEL-7402, SGC-7901, and K-562	SPC-A-1 (0.24 µM), BEL-7402 (3.89 µM), and SGC-7901 (5.59 µM)	Cytotoxic	[208]

3.4. *Anticancer Effects of Euphorbiaceae Extracts and Pure Compounds In Vivo Studies*

The anticancer effects of both extracts and pure compounds have been tested in vivo using various animal models. Many studies are available on in vivo experiments on a number of plants from the Euphorbiaceae family. de Abrantes et al. [209] showed that Tonantzitlolone B (TNZ-B), a diterpene from *Stillingia loranthacea*, exhibits antitumor activity (1.5 or 3 mg/kg i.p.) in a mouse model of Ehrlich ascites carcinoma. The LD50 was estimated to be approximately 25 mg/kg (i.p.). TNZ-B reduced Ehrlich tumor volume and the total number of viable tumor cells. In addition, TNZ-B reduced the density of peri-tumor microvessels, suggesting an anti-angiogenic effect. Gowrav Adiga et al. [210] investigated the anticancer activity of a methanol extract of the stem bark of *Croton oblongifolius* in Sprague-Dawley rats. The rats were tumor-induced with dimethylbenz(a)anthracene (DMBA), administered orally and intramammarily, and with a plant extract. After obtaining the appropriate tumor mass, the extract was administered to the rats by gavage at 200, 500, and 800 mg/kg, which showed a dose-dependent reduction in mammary tumor volume, as confirmed by histopathological observations in the treated groups. In other studies, using a mouse model of breast cancer induced by 4T1 cells, Majumder et al. [211] demonstrated the effect of *Ricinus communis* fruit extract, rich in ricinine, *p*-coumaric acid, epigallocatechin, and ricinoleic acid, on breast cancer progression in vivo. Tumors were induced in female Balb/c mice by injecting 4T1 cells subcutaneously into the mammary fat pad. After 10 days, one group of animals received 4 i.p. doses of the extract (5 mg/kg body weight), while the other group received only the vehicle (0.9% saline). The tumor in the control group continued to grow, and animals treated with the extract showed a significant reduction in tumor volume over time. Tumors removed from the animals after 22 days showed a reduction in tumor volume of over 88% compared to the control group. Table 3 shows in vivo studies.

Table 3. Cytotoxic properties of selected extracts or pure compounds from the Euphorbiaceae family against in vivo models.

Name of the Species	Part of the Plant	Type of Extract	Class of Compounds/Compounds Identified in Extract	Animal Model	Treatment	Activity/Mechanism/Effect	Ref.
Cnidosculos quercifolius Pohl	Root bark	Methanol, chloroform fraction (Favelin rich fraction)	Favelin, Methyl-faveline, Deoxofavelin, Neofavelanone and Coumarin	Mice	250 and 500 mg/kg/day of favelin rich fraction.	Inhibition rates of tumor growth were 58.08 and 48.71% for the 250 mg/kg and 500 mg/kg treatment groups, respectively.	[212]
Croton crassifolius Geiseler	Roots	Ethanol	Penduliflaworosin	Mice and Rats	12.5–50 μM	Exerts its anti-angiogenic effect via the VEGF receptor-2 signaling pathway	[213]
Euphorbia fischeriana S. + *Ziziphus jujuba* M.	-	Water	Jokinolide B and 2,4-dihydroxy-6-methoxy-acetophenone	Mice	2.5, 5.0, and 10.0 g/kg groups of ESZM extract	PI3k/Akt pathway regulation of apoptosis.	[214]
Euphorbia helioscopia L.	Whole plant	Ethyl acetate	-	Mice	50 μg/mL, 100 μg/mL, and 200 μg/mL	Growth inhibition and Cyclin D1 protein expression decreased. Cell apoptosis by changing Bcl-2, Bax, and caspase-3 protein expressions.	[215]
Euphorbia royleana Boiss.	-	Hexane	-	Mice	10 mg/kg.	Tumor volumes were decreased. Necrotic areas in tumor tissue.	[216]

Table 3. *Cont.*

Name of the Species	Part of the Plant	Type of Extract	Class of Compounds/Compounds Identified in Extract	Animal Model	Treatment	Activity/Mechanism/Effect	Ref.
Excoecaria agallocha L.	Bark	Methanol	Quercetin-3-O-rutinoside, Quercetin 3-O- α -L-rhamnoside, Kaempferol-3-O-(2-O-acetyl-α-Lrhamnopyranoside), Kaempferol 3-O-α-Lrhamnopyranoside, Excoecarin A, Excoecarin G1, Excoecarin G2, Taraxerone, 3beta-[(2E,4E)-6-oxo-decadienoyloxy]-olean-12-ene, 2,3-secoatisane, Exoecarin B, Exoecarin C, Exoecarin D, Excoecarin E, Exoecarin F, Exoecarin H	Mice	Different doses up to 200 mg/kg	Normal hemaetological values.	[217]
Tragia involucrata L.	Whole plant	Ethanol	Phenylacetaldehyde-diethylacetal, Neophytadiene, (E)-Phytol, Ethyl palmitate, Phytol, Ethyl linolate, Ethyl elaidate, Linolenic acid, Ethyl octadecanoate, 2-Ethylhexyl phthalate, Squalene, Vitamin E, Clionasterol, Viminalol, Agathisflavone, Loquatoside, Leufolin A, Quercetin, Echinacin, Apigetrin, Cynaroside, 1,2,36-tetrakis-O-galloyl-B-D-glucose, Isoquercetin and Corilagin	Mice	200 mg/kg and 400 mg/kg	Reduction of tumors	[144]

Data not reported are represented by "-".

3.5. Anticancer and Cytotoxic Effects of Nanoparticles Prepared from Euphobiaceae Extracts and Pure Compounds

Nanoparticles (NP) combined with extracts or pure compounds of plant origin are currently a well-known method for biological research and enhancing the effects of various substances in in vitro or in vivo models. In the research by Ghramh et al. [218], an ethanolic leaf extract of *Ricinus communis* with gold nanoparticles (AuNPs) demonstrated a cytotoxic effect. Studies have shown that the extract in combination with AuNPs has a stronger effect on HeLa and HepG2 lines than the *Ricinus communis* extract alone. In turn, Alqahtani et al. [219] also demonstrated a stronger cytotoxic effect of *Jatropha pelargoniifolia* extract in combination with chitosan nanoparticles against human lung adenocarcinoma (A549) than the extract alone. The same author revealed that Euphorbia retusa with a combination of zinc oxide NPs (ZnONPs) exhibited cytotoxic activity against A549 (IC_{50} = 22.3 μg/mL), HepG2 (IC_{50} = 25.6), Huh-7 (IC_{50} = 25.7), MCF-7 (IC_{50} = 37.7), and MDA-MB-231 (IC_{50} = 37) [220]. Similarly, Aboulthana et al. [221] showed that the cytotoxic activity of *Croton tiglium* seed extract increased after the incorporation of ZnONPs against human colon cancer cells (CACO-2). Additionally, the extract combined with ZnONPs stopped the increase of CACO-2 in G2/M and increased the percentage of total apoptotic cells and necrosis. A novel approach using *Excoecaria agallocha* leaf extract for the synthesis of silver NPs (AgONPs) was demonstrated by Banerjee et al. [222] AgONPs exerted initial cytotoxicity specifically against all experimental malignant cells (murine melanoma (B16F10), murine colon cancer (CT26), murine lung adenocarcinoma (3LL), and murine Ehrlich ascites carcinoma (EAC)), while sparing normal cell lines. Furthermore, both in vitro and ex vivo, AgONPs are equally effective in inducing apoptosis in all cancer cells. Studies on nanoparticles are presented in Table 4 below.

Table 4. Nanoparticles made using constituents from the plants of the Euphobiaceae family.

Tested Plant	Components	Type of Nanoparticles	Cells	Effect	Ref.
Acalypha wilkesiana Müll.Arg.	Flowers	Ag NPs	MCF-7 (4.00 μg/mL) and PC-3 (3.60 μg/mL)	Cytotoxicity	[223]
Alchornea cordifolia (Schumach. & Thonn.) Müll.Arg.	Leaves	CuO–ZnO, ZnO, and CuO NPs	HeLa treatment with 100 μg/mL—CuO–ZnO (39.94 ± 5.01). ZnO (44.05 ± 0.91) and CuO NPs (63.64 ± 8.34)	Cytotoxicity	[224]
Baliospermum montanum (Willd.) Müll.Arg.	Roots	Nanoparticles	Aqueous NPS (22%) and Ethanol NPs (6%)	Cytotoxicity	[225]
Croton sparsiflorus Morong	Leaves	AuNPs	HepG2 (116.7 μg/mL)	Cytotoxicity	[226]
Euphorbia dendroides L.	Aerial parts	AuNPs	HepG2 (41.72 ± 1.26 mg/mL) and HCT-116 (44.96 ± 3.23 mg/mL)	Cytotoxicity	[227]
Euphorbia heterophylla L.	Leaves	rGO	A549 (297.81 mg/mL) and HepG2 (357.53 mg/mL)	Cytotoxicity	[228]
Euphorbia peplus L.	Leaves	AuNPs	HepG2 and Hela cells	Inhibitory effect	[229]
Euphorbia royleana Boiss.	Pulp	Ag NPs and Cu_2O NPs	HCT-116 Ag NPs (50.12 μg/mL) and Cu_2O NPs (61.93 μg/mL)	Cytotoxicity	[230]
Excoecaria agallocha L.	Leaves	AgNPs	1.00 lg/mL AgNPs in MCF-7 (8.00% viability)	Cytotoxicity	[231]

4. Potential Anticancer Mechanism of Action of Euphorbiaceae Extracts and Isolated Compounds

The cytotoxic activity reported by several authors in cancer cell lines treated with Euphorbiaceae extracts or isolated compounds may be due to different mechanisms of action. It is known that these extracts and compounds can activate the intrinsic pathway and the extrinsic pathway of apoptosis. The chemical structures of the main isolated compounds with anticancer activity and their underlying mechanisms of action are presented in Figure 2 below.

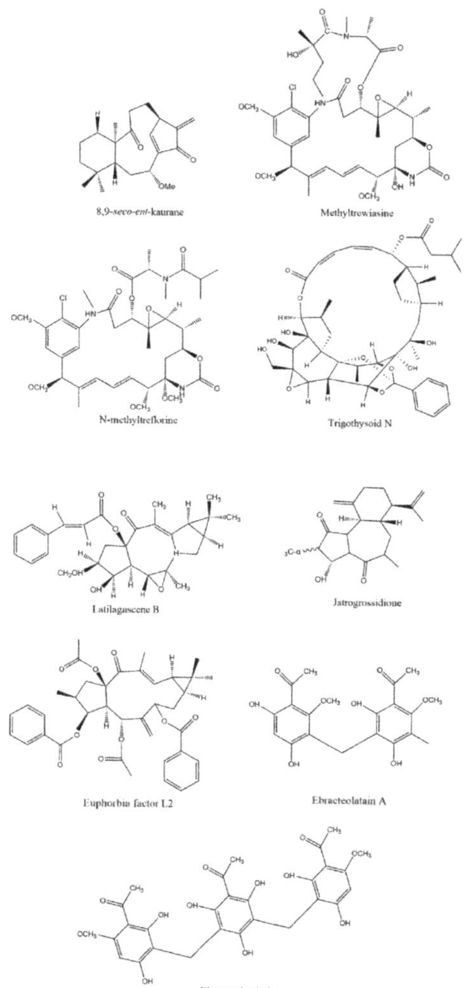

Figure 2. Chemical structure of isolated compounds from Euphorbiaceae plants with anticancer potential.

To activate the intrinsic pathway, the extract or compound could act as a ROS inductor. For example, *Croton gratissimus* Burch, *Drypetes sepiaria* (Wight & Arn.) Pax & K. Hoffm., *Euphorbia cactus* Ehrenb. ex Boiss., *Euphorbia hirta* L., *Euphorbia ingens* E. Mey. ex Boiss., *Euphorbia lathyrism* L., *Excoecaria agallocha* L., *Euphorbia helioscopia* L., and *Ricinus communis* L. extracts [67,68,70,94,95,115,211,215], and the pure compounds Euphorbia Factor L2, Ebracteolatain A, and Ebracteolatain B [147,232], activate the intrinsic pathway at some point. DNA damage promotes the liberation of cytochrome C by mitochondria. Then, cytochrome c and the APAF-1 (Apoptotic Protease Activating Factor-1) protein join together to activate casp-9. In this stage, it becomes a cascade release of different caspases activating each other from an inactive form to an active form and, at the end, activating casp-3, leading, finally, to apoptosis [67,70,94,136]. During this process, mitochondria also release SMAC/DIABLO (Second Mitochondria-Derived Activator of Caspase), an inhibitor of the XIAP (X-linked inhibitor of apoptosis) protein [233,234]. The caspases also cleave PARP (Poly ADP-Ribose Polymerase); this process is considered a hallmark of apoptosis [233].

The extrinsic pathway could be activated too, increasing the expression of casp-2/casp-8. For example, some authors have reported this activity with *Croton gratissimus* Burch, *Drypetes sepiaria* (Wight & Arn.) Pax & K.Hoffm, and *Euphorbia lathyrism* L *extracts* [67,70,94].

The expression of p53 could also be affected by this family of plants. Several authors have reported higher levels of p53 after treatment with *Euphorbia pulcherrima* Willd. ex Klotzsch, *Euphorbia heterophylla* L., *Euhporbia ingens* E.Mey. ex Boiss, and *Excoecaria agallocha* L. in cancer cell lines [68,105,115]. p53 is a tumor-suppressive protein with the ability to induce cell death, including through apoptotic mechanisms and other transcription-dependent mechanisms or independent mechanisms [235]. Zhou et al. [232] also found that the activity of the pure compounds Ebracteolatain A and Ebracteolatain B increased p53 levels and decreased survivin levels. Survivin is a survival protein that inhibits caspases and blocks cell death [236]. Sultana et al. [68] found an altered expression on the levels of p21, the main target protein of p53. This protein, also known as CDKN1A (cyclin-dependent kinase inhibitor 1A), regulates the progression of the cell cycle with cyclin B. The balance of Bax/Bcl family protein expression can also be regulated through p53.

Changing the Bcl2/Bax (antiapoptotic/proapoptotic) protein balance could also be regulated by Euphorbiaceae plants through the STAT3 gene transcription pathway [146]. This balance is reported to be higher for Bax proteins than Bcl2 proteins when cancer cells are treated with *Croton tiglium* L., *Euphorbia cactus* Ehrenb. ex Boiss., *Euphorbia pulcherrima* Willd. ex Klotzsch, *Euphorbia heterophylla* L., *Euphorbia helioscopia* L., *Euphorbia hierosolymitana* Boiss., and *Ricinus communis* L. extracts [13,95,105,106,211,215]. Proapoptotic protein Bax is higher when cancer cells receive treatment with Trigothysoid N, Ebracteolatain A, and Ebracteolatain B also [146,232].

Li et al. [146] reported that cell invasion and migration could be regulated by Trigothysoid N through the FAK pathway. Once the compound inhibits FAK, the transcription of metalloproteinase (MMP)-2 and MMP-9 is downregulated, and the cells are not able to invade or migrate to other tissues.

The Euphorbiaceae extracts and isolated compounds could modulate the level of citoplasmatic proteins, acting as inhibitors or downregulating/upregulating them. For example, Okpako et al. [115] reported a downregulation in androgen receptors after the treatment of prostate cancer cells DU-145 with *Euphorbia ingens* E.Mey. ex Boiss extract. Lei et al. [206] reported inhibited tubulin polymerization after treatment with Methyltrewiasine and *N*-methyltreflorine. Tubulin polymerization/despolimerization plays a critical role in the cell cycle, and some important anticancer drugs are microtubule stabilizers of vegetal origin, for example, paclitaxel and docetaxel. Another example of protein regulation was reported by Shi et al. [237]. Using 8,9-seco-*ent*-kaurane diterpenoid isolated from *Croton kongensis* Gagnep in TNBC cells, the compound acted like an Akt inhibitor, which could induce apoptosis, autophagy, cell G2/M circle arrest, and inhibit cell migration. Latilagascene B was reported to be a *p*-glycoprotein inhibitor (Multidrug-resistant receptor) [145]. The cell cycle is regulated differently depending on the extract or pure compound used in cancer cells. In such a way that we can find stops in phase G1 [58,146], in phase G2/M [68,85], or in phase S [58] after the treatment with Euphorbiaceae. The anticancer potential mechanism of action of extracts and compounds from the Euphorbiaceae family is shown in Figure 3 below.

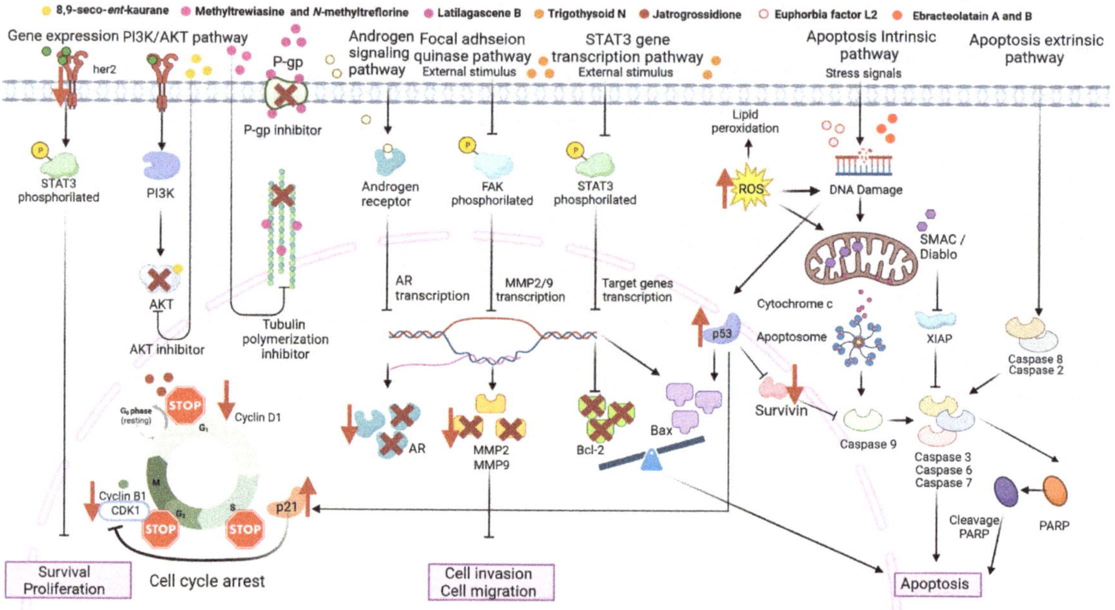

Figure 3. Potential anticancer mechanisms of action of Euphorbiaceae extracts and isolated compounds (created by BioRender).

5. Conclusions and Future Perspectives

Research into the anticancer properties of plants in the Euphorbiaceae family shows promising potential. Cancer continues to be a global health problem, both in terms of health and economy. The lack of effectiveness and selectivity of the currently most used anticancer drugs makes it necessary to continue the search for new drugs. Nature continues to be an inexhaustible source of useful molecules to cure or alleviate diseases. It is for this reason that it is necessary to continue investigating the molecules present in living beings that surround us, including plants, algae, fungi, and marine organisms. In this review, we emphasize the usefulness of the various compounds present in the Euphorbiaceae family. This family of vascular plants is a very diverse family, both in genera and species and in secondary metabolites. The presence of different types of terpenoids, flavonoids, and alkaloids with cytotoxic activity against cancer makes us think about the number of possibilities that these compounds could offer alone or through the synthesis of different derivatives from them. All these active compounds represent an opportunity for the treatment of cancer; however, from a future perspective, it is necessary to continue researching all these molecules. Greater funding is necessary for the research of new molecules to be able to advance them more quickly from the process of discovery to the regulation and approval process for the market and patients. In this context, preclinical and clinical studies in animal models, followed by human clinical trials to evaluate their efficacy, safety, and dosage in different types of cancer, seem to play a very important role in this field.

Author Contributions: Conceptualization, V.J.-G. and P.S.; methodology, V.J.-G., P.S. and T.K.; investigation, V.J.-G., P.S. and T.K.; writing—original draft preparation, V.J.-G., P.S., T.K., J.S. and J.P.; writing—review and editing, V.J.-G., P.S., T.K., J.P., J.S. and P.R.; visualization, V.J.-G.; supervision, P.S. and P.R. All authors have read and agreed to the published version of the manuscript.

Funding: This research received no external funding.

Acknowledgments: The authors would like to express their gratitude to Alexander Harrison for reviewing scientific English.

Conflicts of Interest: The authors declare no conflict of interest.

Abbreviations

AgONPs	Silver oxide nanoparticles
Akt	Protein kinase B
APAF	Apoptotic Protease-Activating Factor-1
AuNPs	Gold nanoparticles
Bax	Apoptosis regulator or bcl-2-like protein 4
Bcl-2	B-cell lymphoma 2 protein
Casp-3	Caspase 3
Casp-6	Caspase 6
Casp-7	Caspase 7
Casp-8	Caspase 8
Casp-9	Caspase 9
CuONPs	Cupper oxide nanoparticles
MAPK	Mitogen-activated protein kinase
MMP-2	Metalloproteinase 2
MMP-9	Metalloproteinase 9
NP	Nanoparticles
P53	Tumor protein P53
PARP	Poly ADP-Ribose Polymerase
PI3K	Phosphoinositide 3-kinases
ROS	Reactive oxygen species
SMAC/DIABLO	Second Mitochondria-Derived Activator of Caspase
STAT3	Signal transducer and activator of transcription 3
TNBC	Triple negative breast cancer
TNB-Z	Tonantzitlolone B
XIAP	X-linked inhibitor of apoptosis
ZnONPs	Zinc oxide nanoparticles

References

1. Sarkar, S.; Horn, G.; Moulton, K.; Oza, A.; Byler, S.; Kokolus, S.; Longacre, M. Cancer Development, Progression, and Therapy: An Epigenetic Overview. *Int. J. Mol. Sci.* **2013**, *14*, 21087–21113. [CrossRef]
2. Bremnes, R.M.; Camps, C.; Sirera, R. Angiogenesis in Non-Small Cell Lung Cancer: The Prognostic Impact of Neoangiogenesis and the Cytokines VEGF and BFGF in Tumours and Blood. *Lung Cancer* **2006**, *51*, 143–158. [CrossRef]
3. World Health Organization (WHO). *WHO-Cancer Report-2020-Global Profile*; World Health Organization (WHO): Geneva, Switzerland, 2020.
4. Sung, H.; Ferlay, J.; Siegel, R.L.; Laversanne, M.; Soerjomataram, I.; Jemal, A.; Bray, F. Global Cancer Statistics 2020: GLOBOCAN Estimates of Incidence and Mortality Worldwide for 36 Cancers in 185 Countries. *CA Cancer J. Clin.* **2021**, *71*, 209–249. [CrossRef]
5. Voda, A.I.; Bostan, I. Public Health Care Financing and the Costs of Cancer Care: A Cross-National Analysis. *Cancers* **2018**, *10*, 117. [CrossRef]
6. Pucci, C.; Martinelli, C.; Ciofani, G. Innovative Approaches for Cancer Treatment: Current Perspectives and New Challenges. *Ecancermedicalscience* **2019**, *13*, 961. [CrossRef]
7. Newman, D.J.; Cragg, G.M. Natural Products as Sources of New Drugs over the Nearly Four Decades from 01/1981 to 09/2019. *J. Nat. Prod.* **2020**, *83*, 770–803. [CrossRef]
8. Cragg, G.M.; Newman, D.J. Plants as a Source of Anti-Cancer Agents. *J. Ethnopharmacol.* **2005**, *100*, 72–79. [CrossRef]
9. Kingston, D.G.I.; Newman, D.J. The Search for Novel Drug Leads for Predominately Antitumor Therapies by Utilizing Mother Nature's Pharmacophoric Libraries. *Curr. Opin. Drug Discov. Dev.* **2005**, *8*, 207–227.
10. Ernst, M.; Grace, O.M.; Saslis-Lagoudakis, C.H.; Nilsson, N.; Simonsen, H.T.; Rønsted, N. Global Medicinal Uses of Euphorbia L. (Euphorbiaceae). *J. Ethnopharmacol.* **2015**, *176*, 90–101. [CrossRef]
11. Saleh, Z.M.; Abdel Azeiz, A.Z.; Mehany, A.B.M.; El-Swaify, Z.A.S. Anticancer and Antimicrobial Activity of Jatropha's Leaves Extracts. *Egypt. J. Bot.* **2023**, *63*, 621–634. [CrossRef]
12. Prakash, E.; Gupta, D.K. Cytotoxic Activities of Extracts of Medicinal Plants of Euphorbiacae Family Studied on Seven Human Cancer Cell Lines. *Univ. J. Plant Sci.* **2013**, *1*, 113–117. [CrossRef]

13. Li, C.; Wu, X.; Sun, R.; Zhao, P.; Liu, F.; Zhang, C. *Croton tiglium* Extract Induces Apoptosis via Bax/Bcl-2 Pathways in Human Lung Cancer A549 Cells. *Asian Pac. J. Cancer Prev.* **2016**, *17*, 4893–4898. [CrossRef]
14. Vasas, A.; Hohmann, J. Euphorbia Diterpenes: Isolation, Structure, Biological Activity, and Synthesis (2008–2012). *Chem. Rev.* **2014**, *114*, 8579–8612. [CrossRef]
15. Block, S.; Baccelli, C.; Tinant, B.; Van Meervelt, L.; Rozenberg, R.; Habib Jiwan, J.-L.; Llabrès, G.; De Pauw-Gillet, M.-C.; Quetin-Leclercq, J. Diterpenes from the Leaves of *Croton zambesicus*. *Phytochemistry* **2004**, *65*, 1165–1171. [CrossRef]
16. Kemboi, D.; Siwe-noundou, X.; Krause, R.W.M.; Langat, M.K.; Tembu, V.J. Euphorbia Diterpenes: An Update of Isolation, Structure, Pharmacological Activities and Structure—Activity Relationship. *Molecules* **2021**, *26*, 5055. [CrossRef]
17. Subramanian, S.S.; Nagarajan, S.; Sulochana, N. Flavonoids of the Leaves of *Jatropha gossypifolia*. *Phytochemistry* **1971**, *10*, 1690. [CrossRef]
18. Šmejkal, K. Cytotoxic Potential of C-Prenylated Flavonoids. *Phytochem. Rev.* **2014**, *13*, 245–275. [CrossRef]
19. Megawati, M.; Saepudin, E.; Hanafi, M.; Darmawan, A.; Lotulung, P.D.N. Identification and Bioactivity Studies of Flavonoid Compounds from *Macaranga hispida* (Blume) Mull.Arg. *Makara J. Sci.* **2015**, *19*, 96–100. [CrossRef]
20. Coelho, P.L.C.; Oliveira, M.N.; da Silva, A.B.; Pitanga, B.P.S.; Silva, V.D.A.; Faria, G.P.; Sampaio, G.P.; Costa, M.d.F.D.; Braga-de-Souza, S.; Costa, S.L. The Flavonoid Apigenin from *Croton betulaster* Mull Inhibits Proliferation, Induces Differentiation and Regulates the Inflammatory Profile of Glioma Cells. *Anticancer Drugs* **2016**, *27*, 960–969. [CrossRef]
21. Novello, C.R.; Marques, L.C.; Pires, M.E.; Kutschenco, A.P.; Nakamura, C.V.; Nocchi, S.; Sarragiotto, M.H.; Mello, J.C.P. Bioactive Indole Alkaloids from *Croton echioides*. *J. Braz. Chem. Soc.* **2016**, *27*, 2203–2209. [CrossRef]
22. Euphorbiaceae. *Plants of the World Online*; Kew Royal Botanical Garden: Richmond, UK, 2023.
23. GBIF. *Euphorbiaceae in Global Biodiversity Information Facility*; GBIF: Copenhagen, Denmark, 2023. [CrossRef]
24. Valdés, B.; Talavera, S.; Fernández-Galiano, E. (Eds.) *Flora Vascular de Andalucía Occidental*; Flora Vascular: Barcelona, Spain, 1987.
25. Blanca, G.; Cabezudo, B.; Cueto, M.; Salazar, C.; Morales Torres, C. (Eds.) *Flora Vascular de Andalucía Oriental*, 2nd ed.; Corregida y Aumentada; Conserjería de Medio Ambiente, Junta de Andalucía: Granada, Spain, 2011.
26. Cueto, M.; Melendo, M.; Giménez, E.; Fuentes, J.; Carrique, E.L.; Blanca, G. *First Updated Checklist of the Vascular Flora of Andalusia (S of Spain), One of the Main*; Biodiversity Centres in the Mediterranean Basin: Auckland, New Zealand, 2018; Volume 339; ISBN 9781776703104.
27. FAO. *Save and Grow: Cassava*; FAO: Rome, Italy, 2013.
28. Mohidin, S.R.N.S.P.; Moshawih, S.; Hermansyah, A.; Asmuni, M.I.; Shafqat, N.; Ming, L.C. Cassava (*Manihot esculenta* Crantz): A Systematic Review for the Pharmacological Activities, Traditional Uses, Nutritional Values, and Phytochemistry. *J. Evid.-Based Integr. Med.* **2023**, *28*, 2515690X231206227. [CrossRef] [PubMed]
29. FAOSTAT Cassava. Available online: https://www.fao.org/faostat/es/#data/qv (accessed on 15 September 2023).
30. Marwat, S.K.; Rehman, F.; Khan, E.A.; Baloch, M.S.; Sci, P.J.P.; Sadiq, M.; Ullah, I.; Javaria, S.; Shaheen, S. Ricinus communis: Ethnomedicinal Uses and Pharmacological Activities. *Pak. J. Pharm. Sci.* **2017**, *30*, 1815–1827. [PubMed]
31. Johnson, W. Final Report on the Safety Assessment of *Ricinus communis* (Castor) Seed Oil, Hydrogenated Castor Oil, Glyceryl Ricinoleate, Glyceryl Ricinoleate SE, Ricinoleic Acid, Potassium Ricinoleate, Sodium Ricinoleate, Zinc Ricinoleate, Cetyl Ricinoleate, Ethyl Ricinoleate, Glycol Ricinoleate, Isopropyl Ricinoleate, Methyl Ricinoleate, and Octyldodecyl Ricinoleate. *Int. J. Toxicol.* **2007**, *26*, 31–77.
32. Kelly, A.J.; Kavanagh, J.; Thomas, J. Castor Oil, Bath and/or Enema for Cervical Priming and Induction of Labour. *Cochrane Database Syst. Rev.* **2013**, *2013*, CD0030992013. [CrossRef] [PubMed]
33. Elkousy, R.H.; Said, Z.N.A.; El-Baseer, M.A.A.; El Wafa, S.A.A. Antiviral Activity of Castor Oil Plant (*Ricinus communis*) Leaf Extracts. *J. Ethnopharmacol.* **2021**, *271*, 113878. [CrossRef] [PubMed]
34. Fitranda, M.I.; Sutrisno; Marfu'ah, S. Physicochemical Properties and Antibacterial Activity of Castor Oil and Its Derivatives. In *Proceedings of the IOP Conference Series: Materials Science and Engineering, Malang, Indonesia, 2–3 November 2019*; Institute of Physics Publishing: Bristol, UK, 2020, Volume 833.
35. Ogunniyi, D.S. Castor Oil: A Vital Industrial Raw Material. *Bioresour. Technol.* **2006**, *97*, 1086–1091. [CrossRef] [PubMed]
36. Neuwinger, H.D. Plants Used for Poison Fishing in Tropical Africa. *Toxicon* **2004**, *44*, 417–430. [CrossRef]
37. Lai, X.Z.; Yang, Y.B.; Shan, X.L. The Investigation of Euphorbiaceous Medicinal Plants in Southern China. *Econ. Bot.* **2004**, *58*, S307–S320. [CrossRef]
38. Polygenis-bigendako, M.J.; Lejoly, J. Plantes employées dans le traitement des diarrhées en médecine traditionnelle au burundi occidental. *Bull. Soc. R. Bot. Belg./Bull. Van K. Belg. Bot. Ver.* **1989**, *122*, 87–97.
39. Gaioni, D.T. Medical Choices in a Philippine Highland Community. Ethnomedical and Biomedical Dimensions of Bauko Clinical Reality. *Anthropos* **2002**, *97*, 505–518.
40. Bard, C.L. *A Contribution to the History of Medicine in Southern California*; Hansebooks: Norderstedt, Germany, 1894.
41. Hargreaves, B.J. The Spurges of Botswana. *Botsw. Notes Rec.* **1991**, *23*, 115–130.
42. Safford, W.E. *The Useful Plants of the Island of Guam*; Bulletin (United States National Museum); U.S. Government Printing Office: Washington, DC, USA, 1905; ISBN 9780598582195.
43. Manandhar, N.P. An Inventory of Some Herbal Drugs of Myagdi District, Nepal. *Econ. Bot.* **1995**, *49*, 371–379. [CrossRef]
44. Zhan, Z.J.; Li, S.; Chu, W.; Yin, S. Euphorbia Diterpenoids: Isolation, Structure, Bioactivity, Biosynthesis, and Synthesis (2013–2021). *Nat. Prod. Rep.* **2022**, *39*, 2132–2174. [CrossRef] [PubMed]

45. Xu, Y.; Tang, P.; Zhu, M.; Wang, Y.; Sun, D.; Li, H.; Chen, L. Diterpenoids from the Genus Euphorbia: Structure and Biological Activity (2013–2019). *Phytochemistry* **2021**, *190*, 112846. [CrossRef] [PubMed]
46. Moremi, M.P.; Makolo, F.; Viljoen, A.M.; Kamatou, G.P. A Review of Biological Activities and Phytochemistry of Six Ethnomedicinally Important South African Croton Species. *J. Ethnopharmacol.* **2021**, *280*, 114416. [CrossRef]
47. Zhu, Q.F.; Xu, G.B.; Liao, S.G.; Yan, X.L. Ent-Abietane Diterpenoids from *Euphorbia fischeriana* and Their Cytotoxic Activities. *Molecules* **2022**, *27*, 7258. [CrossRef]
48. Zhang, Z.; Zhu, P.; Ma, J.; Li, X.; Yuan, W. A New Diterpenoid with Cytotoxic Activities from the Roots of *Euphorbia fischeriana*. *Chem. Nat. Compd.* **2023**, *59*, 701–705. [CrossRef]
49. Wang, W.; Zhang, X.J. Cytotoxic *Ent*-Abietane Diterpenoids from the Leaves of *Croton lachnocarpus* Benth. *J. Asian Nat. Prod. Res.* **2023**, *25*, 309–315. [CrossRef]
50. Sabandar, C.W.; Ahmat, N.; Jaafar, F.M.; Sahidin, I. Medicinal Property, Phytochemistry and Pharmacology of Several Jatropha Species (Euphorbiaceae): A Review. *Phytochemistry* **2013**, *85*, 7–29. [CrossRef]
51. Yuan, H.-T.; Li, Q.-F.; Tian, T.; Zhang, C.-Y.; Huang, Z.-Q.; Fan, C.-X.; Mei, K.; Zhou, J.; Zhai, X.-X.; Li, S.-B.; et al. Lathyrane Diterpenoids from *Jatropha podagrica* and Their Antitumor Activities in Human Osteosarcoma Cells. *Nat. Prod. Res.* **2021**, *35*, 5089–5095. [CrossRef]
52. Kemboi, D.; Peter, X.; Langat, M.; Tembu, J. A Review of the Ethnomedicinal Uses, Biological Activities, and Triterpenoids of Euphorbia Species. *Molecules* **2020**, *25*, 4019. [CrossRef] [PubMed]
53. Hassan, A.R.; Ashour, A.; Amen, Y.; Nagata, M.; El-Toumy, S.A.; Shimizu, K. A New Cycloartane Triterpene and Other Phytoconstituents from the Aerial Parts of *Euphorbia dendroides*. *Nat. Prod. Res.* **2022**, *36*, 828–836. [CrossRef] [PubMed]
54. Ngadjui, B.T.; Folefoc, G.G.; Keumedjio, F.; Dongo, E.; Sondengam, B.L.; Connolly, J.D. Crotonadiol, a Labdane Diterpenoid from the Stem Barkof *Croton zambesicus*. *Phytochemistry* **1999**, *51*, 171–174. [CrossRef]
55. Kapingu, M.C.; Mbwambo, Z.H.; Moshi, M.J.; Magadula, J.J. Brine Shrimp Lethality of Alkaloids from *Croton sylvaticus* Hoechst. *East Cent. Afr. J. Pharm. Sci.* **2012**, *15*, 35–37.
56. Prozesky, E.A. *Antiplasmodial-and Chloroquine Resistance Reversal Properties of a New Diterpene from Croton steenkampianus*; University of Pretoria (South Africa) ProQuest Dissertations Publishing: Ann Arbor, MI, USA, 2005.
57. Mohamed, I.E.; El Nur, E.B.E.; Choudhary, M.I.; Khan, S.N. Bioactive Natural Products from Two Sudanese Medicinal Plants *Diospyros mespiliformis* and *Croton zambesicus*. *Rec. Nat. Prod.* **2009**, *3*, 198–203.
58. Zhang, C.-Y.; Zhang, R.-R.; Zhu, J.Y. New Tetracyclic Triterpenoids from *Jatropha* gossypiifolia Induce Cell-Cycle Arrest and Apoptosis in RKO Cells. *Fitoterapia* **2018**, *130*, 145–151. [CrossRef]
59. Cavalcante, N.B.; da Conceição Santos, A.D.; da Silva Almeida, J.R.G. The Genus Jatropha (Euphorbiaceae): A Review on Secondary Chemical Metabolites and Biological Aspects. *Chem. Biol. Interact.* **2020**, *318*, 108976. [CrossRef]
60. Salehi, B.; Iriti, M.; Vitalini, S.; Antolak, H.; Pawlikowska, E.; Kręgiel, D.; Sharifi-Rad, J.; Oyeleye, S.I.; Ademiluyi, A.O.; Czopek, K.; et al. Euphorbia-Derived Natural Products with Potential for Use in Health Maintenance. *Biomolecules* **2019**, *9*, 337. [CrossRef]
61. Azizi, K.; Hamedi, A.; Azarpira, N.; Hamedi, A.; Shahini, M.; Pasdaran, A. A New Cytotoxic Sesquiterpene Lactone from *Euphorbia microsphaera* Boiss against Human Breast Cancer (MCF-7) and Human Fibrosarcoma (HT1080) Cells. *Toxicon* **2021**, *202*, 60–66. [CrossRef]
62. Kopustinskiene, D.M.; Jakstas, V.; Savickas, A.; Bernatoniene, J. Flavonoids as Anticancer Agents. *Nutrients* **2020**, *12*, 457. [CrossRef]
63. Gálvez, J.; Crespo, M.E.; Jiménez, J.; Suárez, A.; Zarzuelo, A. Antidiarrhoeic Activity of Quercitrin in Mice and Rats. *J. Pharm. Pharmacol.* **1993**, *45*, 157–159. [CrossRef] [PubMed]
64. Fajriah, S.; Darmawan, A. Apigenin, an Anticancer Isolated from *Macaranga gigantifolia* Leaves. *J. Trop. Life Sci.* **2016**, *6*, 7–9.
65. Mondal, A.; Gandhi, A.; Fimognari, C.; Atanasov, A.G.; Bishayee, A. Alkaloids for Cancer Prevention and Therapy: Current Progress and Future Perspectives. *Eur. J. Pharmacol.* **2019**, *858*, 172472. [CrossRef] [PubMed]
66. Vendruscolo, I.; Venturella, S.R.T.; Bressiani, P.A.; Marco, I.G.; Novello, C.R.; Almeida, I.V.; Vicentini, V.E.P.; Mello, J.C.P.; Düsman, E. Cytotoxicity of Extracts and Compounds Isolated from *Croton echioides* in Animal Tumor Cell (HTC). *Braz. J. Biol.* **2022**, *82*, e264356. [CrossRef]
67. Mesas, C.; Martínez, R.; Ortíz, R.; Galisteo, M.; López-Jurado, M.; Cabeza, L.; Perazzoli, G.; Melguizo, C.; Porres, J.M.; Prados, J. Antitumor Effect of the Ethanolic Extract from Seeds of *Euphorbia lathyris* in Colorectal Cancer. *Nutrients* **2021**, *13*, 566. [CrossRef]
68. Sultana, T.; Mitra, A.K.; Das, S. Evaluation of Anti-Cancer Potential of *Excoecaria agallocha* (L.) Leaf Extract on Human Cervical Cancer (SiHa) Cell Line and Assessing the Underlying Mechanism of Action. *Futur. J. Pharm. Sci.* **2022**, *8*, 3. [CrossRef]
69. Kwan, Y.P.; Saito, T.; Ibrahim, D.; Al-Hassan, F.M.S.; Oon, C.E.; Chen, Y.; Jothy, S.L.; Kanwar, J.R.; Sasidharan, S. Evaluation of the Cytotoxicity, Cell-Cycle Arrest, and Apoptotic Induction by *Euphorbia hirta* in MCF-7 Breast Cancer Cells. *Pharm. Biol.* **2016**, *54*, 1223–1236. [CrossRef]
70. Njoya, E.M.; Eloff, J.N.; McGaw, L.J. *Croton gratissimus* Leaf Extracts Inhibit Cancer Cell Growth by Inducing Caspase 3/7 Activation with Additional Anti-Inflammatory and Antioxidant Activities. *BMC Complement. Altern. Med.* **2018**, *18*, 305. [CrossRef]
71. Vargas-Madriz, Á.F.; Luzardo-Ocampo, I.; Moreno-Celis, U.; Roldán-Padrón, O.; Chávez-Servín, J.L.; Vergara-Castañeda, H.A.; Martínez-Pacheco, M.; Mejía, C.; García-Gasca, T.; Kuri-García, A. Comparison of Phytochemical Composition and Untargeted

Metabolomic Analysis of an Extract from *Cnidoscolus aconitifolius* (Mill.) I. I. Johnst and *Porophyllum ruderale* (Jacq.) Cass. and Biological Cytotoxic and Antiproliferative Activity In Vitro. *Plants* **2023**, *12*, 1987. [CrossRef]
72. Al-Massarani, S.; El-Sayed, M.-I.K.; El-Shaibany, A. Antioxidant and Anti-Proliferative Activities of *Acalypha fruticosa:* Possible Elucidated Mechanism. *Pak. J. Pharm. Sci.* **2019**, *32*, 2041–2050.
73. Chekuri, S.; Panjala, S.; Anupalli, R.R. Cytotoxic Activity of *Acalypha Indica* L. Hexane Extract on Breast Cancer Cell Lines (MCF-7). *J. Phytopharm.* **2017**, *6*, 264–268. [CrossRef]
74. Guillén-Meléndez, G.A.; Villa-Cedillo, S.A.; Pérez-Hernández, R.A.; Castillo-Velázquez, U.; Salas-Treviño, D.; Saucedo-Cárdenas, O.; Montes-De-oca-luna, R.; Gómez-Tristán, C.A.; Garza-Arredondo, A.J.; Zamora-ávila, D.E.; et al. Cytotoxic Effect in Vitro of *Acalypha monostachya* Extracts over Human Tumor Cell Lines. *Plants* **2021**, *10*, 2326. [CrossRef] [PubMed]
75. Radhakrishna, S. In-Vitro Anticancer Activity of *Baliospermum montanum* on T Cell Leukemia-Jurkat Cell Line and Human Breast Cancer-MCF-7. *IAETSD J. Adv. Sci. Appl. Sci.* **2018**, *5*, 173–179.
76. Pipatrattanaseree, W.; Itharat, A.; Mukkasombut, N.; Saesiw, U. Potential in Vitro Anti-Allergic, Anti-Inflammatory and Cytotoxic Activities of Ethanolic Extract of *Baliospermum montanum* Root, Its Major Components and a Validated HPLC Method. *BMC Complement. Altern. Med.* **2019**, *19*, 45. [CrossRef] [PubMed]
77. Adi, A.S.; Elya, B.; Hanafi, M. Antioxidant and Cytotoxic Bioassay on *Blumeodendron toxbrai* (Blume.) Stem Bark Hexane, Dichloromethane, and Methanolic Ekstract. *Pharmacogn. J.* **2021**, *13*, 139–141. [CrossRef]
78. Ramadan Kamel, M.; Nafady, A.; Hassanein, A.; Ragaey, R.; Haggag, E. Phytochemical Investigation and Assessment of Antioxidant, Antimicrobial and Cytotoxic Activities of the Root Bark *Chrozophora oblongifolia* (Delile) Spreng. (Euphorbiaceae). *J. Adv. Pharm. Res.* **2019**, *3*, 200–208. [CrossRef]
79. Sunil Kumar, K.; Rao, A.S. Evaluation of Hepatoprotective and Invitro Cytotoxic Activity of Leaves of *Chrozophora plicata* Linn. *Res. J. Pharmacol. Pharmacodyn.* **2017**, *9*, 19–26. [CrossRef]
80. Ikpefan, E.O.; Ayinde, B.A.; Mudassir, A.; Farooq, A.D. Comparative in Vitro Assessment of the Methanol Extracts of the Leaf, Stem, and Root Barks of *Cnidoscolus aconitifolius* on Lung and Breast Cancer Cell Lines. *Turk. J. Pharm. Sci.* **2019**, *16*, 375–379. [CrossRef]
81. Kumarasamy, K.P.; Nallaperumal, N.; Natarajan, C.; Nallamadan, J. An in vitro cytotoxicity study of Cnidoscolus chayamansa McVaugh on selected cell lines. *World J. Pharm. Pharm. Sci.* **2014**, *3*, 1110–1116.
82. Sánchez-Aguirre, O.A.; Juárez-Aguilar, E.; Montoya-Hernández, E.L.; Vázquez-Hernández, M.; Colorado-Peralta, R.; Sánchez-Medina, A.; Márquez-López, M.E.; Hernández-Romero, D. Antioxidant Potential of *Cnidoscolus multilobus* (Pax) I.M. Johnst and Its Antiproliferative and Cytotoxic Effect on Cervical Cancer Cells. *Eur. J. Integr. Med.* **2022**, *53*, 102134. [CrossRef]
83. Paredes, P.F.M.; De Morais, S.M.; Brito, F.C.R.; Moura, L.F.W.G.; De Rodrigues, P.A.; Benjamin, S.R.; Magalhães, F.E.A.; Florean, E.O.P.T.; Guedes, M.I.F. Characterization of *Cnidoscolus quercifolius* Pohl Bark Root Extract and Evaluation of Cytotoxic Effect on Human Tumor Cell Lines. *Asian Pac. J. Trop. Biomed.* **2018**, *8*, 345–351. [CrossRef]
84. Worarat, C.; Pompimon, W.; Udomputtimekakul, P.; Sukdee, S.; Sombutsiri, P.; Kuanmuang, N.; Suwan, I.; Khamyong, Y.; Suksabai, C.; Artkla, W.; et al. In Vitro Screening for Cytotoxic, Anti-Bacterial, Anti-HIV1-RT Activities and Chemical Constituents of *Croton fluviatilis*, *Croton acutifolius*, and *Croton thorelii*. *Nat. Prod. J.* **2021**, *12*, 92. [CrossRef]
85. Bhavana, J.; Mk, K.; Sumathy, A. *Cytotoxic and Pro-Apoptotic Activities of Leaf Extract of Croton bonplandianus Baill. against Lung Cancer Cell Line A549*; NISCAIR-CSIR: New Delhi, India, 2016; Volume 54.
86. Shantabi, L.; Jagetia, G.C.; Moirangthem, D.S.; Nongalleima, K. Anticancer Activity of an Ehnomedicinal Plant *Croton caudatus* Geiseler, Kam Sabut in Cultured HeLa Cells. *Biocatal. Agric. Biotechnol.* **2020**, *23*, 101500. [CrossRef]
87. Rosangkima, G.; Jagetia, G. Anticancer, Antioxidant and Analgesic Properties of *Croton caudatus*. *Int. J. Curr. Res.* **2015**, *7*, 20640–20646.
88. De, B.; Mitra, I.; Choudhury, M.D.; Paul, S.B.; Deb, L.; De, A.; Nath, R. In Vitro Cytotoxic Study of *Croton caudatus* Geiseler—A Traditionally Known Anticancerous Plant in North-East India. *Pleione* **2018**, *12*, 165. [CrossRef]
89. Jéssica, d.A.G.S.; Gibbelly, C.d.S.; Marilia, G.d.F.S.; Vanessa, F.d.S.; Jaciana, d.S.A.; Teresinha, G.d.S.; Sônia, P.L. Physicochemical Characteristics and Cytotoxic Effect of the Methanolic Extract of *Croton heliotropiifolius* Kunth (Euphorbiaceae). *Afr. J. Pharm. Pharmacol.* **2017**, *11*, 321–326. [CrossRef]
90. Ernandes, P.A.D.S.; Silva, J.C.P.D.; Sales, D.L.; Ribeiro, P.R.V.; de Brito, E.S.; Kerntopf, M.R.; Delmondes, G.D.A.; Pinheiro, J.C.A.; Salazar, G.J.T.; Batista, F.L.A.; et al. Chemical Constituents and Biological Activities of *Croton heliotropiifolius* Kunth. *Antibiotics* **2021**, *10*, 1074. [CrossRef]
91. Yeboah, K.O.; Emosivbe, M.; Ntim, E.A.; Sam, G.H.; Ainooson, G. The Antiproliferative, Antimigratory and Anticlonogenic Effects of *Croton membranaceus* Müll. Arg. (Euphorbiaceae) Hydroethanolic Root Extract in Human 22Rv1 Castration-Resistant Prostate Cancer Cells. *Acta Pharm. Sci.* **2023**, *61*, 121–140. [CrossRef]
92. Motta, L.B.; Furlan, C.M.; Santos, D.Y.A.C.; Salatino, M.L.F.; Negri, G.; de Carvalho, J.E.; Monteiro, P.A.; Ruiz, A.L.T.G.; Caruzo, M.B.; Salatino, A. Antiproliferative Activity and Constituents of Leaf Extracts of *Croton sphaerogynus* Baill. (Euphorbiaceae). *Ind. Crops Prod.* **2013**, *50*, 661–665. [CrossRef]
93. Vieira, G.T.; Oliveira, T.T.d; Monteiro, L.P.; Kanashiro, M.M.; Costa, M.R.d; Pereira, W.L. Atividade citotóxica do extrato de *Croton urucurana* Baill contra linhagens de células leucêmicas humanas U937 e THP1. *Ciênc. Nat.* **2017**, *39*, 512. [CrossRef]

94. Gadamsetty, G.; Maru, S.; Tyagi, A.; Chakravarthula, S.N. Anti-Inflammatory, Cytotoxic and Antioxidant Effects of Methanolic Extracts of *Drypetes sepiaria* (Euphorbiaceae). *Afr. J. Tradit. Complement. Altern. Med. AJTCAM/Afr. Netw. Ethnomed.* **2013**, *10*, 274–282. [CrossRef] [PubMed]
95. Al-Hamoud, G.A.; Fantoukh, O.I.; Amina, M.; Nasr, F.A.; Al Musayeib, N.M.; Ahmed, M.Z.; Noman, O.M.; Al-Sharidah, R.E.; Alasmari, F.; Alqahtani, A.S. Unprecedented Insights on Chemical and Biological Significance of *Euphorbia cactus* Growing in Saudi Arabia. *Plants* **2022**, *11*, 681. [CrossRef] [PubMed]
96. Bano, S.; Siddiqui, B.S.; Farooq, A.D.; Begum, S.; Siddiqui, F.; Kashif, M. In vitro growth inhibition and cytotoxicity of *Euphorbia caducifolia* against four human cancer cell lines and its phytochemical characterisation. *Nat. Prod. Res.* **2017**, *31*, 2936–2940. [CrossRef] [PubMed]
97. Rédei, D.; Kúsz, N.; Szabó, M.; Pinke, G.; Zupkó, I.; Hohmann, J. First Phytochemical Investigation of Secondary Metabolites of *Euphorbia davidii* Subils. and Antiproliferative Activity of Its Extracts Short Communication. *Acta Biol. Hung.* **2015**, *66*, 464–467. [CrossRef] [PubMed]
98. Ali, F.T.; Yousef, A.K.; Ahmed, F.A.; Elgneady, F.M.; El-Adl, K.; Elhady, M.M. In Silico ADMET, Docking, Anti-Proliferative and Antimicrobial Evaluations of Ethanolic Extract of *Euphorbia dendroides* L. *S. Afr. J. Bot.* **2022**, *150*, 607–620. [CrossRef]
99. Ikpefan, E.O.; Ayinde, B.A.; Mudassar, A.; Farooq, A.D. In Vitro Antiproliferative and Antioxidant Assessment of the Extract and Partitioned Fractions of Leaves of *Euphorbia graminea* Jacq. (Euphorbiaceae). *Niger. J. Pharm.* **2021**, *55*, 26–31. [CrossRef]
100. Kemboi, D.; Langat, M.K.; Siwe-Noundou, X.; Krause, R.W.M.; Isaacs, M.L.; Tembu, V.J. In Vitro Antibacterial and Cytotoxic Effects of *Euphorbia grandicornis* Blanc Chemical Constituents. *BMC Complement. Med. Ther.* **2022**, *22*, 90. [CrossRef]
101. Magozwi, D.K.; Peter, X.; Langat, M.K.; Mhlanga, R.; Vukea, N.; Mare, J.A.d.L.; Siwe-Noundou, X.; Krause, R.W.M.; Tembu, V.J. In Vitro Cytotoxic Effects of Chemical Constituents of *Euphorbia grandicornis* Blanc against Breast Cancer Cells. *Sci. Afr.* **2021**, *14*, e01002. [CrossRef]
102. Radi, M.H.; El-Shiekh, R.A.; El-Halawany, A.M.; Al-Abd, A.M.; Abdel-Sattar, E. In Vitro Cytotoxic Study of *Euphorbia grantii* Oliv. Aerial Parts against MCF-7 and MCF-7ADRBreast Cancer Cell Lines: A Bioactivity-Guided Isolation. *ACS Omega* **2023**, *8*, 18299–18305. [CrossRef]
103. Al-Robai, S.A.; Ahmed, A.A.; Ahmed, A.A.E.; Zabin, S.A.; Mohamed, H.A.; Alghamdi, A.A.A. Phenols, Antioxidant and Anticancer Properties of *Tagetes minuta, Euphorbia granulata* and *Galinsoga parviflora*: In Vitro and in Silico Evaluation. *J. Umm Al-Qura Univ. Appl. Sci.* **2023**, *9*, 15–28. [CrossRef]
104. Deveci, E.; Çayan, G.T.; Karakurt, S.; Duru, M.E. Anti-Colorectal Cancer Effects of Medicinal Plants: *Euphorbia helioscopia, Ferula elaeochytris,* and *Sideritis albiflora*. *Commagene J. Biol.* **2021**, *5*, 73–77. [CrossRef]
105. El-Hallouty, S.M.; Gohar, L.H.; Elgazzar, E.M. Enhancement of Radiation-Induced Cytotoxicity in Hepatocellular Carcinoma Cells by Some Plant Extracts In Vitro. *Egypt. J. Radiat. Sci. Appl.* **2022**. [CrossRef]
106. EL-Hallouty, S.; Batawi, A.; Shafi, M.; Rashwan, E.; Elhawary, E.; Abdelaal, N. Cytotoxicity of five plant extracts against different human cancer cell lines and their molecular mechanism. *Asian J. Pharm. Clin. Res.* **2020**, *13*, 194–198. [CrossRef]
107. Al-Saraireh, Y.M.; Youssef, A.M.M.; Za'al Alsarayreh, A.; Al Hujran, T.A.; Al-Sarayreh, S.; Al-Shuneigat, J.M.; Alrawashdeh, H.M. Phytochemical and Anti-Cancer Properties of *Euphorbia hierosolymitana* Boiss. Crude Extracts. *J. Pharm. Pharmacogn. Res.* **2021**, *9*, 13–23. [CrossRef] [PubMed]
108. Anitha, P.; Geegi, P.G.; Yogeswari, J.; Anthoni, S.A. In Vitro Anticancer Activity of Ethanolic Extract of *Euphorbia hirta* (L.). *Sci. Technol. Arts Res. J.* **2014**, *3*, 1. [CrossRef]
109. Rashmi; Gupta, P. In Vitro Anti-Inflammatory and Anti-Proliferative Potential of Roots Extract of *Euphorbia hirta* Linn. *J. Phytopharm.* **2021**, *10*, 7–9. [CrossRef]
110. Sharma, N.; Samarakoon, K.W.; Gyawali, R.; Park, Y.H.; Lee, S.J.; Oh, S.J.; Lee, T.H.; Jeong, D.K. Evaluation of the Antioxidant, Anti-Inflammatory, and Anticancer Activities of *Euphorbia hirta* Ethanolic Extract. *Molecules* **2014**, *19*, 14567–14581. [CrossRef]
111. Senniappan, P.; Srinivas, K.; Venkata, M.; Rao, B. In-Vitro Antioxidant and Cytotoxicity Activity of *Euphorbia hirta* Petroleum Ether, Chloroform Extracts. *Eur. Chem. Bull.* **2023**, *12*, 2949–2960.
112. Mali, P. Evaluation of Cytotoxicity of Aqueous Extract of *Euphorbia hirta* Using Human Colon Adenocarcinoma and Vero Cell Line. *Toxicol. Int.* **2017**, *24*, 17–21. [CrossRef]
113. De Sousa, A.S.; Fernandes, T.C.C.; Cardona, Y.T.; Almeida, P.M.D.; Marin-Morales, M.A.; Dos Santos, A.V.; Randau, K.P.; Benko-Iseppon, A.M.; Brasileiro-Vidal, A.C. Cytotoxic and Genotoxic Effects of Ethanolic Extract of *Euphorbia hyssopifolia* L. on HepG2 Cells. *J. Ethnopharmacol.* **2015**, *170*, 16–19. [CrossRef]
114. Alghamdi, A.A.A.; Ali, N.M.; Alam, M.M.; Nazreen, S.; Mahzari, A. HPLC Profile, Anticancer, Anti-Inflammatory and Antioxidant Activities of *Euphorbia inarticulata* Ethanolic Extract. *Adv. Pharmacol. Pharm.* **2023**, *11*, 156–167. [CrossRef]
115. Okpako, I.O.; Ng, F.A.; Kyama, C.M.; Oyem, J.C.; Njeru, S.N. Antiproliferative Activity of Euphorbia ingens Extract against Prostate Cancer Cell Line: An in Silico and in Vitro Analysis. *Preprints* **2023**. [CrossRef]
116. Wongprayoon, P.; Charoensuksai, P. Cytotoxic and anti-migratory activities from hydroalcoholic extract of *Euphorbia lactea* Haw. Against HN22 cell line. *Thai Bull. Pharm. Sci.* **2018**, *13*, 69–77.
117. Taş, A.; Şahin-Bölükbaşı, S.; Çevik, E.; Özmen, E.; Gümüş, E.; Siliğ, Y. An in Vitro Study of Cytotoxic Activity of *Euphorbia macroclada* Boiss on MCF-7 Cells. *Indian J. Pharm. Educ. Res.* **2018**, *52*, S119–S123. [CrossRef]
118. Ebrahim, H.Y.; Osman, S.A.; Haffez, H.R.; Hassan, Z.A. In-vitro screening of some plant extracts for their potential anticancer activity. *Afr. J. Tradit. Complement. Altern. Med.* **2020**, *17*, 1–8. [CrossRef]

119. Younus, M.; Hasan, M.M.; Hanif, M.; Sarwar, G.; Ahmad, K.; Ur Rehman, S.M.; Shirazi, J.H.; Jamil, Q.A.; Khan, K.R.; Syed, S.K.; et al. Botanical Features and Anti-Cancerous Potential of *Euphorbia nivulia* Buch.-Ham. *Trop. J. Nat. Product. Res.* **2021**, *5*, 1591–1596. [CrossRef]
120. Al-Yousef, H.M.; Alqahtani, A.S.; Ghani, A.S.A.; El-Toumy, S.A.; El-Dougdoug, W.I.A.; Hassan, W.H.B.; Hassan, H.M. Nephroprotective, Cytotoxic and Antioxidant Activities of *Euphorbia paralias*. *Saudi J. Biol. Sci.* **2021**, *28*, 785–792. [CrossRef] [PubMed]
121. Aslantürk, Ö.S.; Aşkin Çelik, T. Antioxidant, Cytotoxic and Apoptotic Activities of Extracts from Medicinal Plant *Euphorbia platyphyllos* L. *J. Med. Plants Res.* **2013**, *7*, 1293–1304. [CrossRef]
122. Aslantürk, Ö.S.; Yılmaz, E.Ş.; Aşkın Çelik, T.; Güzel, Y. Evaluation of the Antioxidant and Cytotoxic Potency of *Euphorbia rigida* and *Arbutus andrachne* Methanol Extracts in Human Hepatocellular Carcinoma Cell Lines In Vitro. *Beni Suef Univ. J. Basic. Appl. Sci.* **2021**, *10*, 51. [CrossRef]
123. de Souza, L.S.; Tosta, C.L.; de Oliveira, B.J.R.P.; Varricchio, M.C.B.N.; Kitagawa, R.R.; Filgueiras, P.R.; Kuster, R.M. Chemical Profile and Cytotoxic Evaluation of Aerial Parts of *Euphorbia tirucalli* L. on Gastric Adenocarcinoma (AGS Cells). *Nat. Prod. Res.* **2023**, *37*, 4267–4273. [CrossRef]
124. Archanjo, A.B.; De, F.; Careta, P.; Costa, A.V.; Nunes, C. Evaluation of cytotoxicity and expression of caspase-3 and p53 in HCT-116 cells of lineage treated with different extracts of *Euphorbia tirucalli* L. *Arch. Vet. Sci.* **2016**, *21*, 35–45. [CrossRef]
125. Al-Faifi, Z.I.A.; Masrahi, Y.S.; Aly, M.S.; Al-Turki, T.A.; Dardeer, T. Evaluation of Cytotoxic and Genotoxic Effects of *Euphorbia triaculeata* Forssk. Extract. *Asian Pac. J. Cancer Prev.* **2017**, *18*, 771–777. [CrossRef] [PubMed]
126. Aliomrani, M.; Jafarian, A.; Zolfaghari, B. Phytochemical Screening and Cytotoxic Evaluation of *Euphorbia turcomanica* on Hela and HT-29 Tumor Cell Lines. *Adv. Biomed. Res.* **2017**, *6*, 68. [CrossRef]
127. Campos, A.; Vendramini-Costa, D.B.; Longato, G.B.; Zermiani, T.; Ruiz, A.L.T.G.; De Carvalho, J.E.; Pandiella, A.; Filho, V.C. Antiproliferative Effect of *Synadenium grantii* Hook f. Stems (Euphorbiaceae) and a Rare Phorbol Diterpene Ester. *Int. J. Toxicol.* **2016**, *35*, 666–671. [CrossRef] [PubMed]
128. Kanunfre, C.C.; Leffers, T.; Cruz, L.S.; Luz, L.E.C.; Crisma, A.R.; Wang, M.; Avula, B.; Khan, I.A.; Beltrame, F.L. *Euphorbia umbellata* Bark Extracts—An in Vitro Cytotoxic Study. *Rev. Bras. Farmacogn.* **2017**, *27*, 206–213. [CrossRef]
129. Ali, M.M.; Khattab, M.; Mohamed, M.A.; Abdelsalam, R.M.; Mahmoud, K.; Soliman, S.; Barghash, M.F. The Cytotoxic Effect of *Synadenium grantii* Extract against Human Lung Carcinoma A549 Cells and Its Role in Improvement of Histopathological and Biomarkers Changes in Benzo(a)Pyrene-Induced Lung Cancer in Rats. *Int. J. Res. Pharm. Sci.* **2020**, *11*, 962–971. [CrossRef]
130. Periyasamy, K.; Pharm, I.J.; Sci, B.; Batsa, A.J.S. Anticancer activity of *Excoecaria agallocha* leaf extract in cell line model. *Int. J. Pharm. Biol. Sci.* **2013**, *3*, 392–398.
131. Mohapatra, R. The in Vitro Anti-Tumor Efficacy of Methanolic Leaf Extract of *Exoecaria agallocha* in Cancer Cell Lines of Different Tissue Origin. *Int. J. Innov. Res. Technol.* **2021**, *8*, 1348.
132. Hettihewa, L.M.; Munasinghe, M.M.A.B.; Bulugahapitiya, V.B.; Kihara, N. Dose dependent anti proliferative and cytotoxic effects of Flueggea leucopyrus Willd against human ovarian carcinoma; MTS and human telomerase enzyme inhibition. *EJBPS* **2015**, *2*, 14–18.
133. Vassallo, A.; Armentano, M.F.; Miglionico, R.; Caddeo, C.; Chirollo, C.; Gualtieri, M.J.; Ostuni, A.; Bisaccia, F.; Faraone, I.; Milella, L. *Hura crepitans* L. Extract: Phytochemical Characterization, Antioxidant Activity, and Nanoformulation. *Pharmaceutics* **2020**, *12*, 553. [CrossRef]
134. Mongalo, N.; Soyingbe, O.; Makhafola, T. Antimicrobial, Cytotoxicity, Anticancer and Antioxidant Activities of *Jatropha zeyheri* Sond. Roots (Euphorbiaceae). *Asian Pac. J. Trop. Biomed.* **2019**, *9*, 307–314. [CrossRef]
135. Cruz, A.J.D.P.; Raymundo, J.K.G.; Jacinto, S.D.; Tolentino, J.E.; Ipulan-Colet, L.A.D.G. Combining in vitro and in ovo assays to screen for anti-cancer and anti-angiogenic effects of the leaf extracts of *Mallotus cumingii* Müll.Arg. (Euphorbiaceae). *Malays. Appl. Biol.* **2022**, *51*, 73–82. [CrossRef]
136. Benny, B.; Krishna, A.S.; Samraj, S.; John, P.; Radhakrishnan, U. Cytotoxic and Antiproliferative Potential of Methanolic Extract of *Mallotus phillippensis* in MCF-7 Cell Line. *J. Phytopharm.* **2022**, *11*, 60–63. [CrossRef]
137. Chen, X.-M.; Zhang, Z.-J.; Liu, A.-L.; Lv, F.-J.; Li, S.-F. Cholinesterase and Human Lung Cancer Cells (A-549) Inhibitory Activity of the Cassava Peel of Euphorbiaceae In Vitro. In *International Conference on Food Science and Engineering (ICFSE 2016)*; Trans Tech Publications Ltd.: Stafa-Zurich, Switzerland, 2016; ISBN 978-1-60595-390-8.
138. Al-Douri, N.; Al-Jaidi, B.A.; Hammad, H.M.; Shakya, A.K.; Alkhalailah, T.J.M.; Shilbayeh, S.A.R.; Ibrahim, A.A.; Venugopala, K.N.; Kamal, Y.T. Biological Evaluation of *Mercurialis annua* Extracts for Possible Antioxidant, Antiproliferative and Cytotoxic Activity. *Indian. J. Pharm. Educ. Res.* **2022**, *56*, S479–S486. [CrossRef]
139. Nascimento, A.K.L.; Melo-Silveira, R.F.; Dantas-Santos, N.; Fernandes, J.M.; Zucolotto, S.M.; Rocha, H.A.O.; Scortecci, K.C. Antioxidant and Antiproliferative Activities of Leaf Extracts from *Plukenetia volubilis* Linneo (Euphorbiaceae). *Evid.-Based Complement. Altern. Med.* **2013**, *2013*, 950272. [CrossRef] [PubMed]
140. Islam Shah, T.; Sharma, E.; Shah, G.A. Inhibitory Property of Aqueous Extract of *Ricinus communis* Leaves on Proliferation of Melanoma Treated against A375 Cell Lines. *World J. Pharm. Sci.* **2015**, *3*, 758–761.
141. Prakash, E.; Gupta, D.K. In Vitro Study of Extracts of *Ricinus communis* Linn on Human Cancer Cell Lines. *J. Med. Sci. Public Health* **2014**, *2*, 15–20.
142. Albino, R.C.; Antoniassi, R.; de Faria-Machado, A.F.; Ferraris, F.K.; Amendoeira, F.C.; Ramos, D.F.; Silva, P.E.A.; Leitão, S.G.; Oliveira, D.R. Traditional Detoxification of *Jatropha curcas* L. Seeds. *J. Ethnopharmacol.* **2019**, *241*, 111970. [CrossRef]

143. Florence, D. An Investigation into The Antineoplastic Properties of *Schinziophyton rautanenii* and *Colophospermum mopane* . Ph.D. Thesis, The University of Namibia, Windhuk, Namibia, 2008.
144. Menon, M.; Varghese, L. Evaluation of the Phytochemical Constituents and Tumor Reduction Potentials of *Tragia involucrata* Linn. *J. Appl. Biol. Biotechnol.* **2023**, *11*, 84–91. [CrossRef]
145. Euphorbia Species-Derived Diterpenes and Coumarins as Multidrug Resistance Modulators in Human Colon Carcinoma Cells. *Anticancer. Res.* **2016**, *36*, 2259–2264.
146. Li, Y.; Liu, Y.; Li, Y.; Liu, F.; Zhao, Y.; Xu, J.; Guo, Y. Trigothysoid, N. Inhibits Tumor Proliferation and Migration by Targeting Mitochondria and the STAT3/FAK Pathway. *Arab. J. Chem.* **2023**, *16*, 104930. [CrossRef]
147. Lin, M.; Tang, S.; Zhang, C.; Chen, H.; Huang, W.; Liu, Y.; Zhang, J. Euphorbia Factor L2 Induces Apoptosis in A549 Cells through the Mitochondrial Pathway. *Acta Pharm. Sin. B* **2017**, *7*, 59–64. [CrossRef] [PubMed]
148. Fan, R.Z.; Chen, L.; Su, T.; Li, W.; Huang, J.L.; Sang, J.; Tang, G.H.; Yin, S. Discovery of 8,9-*Seco-Ent*-Kaurane Diterpenoids as Potential Leads for the Treatment of Triple-Negative Breast Cancer. *J. Med. Chem.* **2021**, *64*, 9926–9942. [CrossRef] [PubMed]
149. Wongprayoon, P.; Leelasart, S.; Jantham, J.; Pootaeng-on, Y.; Oekchuae, S.; Limpachayaporn, P.; Rayanil, K.O.; Charoensuksai, P. A Triterpenoid Friedelan-3β-Ol Isolated from *Euphorbia lactea* Exhibited Cytotoxic Activity against HN22 Cells by Inducing an S-Phase Cell Cycle Arrest. *J. Appl. Pharm. Sci.* **2022**, *12*, 31–48. [CrossRef]
150. Li, H.H.; Qi, F.M.; Dong, L.L.; Fan, G.X.; Che, J.M.; Guo, D.D.; Zhang, Z.X.; Fei, D.Q. Cytotoxic and Antibacterial Pyran-2-One Derivatives from *Croton crassifolius*. *Phytochem. Lett.* **2014**, *10*, 304–308. [CrossRef]
151. Cui, J.J.; Ji, K.L.; Liu, H.C.; Zhou, B.; Liu, Q.F.; Xu, C.H.; Ding, J.; Zhao, J.X.; Yue, J.M. Cytotoxic Tigliane Diterpenoids from *Croton damayeshu*. *J. Nat. Prod.* **2019**, *82*, 1550–1557. [CrossRef]
152. Karina, P.; Uchôa, S.; Nunes Da Silva, J.; Silveira, R.; Anne, M.; Lima, S.; Braz-Filho, R. Trachylobane and kaurane diterpenes from *Croton floribundus* Spreng. *Quim. Nova* **2013**, *36*, 778–782.
153. Liu, C.-P.; Xu, J.-B.; Zhao, J.-X.; Xu, C.-H.; Dong, L.; Ding, J.; Yue, J.-M. Diterpenoids from *Croton laui* and Their Cytotoxic and Antimicrobial Activities. *J. Nat. Prod.* **2014**, *77*, 1013–1020. [CrossRef]
154. Zhao, B.Q.; Peng, S.; He, W.J.; Liu, Y.H.; Wang, J.F.; Zhou, X.J. Antitubercular and Cytotoxic Tigliane-Type Diterpenoids from *Croton tiglium*. *Bioorg Med. Chem. Lett.* **2016**, *26*, 4996–4999. [CrossRef]
155. Zhang, X.L.; Wang, L.; Li, F.; Yu, K.; Wang, M.K. Cytotoxic Phorbol Esters of *Croton tiglium*. *J. Nat. Prod.* **2013**, *76*, 858–864. [CrossRef]
156. Wang, J.F.; Yang, S.H.; Liu, Y.Q.; Li, D.X.; He, W.J.; Zhang, X.X.; Liu, Y.H.; Zhou, X.J. Five New Phorbol Esters with Cytotoxic and Selective Anti-Inflammatory Activities from *Croton tiglium*. *Bioorg Med. Chem. Lett.* **2015**, *25*, 1986–1989. [CrossRef] [PubMed]
157. Du, Q.; Zhao, Y.; Liu, H.; Tang, C.; Zhang, M.; Ke, C.; Ye, Y. Isolation and Structure Characterization of Cytotoxic Phorbol Esters from the Seeds of *Croton tiglium*. *Planta Med.* **2017**, *83*, 1361–1367. [CrossRef] [PubMed]
158. Cândido-Bacani, P.D.M.; Figueiredo, P.D.O.; Matos, M.D.F.C.; Garcez, F.R.; Garcez, W.S. Cytotoxic Orbitide from the Latex of *Croton urucurana*. *J. Nat. Prod.* **2015**, *78*, 2754–2760. [CrossRef] [PubMed]
159. Abreu, L.S.; do Nascimento, Y.M.; do Espirito-Santo, R.F.; Meira, C.S.; Santos, I.P.; Brandão, R.B.; Souto, A.L.; Guedes, M.L.S.; Soares, M.B.P.; Villarreal, C.F.; et al. Phenylpropanoids from *Croton velutinus* with Cytotoxic, Trypanocidal and Anti-Inflammatory Activities. *Fitoterapia* **2020**, *145*, 104632. [CrossRef] [PubMed]
160. Chen, D.; Cheng, X.; Sun, Y.; Liu, P. A new friedelane triterpenoid possessing cytotoxicity from the leaves and stems of *Drypetes hainanensis*. *Chem. Nat. Compd.* **2014**, *50*, 93–96. [CrossRef]
161. Abdel-Sattar, E.; Abou-Hussein, D.; Petereit, F. Chemical Constituents from the Leaves of Euphorbia Ammak Growing in Saudi Arabia. *Pharmacogn. Res.* **2015**, *7*, 14–17. [CrossRef]
162. Aljubiri, S.M.; Mahgoub, S.A.; Almansour, A.I.; Shaaban, M.; Shaker, K.H. Isolation of Diverse Bioactive Compounds from *Euphorbia balsamifera*: Cytotoxicity and Antibacterial Activity Studies. *Saudi J. Biol. Sci.* **2021**, *28*, 417–426. [CrossRef]
163. Shadi, S.; Saeidi, H.; Ghanadian, M.; Rahimnejad, M.R.; Aghaei, M.; Ayatollahi, S.M.; Iqbal Choudhary, M. New Macrocyclic Diterpenes from *Euphorbia connata* Boiss. with Cytotoxic Activities on Human Breast Cancer Cell Lines. *Nat. Prod. Res.* **2015**, *29*, 607–614. [CrossRef]
164. Foda, S.M.; Zaghloul, M.G.; Marzouk, A.M.; Shaker Mansour, E.-S. Phytochemical Investigation and Biological Studies of *Euphorbia tithymaloides* L. Family Euphorbiaceae. *Delta Univ. Sci. J.* **2022**, *5*, 260–271. [CrossRef]
165. Shamsabadipour, S.; Zarei, S.M.; Ghanadian, M.; Ayatollahi, S.A.; Rahimnejad, M.R.; Saeedi, H.; Aghaei, M. A New Taraxastane Triterpene from *Euphorbia denticulata* with Cytotoxic Activity against Prostate Cancer Cells. *Iran. J. Pharm. Res. IJPR* **2018**, *17*, 336.
166. Yuan, W.J.; Yang, G.P.; Zhang, J.H.; Zhang, Y.; Chen, D.Z.; Li, S.L.; Di, Y.T.; Hao, X.J. Three New Diterpenes with Cytotoxic Activity from the Roots of *Euphorbia ebracteolata* Hayata. *Phytochem. Lett.* **2016**, *18*, 176–179. [CrossRef]
167. Chen, G.; Ma, T.; Ma, Y.; Han, C.; Zhang, J.; Sun, Y. Chemical Composition, Anti-Breast Cancer Activity and Extraction Techniques of *Ent*-Abietane Diterpenoids from *Euphorbia fischeriana* Steud. *Molecules* **2022**, *27*, 4282. [CrossRef] [PubMed]
168. Zhong, N.F.; Huang, H.H.; Wei, J.C.; Yang, Y.C.; Gao, X.X.; Wei, X.Y.; Wang, A.H.; Jia, J.M. Euphorfiatnoids A–I: Diterpenoids from the Roots of *Euphorbia fischeriana* with Cytotoxic Effects. *Phytochemistry* **2022**, *203*, 113372. [CrossRef] [PubMed]
169. Meng, J.; Li, B.T.; Sheng, G.; Zhang, A.L.; Li, X.C.; Tian, J.M. Cytotoxic Diterpenoids from *Euphorbia fischeriana*. *Chem. Biodivers.* **2021**, *18*, e2000919. [CrossRef] [PubMed]
170. Fu, X.; Yu, D.; Zhu, G.; Xu, J. Three New Abietane Diterpenoids from the Aerial Parts of *Euphorbia fischeriana* and Their Cytotoxic Effects. *Phytochem. Lett.* **2023**, *55*, 56–60. [CrossRef]

171. Zhou, M.; Ma, Q.; He, L.; Chen, Y.H.; Zhu, B.Y.; Wang, J.H.; Yang, Q.; Liu, S.; Ma, L.M. Cytotoxic Jatrophane Diterpenoids from the Aerial Parts of *Euphorbia helioscopia*. *J. Asian Nat. Prod. Res.* **2021**, *23*, 731–737. [CrossRef]
172. Lu, Y.B.; Luo, S.; Wang, Y.X.; Feng, Z.Y.; Gao, K.; Chen, J.J. Jatrophane Diterpenoids with Cytotoxic Activity from the Whole Plant of *Euphorbia heliosocpia* L. *Phytochemistry* **2022**, *203*, 113420. [CrossRef]
173. Adedoyin, B.A. In Vitro Cytotoxicity of *Euphorbia heterophylla* against Human Cancer Cell Lines. *Afr. J. Eng. Environ. Res.* **2022**, *3*, 1.
174. Hu, R.; Sang, J.; Li, W.; Tian, Y.; Zou, M.F.; Tang, G.H.; Yin, S. Structurally Diverse Triterpenoids with Cytotoxicity from *Euphorbia hypericifolia*. *Fitoterapia* **2021**, *151*, 104888. [CrossRef]
175. Hegazy, M.E.F.; Hamed, A.R.; Ibrahim, M.A.A.; Talat, Z.; Reda, E.H.; Abdel-Azim, N.S.; Hammouda, F.M.; Nakamura, S.; Matsuda, H.; Haggag, E.G.; et al. Euphosantianane A–D: Antiproliferative Premyrsinane Diterpenoids from the Endemic Egyptian Plant *Euphorbia sanctae-catharinae*. *Molecules* **2018**, *23*, 2221. [CrossRef]
176. Jia, H.Y.; Liao, Z.X.; Liu, F.Y.; Wu, L.; Xu, C.; Zuo, B. A New Phenylpropanoid from the Roots of *Euphorbia nematocypha*. *Nat. Prod. Res.* **2015**, *29*, 650–655. [CrossRef] [PubMed]
177. Xu, C.; Jia, H.-Y.; Zuo, B.; Liao, Z.-X.; Ji, L.-J.; Sun, H.-F.; Wang, Q. Chemical Constituents of the Aerial Parts of *Euphorbia nematocypha*. *Nat. Prod. Commun.* **2016**, *11*, 1934578X1601100210. [CrossRef]
178. Song, N.; Zheng, X.; Wang, J.; Zhu, L.; Wang, C.; Cai, L.; Ding, Z. Cytotoxicity and Molecular-Docking Approach of a New Rosane-Type Diterpenoid from the Roots of *Euphorbia nematocypha*. *Front. Chem.* **2022**, *10*, 912738. [CrossRef] [PubMed]
179. Gao, Y.; Zhou, J.S.; Liu, H.C.; Zhang, Y.; Yin, W.H.; Liu, Q.F.; Wang, G.W.; Zhao, J.X.; Yue, J.M. Phonerilins A–K, Cytotoxic Ingenane and Ingol Diterpenoids from *Euphorbia neriifolia*. *Tetrahedron* **2022**, *123*, 132955. [CrossRef]
180. Ghanadian, M.; Saeidi, H.; Aghaei, M.; Rahiminejad, M.R.; Ahmadi, E.; Ayatollahi, S.M.; Choudhary, M.I.; Bahmani, B. New Jatrophane Diterpenes from *Euphorbia osyridea* with Proapoptotic Effects on Ovarian Cancer Cells. *Phytochem. Lett.* **2015**, *12*, 302–307. [CrossRef]
181. Wang, K.; Yu, H.; Wu, H.; Wang, X.; Pan, Y.; Chen, Y.; Liu, L.; Jin, Y.; Zhang, C. A New Casbane Diterpene from *Euphorbia pekinensis*. *Nat. Prod. Res.* **2015**, *29*, 1456–1460. [CrossRef] [PubMed]
182. Hou, P.; Zeng, Y.; Ma, B.; Bi, K.; Chen, X. A New Cytotoxic Cembrane Diterpene from the Roots of *Euphorbia pekinensis* Rupr. *Fitoterapia* **2013**, *90*, 10–13. [CrossRef] [PubMed]
183. Chen, Y.Y.; Zeng, X.T.; Xu, D.Q.; Yue, S.J.; Fu, R.J.; Yang, X.; Liu, Z.X.; Tang, Y.P. Pimarane, Abietane, and Labdane Diterpenoids from *Euphorbia pekinensis* Rupr. and Their Anti-Tumor Activities. *Phytochemistry* **2022**, *197*, 113113. [CrossRef]
184. Ismail, M.; Ahmed, M.H.; Zaki, M.; Moawad, A.; Mohammed, R. Colorectal Cytotoxic Activities of Phenolic Constituents Isolated from *Euphorbia pseudocactus* Cultivated in Egypt. *J. Appl. Pharm. Sci.* **2022**, *12*, 97–102. [CrossRef]
185. Wu, S.; Gan, L.; Su, T.; Wei, X.; Yin, S. New Ingenane and Ingol Diterpenoids from *Euphorbia royleana*. *Nat. Prod. Res.* **2023**, *37*, 1130–1137. [CrossRef]
186. Banjar, M.F.S.; Mohamed, G.A.; Shehata, I.A.; Abdallah, H.M.; Shati, A.A.; Alfaifi, M.Y.; Elbehairi, S.E.I.; Koshak, A.E.; Ibrahim, S.R.M. Cycloschimperols A and B, New Cytotoxic Cycloartane Triterpenoids from *Euphorbia schimperi*. *Phytochem. Lett.* **2019**, *32*, 90–95. [CrossRef]
187. Aljubiri, S.M.; Mahmoud, K.; Mahgoub, S.A.; Almansour, A.I.; Shaker, K.H. Bioactive Compounds from *Euphorbia schimperiana* with Cytotoxic and Antibacterial Activities. *S. Afr. J. Bot.* **2021**, *141*, 357–366. [CrossRef]
188. Zolfaghari, B.; Yazdiniapour, Z.; Ghanadian, M.; Lanzotti, V. Cyclomyrsinane and Premyrsinane Diterpenes from *Euphorbia sogdiana* Popov. *Tetrahedron* **2016**, *72*, 5394–5401. [CrossRef]
189. Zhu, H.; Ren, X.; Huang, Y.; Su, T.; Yang, L. Chemical Constituents of *Euphorbia stracheyi* Boiss (Euphorbiaceae). *Metabolites* **2023**, *13*, 852. [CrossRef] [PubMed]
190. Ye, Y.; Liu, G.H.; Dawa, D.; Ding, L.S.; Cao, Z.X.; Zhou, Y. Cytotoxic Diterpenoids from the Roots of *Euphorbia stracheyi*. *Phytochem. Lett.* **2020**, *36*, 183–187. [CrossRef]
191. Rédei, D.; Kúsz, N.; Sátori, G.; Kincses, A.; Spengler, G.; Burián, K.; Barina, Z.; Hohmann, J. Bioactive Segetane, Ingenane, and Jatrophane Diterpenes from *Euphorbia Taur*. *Planta Med.* **2018**, *84*, 729–735. [CrossRef]
192. Silva, V.A.O.; Rosa, M.N.; Tansini, A.; Oliveira, R.J.S.; Martinho, O.; Lima, J.P.; Pianowski, L.F.; Reis, R.M. In Vitro Screening of Cytotoxic Activity of Euphol from *Euphorbia tirucalli* on a Large Panel of Human Cancer-Derived Cell Lines. *Exp. Ther. Med.* **2018**, *16*, 557–566. [CrossRef]
193. Liu, G.; Zhang, Z.; Wang, Y.; Li, X. Highly Oxygenated Ent-Atisane and Podocarpane Diterpenoids from *Excoecaria agallocha*. *Nat. Prod. Res.* **2022**, *36*, 3924–3930. [CrossRef]
194. Asep, S.; Hening, H.; Gema, S.P.; Gigih, S.; Widya, M.C. Sahidin Anticancer Activity of Jatrophone an Isolated Compound from *Jatropha gossypifolia* Plant against Hepatocellular Cancer Cell Hep G2 1886. *Biomed. Pharmacol. J.* **2017**, *10*, 667–673. [CrossRef]
195. Byrappa, M.; Viswanathan, G.; Doss, J.; Ananthi, J.; Rajan, N.; Raja, L.; Venkateshan, N. Cytotoxic Pyrrolidinone from Leaves of *Jatropha tanjorensis*. *Int. J. Res. Sci. Innov.* **2018**, *5*, 45–50.
196. Segun, P.A.; Ogbole, O.O.; Ismail, F.M.D.; Nahar, L.; Evans, A.R.; Ajaiyeoba, E.O.; Sarker, S.D. Bioassay-Guided Isolation and Structure Elucidation of Cytotoxic Stilbenes and Flavonols from the Leaves of *Macaranga barteri*. *Fitoterapia* **2019**, *134*, 151–157. [CrossRef] [PubMed]
197. Wanandri, R.; Rewa, S.; Saputri, R.D.; Tjahjandarie, S.; Tanjung, M. Cytotoxic Activity of Flavonols from *Macaranga gigantea*. *Pharm. J. Farm. Indones.* **2020**, *17*, 360–367.

198. Yang, D.S.; Wei, J.G.; Peng, W.B.; Wang, S.M.; Sun, C.; Yang, Y.P.; Liu, K.C.; Li, X.L. Cytotoxic Prenylated Bibenzyls and Flavonoids from Macaranga Kurzii. *Fitoterapia* **2014**, *99*, 261–266. [CrossRef] [PubMed]
199. Tanjung, M.; Tjahjandarie, T.S. Dihydroflavonols from the Leaves of *Macaranga recurvata* and Their Cytotoxic and Antioxidant Activities. *J. Chem. Pharm. Res.* **2014**, *6*, 90–95.
200. Zhang, Y.; Zhou, D.; Liu, W.; Li, C.; Hao, L.; Zhang, G.; Deng, S.; Yang, R.; Qin, J.; Li, J.; et al. Cytotoxic Activity and Related Mechanisms of Prenylflavonoids Isolated from *Mallotus conspurcatus* Croizat. *Chem. Biodivers.* **2019**, *16*, e1800465. [CrossRef]
201. Mbeunkeu, A.B.D.; Azebaze, A.G.B.; Tala, M.F.; Teinkela, J.E.M.; Noundou, X.S.; Krause, R.W.M.; Vardamides, J.C.; Laatsch, H. Three New Pentacyclic Triterpenoids from Twigs of *Manniophyton fulvum* (Euphorbiaceae). *Phytochem. Lett.* **2018**, *27*, 1–8. [CrossRef]
202. Toussaint-Douhoré, G.Y.; Soro, Y.; Ouédraogo, N.; Vaca-Garcia, C.; Koffi-Attioua, B.; Carraz, M. Liver Cancer Antiproliferative Activity of a New Nor-Cucurbitacin from *Mareya micrantha* Müll. Arg. *Fitoterapia* **2023**, *166*, 105471. [CrossRef]
203. Johnson-Ajinwo, O.R.; Richardson, A.; Li, W.W. Cytotoxic Effects of Stem Bark Extracts and Pure Compounds from *Margaritaria discoidea* on Human Ovarian Cancer Cell Lines. *Phytomedicine* **2015**, *22*, 1–4. [CrossRef]
204. Yakubu, O.F.; Adebayo, A.H.; Dokunmu, T.M.; Zhang, Y.J.; Iweala, E.E.J. Cytotoxic Effects of Compounds Isolated from *Ricinodendron heudelotii*. *Molecules* **2019**, *24*, 145. [CrossRef]
205. Mangisa, M.; Tembu, V.J.; Fouche, G.; Nthambeleni, R.; Peter, X.; Langat, M.K. Ent-Abietane Diterpenoids from *Suregada zanzibariensis* Baill. (Euphorbiaceae), Their Cytotoxic and Anticancer Properties. *Nat. Prod. Res.* **2019**, *33*, 3240–3247. [CrossRef]
206. Lei, C.; Li, Y.N.; Li, J.N.; Zhou, Y.B.; Cui, M.J.; Fu, K.C.; Li, J.; Hou, A.J. Two New Cytotoxic Maytansinoids Targeting Tubulin from *Trewia nudiflora*. *Planta Med.* **2021**, *88*, 678–684. [CrossRef] [PubMed]
207. Liu, Y.P.; Hu, S.; Wen, Q.; Ma, Y.L.; Jiang, Z.H.; Tang, J.Y.; Fu, Y.H. Novel γ-Lactone Derivatives from *Trigonostemon heterophyllus* with Their Potential Antiproliferative Activities. *Bioorg. Chem.* **2018**, *79*, 107–110. [CrossRef] [PubMed]
208. Yang, B.; Chen, G.Y.; Song, X.P.; Yang, L.Q.; Han, C.R.; Wu, X.Y.; Zheng, C.J.; Ran, X.; Tang, R.F. Trigoxyphins O-T, Six New Heterodimers from *Trigonostemon xyphophylloides*. *Tetrahedron Lett.* **2013**, *54*, 6434–6438. [CrossRef]
209. de Abrantes, R.A.; Batista, T.M.; Mangueira, V.M.; de Sousa, T.K.G.; Ferreira, R.C.; Moura, A.P.G.; Abreu, L.S.; Alves, A.F.; Velozo, E.S.; Batista, L.M.; et al. Antitumor and Antiangiogenic Effects of Tonantzitlolone B, an Uncommon Diterpene from *Stillingia loranthacea*. *Naunyn Schmiedebergs Arch. Pharmacol.* **2022**, *395*, 267–274. [CrossRef] [PubMed]
210. Adiga, P.G.; Shridhar, N.B.; Sanganal, J.S.; Rao, S.; Shilpa, N.; Aparna, V.; Santhosh, I.M.; Tirumala, M.; Sindhu, B.M. In Vivo Anti-Tumor Efficacy of *Croton oblongifolius* in DMBA Induced Mammary Tumor in Rats. *Indian J. Anim. Res.* **2018**, *52*, 144–147. [CrossRef]
211. Majumder, M.; Debnath, S.; Gajbhiye, R.L.; Saikia, R.; Gogoi, B.; Samanta, S.K.; Das, D.K.; Biswas, K.; Jaisankar, P.; Mukhopadhyay, R. *Ricinus communis* L. Fruit Extract Inhibits Migration/Invasion, Induces Apoptosis in Breast Cancer Cells and Arrests Tumor Progression in Vivo. *Sci. Rep.* **2019**, *9*, 14493. [CrossRef]
212. De Castro, J.B.R.; Wemmenson, F.; Moura, G.; Solheiro Bezerra, A.; De, P.; Rodrigues, A.; Da Costa, H.P.S.; Do, N.; Canabrava, V.; Matheus, C.; et al. Antitumoral activity and in vivo toxicity of *Cnidoscolus quercifolius* pohl (euphorbiaceae). *Int. J. Dev. Res.* **2020**, *10*, 20359. [CrossRef]
213. Liang, Y.; Zhang, Y.; Wang, G.; Li, Y.; Huang, W. Penduliflaworosin, a Diterpenoid from *Croton crassifolius*, Exerts Anti-Angiogenic Effect via VEGF Receptor-2 Signaling Pathway. *Molecules* **2017**, *22*, 126. [CrossRef]
214. Ma, L.; Chen, Z.; Wang, W.; Zhang, J.; Zhang, H.; Liu, J. The Molecular Mechanism of ESZM Extract on Treatment ER(−) Breast Cancer in Vivo: Application of "Combat Poison with Poison" Theory. *Preprint* **2021**. [CrossRef]
215. Cheng, J.; Han, W.; Wang, Z.; Shao, Y.; Wang, Y.; Zhang, Y.; Li, Z.; Xu, X.; Zhang, Y. Hepatocellular Carcinoma Growth Is Inhibited by *Euphorbia helioscopia* L. Extract in Nude Mice Xenografts. *Biomed. Res. Int.* **2015**, *2015*, 601015. [CrossRef]
216. Huang, Y.Y.; Chen, C.H.; Hsu, C.H.; Kuo, T.Y.; Liu, C.C.; Liao, A.T.C.; Lin, C.S. Inhibiting Autophagy Potentiates the Antitumor Efficacy of *Euphorbia royleana* for Canine Mammary Gland Tumors. *BMC Vet. Res.* **2020**, *16*, 193. [CrossRef] [PubMed]
217. Sultana, S. Evaluation of the Antioxidant and In Vivo Anticancer Activity of *Excoecaria agallocha* Bark Extrac. Ph.D. Thesis, Brac University, Dhaka, Bangladesh, 2019.
218. Ghramh, H.A.; Khan, K.A.; Ibrahim, E.H.; Setzer, W.N. Synthesis of Gold Nanoparticles (AuNPs) Using *Ricinus communis* Leaf Ethanol Extract, Their Characterization, and Biological Applications. *Nanomaterials* **2019**, *9*, 765. [CrossRef] [PubMed]
219. Alqahtani, M.S.; Al-Yousef, H.M.; Alqahtani, A.S.; Tabish Rehman, M.; AlAjmi, M.F.; Almarfidi, O.; Amina, M.; Alshememry, A.; Syed, R. Preparation, Characterization, and in Vitro-in Silico Biological Activities of *Jatropha pelargoniifolia* Extract Loaded Chitosan Nanoparticles. *Int. J. Pharm.* **2021**, *606*, 120867. [CrossRef] [PubMed]
220. Alqahtani, A.A.; Attia, G.H.; Elgamal, A.; Aleraky, M.; Youns, M.; Ibrahim, A.M.; Abdou, R.; Shaikh, I.A.; El Raey, M.A. Cytotoxic Activity of Zinc Oxide Nanoparticles Mediated by *Euphorbia retusa*. *Crystals* **2022**, *12*, 903. [CrossRef]
221. Aboulthana, W.M.; Omar, N.I.; El-Feky, A.M.; Hasan, E.A.; Ibrahim, N.E.S.; Youssef, A.M. In Vitro Study on Effect of Zinc Oxide Nanoparticles on the Biological Activities of *Croton tiglium* L. Seeds Extracts. *Asian Pac. J. Cancer Prev.* **2022**, *23*, 2671–2686. [CrossRef] [PubMed]
222. Banerjee, K.; Das, S.; Choudhury, P.; Ghosh, S.; Baral, R.; Choudhuri, S.K. A Novel Approach of Synthesizing and Evaluating the Anticancer Potential of Silver Oxide Nanoparticles in Vitro. *Chemotherapy* **2017**, *62*, 279–289. [CrossRef] [PubMed]

223. El Raey, M.A.; El-Hagrassi, A.M.; Osman, A.F.; Darwish, K.M.; Emam, M. *Acalypha wilkesiana* Flowers: Phenolic Profiling, Cytotoxic Activity of Their Biosynthesized Silver Nanoparticles and Molecular Docking Study for Its Constituents as Topoisomerase-I Inhibitors. *Biocatal. Agric. Biotechnol.* **2019**, *20*, 101243. [CrossRef]
224. Elemike, E.E.; Onwudiwe, D.C.; Singh, M. Eco-Friendly Synthesis of Copper Oxide, Zinc Oxide and Copper Oxide–Zinc Oxide Nanocomposites, and Their Anticancer Applications. *J. Inorg. Organomet. Polym. Mater.* **2020**, *30*, 400–409. [CrossRef]
225. Cherian, A.M.; Snima, K.S.; Kamath, C.R.; Nair, S.V.; Lakshmanan, V.K. Effect of *Baliospermum montanum* Nanomedicine Apoptosis Induction and Anti-Migration of Prostate Cancer Cells. *Biomed. Pharmacother.* **2015**, *71*, 201–209. [CrossRef]
226. Boomi, P.; Poorani, G.P.; Selvam, S.; Palanisamy, S.; Jegatheeswaran, S.; Anand, K.; Balakumar, C.; Premkumar, K.; Prabu, H.G. Green Biosynthesis of Gold Nanoparticles Using *Croton sparsiflorus* Leaves Extract and Evaluation of UV Protection, Antibacterial and Anticancer Applications. *Appl. Organomet. Chem.* **2020**, *34*, e5574. [CrossRef]
227. Abd El-Moaty, H.I.; Ismail, E.H.; Abu-Khudir, R.; Soliman, N.A.; Sabry, D.Y.; Al Abdulsalam, N.K.; Sorour, W.A.; Khalil, M.M.H. Characterization and Evaluation of Multiple Biological Activities of Phytosynthesized Gold Nanoparticles Using Aqueous Extract of *Euphorbia dendroides*. *Nanomater. Nanotechnol.* **2022**, *12*, 18479804221141266. [CrossRef]
228. Lingaraju, K.; Naika, H.R.; Nagaraju, G.; Nagabhushana, H. Biocompatible Synthesis of Reduced Graphene Oxide from *Euphorbia heterophylla* (L.) and Their in-Vitro Cytotoxicity against Human Cancer Cell Lines. *Biotechnol. Rep.* **2019**, *24*, e00376. [CrossRef] [PubMed]
229. Ghramh, H.A.; Khan, K.A.; Ibrahim, E.H. Biological Activities of *Euphorbia peplus* Leaves Ethanolic Extract and the Extract Fabricated Gold Nanoparticles (AuNPs). *Molecules* **2019**, *24*, 1431. [CrossRef] [PubMed]
230. Kumari, A.; Naveen; Dhatwalia, J.; Thakur, S.; Radhakrishnan, A.; Chauhan, A.; Chandan, G.; Choi, B.H.; Neetika; Nidhi. Antioxidant, Antimicrobial, and Cytotoxic Potential of *Euphorbia royleana* Extract-Mediated Silver and Copper Oxide Nanoparticles. *Chem. Pap.* **2023**, *77*, 4643–4657. [CrossRef]
231. Bhuvaneswari, R.; Xavier, R.J.; Arumugam, M. Facile Synthesis of Multifunctional Silver Nanoparticles Using Mangrove Plant *Excoecaria agallocha* L. for Its Antibacterial, Antioxidant and Cytotoxic Effects. *J. Parasit. Dis.* **2017**, *41*, 180–187. [CrossRef] [PubMed]
232. Zhou, J.B.; Peng, G.; Wang, J.; Nie, S.; Li, J.; Jia, Y.C.; Zhang, Q.Y. Ebracteolatain A and Ebracteolatain B Induce Apoptosis of Human Hepatoma Cell Line (HepG2). *Trop. J. Pharm. Res.* **2015**, *14*, 1821–1828. [CrossRef]
233. Chaitanya, G.V.; Alexander, J.S.; Babu, P.P. PARP-1 Cleavage Fragments: Signatures of Cell-Death Proteases in Neurodegeneration. *Cell Commun. Signal.* **2010**, *8*, 31. [CrossRef] [PubMed]
234. Shi, Y. Mechanisms of Caspase Activation and Inhibition during Apoptosis. *Mol. Cell* **2002**, *9*, 459–470. [CrossRef]
235. Hao, Q.; Chen, J.; Lu, H.; Zhou, X. The ARTS of P53-Dependent Mitochondrial Apoptosis. *J. Mol. Cell Biol.* **2023**, *14*, mjac074. [CrossRef]
236. Jaiswal, P.L.; Goel, A.; Mittal, R.D. Survivin: A Molecular Biomarker in Cancer. *Indian J. Med. Res.* **2015**, *141*, 389.
237. Shi, S.-Q.; Fan, Y.-Y.; Xu, C.-H.; Ding, J.; Wang, G.-W.; Yue, J.-M. Supporting Information Cytotoxic 8,9-*Seco*-Ent-Kaurane Diterpenoids from *Croton kongensis*. *J. Asian Nat. Prod. Res.* **2018**, *20*, 920–927. [CrossRef] [PubMed]

cancers

Review

Targeting Cell Signaling Pathways in Lung Cancer by Bioactive Phytocompounds

Neeraj Choudhary [1,†], Sweta Bawari [2,†], Jack T. Burcher [3], Dona Sinha [4], Devesh Tewari [5,*] and Anupam Bishayee [3,*]

1 Department of Pharmacognosy, GNA School of Pharmacy, GNA University, Phagwara 144 401, India
2 Amity Institute of Pharmacy, Amity University, Noida 201 301, India
3 College of Osteopathic Medicine, Lake Erie College of Osteopathic Medicine, Bradenton, FL 34211, USA
4 Department of Receptor Biology and Tumor Metastasis, Chittaranjan National Cancer Institute, Kolkata 700 026, India
5 Department of Pharmacognosy and Phytochemistry, School of Pharmaceutical Sciences, Delhi Pharmaceutical Sciences and Research University, New Delhi 110 017, India
* Correspondence: devesh.tewari@dpsru.edu.in or dtewari3@gmail.com (D.T.); abishayee@lecom.edu or abishayee@gmail.com (A.B.)
† These authors contributed equally to this work.

Simple Summary: Lung cancer is the leading cause of mortality in cancer patients, causing an estimated 1.8 million deaths in the year 2020. However, the available therapeutic options exert numerous adverse effects and adequate therapeutic activity is still to be achieved. Therefore, there is a need for the development of safe and effective treatment for lung cancer. Phytochemicals are well documented for their anticancer potential against lung cancer and have a strong rationale for further investigation as a potential chemotherapeutic agent. Notably, phytochemicals act by modulating several signaling pathways, promoting apoptosis, oxidative stress, and disruption of the mitochondrial membrane, inhibiting angiogenesis, and regulating transcription factors. Therefore, an exhaustive and detailed review was carried out to establish the potential role of phytochemicals by conducting a critical analysis of in vitro, in vivo, and clinical evidence in mitigating lung cancer, with emphasis on their impact on signaling pathways.

Abstract: Lung cancer is a heterogeneous group of malignancies with high incidence worldwide. It is the most frequently occurring cancer in men and the second most common in women. Due to its frequent diagnosis and variable response to treatment, lung cancer was reported as the top cause of cancer-related deaths worldwide in 2020. Many aberrant signaling cascades are implicated in the pathogenesis of lung cancer, including those involved in apoptosis (B cell lymphoma protein, Bcl-2-associated X protein, first apoptosis signal ligand), growth inhibition (tumor suppressor protein or gene and serine/threonine kinase 11), and growth promotion (epidermal growth factor receptor/proto-oncogenes/phosphatidylinositol-3 kinase). Accordingly, these pathways and their signaling molecules have become promising targets for chemopreventive and chemotherapeutic agents. Recent research provides compelling evidence for the use of plant-based compounds, known collectively as phytochemicals, as anticancer agents. This review discusses major contributing signaling pathways involved in the pathophysiology of lung cancer, as well as currently available treatments and prospective drug candidates. The anticancer potential of naturally occurring bioactive compounds in the context of lung cancer is also discussed, with critical analysis of their mechanistic actions presented by preclinical and clinical studies.

Keywords: lung cancer; phytochemicals; signaling pathways; preclinical; clinical studies

1. Introduction

Lung cancer represents one of the most frequently diagnosed malignancies globally, falling behind only prostate cancer in males and breast cancer in females [1,2]. As most cases are discovered as locally advanced or metastatic disease, lung cancer has a notoriously poor five-year survival rate (18.6%) compared with other cancers, such as colorectal (64.5%), breast (89.6%), and prostate (98.2%) [2–4]. Depending on disease progression and patient goals, several treatment options may be used against lung cancer, including chemotherapy, radiotherapy, immunotherapy, and surgical intervention [5]. Historically, broad-spectrum chemotherapy has been the mainstay of treatment, but targeted therapies have begun to emerge as highly efficacious options, thereby shifting focus towards personalized medicine. This advancement is made possible by extensive and ongoing research on the cellular signal transduction pathways disrupted in lung malignancies [6].

Despite new therapies and ongoing developments, cancer of the lung was deemed the number one cause of cancer-related deaths worldwide in 2020, claiming an estimated 1.8 million lives [7]. Unfortunately, current therapeutic options are not providing adequate response and are frequently accompanied by significant adverse effects [2]. Approved agents routinely used in medical oncology for the treatment of lung cancer are notorious for their toxic effects. Many first-line drugs are documented to have toxicity such as celecoxib [8], carboplatin, or cisplatin in combination with oxaliplatin [9] and docetaxel [10]. The need for novel, safe, and effective treatments for lung cancer is further underscored in the setting of recurrent and drug-resistant cancers [3,4]. Ultimately, the high mortality and frequent adverse effects of classic treatments serve as an impetus to explore medicinal plants for their pharmacological beneficence.

Plant-based metabolites have been shown to possess anticancer activity in the context of lung malignancies [11]. Furthermore, various challenges associated with the effective and safe use of plant metabolites have been overcome due to the new approaches used in the pharmaceutical industry [12–14]. Specialized plant-derived metabolites are strong contenders as anticancer drugs due to their reduced toxicity and high efficacy against lung cancer [15]. Plant metabolites exert their anticancer activity via different mechanisms in lung cancer but act primarily by inhibiting cellular metabolism, thereby preventing tumor cell proliferation [16,17]. Previous reviews have attempted to capture the broad scope of phytochemicals in the context of lung cancer. One review highlights the structure–activity relationship of various bioactive compounds in regard to non-small cell lung cancer (NSCLC) only and failed to provide significant insight on mechanisms of action [18]. In another review, the role of natural products was discussed in the context of lung cancer, but this study's discussion of phytochemicals was limited to their targeting of the tumor microenvironment [17]. Another article discusses the anticancer effects of various phytochemicals in lung cancer stem cells but was limited in scope by its selection of only nine phytochemicals and emphasis on stem cells [19]. In one more publication, the roles of a few phytochemicals were discussed against lung cancer biomarkers [20]. Still, limitations in scope are seen in other publications by narrowing inclusion criteria to only one group of phytochemicals, e.g., phenolics [21]. Numerous phytochemicals were recognized, and their mechanisms of action were explained. However, the review was not utterly comprehensive, and since then, several in vitro, in vivo, and clinical studies were conducted in the past few years, which have identified numerous additional phytochemicals that displayed anticancer effects in lung cancer [16]. An exhaustive and detailed review of the role of phytochemicals against lung cancer, including a focused discussion of their mechanistic action as presented in preclinical and clinical studies, is still lacking. Therefore, this review is an attempt to provide an up-to-date discussion of all phytochemicals relevant to the treatment or prevention of lung cancer, with emphasis on their impact on signaling pathways.

2. Pathophysiology of Lung Cancer

The World Health Organization (WHO) broadly divides lung cancers into two major categories: small cell lung cancer (SCLC) and NSCLC [22]. Of the two, NSCLC is more prevalent and constitutes approximately 80% of lung cancers. SCLC, however, is more aggressive, develops rapidly, and is more prone to metastasis compared to NSCLC [23,24]. Whereas SCLC is more central in location with its common site of origin in the bronchial epithelium [22], NSCLC is more peripheral and essentially originates in the epithelium of either bronchioles or alveoli [25]. Moreover, SCLC originates from neuroendocrine cells, whereas NSCLC originates from various types of epithelial cells [26]. NSCLC is further divided into three histological groups, including centrally located squamous cell carcinoma, distally located adenocarcinoma, and large cell lung cancer, which is variable in its location [3,26,27]. Similarly, SCLC is categorized into limited and extensive types based on if the confined borders of SCLC are limited to the ipsilateral hemithorax and the associated lymph nodes or if there is any spread of the malignancy to areas beyond the thorax [24,28] (Figure 1). Regardless of the varying subtypes, all lung cancers follow a similar course of events stemming from genetic mutations which usually occur following exposure to carcinogens, eventually followed by clonal expansion of the implicated cells [29].

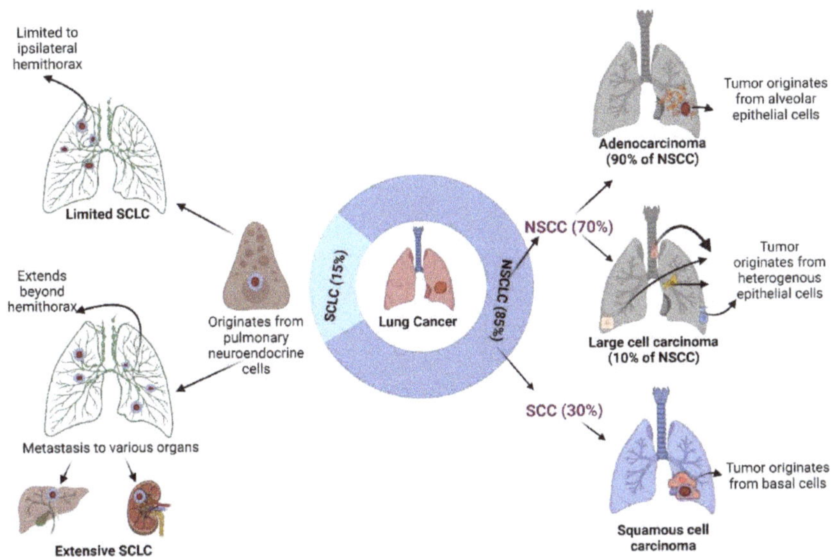

Figure 1. Various types of lung cancer. Lung cancer is categorized into small cell lung cancer (SCLC) which accounts for 15% of all lung cancers and non-small cell lung cancer (NSCLC) which accounts for the remaining 85%. SCLC originates from pulmonary neuroendocrine cells and is further categorized into limited SCLC, characterized by involvement of the ipsilateral hemithorax, and extensive SCLC, which extends to the contralateral hemithorax or beyond. NSCLC is subdivided into squamous cell carcinoma (SCC), which comprises 30% of all NSCLC cases and originates from lung basal cells, and non-squamous cell carcinoma (NSCC) that encompasses 70% of all NSCLC incidences. Ninety percent of cases of NSCC are those of adenocarcinoma that originates from alveolar epithelial cells; only 10% of cases of NSCC are those of large cell carcinoma which exhibits tremendous heterogenicity in its origin.

Two major hypotheses have been put forth to best describe the pathogenesis of lung cancer, namely "the field of cancerization" and "the field of injury" theories (Figure 2) [27]. Field of cancerization is based upon observations made by Slaughter in the year 1944 [30], later expanded upon by Auerbach et al. [31] who reported serious histological changes in the bronchial epithelium as a result of cigarette smoking in 1957. According to this theory, carcinogens induce extensive genetic aberrations that can be seen in the regions with a neoplasm and immediately adjoining respiratory epithelium, more like involving a patch or field of histological changes that develop into cancer [29]. Although there may be no apparent morphological changes, the normal cells in a field of cancerization are replaced by tumorigenic cells owing to carcinogen-induced genetic mutations long before an actual cancerous lesion develops [32]. Therefore, even after the tumor develops and is surgically removed, the field of cancerization remains, resulting in secondary tumorigenesis [33]. The field of injury describes extensive histological changes that occur throughout the carcinogen-exposed areas of the respiratory tract, including the epithelial tissues in the airway, as well as the lungs, suggesting host response upon carcinogen encounter [34]. This host response is responsible for inflammation and genetic aberrations which may result in the genesis of a neoplasm [30].

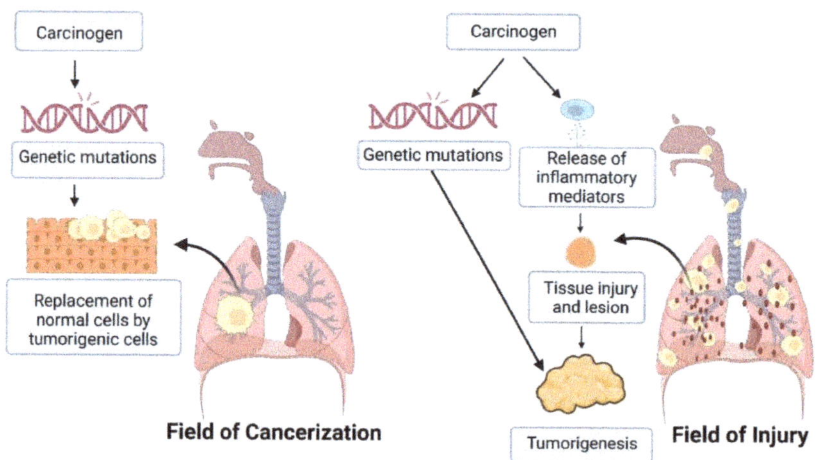

Figure 2. Field of cancerization and field of injury theories of lung cancer development. Field of cancerization is based upon the replacement of normal pulmonary cells by tumorigenic cells upon exposure to carcinogens. These cells go on to produce genetic aberrations, ultimately leading to carcinogenesis in the exposed areas of the lungs. Field of injury-mediated tumorigenesis is an outcome of carcinogen-induced genetic mutations and tissue injury as a result of extensive host response. These carcinogen-induced tumorigenic lesions are not restricted to a particular region or field (as in field of cancerization) but are widespread in the entire respiratory tract and lungs.

NSCLC is majorly an outcome of Kirsten rat sarcoma viral oncogene (KRAS) mutations and epidermal growth factor receptor (EGFR) mutations. Other genes which may harbor mutations and contribute to NSCLC in some capacity include anaplastic lymphoma kinase (ALK), mesenchymal epithelial transition factor (MET), V-Raf murine sarcoma viral oncogene homolog B (BRAF), mitogen-activated protein kinase (MAPK) or extracellular signal-related kinase (ERK) kinase (MEK), and rearranged during transfection (RET) mutations. In contrast, gene alterations most typically seen in the setting of SCLC include mutations of phosphatidylinositol-4,5-bisphosphate 3-kinase catalytic subunit alpha (PIK3CA), fibroblast growth factor receptor 1 (FGFR1), and phosphatase and TENsin homolog gene (PTEN) [35], which are addressed in subsequent sections. Inactivating mutations in the tumor suppressor TP53 and retinoblastoma (RB) 1 genes are witnessed ubiquitously in approximately 90% of the cases of SCLC [36,37]. Similarly, inactivation of RB tumor suppressor gene is also a very common finding in SCLC [38]. These genetic mutations in NSCLC and SCLC are considered to be the major oncogenic drivers due to their ability to affect various upstream and downstream signaling molecules of numerous pathways, including the phosphatidylinositol-3-kinase (PI3K)/protein kinase B (Akt)/mammalian target of rapamycin (mTOR) pathway (PI3K/Akt/mTOR pathway); rat sarcoma virus gene (RAS)/rapidly accelerated fibrosarcoma (RAF)/MAPK or ERK kinase (MEK)/ERK pathway (RAF/MEK/ERK pathway); and Janus kinase (JAK)/signal transducer and activator of transcription (STAT) transduction pathway (JAK/STAT pathway) [35].

3. Cell Signaling Pathways in Lung Cancer

Lung cancer is a product of aberrations in normal cell function, including oxidative stress, genetics, and multiple signaling pathways [39,40]. Of the signaling pathways implicated in lung cancer, receptor tyrosine kinases (RTKs) are most frequently involved in carcinogenesis. These transmembrane receptors are further involved in triggering a multitude of signaling cascades that ultimately result in activation of prosurvival oncogenes, such as X-linked inhibitor of apoptosis protein (XIAP), myeloid cell leukemia sequence 1 (Mcl-1), survivin, and B cell lymphoma protein-2 (Bcl-2). Additionally, RTKs promote the inactivation of the proapoptotic genes, such as Forkhead box O (FOXO), further promoting cell proliferation, survival, and cell cycle progression [41,42]. The major signaling pathways implicated in the pathogenesis of lung cancer include RAF/MEK/ERK, PI3K/Akt/mTOR, and JAK/STAT signaling. The detailed role of these pathways is presented in the present section.

3.1. RAS/RAF/MEK/ERK Pathway

The RAF/MEK/ERK signal transduction pathway is a major player involved in cell proliferation, apoptosis, and senescence [43,44] and has been shown to be an active participant in both NSCLC [45] and SCLC [46]. RAS encodes a G protein with guanosine triphosphatase activity [47] and acts as a crucial scaffold between the cell surface receptors and various downstream signaling pathways responsible for cell survival and cell proliferation. These cell surface receptors include EGFR and fibroblast growth factor receptor (FGFR). Downstream signaling cascades include the PI3K/Akt/mTOR pathway; RAS/RAF/MEK/ERK pathway [48]; and Ras-like (Ral) guanine nucleotide exchange factors (GEFs)/Ral [49]. Upon binding of growth factors to their respective receptors, RAS is activated with the aid of the growth factor receptor-bound protein 2 (Grb2)/son of sevenless (SOS) coupling complex [50]. RAS then undergoes a conformational change, binds GTP, and further recruits RAF (A-RAF, B-RAF, or RAF-1). Upon binding to the cell membrane, RAF undergoes dimerization, allowing removal of the inhibitory actions of RAF kinase. RAF further associates with proteins such as heat shock protein 90 (HSP90) which aids in stabilizing the RAF dimer [49]. RAF dimer then triggers phosphorylation–activation of downstream MEK (MEK1 or MEK2), which activates ERK (ERK1 or ERK2). ERK undergoes dimerization and translocates to the nucleus to regulate the transcription of genes like c-Fos, c-Jun, c-Myc, CREB, MSK, and ELK-1. These genes are crucial regulators of cell cycle progression and proliferation.

Mutations in KRAS, Harvey rat sarcoma virus (HRAS), and neuroblastoma rat sarcoma viral oncogene homolog (NRAS) oncoproteins of the RAS superfamily have been reported in various cases of NSCLC. Amongst these genes, KRAS is the most frequently mutated, primarily in adenocarcinomas and to a lesser extent in squamous cell carcinoma [48]. Contrarily, KRAS mutations are a rare finding in SCLC [38]. Missense mutation resulting in replacement of glycine with cysteine at codon 12 (KRAS G12C mutation) is the most commonly recorded mutation of KRAS in NSCLC. KRAS mutations are strongly associated with smoking [47]. Unlike KRAS mutations, mutations in BRAF are less frequent and usually found in NSCLC patients who are non-smokers [51].

3.2. PI3K/Akt/mTOR Pathway

The PI3K/Akt/mTOR pathway is chiefly responsible for the development and exacerbation of lung cancers. PI3K/Akt/mTOR signal transduction is initiated upon binding of growth factors to the cell surface receptor tyrosine kinases (RTKs). These RTKs include vascular endothelial growth factor receptor (VEGFR), human epidermal growth factor receptor-2 (HER2), insulin-like growth factor receptor (IGFR), epidermal growth factor receptor (EGFR), and platelet-derived growth factor receptor (PDGFR). This ligand–receptor binding triggers localization of PI3K to the plasma membrane via the p85 (regulatory) subunit of PI3K, which binds to the RTK. This is followed by phosphorylation and dimerization of PI3K. Upon binding of the regulatory p85 subunit, the p110 (catalytic) subunit of PI3K is exposed. This p110 subunit then catalyzes the formation of phosphatidylinositol 3,4,5-trisphosphate (PIP3) upon phosphorylation of phosphatidylinositol 4,5-bisphosphate (PIP2). PIP3 serves as a secondary messenger and commences the recruitment of Akt to plasma membrane and its phosphorylation and activation by 3-phosphoinositide-dependent kinase 1 (PDK1) and subsequently by mTOR complex-2. This phosphorylation and activation of Akt results in the dissociation of Akt from the plasma membrane into the cytoplasm where it serves as a crucial mediator of cell proliferation, growth, and survival. Akt produces these effects by phosphorylating and activating downstream effector proteins like mTOR complex-1, 4E-binding protein 1 (4EBP1), and p70S6 kinase 1 (p70S6K). Akt also upregulates prosurvival proteins like X-linked inhibitor of apoptosis protein (XIAP) and Bcl-2 and downregulates proapoptotic proteins, fostering cancer progression and exacerbation. Normally, this is kept in check by phosphatase and tensin homolog (PTEN) tumor suppressor protein in healthy cells, which inhibits the activation of Akt by negatively regulating PIP3, thus halting the PI3K/Akt/mTOR signaling cascade [41,52,53]. But, the PI3K/Akt/mTOR signaling pathway has been reported to be majorly dysregulated in NSCLC [54,55]. This has been witnessed to be the outcome of inactivating mutations of PTEN [56,57]. Also, overexpression of PIK3CA has been reported to be a major driving event in NSCLC development and progression [58–61]. Over activity of the p110α catalytic subunit of PIP3 as a result of activating mutations majorly in the helical and kinase domain of the PIK3CA gene was found to be a main culprit in lung cancer progression [62].

3.3. *JAK-STAT Pathway*

Janus kinase of the JAK-STAT pathway is constitutively present intracellularly in association with the transmembrane receptors such as interleukin-6 receptor, granulocyte colony-stimulating factor receptor, and erythropoietin receptor [63]. JAK proteins (JAK1-3, tyrosine kinase-2) possess four functional domains, including the FERM domain which serves as a binding site to bind to the receptors; the SH2 unit to bind to phosphorylated tyrosine residues; a phosphorylating JH1 domain; and a regulatory JH2 unit [63,64]. STAT proteins (STAT1-4, STAT5A, STAT5B, and STAT6) possess an N-terminal domain that promotes dimerization for binding to transcription factors; a regulatory coiled-coil domain; DNA-binding domain; an SH2 domain to bind to phosphorylated tyrosine residues; a linker domain that links the DNA-binding domain to the SH2 domain; and a transcription–activation domain [64]. Upon binding of a ligand to the extracellular domain of the JAK-associated receptor, receptor dimerization and conformational changes lead to phosphorylation and activation of JAK. Activated JAK then phosphorylates the tyrosine residues in the intracellular domains of the bound receptor that recruits STAT and induces its phosphorylative activation. STAT, upon activation, dissociates and dimerizes through its SH2 domain and translocate to the nucleus where it regulates the transcription of numerous target genes [63,64] involved in cell proliferation, differentiation, inflammation, and apoptosis [65,66].

The JAK-STAT pathway is kept under check by regulatory proteins. Protein inhibitor of activated STAT (PIAS) blocks STAT-mediated transcription of target genes by inhibiting STAT–DNA interaction. Protein tyrosine phosphatase (PTP) promotes dephosphorylation inactivation of the tyrosine residues of the receptor, JAK, and STAT, whereas suppressor of cytokine signaling (SOCS) is involved in blocking binding sites for STAT at the receptor, in addition to promoting proteasomal degradation of STAT via ubiquitination [63–65,67].

3.4. NRF2-KEAP1-ARE Pathway

The nuclear factor erythroid 2-related factor 2 (NRF2)–Kelch-like ECH-associated protein 1 (KEAP1)–antioxidant responsive elements (AREs) pathway is basically a protective measure of the cells against reactive oxygen species (ROS) and electrophilic stress signals [68]. NRF2 is a redox regulator from the basic leucine zipper protein family, whereas KEAP1 is an adaptor protein. Under normal conditions, NRF2 undergoes ubiquitination through interaction with Cullin-3 carrying a ubiquitin E3 ligase complex mediated through a KEAP1 scaffold. This marks NRF2 for proteasomic degradation. Under conditions of oxidative and electrophilic stress, KEAP1 sequestration of NRF2 is halted, and released NRF2 then translocates to the nucleus [68,69]. In the nucleus, NRF2 mediates the upregulation of antioxidant and cytoprotective genes by binding to AREs [68–70]. Constitutive activation of NRF2 leads to oncogenesis via activation of Myc, KRAS, PI3K, and BRAF oncogenes [69]. Moreover, NRF2-regulated production of antioxidants, such as glutathione reductase, glutathione S-transferase, and glutathione and glutathione peroxidase, confers chemoresistance to cancer cells [71] against anticancer drugs, including cisplatin via thiol-cisplatin adduct-mediated inactivation of cisplatin [72]. Apart from cell proliferation, NRF2 also mediates cellular motility and invasion by dysregulating the mediator of cellular contractility RhoA/Rho-associated coiled-coil-forming kinase (ROCK1) signaling [73]. Mutations resulting in gain of function of NRF2 [26,74] and loss of functions of KEAP1 resulting in higher levels of free NRF2 have been witnessed in NSCLC and mediate metastasis [74,75] and metabolic remodeling in lung cancer cells [76].

3.5. PD-1/PD-L1 Pathway

The programmed cell death protein-1 (PD-1)/programmed cell death ligand-1 (PD-L1) signaling pathway in lung cancer cells is a form of immunosuppressive signaling which helps to null the T cell response against lung cancer cells [77]. The PD-1 receptor and its ligand, PD-L1, are transmembrane proteins expressed on the surface of immune cells, such as T cells, B cells, and antigen-presenting cells [78,79]. PD-L1 is frequently expressed on the surface of malignant cells. Physiological binding of PD-L1 to PD-1 on an activated T cell results in phosphorylative activation of the PD-1, which causes suppression of PI3/Akt signaling in T cells [80]. This inactivation of the PI3K/Akt signaling pathway further downregulates prosurvival proteins, such as Bcl-xL, and results in apoptosis of T cells, thus sparing cancer cells from immune intervention [81].

4. Potential Therapeutic Targets for Lung Cancer

A surge of potential therapeutic targets of lung cancer such as ALK, EGFR, BRAF, c-Ros oncogene 1 (ROS1) [82], MET, and RET came to light in the last decade [83]. EGFR is a receptor tyrosine kinase which possesses an extracellular ligand-binding domain [84,85], with its major ligands being epidermal growth factor and transforming growth factor alpha [84], and a cytoplasmic domain rich in tyrosine residues. These two domains are linked by a transmembrane scaffold. Upon ligand-mediated stimulation, EGFR undergoes dimerization and a conformational change conferring autophosphorylation of its intracellular tyrosine residues. This triggers signal transduction through the RAS/RAF/MEK/ERK pathway, or PI3K/Akt/mTOR pathway, or through stimulation of STAT [86,87] which is implicated in cell proliferation and inhibition of apoptosis [86]. After discovering the link between NSCLC and mutations in EGFR, small molecule tyrosine kinase inhibitors were developed and are currently being utilized for targeted therapy in EGFR mutant-positive cases [84]. The most frequently encountered EGFR mutations in NSCLC include substitution of leucine for arginine at codon 858 of exon 21 (L858R), as well as exon 19 deletions [87,88]. A wide repertoire of receptor, signaling, and effector proteins in these pathways serve as potential targets in the treatment of lung cancer [89].

Yet another valuable target for lung cancer is ALK. Like EGFR, ALK is also a tyrosine kinase receptor belonging to the insulin receptor family [90]. In NSCLC, ALK is basically present as a fusion kinase, with ALK being the cytoplasmic domain of the transmembrane receptor rich in tyrosine residues. The extracellular domain consists of the echinoderm microtubule-associated protein-like 4 (EML4) [91–93]. Even without stimulation by ligands, this fusion complex undergoes dimerization and autophosphorylation in a manner identical to receptor-bound EGFR. This phosphorylation activation then triggers a signaling cascade through either the RAS/RAF/MEK/ERK pathway, PI3K/Akt/mTOR pathway, or JAK-STAT pathways, or by phospholipase C-γ stimulation which mediates ALK-triggered cell proliferation and survival [90]. Similar ligand-independent signaling in NSCLC tumorigenesis has been witnessed with RET mutations, another tyrosine kinase receptor and novel target for NSCLC treatment. RET is reported to be associated with chimeric kinase protein resulting in an auto-triggering fusion complex, alike to that witnessed with ALK in NSCLC [94].

Another potential target for lung cancer treatment is MET. This oncogene encodes for receptor tyrosine kinase (RTK), which triggers a multitude of signaling cascades, including the PI3K/Akt/mTOR pathway, MAPK/ERK pathway, and JAK/STAT transduction pathway. Although these signaling cascades require ligand-mediated stimulation of the RTK receptor under normal conditions, activating mutations such as METex-14 abolish this prerequisite [82]. Accordingly, MET inhibitors are currently being explored as targeted therapies mitigating lung cancer.

In addition to signaling molecules, microRNAs are emerging as mediators of either tumorigenesis or tumor suppression. They serve as crucial biomarkers as well as therapeutic targets for lung cancers [95]. Certain microRNAs, like microRNA-148a-3p, microRNA-129-5p, and microRNA-218-5p, have been shown to be associated with the radiosensitivity of NSCLC cells. MicroRNA-148a-3p has emerged as a crucial target in catering to patients with radiation-resistant NSCLC; upregulation of microRNA-148a-3p is proposed to enhance radiosensitivity [96]. Also, microRNA-148a-3p acts as a tumor suppressor. It inhibits salt overly sensitive2 (SOS2) and thus prevents the activation of RAS, further obstructing tumor progression [95].

5. Current Therapeutic Strategies for Mitigating Lung Cancer and Associated Adversities

The choice of treatment for NSCLC is surgical resection in patients without comorbidities or radiation therapy in patients with existing comorbidities [97]. Additionally, surgery is limited to early-stage lung cancer patients and the majority of the advanced cases are treated either with chemotherapy or radiotherapy or concurrent chemo- and radiotherapy. Radiation therapy, however, is damaging to non-cancerous cells in the vicinity, which may result in side effects like esophagitis, pneumonitis [98], and compromised lung functionality [99]. Surgical options like pneumonectomy are associated with postoperative pulmonary hypertension, acute respiratory distress syndrome (ARDS), and mortality, which was reported to be 8.5% amongst the 294 patients of malignant lung cancer subjected to pneumonectomy in a study carried out by Daffré and colleagues [100]. For both limited and extensive SCLC, platinum-based combination chemotherapy is the first line of treatment [97,101], although lobectomy and radiotherapy are also employed in mitigating limited SCLC [102]. However, given the associated risks and limited response, benefits of surgical resection in the management of SCLC are subject to debate [101].

A multitude of chemotherapeutic agents are available for treating lung cancer (Table 1). The drug combinations cisplatin and paclitaxel, cisplatin and docetaxel, cisplatin and gemcitabine, and carboplatin and paclitaxel are commonly employed for the treatment of NSCLC. Each of these combinations has similar efficacy against NSCLC and is proven to enhance life expectancy by as much as 1 to 2 years. The combination carboplatin and paclitaxel, however, is generally preferred over other options due to its relatively low toxicity [103]. For SCLC, etoposide in combination with either carboplatin or cisplatin is preferred [104].

Table 1. Currently available drugs for lung cancer treatment.

Drug/Chemical Moiety	Mechanism of Action	Dose, Frequency, and Route	References
Gemcitabine	Inhibits ribonucleotide reductase resulting in inhibition of DNA synthesis	1000 mg/m^2, weekly, i.v.	[105–107]
Docetaxel	Binds to tubulin protein of microtubules, promotes its polymerization and stabilization, resulting in cell arrest in G2/M phase	75 mg/m^2, daily, i.v.	[108,109]
Carboplatin	Forms adducts with purine bases, resulting in inhibition of DNA replication and subsequent apoptosis of cancer cells owing to damaged DNA	25 mg/m^2, daily, i.v.	[110,111]
Cisplatin	Forms adducts with purine, resulting in inhibition of DNA replication and subsequent apoptosis of cancer cells owing to damaged DNA	75 mg/m^2, daily, i.v.	[108,110]
Trametinib	Inhibits MEK 1/2, resulting in obstruction of the RAS/RAF/MEK/ERK oncogenic pathway and cell cycle arrest	2 mg, daily, orally	[112,113]
Dabrafenib	Inhibits of RAF, resulting in obstruction of the RAS/RAF/MEK/ERK oncogenic pathway and cell cycle arrest	150 mg, twice daily, orally	[112,113]
Atezolizumab	Reverses immunosuppression within the tumor by blocking PD-L1 by binding to its receptor	1200 mg, every 3 weeks, orally	[114,115]
Pembrolizumab	Reverses immunosuppression within the tumor by blocking PD-L1 by binding to its receptor	250 mg, every 3 weeks, orally	[116]
Nivolumab	Reverses immunosuppression within the tumor by blocking PD-L1 by binding to its receptor	240 mg, every 2 weeks, orally	[117]
Selumitinib	Inhibits MEK 1/2, resulting in obstruction of the RAS/RAF/MEK/ERK oncogenic pathway and cell cycle arrest	75 mg, twice daily, orally	[118,119]
Navitoclax (ABT-263)	Blocks binding of Bcl-2 and BCL-XL to BIM, halting the antiapoptotic outcome	150 mg, daily, orally	[37,118,120]
Selpercatinib	Inhibits multiple altered RET kinase isoforms, thus inhibiting oncogenic signaling	20 mg, twice daily, orally	[94,121]
Crizotinib	Induces apoptosis in tumor cells and produces G1/S phase arrest by inhibiting ALK, MET, and ROS1 and downregulating JAK and STAT	250 mg, twice daily, orally	[66,122,123]
Alectinib	Induces apoptosis in tumor cells by inhibiting ALK	300 mg, twice daily, orally	[124]
Ceritinib	Inhibits ALK tyrosine kinase	400 mg, daily orally	[125,126]
Ensartinib	Inhibits ALK tyrosine kinase and oncogenic triggers from MET, ROS1, SLK, ABL, LTK, anexelekto (Axl), and EPHA2	225 mg, daily orally	[127–129]
Bevacizumab	Inhibits VEGF, resulting in angiogenesis	15 mg/kg, every three weeks, i.v.	[130,131]

Table 1. *Cont.*

Drug/Chemical Moiety	Mechanism of Action	Dose, Frequency, and Route	References
Buparlisib	Inhibits PI3K, resulting in downregulation of PI3K/Akt/mTOR signaling and downstream cancer cell proliferation and angiogenesis	100 mg/day, orally	[132,133]
Cabozantinib	Inhibits c-MET, RET, and VEGFR2 tyrosine kinase receptors, thus obstructing the stimulation of downstream signaling molecules involved in tumor proliferation and angiogenesis	60 mg, daily, orally	[134,135]
Capmatinib	Inhibits c-MET, thus obstructing the stimulation of downstream signaling molecules involved in tumor proliferation	400 mg, twice daily, orally	[136]
Erlotinib	Inhibits EGFR tyrosine kinase, resulting in obstruction of cancer cell proliferation by arresting cells in G0/G1 phase of cell cycle	150 mg, daily, orally	[84,137]
Gefitinib	Inhibits EGFR tyrosine kinase blocking oncogenic signals from EGFR-activating mutations	250 mg, daily, orally	[137]
Afatinib	Inhibits EGFR tyrosine kinase blocking oncogenic signals from EGFR-activating mutations	40 mg, daily, orally	[138]
Rociletinib	Inhibits EGFR tyrosine kinase blocking oncogenic signals from EGFR-activating mutations	625 mg, twice daily, orally	[139,140]
Cetuximab	EGFR inhibition and downregulation, antibody-mediated and complement-mediated cytotoxicity in lung cancer cells	400 mg/m^2 loading dose followed by 250 mg/m^2 dose weekly, i.v.	[141]
Emibetuzumab	Inhibits ligand-dependent and ligand-independent MET oncogenic signaling	750 mg, every two weeks, orally	[88]
Napabucasin	Inhibits STAT3 and promotes its downregulation, resulting in the inhibition of oncogenic transducer signaling and triggering apoptosis	240 mg, twice daily, orally	[142,143]

Abbreviations: ABL, Abelson murine leukemia viral oncogene; ALK, anaplastic lymphoma kinase; Axl, anexelekto; Bcl-2, B cell lymphoma 2; BCL-XL, B cell lymphoma-extra-large; BIM, Bcl-2-interacting mediator of cell death; c-MET, c-mesenchymal–epithelial transition factor; EGFR, epidermal growth factor receptor; EPHA2, ephrin type-A receptor 2; ERK, extracellular signal-related kinase; JAK, Janus kinase; LTK, leukocyte receptor tyrosine kinase; MEK, mitogen-activated protein kinase; MET, mesenchymal–epithelial transition factor; mTOR, mammalian target of rapamycin; PD-L1, programmed death ligand-1; PI3K, phosphatidylinositol 3-kinase; RAS, rat sarcoma virus gene; RAF, rapidly accelerated fibrosarcoma; RET, rearranged during transfection; ROS1, c-Ros oncogene 1; SLK, Ste20-like kinase; STAT, signal transducer and activator of transcription; STAT3, signal transducer and activator of transcription 3; VEGF, vascular endothelial growth factor; VEGFR2, vascular endothelial growth factor receptor 2.

Chemotherapy with platinum coordination complexes, such as cisplatin, has been proven to be efficacious in completely resected and excision repair cross-complementation group 1 (ERCC1) protein-negative NSCLC [144]. ERCC1 is a major player involved in repairing cisplatin–DNA complexes [145]. A prolonged survival rate was witnessed when cisplatin plus gemcitabine was given in ERCC1-negative advanced NSCLC. As mentioned above, platinum coordination complexes such as carboplatin and cisplatin, as well as etoposide, are mainstay treatments of SCLC [146]. These compounds have been shown to be highly efficacious in mitigating limited SCLC when combined with thoracic radiation. Despite being first-line treatment against SCLC, a high relapse rate and high overall mortality are seen [147]. Apart from this, all platinum-based anticancer agents pose a risk of causing adverse effects ranging from anorexia, vomiting, diarrhea, alopecia, and stomatitis to ototoxicity [110,148], as well as hepatotoxicity, nephrotoxicity, cardiotoxicity, neurotoxicity, myelosuppression [149], and anaphylaxis [150].

Bevacizumab, a recombinant humanized monoclonal antibody targeting vascular endothelial growth factor (VEGF), has shown promising outcomes in the survival of patients with non-squamous NSCLC when given alone or in combination with platinum-based chemotherapy [151,152]. Bevacizumab is associated with increased risk of developing hypertension, pulmonary hemorrhage, and thromboembolism [35,130]. Cetuximab, a chimeric monoclonal antibody against EGFR, not only blocks EGFR–ligand interaction, but also promotes the internalization and degradation of EGFR, resulting in its downregulation [141]. It is employed for the treatment of advanced NSCLC. Yet another category of drugs that target EGFR include gefitinib, erlotinib, and rociletinib. These drugs act by inhibiting EGFR tyrosine kinase [85]. All agents within this class of EGFR-targeting drugs have been reported to put patients at risk of skin rashes and diarrhea [141,153]. Gefitinib is also known to cause appetite loss, anemia, and sensory neuropathy [154], whereas rociletinib is prone to cause QT prolongation and hyperglycemia [139].

Targeted therapies for mitigating mutation-associated malignancies have been introduced lately. Concurrent administration of dabrafenib (150 mg, twice daily, orally) and trametinib (2 mg, daily, orally) have been approved by the United States Food and Drug Administration (FDA) for treating BRAF V600E mutation-positive metastatic NSCLC. An open-label, multicenter, and multicohort trial of 93 patients found this combination to be effective, but not free of adverse effects. Dabrafenib–trametinib combination therapy has been reported to cause vomiting, diarrhea, pyrexia, dyspnea, edema, and hemorrhage [112]. It is also associated with an increase in alanine aminotransferase and aspartate aminotransferase, as witnessed in phase II trials [155]. In addition to trametinib, other MEK1/2 inhibitors are undergoing trials for the treatment of lung cancer. One of these compounds is selumetinib (75 mg, twice daily, orally), which was reported to be efficacious in treating *KRAS* mutation-positive advanced NSCLC when paired with docetaxel but failed to promote survival in lung cancer patients in phase III trials [119,156].

Sotorasib recently received FDA approval in May 2021 for use in *KRAS* G12C mutation-associated NSCLC [157]. It has been reported to be clinically effective and safe at a tested dose of 960 mg, daily in phase II trials carried out on 126 patients with KRAS G12C mutation-positive NSCLC [158]. Atezolizumab, a monoclonal antibody against programmed death ligand-1 (PD-L1), has shown highly promising outcomes in enhancing survival rates in patients with metastatic lung cancer with EGFR or ALK aberrations and PD-L1 expression, as well as in resected patients diagnosed with stage II or IIIA NSCLC [114]. Similar survival outcomes have also been witnessed for pembrolizumab, yet another approved monoclonal antibody against PD-L1 [116]. Adversities encountered with atezolizumab and pembrolizumab range from pruritis, cough, pyrexia, and gastrointestinal disturbances like vomiting and diarrhea to peripheral edema, dyspnea, and anemia [116,159].

ALK inhibitors like alectinib, brigatinib, ceritinib, and lorlatinib are first-line therapies in advanced ALK-positive NSCLC [160]. Crizotinib is another an inhibitor of ALK phosphorylation which also inhibits c-MET [123] and ROS1 [122]. Crizotinib has received "breakthrough" designation for its remarkable outcomes in NSCLC with METex-14 mutations [161] but has also been reported to cause serious visual impairment [162], hepatotoxicity [163], bradycardia [164], hypogonadism in males [165], and gastrointestinal disturbances [123].

Other treatment options for lung cancer exist, including chemotherapeutic and radiotherapeutic options. A STAT3 inhibitor, napabucasin, has been shown to exhibit synergism with paclitaxel in promoting tumor regression and patient survival in extensively pretreated NSCLC. Reported side effect include diarrhea and hyponatremia [142]. Lung cancer is often treated using a combination of external beam radiation therapy with adjuvant chemotherapy. However, brachytherapy has emerged as a better therapeutic strategy compared to external beam radiation due to its ability to deliver a higher dose of radiation with greater precision, thereby sparing more healthy tissue [166,167].

6. Literature Search and Selection Process

The Preferred Reporting Items for Systematic Reviews and Meta-Analyses (PRISMA) criteria [168,169] for methodical reviews were employed when evaluating literature. Searches were conducted in PubMed using keywords and phrases to identify relevant articles. Search criteria consisted of combinations of the following words and phrases: lung cancer; lung carcinoma; phytochemicals; cell metabolism; phenolics; terpenoids; alkaloids; sulfur-containing compounds; secondary metabolites; prevention; treatment. Following identification, articles were evaluated for their content. Reviews and letters, articles not in English, and those concerning phytochemicals outside the context of lung cancer were excluded. Additionally, weak methodology articles and those with little relevance or limited presentation of findings were excluded. A breakdown of the article selection process according to the PRISMA guidelines is represented in Figure 3.

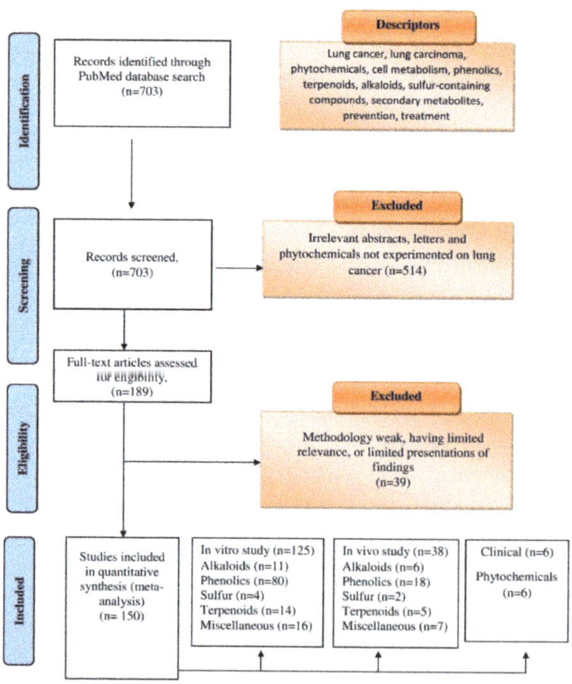

Figure 3. PRISMA flowchart detailing the selection process for included studies. The total quantity of in vitro, in vivo, and clinical experiments (169) is larger than the number of unique studies included in this systematic analysis (150) because several publications contain more than one type of experiment.

7. Anticancer Potential of Bioactive Phytocompounds in Lung Cancer

7.1. Preclinical Studies

Plant secondary metabolites are considered safe and effective in the treatment of cancer [170] and act primarily by modulation of numerous signaling pathways [171] Phytochemicals may be classified into four broad groups, such as alkaloids, phenolics, sulfur-containing compounds, and terpenoids. In the recent past, various in vitro and in vivo studies were conducted to elucidate the role of plant phytocompounds in the context lung cancer which are presented in the following subsections.

7.1.1. Alkaloids

Alkaloids represent a large group of organic compounds distinguished by their nitrogen-containing structures. They are present in a wide variety of plants and are known for their cancer preventive and anticancer activities [172]. Their wide-ranging biological activities have prompted extensive research into their potential therapeutic applications in drug discovery and development [173].

Acutiaporberine

Acutiaporberine (Figure 4) is a bisalkaloid derived from *Thalictrum acutifolium*. Very limited research has been conducted on acutiaporberine since its discovery approximately 20 years ago. In one such study, researchers determined that application of acutiaporberine to 95-D lung cancer cells resulted in upregulation of apoptosis (Table 2). The researchers reported these effects to be mediated by enhancing the Bak/Bcl-2 ratio [174].

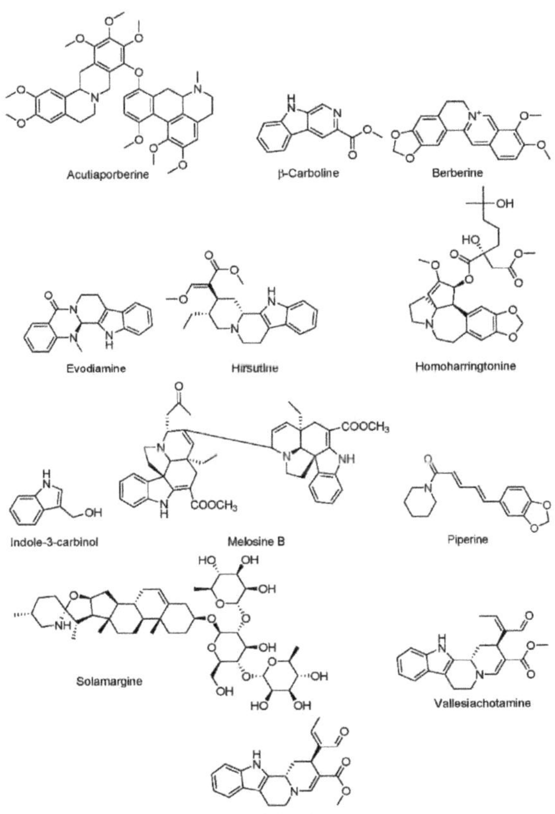

Figure 4. Chemical structures of alkaloids with anticancer activity in lung cancer.

Table 2. In vitro studies of plant-based bioactive compounds in lung cancer.

Phytochemicals	Cell Lines	Conc.	IC_{50}	Anticancer Effect	Mechanisms	References
			Alkaloids			
Acutiaporberine	95-D	0.003 μM	Not reported	Increased cell death	↑Bak/Bcl-2 ratio	[174]
β-Carboline	A549	1.80 μM	Not reported	Showed cytotoxic activity	↑ERK1/2; ↓Akt/mTOR	[175]
Berberine	A549 and H1299	25, 50, 75, and 100 μM	Not reported	Suppressed tumor cell growth and increased cell death	↓Bcl-2; ↑caspase-3; ↑Bax	[176]
Homoharringtonine	A549 and H1975	2–4 μM	3.7 μM(A549) and 0.7 μM (H1975)	Inhibited tumor cell metastasis	↓JAK1/STAT3	[177]
	A549 and H1299	2 μM	Not reported	Inhibited tumor cell growth and metastasis	↓KRAS; ↓ERK; ↓Akt; ↓STAT3; ↓CDK4; ↓CDK6; ↓p21; ↓RB	[178]
Indole-3-carbinol	H1299	400 μM	449.5 μM	Increased cell death and oxidative stress	↑ROS; ↑caspase-3; ↑caspase-7; ↑caspase-9; ↓Bcl-2	[179]
Melosine B	A549	0.064, 0.32, 1.6, 8, and 40 μM	8.1 μM	Exhibited cytotoxicity and increased cell death	Not reported	[180]
Piperine	A549	50, 100, and 200 μg/mL	122 μg/mL	Inhibited tumor cell growth	↑Bax/Bcl-2 ratio; ↑caspase-3; ↑caspase-9	[181]
	A549	20, 40, 80, 160, and 320 μM	198 μM	Inhibited tumor cell migration and invasion	↓ERK 1/2; ↓SMAD 2; ↓TGF-β	[182]
Solamargine	H1650, H1975, PC9, A549, and H1299	2, 4, and 6 μM	Not reported	Reduced tumor cell growth and increased DNA damage	↑ERK1/2; ↓prostaglandin E2; ↓DNMT1; ↓c-Jun	[183]
Vallesiachotamine and iso-vallesiachotamine	H1299	12.5, 25, 50, 100, and 200 μM	4.24 μM (vallesiachotamine) and 3.79 μM (iso-vallesiachotamine)	Suppressed tumor cell growth and caused DNA damage	↑Apoptosis	[184]
			Phenolics			
Acacetin	A549	1–5 μM	Not reported	Decreased tumor cell growth and viability	↓Activator protein-1; ↓NF-κB; ↓MLK3; ↓MAPK3/6; ↓p38a; ↓MAPK	[185]
Apocynin	A549	50–1000 μM	890 μM	Decreased tumor cell growth and enhanced cell death	↓Cellular microtubule network	[186]
Baicalein	A549 and H1299	2.5, 10, and 40 μM	Not reported	Reduced tumor cell growth, metastasis, and invasion	↓Cellular ezrin S-nitrosylation	[187]
Batatasin III	H460	25–100 μM	Not reported	Inhibited tumor cell migration and invasion	↓EMT; ↓N-cadherin; ↓vimentin; ↓Akt; ↑E-cadherin	[188]
Caffeic acid	A549	50–1000 μM	Not reported	Reduced tumor cell growth	↓Superoxide level	[189]
Cardamonin	A549 and H460	40 μM	Not reported	Decreased tumor cell growth and increased cell death	↑Caspase-3; ↑Bcl-2; ↑Bax; ↑cyclin D1; ↓CDK4; ↓PI3K; ↓Akt; ↓mTOR	[190]
Cardamonin	A549	0.1, 1, 10, and 30 μM	Not reported	Reduced tumor cell growth and enhanced cell death	↓mTOR; ↓DNA synthesis; ↓p70S6K	[191]

Table 2. *Cont.*

Phytochemicals	Cell Lines	Conc.	IC_{50}	Anticancer Effect	Mechanisms	References
Cardamonin analogs	A549 and NCI-H460	0.05–100 μM	0.445 μM (DHC) and 0.166 μM (DHMC)	Inhibited tumor cell growth	↓NF-κB	[192]
Casticin	A549	1, 5, 10 μM	14.3 μM	Suppressed tumor cell growth and enhanced cell death	↓IL-6; ↓COX-2; ↓MAPK; ↓NF-κB; ↓p65; ↓chemokine gene	[193,194]
Chrysin	A549	25, 50, and 75 μg/mL	55.72 μg/mL	Inhibited tumor cell growth and increased cell death	↑Bax; ↓Bcl-2; ↑caspase-3	[195]
Curcumin	A549	10 μM	Not reported	Decreased tumor cell growth and enhanced cell death	↓Prosurvival antiapoptotic factors; ↓EGFR	[196]
	A-549	10–50 μM	Not reported	Caused DNA damage and G2/M phase cell cycle arrest	↑Caspase-3-induced apoptosis; ↑DNA damage; ↑ER stress	[197]
	NCI-H460	30 μM	Not reported	Suppressed tumor cell growth and enhanced cell death	↑Caspase-3; ↑caspase-8; ↓cyclin-dependent kinase 1	[198]
	CL1-5	1–20 μM	Not reported	Inhibited tumor cell growth and metastasis	↑Activator protein-1; ↓E-cadherin;	[199]
	PC-9	50 μM	Not reported	Enhanced DNA damage, cell death and suppressed tumor cell growth	↑DNA damage; ↓Bcl-2; ↓cyclin D1; ↓CDK2; ↓CDK4; ↓CDK6	[200]
	NCI-H292	5–40 μM	15 μM	Increased cell death and inhibited tumor cell growth	↑Bax; ↑caspase-3; ↑caspase-7	[201]
p-Coumaric acid	A549, NCI-H1299, and HCC827	10–100 μg/mL	37.73 μg/mL (A549); 50.6 μg/mL (H1299); 62.0 μg/mL (HCC827)	Increased cell death	↑Bax; ↓Bcl-2; ↑caspase-3; ↑caspase-9	[202]
	H1993	50–100 μM	Not reported	Reduced tumor cell growth and viability	↓Resistance of tyrosine kinase inhibitor	[203]
EGCG	A549 and H1299	20–300 μM	86.4 μM (A549) and 80.6 μM (H1299)	Inhibited tumor cell proliferation and induced apoptosis	↓NF-κB	[204]
	H1299 and CL-13	10–100 μM	174.9 μM(H1299) and 181.5 μM (CL-13)	Reduced tumor cell proliferation	↑ROS; ↓ NF-κB	[205]
	A549	10, 25, 50, and 100 μM	Not reported	Decreased tumor cell growth	↓Nicotine-induced Akt; ↓ERK1/2	[206]
	A549	12.5, 25, and 50 μM	25 μM	Suppressed tumor cell growth, invasion, migration and increased G2/M phase cell cycle arrest	↑Bax/Bcl-2 ratio	[207]
	A549	0.5 μM	Not reported	Decreased tumor cell growth and increased oxidative stress	↑ Nrf2; ↑ROS	[208]
	A549 and NCI-H23	0.05–500 μM	Not reported	Reduced etoposide resistance and tumor cell growth	↑Nrf2; ↑ROS;	[209]
	H1299, H460 and A549	40 μM	Not reported	Decreased tumor cell growth	↑miR-210	[210]
	H1299 and A549	10, 20, and 40 μM	Not reported	Induced apoptosis	↓PI3K/Akt	[211]
EGCG and luteolin	A549 and H460	30 μM (EGCG) and 10 μM (luteolin)	Not reported	Induced apoptosis	↑p53 mitochondrial translocation; ↑DNA damage	[212]

Table 2. *Cont.*

Phytochemicals	Cell Lines	Conc.	IC_{50}	Anticancer Effect	Mechanisms	References
EGCG and theaflavins	NCI-H460	100 μM	Not reported	Inhibited tumor cell proliferation and promoted apoptosis	↑p53; ↓Bcl-2	[213]
Ferulic acid	A549	50–1000 μM	Not reported	Enhanced oxidative stress and decreased cell viability	↓Superoxide anion	[189]
Fisetin	A549	5–20 μM	Not reported	Decreased cell viability and increased cell death	↓PI3K/Akt; ↓mTOR	[214]
	NCI-H460	75 μg/mL	Not reported	Inhibited tumor cell growth and viability	↓β-cell lymphoma-2; ↑Bcl-2; ↑caspase-9; ↑caspase-3	[215,216]
	HCC827-ER	10, 20, 40, 60, 80, 100, 120 μM	Not reported	Inhibited tumor cell growth, viability and increased cell death	↓Axl; ↓MAPK; ↓Akt	[217]
Gallic acid	Calu-6 and A549	10–200 μM	10–50 μM (Calu-6); 100–200 μM (A549)	Inhibited tumor cell growth and enhanced oxidative stress	↓GSH; ↑ROS	[218]
	H1975 and H1993	50 μM	Not reported	Increased cell death	↓Src-mediated STAT3; ↓Bcl-2; ↓cyclin D; ↓NF-κB; ↓IL-6	[219]
Genistein	A549	10 μM	Not reported	Inhibited tumor cell growth and enhanced cell death	↑Caspase-3	[220]
	H3255, H1650, and H178	25 μM	Not reported	Decreased tumor cell growth and increased cell death	↓DNA binding of NF-κB; ↓COX-2; ↓pAkt; ↓EGFR; ↓PGE2	[221]
	SPC-A-1	20–40 μM	Not reported	Reduced tumor cell growth and increased cell death	↓Bcl-2	[222]
	H460	15–30 μM	Not reported	Suppressed tumor cell growth and increased cell death	↓NF-κB	[223]
Gigantol	A549	25, 50, and 100 μM	Not reported	Inhibited tumor cell growth and increased cell death	↓Ki-67; ↓Bcl-2; ↑Bax; ↑Wnt/β-catenin	[224]
	H460	50 μM	Not reported	Increased tumor cell death	↓EMT	[225]
	H460	20–200 μM	Not reported	Reduced tumor cell proliferation, migration, and invasion	↓PI3K/Akt/mTOR; ↓JAK/STAT	[226]
Hesperidin	A549 and NCI-H358	5–50 μM	50 μM	Increased cell death	↑Apoptosis; ↑mitochondrial disruption; ↑caspase-3; ↑NF-κB	[227]
	H1993	5–100 μM	Not reported	Decreased cell viability and enhanced cell death	↓Resistance of tyrosine kinase inhibitor	[203]
Honokiol	A549 and 95-D	5, 10, or 20 μM	Not reported	Increased cell death	↑Bax; ↑caspase-9; ↑PERK; ↑ER stress; ↓Bcl-2	[228,229]
	A549 and LL/2	10–50 μM	21.1 μM	Reduced tumor cell growth and increased cell death	↓VEGF-A	[230]
Mono-demethylated polymethoxyflavones	H1299	1–30 μM	16.5 μM	Increased cell death	↓iNOS; ↓COX-2; ↓Mcl-1; ↑caspase-3; ↑PARP cleavage	[231]
Indolyl-chalcone derivatives	A549	2.5 μM and 5 μM	2.46 μM	Suppressed tumor cell growth	↑Nrf-2/HO-1	[232]

Table 2. *Cont.*

Phytochemicals	Cell Lines	Conc.	IC_{50}	Anticancer Effect	Mechanisms	References
Isorhamnetin	A549	8 μM and 16 μM	Not reported	Increased cell death and mitochondrial dysfunction	↑Caspase-3	[233]
	A549	25 μM	Not reported	Enhanced mitochondrial dysfunction, cell death and decreased tumor cell growth	↑Caspase-3; ↑PARP	[234]
Kaempferol	A549	10–140 μM	72 μM	Inhibited epithelial–mesenchymal transition and increased cell death	↑EMT; ↓E-cadherin; ↓vimentin	[235]
	A549	25 μM	Not reported	Inhibited tumor cell growth and viability	↓E-Cadherin; ↓vimentin ↓Akt1-mediated phosphorylation; ↓TGF-β1	[236]
	H460	30, 50, and 80 μM	50 μM	Enhanced oxidative stress and cell death	↑Caspase-3; ↑AIF	[237]
Kurarinone	H460	2 μg/mL	5.8 μg/mL	Inhibited tumor cell growth	↓NF-κB; ↓tyrosine kinase	[238]
	H1688 and H146	6.25, 12.5, and 25 μM	12.5 μM (H1688) and 30.4 μM (H146)	Enhanced cell death	↓EMT; ↓MMP-2	[239]
Luteolin	A549	20–80 μM	40.2 μM	Increased G2/M phase cell cycle arrest and cell death	↑Bax; ↑procaspase-9; ↑caspase-3; ↓NF-κB; ↑JNK	[240]
	A549	25–100 μM	42.8 μM	Decreased cell viability and increased cell death	↑Bax; ↑caspase-3; ↑caspase-9; ↑MEK/ERK; ↓Bcl-2	[241]
	A549 and H460	10–100 μM	40 μM	Inhibited tumor cell growth and increased cell death	↑miR-34a-5p via targeting MDM4	[242,243]
	NCI-H460	20–160 μM	Not reported	Decreased cell viability and increased cell death	↓Bad; ↓Bcl-2; ↑caspase-3; ↓Sirt1	[244]
Moscatilin	H460	1 μM	Not reported	Reduced tumor cell growth	↓ERK; ↓EMT; ↓Akt; ↓Cav-1	[245]
Naringenin	A549	25, 50, 100, 200, and 300 μM	Not reported	Reduced tumor cell growth	↓MMP-2; ↓MMP-9; ↓Akt	[246]
	A549	10, 100, and 200 μM	Not reported	Decreased tumor cell growth and enhanced cell death	↑Caspase-3; ↓MMP-3; ↓MMP-9; ↑p38	[247]
Nobiletin	A549 (adriamycin resistant)	50 μM	Not reported	Enhanced cell death	↑Caspase-3; ↓Akt; ↓GSK-3β; ↓β-catenin; ↓MRP1	[248]
Osthol	A549	25, 50, 100, 150, and 200 μM	Not reported	Increased G2/M phase cell cycle arrest and cell death	↑Bax; ↓cyclin B1; ↓p-Cdc2 ↓Bcl-2; ↓PI3K/Akt	[249]
	A549	40 and 80 μM	Not reported	Inhibited tumor cell growth, migration, and invasion	↓MMP-2; ↓MMP-9	[250,251]
	A549	5–80 μM	Not reported	Inhibited tumor cell growth and metastasis	↓TGF-β-induced EMT; ↓NF-κB; ↓Snail	[252]
Phloretin	A549, Calu-1 H838, and H520	25–75 μg/mL	Not reported	Enhanced cell death	↓Bcl-2; ↓MMP-2; ↓MMP-9; ↑caspase-3; ↑caspase-9	[253]
	A549	25, 50, 100, and 200 μM	Not reported	Inhibited tumor cell growth and increased cell death	↑Bax; ↓Bcl-2; ↑caspase-3; ↑caspase-9; ↑ERK; ↑JNK; ↑p38; ↑MAPK; ↑JNK1/2; ↓NF-κB	[254]

Table 2. *Cont.*

Phytochemicals	Cell Lines	Conc.	IC_{50}	Anticancer Effect	Mechanisms	References
Polydatin	A549 and NCI-H1975	50 μM	2.95 μM (A549) and 3.23 μM (NCI-H1975)	Reduced tumor cell growth and increased cell cycle arrest	↑Bak/Bcl-2 ratio	[255]
Pterostilbene	NCI-H460 and SK-MES-1	10–100 μM	Not reported	Decreased cell viability and increased cell death	↑Caspase-3; ↑caspase-7	[256]
Quercetin	A549	0.74–4.40 μM	1.41 μM	Decreased cell growth and increased cell death	↑Bax; ↓Bc1-2	[257]
Resveratrol	A549	20 μM	Not reported	Inhibited tumor cell growth and invasion	↓TGF-β1-induced EMT	[258]
	A549	4–64 μM	8.9 μM	Reduced tumor cell growth and increased cell death	↑Caspase-3	[259]
	H1993	1–10 μM	Not reported	Decreased cell viability and increased cell death	↓Resistance of tyrosine kinase inhibitor	[203]
Salicylic acid	A549	1.5–9.5 mM	6.0 mM	Showed cytotoxicity and suppressed tumor cell growth	Not reported	[260]
Tangeretin derivative	CL1-5, H1299, H226, and A549	2.5 and 5 μM	3.2 μM (CL1-5), 6.7 μM (H1299), 10.2 μM (H226), and 9.8 μM (A549)	Enhanced G2/M phase cell cycle arrest, cell death, mitochondrial dysfunction and reduced tumor cell growth	↑Caspase-3; ↓Bcl-2; ↓survivin; ↓PI3K/Akt/mTOR	[261]
Tatariside B, C, and D	A549	0.001, 0.01, 0.1, 1, 10, and 100 μg/mL	18.31 μg/mL (Tatariside B), 6.44–7.49 μg/mL (Tatariside C), and 2.83 μg/mL (Tatariside D)	Enhanced cytotoxicity, oxidative stress, cell death and reduced tumor cell growth	Not reported	[262]
			Sulfur-containing compounds			
Allicin	A549 and NCI-H460	10–60 μg/mL	25 μg/mL (A549) and 15 μg/mL (NCI-H460)	Inhibited tumor cell growth	↓Cadherin 2; ↑cadherin 1	[263]
Sulforaphane	H1299, 95-C and 95-D	1–5 μM	9.52 μM (H1299), 9.04 μM (95-C), and 17.35 μM (95-D)	Reduced tumor cell growth and increased S/G2–M phase cell cycle arrest	↓miR-616-5p levels; ↓GSK3β/β-catenin	[264]
	A549 and H1299	0, 5, 10, and 15 mM	Not reported	Inhibited tumor cell growth and enhanced G2/M cell cycle arrest	↑Apoptosis; ↓histone deacetylase	[265]
	A549	2.5 and 5 μM	Not reported	Suppressed tumor cell growth and increased G1/S cell cycle arrest	↓miR-21; ↓CDH1; ↓DNMTs	[266]
			Terpenoids			
Abietane diterpene	NCI-H460, and A549	10 and 30 μg/mL	14 μM (NCI-H460) and 30 μM (A549)	Enhanced cell death	↑Caspase-3; ↓caspase-9	[267]
β-Sitosterol	A549	50–200 μg/mL	95.19 μg/mL	Enhanced G2/M phase cell cycle arrest	↑Apoptosis	[268]
Cucurbitacin B	A549	10 μM	Not reported	Reduced tumor cell growth and increased cell death	↓CDK2; ↓CDK4; ↓cyclin D; ↓cyclin E; ↓mortalin; ↓hnRNP-K; ↓MMP-2; ↓fibronectin; ↑p53; ↑CARF	[269]
Dihydroartemisinin	PC-14	1 μg/mL	Not reported	Increased cell death	↑p38 MAPK; ↑Ca^{2+}	[270]
	LLC cells	5, 10, 20, and 40 μg/mL	26.98 μg/mL	Enhanced G0/G1 phase cell cycle arrest	↑p38 MAPK	[271]
	A549 and H1299	0.23–749.90 μM	80.89 uM	Reduced tumor cell growth	↓Transferrin receptor	[272]

Table 2. *Cont.*

Phytochemicals	Cell Lines	Conc.	IC_{50}	Anticancer Effect	Mechanisms	References
Oridonin	H1975	10 µM	Not reported	Decreased tumor cell metastasis and angiogenesis	↓Mesenchymal transition; ↑proapoptotic activity	[273]
	A549	10, 20, and 30 µM	Not reported	Reduced tumor cell metastasis and angiogenesis	↑Bax; ↑cisplatin-induced apoptosis via AMPK/Akt/mTOR; ↑PARP expression	[274]
Soyasapogenol	H-1299	2–10 µM	6 µM	Reduced tumor cell growth, metastasis and increased cell death	↓CDK2; ↓CDK4; ↓cyclin A; ↓cyclin D1; ↓pATR-Chk1 ↓catenin/vimentin/hnRNPK-mediated EMT	[275]
Thymoquinone	LNM35	1–100 µM	50–78 µM	Suppressed tumor cell growth and increased cell death	↑Caspase-3	[276]
Ursolic acid	A549	11, 22, 44, and 88 µM	Not reported	Decreased cell viability and enhanced autophagy	↑LC3-II/LC3-I ratio; ↑p62; ↑PINK1; ↑Nrf2; ↑ROS; ↓p-Akt/mTOR	[277]
	H1975	0.001–0.1 µM	Not reported	Reduced tumor cell growth and angiogenesis	↓N-cadherin; ↓MMP-2; ↓MMP-9; ↓TGF-β1; ↑E-cadherin	[278]
	A549, H460, H1975, H1299, H520, H82, LLC, and H446	5–40 µM	Not reported	Inhibited tumor cell growth and angiogenesis	↓Bcl-2; ↑cleaved PARP; ↑LC3-II; ↓p-S6K T389; ↓p-Akt	[279]
Withaferin A	A549	10 µM	Not reported	Increased cell death, oxidative stress and decreased cell viability	↑ROS	[280]
Miscellaneous compounds						
Cannabidiol	A549 and H460	3 µM	Not reported	Increased cell death	↑ICAM-1	[281,282]
	A549 and H460	1–10 µM	3.47 µM (A549) and 2.80 µM (H460)	Increased cell death	↑ICAM-1; ↑COX-2; ↑PPAR-γ	[283]
	A549	3 µM	Not reported	Enhanced cell death and reduced tumor cell growth	↑MMP-1	[284]
Cypripedin	H23	50 µM	Not reported	Suppressed tumor cell growth	↓N-cadherin; ↓vimentin; ↓Akt/GSK-3β	[285]
	H460	50 µM	Not reported	Inhibited tumor cell growth	↓Bcl-2	[286]
Daucosterol	A549	50–200 µg/mL	17.46 µg/mL	Reduced tumor cell growth and enhanced G2/M phase cell cycle arrest	↓Bcl-2; ↑Bax; ↑caspase-3	[268]
Emodin	A549 and H1299	20, 40, 60, and 80 µM	Not reported	Enhanced cell death	↑ER stress; ↑TRIB3/NF-κB	[287]
Glossogin	A549	12.5 µg/mL	Not reported	Suppressed tumor cell growth	↑Cyt c; ↑caspase-9; ↑caspase-3; ↑Bak/Bcl-2 ratio	[288]
Ouabain	A549 and H1975	25 nM	Not reported	Inhibited tumor cell growth	↑JNK; ↓Bcl-2	[289]
Physalin A	H292, H358, and H1975	5, 10, and 15 µM	Not reported	Decreased tumor cell growth and enhanced cell death	↓JAK/STAT3	[290]

Table 2. *Cont.*

Phytochemicals	Cell Lines	Conc.	IC_{50}	Anticancer Effect	Mechanisms	References
Rhein	A549	25, 50, and 100 µM	45 µM	Enhanced G0/G1 phase cell cycle arrest and cell death	↑ER stress; ↑p53; ↑p21; ↑Bax; ↓Bcl-2; ↓GADD153; ↓cyt c	[291,292]
	A549	25, 50, and 100 µM	100 µM	Inhibited tumor cell growth	↓Bcl-2; ↓p-PI3K; ↓Akt; ↓mTOR	[293]
	PC-9, H460, and A549	30, 60, and 100 µM	24.59 µM (PC-9), 52.88 µM(H460), and 23.9 µM (A549)	Increased G2/M phase cell cycle arrest and cell death	↓Bcl-2; ↑Bax; ↓STAT3	[294]
Withanone	A549	2.5–10 µM	Not reported	Reduced tumor cell growth and increased cell death	↓CDK2; ↓CDK4; ↓cyclin D; ↓cyclin E ↓mortalin; ↓hnRNP-K; ↓MMP-2; ↓fibronectin; ↑p53; ↑CARF	[269]

Symbols and abbreviations: ↑, increased or upregulated; ↓, decreased or downregulated; AIF, apoptosis-inducing factor; Bax, Bcl-2-associated X protein; Bcl-2, B cell lymphoma-2; CARF, calcium-response factor; CDK, cyclin-dependent kinase; COX, cyclooxygenase; DNMT, DNA methyltransferase; EGFR, epidermal growth factor receptor; EMT, epithelial to mesenchymal transition; ERK, extracellular signal-related kinase; GSH, glutathione; GSK3β, glycogen synthase kinase 3β; HO-1, heme oxygenase-1; ICAM-1, intercellular adhesion molecule-1; IL, interleukin; iNOS, inducible nitric oxide synthase; JAK, Janus kinase; MAPK, mitogen-activated protein kinase; Mcl-1, myeloid cell leukemia-1; MEK, mitogen-activated protein kinase; MLK3, mixed lineage kinase 3; MMP-3, matrix metalloproteinase-3; MRP1, multidrug resistance protein 1; mTOR, mammalian target of rapamycin; NF-κB, nuclear factor-κB; PARP, poly (ADP-ribose) polymerase; PERK, protein kinase RNA-like endoplasmic reticulum kinase; PGE2, prostaglandin E2; PI3K, phosphatidylinositol-3-kinase; PPAR-γ, peroxisome proliferator-activated receptor-γ; ROS, reactive oxygen species; STAT, signal transducer and activator of transcription; TGF-β, transforming growth factor-β; VEGF-A, vascular endothelial growth factor-A.

β-Carboline

β-Carboline is an indole alkaloid (Figure 4) derived from *Peganum harmala* and *Nicotiana tobacum* and has been reported to be effective in the treatment of neurodegenerative diseases, such as Parkinson's and Alzheimer's [295]. Investigators observed the role of β-carboline in A549 lung cancer cells and reported cytotoxic effects at a concentration of 1.80 μM. Researchers attributed these anticancer effects to an increase in the expression of ERK1/2 and Akt/mTOR signaling pathways [175].

Berberine

Berberine (Figure 4) is a quaternary alkaloid derived from various plants, including Oregon grape, European barberry, goldenseal, phellodendron, goldthread, and tree turmeric, which is reported to inhibit the cell cycle and induce apoptosis in cancer cells [296,297]. Berberine exerts its anticancer activity against A549 and H1299 lung cancer cell lines by promoting Bcl-2-associated X protein (Bax) and caspase-3 Bcl-2-associated X protein (Bax) and caspase-3-mediated apoptosis [176]. In vivo study furthered these results by demonstrating a reduction of Bcl-2 expression and enhanced the Bax- and caspase-3-mediated apoptosis of cancerous cells in the xenografts of athymic nude mice [176].

Evodiamine

Evodiamine (Figure 4) is a quinolone alkaloid derived from tetradium fruit that is commonly used for its weight management, analgesic, and neuroprotective effects [298–300]. Documented anticancer effects of evodiamine include its ability to inhibit various signaling molecules, such as mTOR, NF-κB, PI3K/Akt, and JAK-STAT [301]. In vivo analysis utilizing nude mice with Lewis lung carcinoma xenografts demonstrated evodiamine's ability to improve host immune response against tumor cells at doses of 10, 20, and 30 mg/kg (Table 3). Mechanistically, evodiamine was found to reduce the transmembrane glycoprotein mucin 1-C (MUC-1)/PD-L1 expression and increase CD8+ T cells [302].

Table 3. In vivo studies of plant-based bioactive compounds in lung cancer.

Phytochemicals	Anticancer Model	Dose (Route)	Anticancer Effects	Mechanisms	References
		Alkaloids			
Berberine	Xenograft athymic nude mouse model	50, 100, and 200 mg/kg (p.o.)	Increased cell death and decreased tumor weight	↓Bcl-2; ↑Bax; ↑caspase-3	[176]
Evodiamine	Xenograft nude mouse model and Lewis lung carcinoma model	10, 20, and 30 mg/kg (p.o.)	Reduction in tumor volume	↑CD8+ T cells; ↓MUC1-C/PD-L1	[302]
Hirsutine	Lung metastasis model in BALB/c mice	25 μM (i.p.)	Decreased tumor weight	↓NF-κB	[303]
Homoharringtonine	Xenograft tumor mouse model	10 mg/kg (p.o.)	Suppressed tumor growth	↓IL-6; ↓JAK1/STAT3	[177]
	Xenograft tumor mouse mode and transgenic carrying the KRAS mutation mode	1.25 and 2.5 mg/kg (i.p.)	Inhibited tumor growth	↓Bcl-2; ↑caspase-3; ↑caspase-9	[178]
Solamargine	Xenograft mouse model	4 and 8 mg/kg (p.o.)	Decreased tumor growth	↑ERK1/2; ↓prostaglandin E2; ↓DNMT1; ↓c-Jun	[183]
		Phenolics			
Apocynin	Xenograft BALB/c mouse model	50 and 100 mg/kg (i.p.)	Suppressed tumor growth	↓Microtubule network	[186]
Baicalein	Xenograft BALB/c nude mice	2.5, 10, and 40 mg/kg (i.g.)	Reduction in tumor volume	↓Cellular ezrin S-nitrosylation	[187]
Cardamonin	Xenograft nude mouse model	5 mg/kg (i.p.)	Enhanced cell death and inhibited tumor cell metastasis	↑Bax; ↓Bcl-2; ↑caspase-3; ↓cyclin D1; ↓CDK4; ↓PI3K; ↓Akt/mTOR	[304]
Chrysin	Tumor reduction model in BALB/c mice	1.3 mg/kg (p.o.)	Increased cell death	Caspase-3	[195]
Curcumin + neoadjuvant radiotherapy	Lung carcinoma model in C57BL/6J mice	100 μg (i.v.)	Inhibited angiogenesis and increased cell death	↓Prosurvival antiapoptotic factors	[196]
p-Coumaric acid	Xenograft model in nude mice	50 mg/kg (i.p.)	Enhanced cell death	↑Bax; ↓Bcl-2; ↑caspase-3; ↑caspase-9	[202]
EGCG	Xenograft BALB/c athymic nude mouse model	20 mg/kg (i.p.)	Inhibited tumor size and induced apoptosis	↓NF-κB	[305]
	Xenograft BALB/c athymic nude mouse model	100 μM (s.c.)	Inhibited tumor number	↓Nicotine-induced Akt; ↓ERK1/2; ↓ HIF-1α; ↓VEGF	[206]
	Xenograft nude mouse model	1.62 mg/kg (i.p.)	Inhibited tumor number and size	↓Cisplatin-induced lung tumorigenesis	[306]
EGCG and luteolin	Xenograft nude mouse model	125 mg/kg (EGCG) and 10 mg/kg (luteolin) (p.o.)	Decreased tumor size, volume and induced tumor cell apoptosis	↑p53 mitochondrial translocation; ↑DNA damage	[212]
Gallic acid	Xenograft tumor mouse model	200 mg/kg (i.p.)	Increased cell death and G2/M phase cell cycle arrest	↓Src-mediated STAT3; ↓Bcl-2; ↓cyclin D	[219]
Gigantol	Xenograft tumor mouse model	Pretreated 20 μM (i.p.)	Inhibited tumor cell growth, migration, and invasion	↓PI3K/Akt/mTOR; ↓JAK/STAT	[226]
Honokiol	Orthotopic model of lung cancer in NOD/SCID mice	7.5, 37.5, and 75 μmol/kg (p.o.)	Decrease in tumor volume	↑ ROS; ↑mitochondrial Prx3 oxidation; ↑AMPK; ↓STAT3	[307]
Kurarinone	Xenograft in BALB/c nude mouse model	100 mg/kg (i.p.)	Increased cell death	↓Bcl-2; ↑caspase-8; ↑caspase-3	[238]
Nobiletin	Xenograft in athymic BALB/c nude mouse model	40 mg/kg (s.c.)	Inhibited tumor growth and enhanced cell death	↑Caspase-3; ↓Akt; ↓GSK3β, β-catenin; ↓MRP1	[248]

Table 3. *Cont.*

Phytochemicals	Anticancer Model	Dose (Route)	Anticancer Effects	Mechanisms	References
Quercetin	Xenograft BALB/c nude mouse model	8 mg/kg (i.v.)	Decreased tumor growth, viability and promoted cell death	↑Bax; ↓Bcl-2	[257]
Resveratrol	Xenograft BALB/c nude mouse model	15, 30, and 60 mg/kg (i.v.)	Inhibited tumor growth and increased cell death	↑Caspase-3	[259]
Tangeretin derivatives	Xenograft BALB/c athymic nude mouse model	20 mg/kg (i.p.)	Increased G2/M cell cycle arrest, mitochondrial disruption, cell death and decreased tumor growth	↓Bcl-2; ↑caspase-3; ↓phophoatidylinositol 3-kinase/Akt/mTOR	[261]
Sulfur-containing compounds					
Sulforaphane	Xenograft nude mouse model	9 µM (p.o.)	Suppressed tumor growth and enhanced G2/M cell cycle arrest	↑Apoptosis; ↓histone deacetylase	[265]
Sulforaphane	Xenograft nude mouse model	25 and 50 mg/kg (i.p.)	Reduction in tumor volume	↑E-cadherin; ↑ZO-1; ↑ERK5; ↓N-cadherin; ↓Snail 1	[308]
Terpenoids					
Thymoquinone	Xenograft nude mouse model	10 mg/kg (i.p.)	Inhibited tumor growth	↑Caspase-3	[276]
Betulinic acid	Xenograft nude mouse model	50 and 75 mg/kg (i.p.)	Suppressed tumor growth	↓Skp2; ↑p27; ↑E-cadherin	[309]
Scabertopin	Xenograft nude mouse model	20 mg/kg (i.p.)	Inhibited tumor growth	↑Apoptosis ↑Bax; ↑ROS	[310]
Soyasapogenol	Xenograft immune-deficient mouse model	15 mg/kg (i.v.)	Suppressed tumor growth and metastasis	↓CDK2; ↓CDK4; ↓cyclin A; ↓cyclin D1; ↓catenin/vimentin/hnRNPK	[275]
Miscellaneous compounds					
Cannabidiol	Xenograft nude mouse model	5 mg/kg (i.p.)	Increased cell death and inhibited tumor proliferation	↑ICAM-1; ↑COX-2; ↑PPAR-γ	[283]
Emodin	Xenograft model in nude mice	20 and 50 mg/kg (i.p.)	Induced cell death	↑ER stress; ↑TRIB3/NF-κB	[287]
Hypericin	Rodent tumor model in BALB/c nude mice	0.1 mg/kg (i.p.)	Displayed antiproliferative effects	↑siRNA; ↓HIF-1α	[168,311]
	Rodent tumor model/W256 tumor rats and mice	2 mg/kg (intra tumor)	Inhibited tumor proliferation and induced cell death	↑Apoptosis	[168,312]
Physalin A	Xenograft mouse model	40 and 80 mg/kg (i.p.)	Decreased tumor growth and increased cell death	↓STAT3; ↓JAK/STAT3	[290]
Rhein	Xenograft mouse model	60 and 100 mg/kg (i.p.)	Increased G2/M phase cell cycle arrest, cell death and reduction in tumor volume	↓Bcl-2; ↑Bax; ↓STAT3	[294]

Symbols and abbreviations: ↑, increased or upregulated; ↓, decreased or downregulated; Bax, Bcl-2-associated X protein; Bcl-2, B cell lymphoma-2; CDK, cyclin-dependent kinase; DNMT, DNA methyltransferase; ERK, extracellular signal-related kinase; GSK3β, glycogen synthase kinase 3β; JAK, Janus kinase; MRP1, multidrug resistance protein 1; mTOR, mammalian target of rapamycin; MUC1, mucin 1; NF-κB, nuclear factor-κB; PI3K, phosphatidylinositol-3-kinase; ROS, reactive oxygen species; STAT, signal transducer and activator of transcription; ZO-1, zonula occludens-1 epithelial marker.

Hirsutine

Hirsutine (Figure 4), an indole alkaloid, is derived from the bark of Uncaria and has been shown to possess antiviral and neuroprotective properties [313]. Hirsutine has proven efficacy against various cancer models, including T cell leukemia and lung cancer [314,315]. In an in vivo lung metastasis model using female BALB/c mice, hirsutine was found to reduce cell invasion and metastasis at an intravenous dose of 25 μM by targeting the NF-κB signaling pathway [303].

Homoharringtonine

Homoharringtonine (Figure 4) is an ester of the cephalotaxine alkaloid that is present in *Cephalotaxus harringtonia* belonging to the family Cephalotaxaceae and has displayed antiviral properties [316] and breast anticancer activity by suppression of the miR-18a-3p/Akt/mTOR signaling pathway [317]. In lung cancer, specifically, homoharringtonine has been reported to decrease JAK1/STAT3 signaling at a concentration of 2–4 μM in A549 cells [177]. In another study, at a concentration of 2 μM, homoharringtonine inhibited the expression of KRAS, ERK, Akt, STAT3, CDK4, and CDK6 in A549 and H1299 lung cancer cells. Somewhat paradoxically, researchers also noted a decrease in the expression of tumor suppressor protein p21 and RB-treated cells [178]. These findings are, in part, supported by in vivo experiments. Utilizing a xenograft tumor mouse model, Cao et al. [177] demonstrated the ability of 10 mg/kg homoharringtonine to reduce the cell proliferation by suppressing IL-6/JAK1/STAT3 signaling. Later, Weng et al. [178] also conducted an experiment investigated the effects of 2.5 mg/kg homoharringtonine on mice bearing KRAS mutation-positive xenograft tumors. The researchers determined that treatment with homoharringtonine elevated the expression of caspase-3 and caspase-9 and downregulated Bcl-2 expression.

Indole-3-Carbinol

Indole-3-carbinol (Figure 4) is an indole alkaloid and glucosinolate derivative, derived from broccoli, cauliflower, cabbage, and other cruciferous vegetables. In vitro analyses have been conducted to evaluate the anticancer effects of indole-3-carbinol. Dadashpour and Emami [318] report the ability of indole-3-carbinol to cause G1/S cell cycle arrest and apoptosis in several cancer models. More specifically, indole-3-carbinol increased oxidative stress and expression of caspase-3, caspase-7, and caspase-9 to ultimately induce apoptosis in H1299 lung cancer cells at a concentration of 400 μM [179].

Melosine B

Melosine B (Figure 4), an indole alkaloid derived from *Melodinus cochinchinensis*, has been demonstrated to be cytotoxic to various cancer cell lines [319]. Researchers report the ability of melosine B to induce apoptosis in A549 lung cancer cells at concentrations of 0.064, 0.32, 1.6, 8, and 40 μM. The investigators did not report any mechanism of action to explain these findings [180].

Piperine

Piperine (Figure 4) is an amide alkaloid, commonly found in black pepper. It has several biological activities, such as hepatoprotective, immunomodulatory, antioxidant, antitumor, antidiabetic, and cardioprotective effects [320]. Piperine was reported to induce cell cycle arrest in the A549 lung cancer cell line at a concentration of 50, 100, and 200 μg/mL by upregulating caspase-3 and caspase-9 cascades and the Bax/Bcl-2 ratio [181]. In another in vitro analysis, piperine demonstrated the ability to suppress A549 cell viability and migration at a concentration of 20, 40, 80, 160, and 320 μM by inhibiting ERK 1/2, SMAD 2 phosphorylation, and the transforming growth factor-β (TGF-β) signaling pathway [182].

Solamargine

Solamargine (Figure 4) is a steroidal alkaloid and cytotoxic compound derived from *Solanum incanum*, a member of the Solanaceae family, and acts by disrupting the growth of cancer cells [321]. Solamargine was found to inhibit the actions of prostaglandin E2 (PGE2), restrict DNA protein expression, and enhance ERK1/2 phosphorylation in H1650, H1975, PC9, A549, and H1299 lung cancer cell lines at a concentration of 2, 4, and 6 μM [183]. In a xenograft mouse model, solamargine again decreased the PGE2 and DNA protein expression at doses of 4 and 8 mg/kg [183].

Vallesiachotamine and Iso-Vallesiachotamine

Vallesiachotamine and iso-vallesiachotamine (Figure 4) are indole alkaloids derived from *Anthocephalus cadamba* which act by promoting apoptosis in cancer cells [322]. In vitro analysis performed by Mishra et al. [184] demonstrated efficacy against the lung cancer cell line H1299 at concentrations of 12.5, 25, 50, 100, and 200 μM. The researchers attribute these anticancer effects to an increase in DNA damage and upregulation of apoptosis.

7.1.2. Phenolics

Phenolics are a diverse group of natural compounds widely distributed in plants. These compounds are characterized by their inclusion of at least one aromatic ring within their chemical structure, which contributes to their antioxidant properties. Plant-derived phenolics play essential roles in numerous biological processes, including defense against pathogens, UV protection, and cell signaling. Based on structural differences, phenolics may be subcategorized primarily into flavonoids and non-flavonoids. Flavonoids are further divided into six major groups: anthocyanidins, flavanols, flavanones, flavones, flavonols, and isoflavonoids. The non-flavonoids may be further subdivided into phenolic acids, stilbenes, and lignans, amongst others. These bioactive compounds have garnered significant interest due to their broad-spectrum biological and pharmacological activities, such as antioxidant, anti-inflammatory, and antineoplastic properties [323–325].

Acacetin

Acacetin (Figure 5) is a flavonoid derived from *Tunera diffusa*, *Dracocephalum moldavica* propolis, *Betula pendula*, *Flos chrysanthemi* indici, *Robinia pseudoacacia* chrysanthemum, Calamintha, safflower, and Linaria species. Generally, anticancer effects of acacetin include inhibition of tumor cell migration and invasion [326]. In lung cancer specifically, acacetin has been shown to inhibit cell viability, invasion, migration, and inflammation and accelerate apoptosis in A549 NSCLC cells. Researchers report these effects to be mediated by suppression of the p38α MAPK signaling pathway [185].

Apocynin

Apocynin (4-hydroxy-3-methoxy-acetophenone (Figure 5), a phenolic compound derived from *Apocynum cannabinum* and *Picrorhiza kurroa*, has been reported to possess anti-inflammatory, antioxidant, and anticancer effects [327]. Paul et al. [186] investigated the role of apocynin against A549 lung cancer cells and observed decrease in the microtubule network of cells, as well as reductions in proliferation, colony formation, and cell invasion. The same group of investigators further studied these effects by conducting an in vivo study using BALB/c mice with xenograft tumors. They found that treatment with apocynin at doses of 50 and 100 mg/kg inhibited cell growth, invasion, colony formation, and microtubule network. They attribute these findings to cellular microtubule depolymerization, resulting in tumor cell apoptosis.

Baicalein

Baicalein (5,6,7-trihydroxyflavone, Figure 5) is a flavonoid derived from the root of *Scutellaria baicalensis* that is known to modulate cardiovascular health [328]. Biacalein has displayed broad anticancer effects by initiating apoptosis via mitochondria and receptor-mediated pathways [329]. In lung cancer cell lines A549 and H1299, baicalein has been shown to suppress the cytoskeleton linker protein ezrin, resulting in decreased cell invasion and metastasis [187]. Researchers validated these findings in an in vivo experiment utilizing BALB/c nude mice with tumor xenografts. Baicalein was also found to inhibit cancer invasion and metastasis at doses of 2.5, 10, and 40 mg/kg [187].

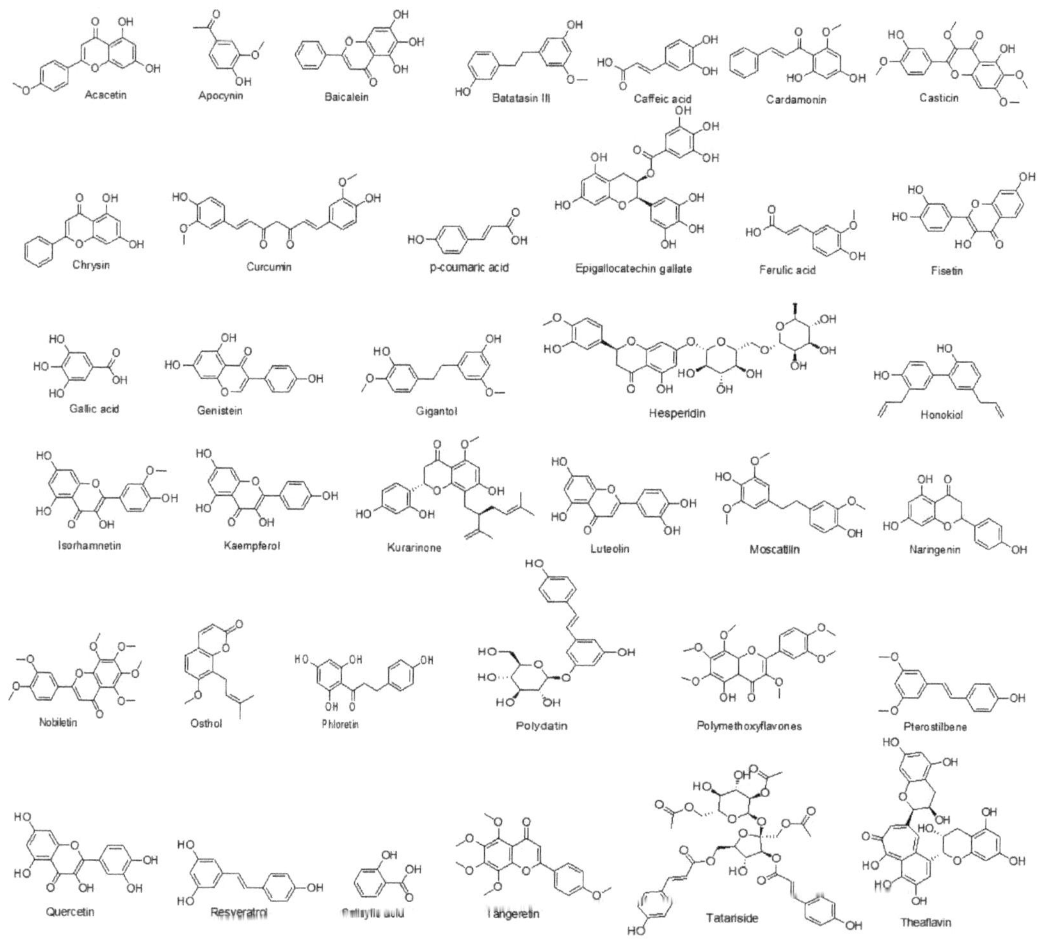

Figure 5. Chemical structures of phenolic compounds with anticancer activity in lung cancer.

Batatasin

Batatasin III (Figure 5) is a stilbenoid compound derived from *Dendrobium draconi, Bulbophyllum reptans*, and *Cymbidium aloifolium*. It has numerous pharmacological actions, including antioxidant, anticancer, anti-inflammatory, antidiabetic, antiapoptotic, anticholinesterase, antioxidant, antiherpetic, and antimalarial activities [330]. In vitro analysis of batatasin against H460 lung cancer cells demonstrated its ability to decrease cell proliferation, invasion, and metastasis. Researchers attribute these findings to a decrease in epithelial–mesenchymal transition (EMT) through downregulation of N-cadherin and vimentin and the Akt pathway and upregulation of E-cadherin [188].

Caffeic Acid

Caffeic acid (Figure 5) is a polyphenol derived from coffee beans, olives, fruits, carrots, potatoes, and propolis. In hepatocellular carcinoma, caffeic acid has been demonstrated to increase reactive oxygen species and DNA oxidation, as well as decrease angiogenesis [331]. In A549 lung cancer cells, caffeic acid was shown to reduce cell proliferation, adhesion, and migration by inhibition of superoxide production [189].

Cardamonin

Cardamonin (Figure 5) is a chalcone compound that is present in cardamom, a spice belonging to the Zingiberaceae family. Anticancer effects displayed by cardamonin include inhibition of the PI3K/Akt pathway in various cancer models [190]. In A549 and H460 lung cancer cells, cardamonin was reported to inhibit the PI3K/Akt pathway and increase the expression of caspase-3, Bcl-2, and Bax at a concentration of 40 μM [190]. In another study, at a concentration of 30 μM, cardamonin inhibited DNA synthesis and promoted apoptosis in A549 cells [191]. Cardamonin analogs, including 4,40-dihydroxylchalcone (DHC) and 4,40-dihydroxy-20-methoxychalcone (DHMC), reduce cell growth and expression of NF-κB at concentrations of 0.445 μM and 0.166 μM, respectively, in A549 and NCI-H460 cell lines [192]. In vivo analysis of the effects of cardamonin demonstrated its ability to inhibit cell proliferation, migration, and angiogenesis in nude mice with xenograft tumors of lung origin. Researchers noted an increase in caspase-3 and Bax expression, with concurrent decreases in the expression of Bcl-2, cyclin D1, CDK4, and PI3K and Akt and mTOR signaling [304].

Casticin

Casticin (Figure 5) is a methoxylated flavonol derived from *Vites trifolia*, *Vites agnus-castus*, and *Vites negundo*. Casticin has been demonstrated to possess antiproliferative and proapoptotic effects in numerous types of cancer, including breast, colon, liver, and others [332]. These anticancer effects have been validated in the setting of lung cancer using A549 cells. Researchers demonstrated the ability of casticin to decrease inflammatory mediators such as IL-6, cyclooxygenase-2 (COX-2), and NF-κB, in addition to downregulating chemokine gene expression [193,194].

Chrysin

Chrysin (5,7-dihydroxyflavone) (Figure 5) is present in propolis, honey, *Passiflora caerulea*, *Passiflora incarnata*, *Alpinia galangal*, and *Oroxylum indicum* and has been reported to exert its anticancer effects by caspase activation and inactivation of Akt signaling [333]. In A549 lung cancer cells, chrysin has been shown to increase apoptosis by elevating caspase-3, Bcl-2, and Bax expression. Investigators also noted decreased cell proliferation following the application of chrysin. In a follow-up in vivo study, researchers treated tumor-bearing BALB/c mice with chrysin at a dose of 1.3 mg/kg and observed an increase in caspase-3-mediated apoptosis [195].

Curcumin

Curcumin (Figure 5) is a spice derived from *Curcuma longa* L. with substantial evidence for its use as a chemotherapeutic agent. Some of the well-established anticancer applications of curcumin include its ability to induce apoptosis and inhibit proliferation of tumor cells by numerous cellular signaling pathways [334]. In A549 lung cancer cells, 10 μM of radiosensitized curcumin was shown to reduce the migration and invasion of tumor cells, likely by suppression of antiapoptotic factors [196]. In another study utilizing A549 cells, curcumin at 10–50 μM increased caspase-3-induced apoptosis by promoting G2/M phase cell cycle arrest and DNA damage and caused stress to the endoplasmic reticulum, resulting in activation of the unfolded protein response and eventual apoptosis in tumor cells [197]. Additional in vitro analysis using HCI-H460 cells also showed that, at a concentration of 30 μM, curcumin induced apoptosis by reducing expression of CDK1 and upregulating caspase-3 and caspase-8 [198]. Moreover, 1–20 μM of curcumin was documented to increase activator protein-1 in the CL1–5 cell lines, thereby reducing cancer cell invasion and metastasis [199]. Curcumin was also shown to cause DNA damage and promote apoptosis in PC-9 cells at a concentration of 50 μM. Researchers attribute these findings to curcumin's role in reducing the expression of Bcl-2 and cyclin D1 and CDK2, CDK4, and CDK6 gene expression [200]. Furthermore, 5–40 μM of curcumin contributed to apoptosis in NCI-H292 cells with measured reductions in the expression of CDK1 and enhanced expression of caspase-3 and caspase-8 [201].

Limited in vivo experimentation has been conducted with curcumin in the context of lung cancer. Sak [196] utilized a C57BL/6J lung carcinoma mouse model to demonstrate that, at a dose of 100 mg/kg, curcumin effectively reduced angiogenesis and cancer cell proliferation and initiated apoptosis by suppression of prosurvival factors.

p-Coumaric Acid

p-Coumaric acid (Figure 5), a hydroxycinnamic acid, belongs to a class of polyphenols found in various edible plants such as tomatoes, carrots, and cereals. It has several biological activities, including anti-inflammatory, analgesic, antioxidant, and antimicrobial properties [335]. p-Coumaric acid was reported to increase apoptosis in A549, NCI-H1299, and HCC827 lung cancer cell lines at a concentration of 10–100 μg/mL by upregulating caspase-3 and caspase-9 [202]. Separate in vitro analysis by Jeong et al. [203] demonstrated the ability of p-coumaric acid to suppress H1993 cell viability at a concentration of 50–100 μM by overcoming the resistance of epidermal growth factor receptor tyrosine kinase inhibitor. Despite promising in vitro studies, the anticancer effect of p-coumaric acid has been relatively understudied in animal models of lung cancer. One available report further describes the proapoptotic effects of p-coumaric acid against a xenograft lung cancer model in nude mice. Researchers found that, at a dose of 50 mg/kg, p-coumaric acid enhanced caspase-3- and caspase-9-mediated apoptosis in xenograft tumors [202].

Epigallocatechin Gallate

Epigallocatechin gallate (EGCG, Figure 5), a green tea-derived polyphenol, has been reported to be effective against several types of cancers, including kidney, colon, lung, brain, and breast, as well as in leukemia [336,337]. In A549 and H1299 lung cancer cells, 20–300 μM of EGCG was shown to decrease the tumor cell proliferation likely by suppression of the NF-κB signaling pathway [204]. In another study, at a concentration of 10–100 μM, EGCG decreased the A549 cell proliferation by inhibiting the NF-κB signaling pathway and increasing oxidative stress [205]. EGCG was also shown to reduce the tumor cell proliferation at a concentration of 10, 25, 50, and 100 μM. Researchers attributed these findings to EGCG's role in reducing nicotine-induced Akt, ERK1/2 signaling, hypoxia-inducible factor 1α (HIF 1α), and vascular endothelial growth factor (VEGF) expression [206]. Moreover, 12.5, 25, and 50 μM of EGCG suppressed tumor cell growth, invasion, and migration with measured reductions in the Bax/Bcl-2 ratio [207]. Datta and Sinha [208] investigated the role of EGCG against A549 lung cancer cells and observed inhibition of tumor cell growth by a decrease in the Nrf2 signaling pathway and increase in the oxidative stress in tumor cells at a concentration of 20–300 μM. The same group of investigators further reported that EGCG reduced the etoposide resistance in A549 and NCI-H23 cells at a concentration of 0.05–500 μM [209]. Moreover, 40 μM of EGCG suppressed the growth of H1299, H460, and A549 cells with measured reductions in miR-210 expressions [210]. Later, in vitro analysis using H1299 and A549 cells also showed that EGCG at a concentration of 10, 20, and 40 μM induced apoptosis by reducing expression of the PI3K/Akt signaling pathway [211]. Additionally, the combination of EGCG (30 μM) and luteolin (10 μM) was documented to induce apoptosis, likely by enhancing p53 mitochondrial translocation and DNA damage, in A549 and H460 cells [212]. Furthermore, theaflavins and EGCG at a concentration of 100 μM suppressed the tumor cell proliferation by enhancing expressions of p53 and inhibiting Bcl-2 expression [213].

In vivo analysis of the effects of EGCG demonstrated its ability to inhibit cell proliferation and promote apoptosis in nude mice with xenograft tumors of lung origin. Researchers noted a simultaneous decrease in nicotine-induced Akt and ERK1/2 signaling [305]. Shi et al. (2015) utilized a xenograft BALB/c athymic nude mouse model to demonstrate that pretreatment of animals with EGCG subcutaneously at 100 μM effectively reduced cancer cell proliferation by suppression of nicotine-induced Akt and ERK1/2 signaling [206]. Researchers validated these findings in an in vivo experiment utilizing a nude mouse model with tumor xenografts. EGCG was also found to inhibit cisplatin-induced lung tumorigenesis at doses of 1.62 mg/kg [306].

Ferulic Acid

Ferulic acid (Figure 5) is a hydroxycinnamic acid derived from fruits and vegetables such as sweet corn, tomatoes, and rice bran, and has been found to have antioxidant and anticancer activity [338,339]. In an in vitro study carried out utilizing A549 lung cancer cells, 200 μM of ferulic acid decreased cell proliferation, adhesion, and migration. Researchers believe these results to be mediated by inhibition of superoxide production [189].

Fisetin

Fisetin (Figure 5) is a flavone present in numerous vegetables and fruit, such as apples, strawberries, grapes, persimmons, cucumbers, and onions. Fisetin is reported to be efficacious in the treatment of numerous malignancies, including breast, cervical, prostate, lung, skin, colon, and gastric cancers, as well as hepatocellular carcinoma, leukemia, and myeloma. Fisetin has displayed anticancer effects by modulating multiple signaling pathways such as Akt/mTOR, Axl, MAPK, PARP, PI3K, and ERK1/2 [340]. In A549 lung cancer cells, fisetin has been shown to induce apoptosis, likely due to its ability to downregulate PI3K/Akt/mTOR signaling [214]. In two studies, Kang et al. [215,216] demonstrated the ability of 75μg/mL of fisetin to decrease cell proliferation in NCI-H460 cells. The investigators believe these results to be mediated by a reduction in the expression of Bcl-2, with increases in the expression of caspase-9 and caspase-3. In a separate study, fisetin was noted to reverse acquired erlotinib resistance of HCC827-ER lung adenocarcinoma cells at concentrations ranging from 10–120 μM. The researchers attributed these findings to fisetin's role in suppressing the Axl, MAPK, and Akt signaling pathways [217].

Gallic Acid

Gallic acid is a phenolic acid (Figure 5), commonly found in bearberry, pomegranate, gallnuts, oak bark, and several other plants, and is well known for its gastrointestinal, cardiovascular, and neuropsychological medicinal properties as well as antioxidant, anti-inflammatory, and antineoplastic properties [341]. In Calu-6 and A549 lung cancer cell lines, gallic acid enhances oxidative stress, decreases the glutathione (GSH) levels, and inhibits cell growth [218]. Researchers attribute these findings to be due to gallic acid's ability to downregulate STAT3-regulated tumor-promoting gene expression, resulting in cell cycle arrest and apoptosis. Furthermore, gallic acid has been shown to induce cell cycle arrest and upregulate apoptosis in H1975 and H1993 cell lines, likely due to its role in decreasing STAT3 phosphorylation but also due to reduced expression of Bcl-2, cyclin D, NF-κB, and IL-6 [219]. In an in vivo study, gallic acid reduced Src-mediated phosphorylation of STAT3, thereby promoting cell cycle arrest and apoptosis in a mouse xenograft tumor model [219].

Genistein

Genistein (Figure 5) is a phytoestrogen primarily derived from legumes and has been proven effective against numerous types of malignancies including liver, breast, prostate, pancreatic, lung, skin, and cervical cancer [342]. In A549 lung cancer cells, genistein has been demonstrated to accelerate trichostatin A-induced caspase-3 activity, thereby causing cell apoptosis [220]. Genistein was also reported to inhibit NF-κB DNA-binding affinity and downregulate expression of COX-2, p-Akt, EGFR, and PGE2, resulting in decreased cell proliferation and upregulation of apoptosis in H3255, H1650, and H1781 lung cancer cell lines [221]. These results have been further validated in two additional studies in which genistein increased apoptosis and cell cycle arrest in the SPC-A-1 line [222] and H460 cell lines [223].

Gigantol

Gigantol (Figure 5) is a bibenzyl phenolic compound derived from orchids and is known to have antioxidative, antinociceptive, antispasmodic, anti-inflammatory, and anticancer activity [343]. In lung cancer cell line A549, gigantol has been shown to suppress cell proliferation and enhance apoptosis in tumor cells at a concentration of 25, 50, and 100 μM. Investigators report these effects to be mediated by inhibition of Bcl-2 expression and upregulation of Bax expression and Wnt/β-catenin signaling [224]. In another study, gigantol has been shown to inhibit cell proliferation in H460 lung cancer cells at a concentration of 50 μM. The investigators noted these findings to be associated with inhibition of EMT transcription factor expression [225]. In H460 lung cancer cells, gigantol was shown to destabilize tumor integrity via suppression of the PI3K/Akt/mTOR and JAK/STAT pathways at concentrations of 20–200 μM [226]. To validate these findings, in vivo experimentation has been conducted with lung cancer utilizing a xenograft tumor mouse model. Researchers found that, pretreated at a dose of 20 μM, gigantol reduced cell proliferation by suppressing PI3K/Akt/mTOR and JAK/STAT pathways [226].

Hesperidin

Hesperidin (Figure 5) is a flavanone glycoside present in citrus fruits with documented antioxidative, anti-inflammatory, cardiovascular, antiobesity, and anticancer activities [344]. Specifically, hesperidin was reported to promote apoptosis in A549 and NCI-H358 lung cancer cells at concentrations of 5–50 μM. Researchers suggest these results are due to hesperidin's ability to promote mitochondrial membrane disruption and production of caspase-3, while also enhancing NF-κB signal transduction pathways [227]. A separate study conducted by Jeong et al. [203] demonstrated that, at a concentration of 100 μM, hesperidin reduced cell proliferation and growth in H1993 cell lines. They believe these results to be mediated by overcoming the resistance of EGFR tyrosine kinase inhibitor.

Honokiol

Honokiol (Figure 5), a lignan belonging to the genus *Magnolia*, has been revealed to exhibit antiproliferative effects against several cancer cells, including bladder, bone, brain, blood, breast, and colon cancer [345]. When 5, 10, or 20 μM of honokiol was applied to A549 and 95-D lung cancer cell lines, researchers observed inhibited cell proliferation and migration, which they attributed to resultant increases in Bax, caspase-9, and PERK phosphorylation [228,229]. Separate analysis using A549 and LL/2 cell lines further demonstrates the anticancer potential of honokiol as researchers found that application of honokiol to these cell lines promoted apoptosis and regulated vascular endothelial growth factor-A (VEGF-A) expression [230]. In an in vivo analysis, honokiol administered at doses of 7.5, 37.5, and 75 μM/kg led to apoptosis of lung cancer cells in an orthotopic model using NOD/SCID mice. The researchers believed that honokiol exerted anticancer effects by enhancing oxidative stress, mitochondrial Prx3 oxidation, and AMPK pathway activation and inhibition of STAT3 phosphorylation [307].

Isorhamnetin

Isorhamnetin (Figure 5), a bioflavonoid that is derived from *Hippophae rhamnoides* L. and *Ginkgo biloba* L., is reported to be efficacious in the management of cerebrovascular and cardiovascular diseases [346]. At a concentration of 16 μM, isorhamnetin was shown to reduce cancer cell proliferation and colony formation and increase apoptosis via caspase activation in A549 cells [233]. In a separate study, 25 μM of isorhamnetin also caused an increase in mitochondrial disruption and caspase-induced apoptosis of A549 cells [234].

Kaempferol

Kaempferol (Figure 5) is a flavonol found abundantly in broccoli, yellow fruits, and grapes. In addition to its documented anticancer activities, kaempferol is said to possess neuroprotective, antimicrobial, antioxidant, and anti-inflammatory properties [347]. In lung cancer, 10–140 μM of kaempferol increased expression of EMT-related protein E-cadherin and reduced expression of vimentin, resulting in reduced cell growth and proliferation of A549 cells [235]. In another study utilizing identical cells, kaempferol was shown to decrease cell proliferation, migration, and invasion at a concentration of 25 μM. The researchers noted the role of kaempferol in reducing Akt1-mediated phosphorylation and expression of transforming growth factor-β1 in treated A549 cells [236]. A separate study found that, at concentrations of 30, 50, and 80 μM, kaempferol was able to increase the oxidative stress and caspase-3-induced apoptosis of H460 cells [237].

Kurarinone

Kurarinone (Figure 5) is a flavanone derived from *Sophora alopecuroides* and is reported to have immunosuppressive effects and antioxidant activity [348]. When 5.8 μg/mL of kurarinone was applied to H460 cells, investigators observed its ability to cause G2/M blockade and enhance apoptosis. These findings are supported by measurable decreases in NF-κB signaling and tyrosine kinase activity [238]. In another in vitro analysis, researchers reported that kurarinone decreased the expression of EMT-related proteins and MMP-2 in H1688 and H146 cell lines at IC_{50} values of 12.5 and 30.4 μM, respectively, thereby decreasing cell viability, invasion, and migration of tumor cells [239]. One in vivo study of kurarinone demonstrated that a dose of 100 mg/kg increased the rate of apoptosis in BALB/c nude mice with xenografted tumors. Researchers believe these effects to be mediated by an increase in caspase-3 expression [238].

Luteolin

Luteolin (Figure 5) is a flavone present in several vegetables and fruits and is reported to have several therapeutic activities, such as antioxidant, antimicrobial, anticancer, neuroprotective, antiviral, cardioprotective, and anti-inflammatory properties [349,350]. Luteolin has been observed to promote apoptosis in A549 cells at a concentration of 20–80 μM. Researchers also noted an increase in G2/M phase cell cycle arrest, Janus kinase (JNK) and Bax expression, procaspase-9 cleavage, and caspase-3 [240]. In another study utilizing A549 cells, 25–100 μM of luteolin decreased cell motility and migration and upregulated apoptosis. The researchers attribute these findings to luteolin's ability to enhance MEK/ERK signaling and upregulate expression of caspase-3 and caspase-9 [241]. Moreover, additional in vitro analysis supported luteolin's role as a proapoptic regulator by its action on A549 and H460 cell lines. At a concentration of 10–100 μM, luteolin enhanced miR-34a-5p via targeting MDM4 expression and induced apoptosis in these cancer cell lines [242,243]. Interestingly, luteolin was discovered to downregulate Bad expression in NCI-H460 cells at concentrations of 20–160 μM. Despite this finding, application of luteolin caused increased apoptosis, which was attributable to more significant upregulation of caspase-3 and suppression of Bcl-2 [244].

Moscatilin

Moscatilin (Figure 5) is a bibenzyl phenolic compound, derived from stems of the orchid *Dendrobium loddigesii*, which is reported to have antimetastatic properties in hepatocellular carcinoma by targeting the Akt/NF-κB signaling pathway [351]. In the H460 lung cancer cell line, moscatilin was shown to possess antiproliferative properties. Researchers noted that application of moscatlin caused decreased expression of ERK, EMT, Akt, and Cav-1 [245].

Naringenin

Naringenin (Figure 5), a flavanone derived from citrus fruits and grapes, has displayed antioxidant, antiviral, antitumor, antibacterial, antiadipogenic, anti-inflammatory, and cardioprotective effects [352]. When applied to A549 cells, naringenin was shown to decrease cell proliferation, invasion, and metastasis via suppression of MMP-2, MMP-9, and the Akt pathway [246]. In another study, naringenin inhibited tumor cell migration and invasion and promoted apoptosis. Researchers again found reduced expression of MMP-2 and MMP-9 but enhanced caspase-3 and p38 MAPK [247].

Nobiletin

Nobiletin (Figure 5) is a flavonoid derived from citrus peels that causes tumor cell apoptosis and prevents myocardial injury via the PI3K/Akt signaling pathway [353]. In A549 lung cancer cells, nobiletin decreased the expression of Akt, GSK3β, β-catenin, and multidrug resistance-associated protein (MRP1) expression, while it increased caspase-3-mediated apoptosis and polymerase cleavage [248]. Researchers expanded upon this study by performing in vivo experiments utilizing a xenografted BALB/c nude mouse model. Again, nobiletin was found to enhance caspase-3-mediated apoptosis and DNA polymerase cleavage, with concurrent downregulation of Akt signaling and MRP1 at a dose of 40 mg/kg [248].

Osthol

Osthol (Figure 5), a coumarin derivative derived from *Angelica pubescens* and *Cnidium monnieri*, is reported to exert antitumor, neuroprotective, anti-inflammatory, osteogenic, antimicrobial, cardiovascular protective, and antiparasitic effects [354]. In A549 lung cancer cells, osthol was shown to decrease cell proliferation, invasion, and metastasis at concentrations of 25, 50, 100, 150, and 200 μM. Researchers credit these anticancer effects to a reduction in the expression of cyclin B1, p-Cdc2, and Bcl-2, with accompanying inhibition of PI3K/Akt signaling [249]. In another study, 80 μM of osthol decreased cell invasion and migration by reducing the MMP-2 and MMP-9 expression in A549 cells [250,251]. In another in vitro study, osthol decreased TGF-β-induced EMT, NF-κB, and Snail signaling pathways, resulting in decreased cell invasion, migration, and metastasis in A549 cells at 5–80 μM concentrations [252].

Phloretin

Phloretin (Figure 5) is a dihydrochalcone derivative present abundantly in strawberries and apples. Reported pharmaceutical applications of phloretin include antioxidant, anticarcinogenic, antidiabetic, and hepatoprotective effects [355]. In lung cancer, 25–75 μg/mL of phloretin was demonstrated to induce apoptosis in several cell lines, including A549, Calu-1, H838, and H520 cells. Researchers report a reduction in Bcl-2, MMP-2, and MMP-9 expression, as well as upregulation of caspase-3 and caspase-9 following treatment [253]. Separate in vitro analysis of phloretin utilizing A549 cells indicated that, at concentrations of 25, 50, 100, or 200 μM, cancer cell migration, invasion, and metastasis were reduced. The investigators noted an increased phosphorylation of p38 MAPK and upregulation of JNK1/2, caspase-3, and caspase-9, with concurrent reductions in the expression of Bcl-2 and NF-κB [254].

Polydatin

Polydatin (Figure 5) is a glycosylated form of resveratrol derived from *Polygonum cuspidatum* and is reported to be an efficacious antioxidant and anti-inflammatory agent. Furthermore, polydatin possesses greater capacity to modify the gut microbiota and enhance lipid metabolism in comparison to resveratrol [356]. At a concentration of 50 μM, polydatin was shown to reduce tumor cell proliferation and colony formation via enhancing the Bak/Bcl-2 ratio in A549 and NCI-H1975 cell lines [255].

Polymethoxyflavones

Monodemethylated polymethoxyflavones derived from the peels of *Citrus sinensis* have been reported to have numerous therapeutic applications, including anticancer, anti-inflammatory, and antiatherogenic properties [357]. In vitro analysis utilizing H1299 cells demonstrated the ability of polymethoxyflavones to induce apoptosis and regulate cancer cell metabolism. Researchers attribute these effects to a reduction in the expression of iNOS, COX-2, and myeloid leukemia cell differentiation protein (Mcl-1), with increased expression of caspase-3 [231].

Pterostilbene

Pterostilbene (Figure 5), a stilbenoid bearing chemical resemblance to resveratrol, is present in *Pterocarpus marsupium* and blueberries. Anticancer applications of pterostilbene are well documented and include discussions of its roles in inhibition of tumor growth, angiogenesis, and metastasis [358]. Application of pterostilbene to NCI-H460 and SK-MES-1 lung cancer cells resulted in increased apoptosis and diminished cell viability, likely due to an upregulation of caspase-3- and caspase-7-induced cell death [256].

Quercetin

Quercetin (Figure 5) is a vastly abundant natural flavonoid, present in berries, apples, vegetables, grapes, onions, tomatoes, red wine, and tea [359]. Medicinal applications of quercetin have been researched greatly and include applications as an anti-inflammatory, antioxidant, and anticancer agent, in addition to a regulator of cardiovascular disease [360,361]. When applied to A549 cells, quercetin was shown to reduce cell growth and promote apoptosis. Researchers also noted an increase in the Bc1-2 gene in treated cells [257]. In an in vivo study, quercetin was shown to enhance cancer cell apoptosis in the xenografts of BALB/c nude mice at a dose of 8 mg/kg. The researchers attributed these findings to quercetin's role in reducing Bcl-2 expression and augmenting Bax gene expression [257].

Resveratrol

Resveratrol (Figure 5) is a stilbenoid compound found in grapes, blueberries, plums, apples, and peanuts which has been reported to exhibit antiproliferative activities against various cancer cells and animal tumor models [362–364]. In lung cancer, resveratrol inhibits TGF-β1-induced EMT at a concentration of 20 μM in A549 cells, thereby preventing cell invasion and metastasis [258]. Another study determined that resveratrol also initiates caspase-3-mediated apoptosis when applied at a concentration of 8.9 μM to A549 cells [259]. Apoptosis was also observed when a lower concentration of resveratrol (1–10 μM) was applied to the H1993 cell line, presumably by disabling the resistance of EGFR tyrosine kinase inhibitor [203]. Limited in vivo data support the proapoptotic effects of resveratrol. Researchers observed an increase in apoptosis of the xenograft tumor cells of BALB/c nude mice when they were treated with 15, 30, or 60 mg/kg resveratrol, probably due to upregulation of caspase-3 [259].

Salicylic Acid

Salicylic acid (Figure 5) is a phenolic compound derived from the bark of the willow tree. It is documented to have anti-inflammatory and analgesic activity, in addition to being used to treat several skin disorders, such as acne, psoriasis, dandruff, seborrheic dermatitis, corns, and warts [365]. When applied to A549 cells, salicylic acid was shown to increase cell cytotoxicity and apoptosis at concentrations from 1.5–9.5 mM. No mechanism of action is suggested by the investigators to explain these findings [260].

Tangeretin Derivative

Tangeretin derivative (5-acetyloxy-6,7,8,4′-tetramethoxyflavone, Figure 5) belongs to the class of flavonoids and is present in citrus peels. This compound possesses various therapeutic activities, such as hepatoprotective, antioxidant, antitumor, anti-inflammatory, and neuroprotective effects [366]. With regard to lung cancer, tangeretin derivative has been shown to decrease tumor cell proliferation, metastasis, and angiogenesis in CL1-5, H1299, H226, and A549 cell lines. Researchers believe these effects to be mediated by an increase in G2/M phase arrest and mitochondrial membrane disruption and by inhibition of the PI3K/Akt/mTOR signaling pathway [261]. In an in vivo study, tangeretin derivative also led to disruption of the mitochondrial membrane and suppressed the Akt/mTOR signaling pathway, resulting in decreased cell proliferation, migration, and angiogenesis in the xenograft tumor cells of BALB/c athymic nude mice. Furthermore, the researchers observed an enhancement of caspase-mediated apoptosis at the given dose of 20 mg/kg [261].

Tatariside

Tatarisides B, C, and D (Figure 5) are flavonoids derived from the roots of Tartary buckwheat. Collectively, these phytochemicals are reported to have antitumor, anti-inflammatory, antioxidant, antidiabetic, and hepatoprotective activities [367]. Concerning lung cancer, Tatarisides B, C, and D have been shown to increase apoptosis and cell cytotoxicity in A549 cells. However, Tatariside C was found to be most potent against A549 cells [262]. Additional efforts are required to elucidate the mechanistic action of these compounds.

7.1.3. Sulfur-Containing Compounds

Sulfur-containing compounds in plants are a diverse group of chemical substances that contain sulfur atoms within their molecular structures. These compounds are essential for the growth, development, and defense mechanisms of plants. Glutathione, for example, plays a crucial role in cellular detoxification and antioxidant defense in both humans and plants. Another important sulfurous group of natural compounds are the glucosinolates, which contribute to the characteristic flavors and odors of certain plants, such as cruciferous vegetables. The study of these compounds in plants is of considerable interest due to their diverse biological functions and their potential applications in health promotion and disease mitigation [368–372].

Allicin

Allicin (Figure 6) is an organosulfur compound derived from garlic and has various biological activities such as anthelmintic, antimicrobial, nematocidal, antioxidant, anticancer, and immunomodulatory actions [373]. In an in vitro study, allicin demonstrated effectiveness against cisplatin-resistant A549 and NCI-H460 cells, evidenced by increased ROS-mediated cell death and decreased proliferation. The researchers noted downregulation of cadherin 2 (N-cadherin) and upregulation of cadherin 1 (E-cadherin), with concurrent suppression of hypoxia-inducible factors (HIF-1α and HIF-2α) [263].

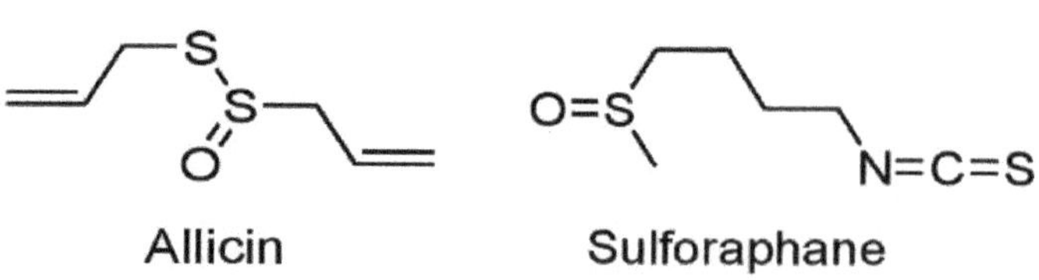

Figure 6. Chemical structures of sulfur compounds with anticancer activity in lung cancer.

Sulforaphane

Sulforaphane (Figure 6) is an organosulfur compound, present in cruciferous vegetables such as broccoli and cabbage, and has displayed broad anticancer activity by inhibiting phase I metabolic enzymes and accelerating cell cycle arrest in G2/M and G1 phases, oxidative stress, cell migration, and proliferation [372,374]. Sulforaphane has been shown to decrease the levels of miR-616-5p and GSK3β/β-catenin signaling and to increase S/G2–M phase cell cycle arrest in lung cancer cell lines H1299, 95-C, and 95-D [264]. In another study, sulforaphane downregulated histone deacetylase and enhanced apoptosis by causing cell cycle arrest in G2/M phase in A549 and H1299 [265]. Additional research conducted on sulforaphane demonstrated its ability to act as an epigenetic modulator of miR-21 and decrease CDH1 and DNMT protein levels in A549 lung cancer cells [266]. In an in vivo study, nude mice with xenograft tumors treated with sulforaphane experienced increased apoptosis of tumor cells. The researchers suggest these effects to be a result of downregulated histone deacetylase and promotion of G2/M phase cell cycle arrest [265]. In another study, sulforaphane at a dose of 50 mg/kg was administered to nude mice with xenograft tumors. The researchers observed decreased tumor cell invasion and migration, which they attribute to sulforaphane's role in enhancing the levels of E-cadherin and ZO-1 and decreasing N-cadherin and Snail 1, thereby causing ERK5 activation [308].

7.1.4. Terpenoids

Terpenoids, also known as isoprenoids, form an extensive and diverse group of compounds found abundantly in natural resources. These compounds are characterized by their structural backbone which is comprised of isoprene units. Terpenoids play crucial roles in various biological processes, including photosynthesis, pigmentation, and defense mechanisms against herbivores and pathogens. Perhaps the most well-known terpenoids include carotenoids, which are responsible for the vibrant colors of fruits and vegetables. Other examples of naturally occurring terpenoids include those present in the essential oils of plants utilized in aromatherapy and traditional medicines. Their historic uses and wide range of purported biological activities have attracted significant interest in pharmaceutical research; in fact, many terpenoids have been shown to exhibit potential therapeutic properties with applications in cancer drug development [375–377].

Abietane Diterpene

Abietane diterpene (6,7-dehydroroyleanone, Figure 7) is derived from the essential oil of *Plectranthus madagascariensis* and exerts several therapeutic properties, such as antimicrobial, antileishmaniasis, antimalarial, antiviral, antiulcer, antioxidant, and anticancer effects [376]. Garcia et al. [267] demonstrated the ability of abietane to upregulate apoptosis in NCI-H460 and A549 lung cancer cells. The researchers noted an increase in caspase activation and metaphase arrest.

β-Sitosterol

β-Sitosterol (Figure 7) is a phytosterol belonging to the class of triterpenoids. Derived from *Grewia tiliaefolia*, β-sitosterol possesses several therapeutic activities, such as antioxidant, antidiabetic, antimicrobial, anticancer, and immunomodulatory effects [377]. β-sitosterol was reported to inhibit the cell cycle at the G2/M phase and initiate apoptosis when applied to A459 cells [268].

Betulinic Acid

Betulinic acid (Figure 7) is a pentacyclic triterpenoid primarily derived from the bark of white birch trees and has been shown to promote mitochondrial oxidative stress, regulate transcription factors, and inhibit STAT and activator of the NF-κB signaling pathway in prostate, breast, colorectal, and lung cancers [378]. In an in vivo model of lung cancer, betulinic acid at a dose of 50 or 75 mg/kg was shown to inhibit the migration and proliferation of cancer cells in nude mice bearing xenograft tumors. The researchers noted that betulinic acid acted as an Skp2-SCF E3 ligase inhibitor, thereby inhibiting cancer cell metastasis and proliferation [309].

Cucurbitacin B

Cucurbitacin B (Figure 7) is a triterpene obtained from the Cucurbitaceae family which possesses several bioactivities, such as anti-inflammatory, anticancer, and hepatoprotective properties [379]. In lung cancer, cucurbitacin B has been shown to reduce cell proliferation, migration, invasion, and metastasis in A549 cells. Researchers report these findings to be associated with reduced expression of CDK2, CDK4, cyclin D, cyclin E, and mortalin and increased p53 and collaborator of ARF (CARF) proteins [269].

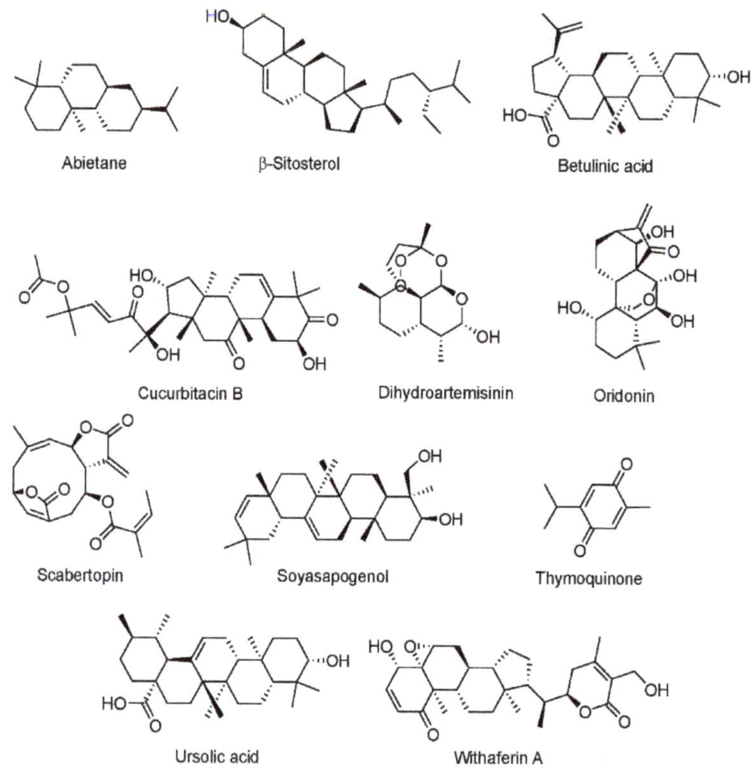

Figure 7. Chemical structures of terpenoids with anticancer activity in lung cancer.

Dihydroartemisinin

Dihydroartemisinin (Figure 7) is a semi-synthetic derivative of artemisinin derived from *Artemisia annua* and is reported to have antimalarial, antiviral, anti-inflammatory, and anticancer activity [380]. In the context of lung cancer, dihydroartemisinin is reported to cause apoptosis by enhancing the p38 MAPK expression in the PC-14 cell line at a concentration of 1 μg/mL [270]. In a similar in vitro analysis, researchers reported that dihydroartemisinin increased the expression of p38 MAPK in LLC cells at concentrations of 5, 10, 20, and 40 μg/mL [271]. Another study found that 0.23–749.90 μM of dihydroartemisinin also caused a decrease in transferrin receptor expression in the A549 and H1299 lung cancer cell lines by causing cell cycle arrest in G1 phase [272].

Oridonin

Oridonin (Figure 7) is a diterpenoid derived from the Chinese herb *Rabdosia rubescens* and has been reported to have antifibrotic, antibacterial, anti-inflammatory, and anticancer effects [381]. In lung cancer, oridonin decreases cell migration, invasion, and metastasis via mesenchymal transition in the H1975 cell line at a concentration of 10 μM [273]. Additional analysis reported that concentrations of 10, 20, and 30 μM of oridonin increased Bax expression in A549 cells, thereby enhancing cisplatin-induced apoptosis by the AMPK/Akt/mTOR pathway [274].

Scabertopin

Scabertopin (Figure 7), a germacrane-type sesquiterpene lactone, is derived from *Elephantopus scaber*. It has displayed an anticancer effect in bladder cancer by modulating ROS and intracellular signaling [382]. In a xenograft mouse model of lung cancer, scabertopin was shown to promote cancer cell death through increased Bax expression and ROS-mediated apoptosis at a dose of 20 mg/kg [310].

Soyasapogenol

Soyasapogenol (Figure 7) is a pentacyclic triterpenoid present in soy-based foods and has been shown to reduce the proliferation, migration, and invasion of H1299 cancer cells, with concurrent upregulation of caspase-mediated apoptosis. Researchers also noted a reduction in CDK2, CDK4, cyclin A, and cyclin D1 expression, as well as suppression of pATR-Chk1 signaling [275]. In an in vivo study, 15 mg/kg of soyasapogenol enhanced apoptosis of xenografted tumor cells in a mouse model. Researchers also noted reduced migration and invasion of cancer cells, further confirming soyasapogenol's role as a potential anticancer pharmaceutical [275].

Thymoquinone

Thymoquinone (Figure 7), a monoterpene derived from the seeds of *Nigella sativa*, is well documented for its role in the management and treatment of numerous types of cancers, such as breast and colon cancers, in addition to osteosarcoma [383,384]. The anticancer activities of thymoquinone are primarily exerted through alterations in several oncogenic pathways, such as regulation of oxidative stress, inflammation, metastasis, and angiogenesis [385,386]. In one in vitro study, thymoquinone was found to promote caspase-3-induced apoptosis of LNM3 lung cancer cells. Building from their in vitro analysis, the researchers believed that thymoquinone increased cell death via caspase-3-mediated apoptosis in a xenografted nude mouse model at a dose of 10 mg/kg [276].

Ursolic Acid

Ursolic acid (Figure 7) is a pentacyclic terpenoid found abundantly in *Ilex paraguarieni*, *Mimusops caffra*, and *Glechoma hederacea*. In addition to its documented anticancer activities, ursolic acid is said to possess anti-inflammatory, antidiabetic, antibacterial, and antioxidant effects [387,388]. At a concentration of 11, 22, 44, and 88 μM, ursolic acid decreased cell viability and enhanced autophagy in A549 lung cancer cell lines. Researchers observed these changes to be associated with augmented ratio of LC3–phosphatidylethanolamine conjugates (LC3-II/LC3-I) and enhanced expression of ubiquitin-binding protein (p62), PTEN-induced kinase 1 (PINK1), and Nrf2, with reductions in p-Akt and p-mTOR expression [277]. A separate study found that, at a concentration of 0.001–0.1 μM, ursolic acid caused inhibition of tumor cell proliferation and angiogenesis in H1975 cells. Investigators found that application of ursolic acid resulted in decreased N-cadherin and TGF-β1 expression, with enhanced expression of E-cadherin, MMP-2, and MMP-9 [278]. In another study utilizing A549, H460, H1975, H1299, H520, H02, LLC, and H446 cell lines, 5–40 μM of ursolic acid decreased cell proliferation and angiogenesis. The researchers attributed these findings to ursolic acid's ability to upregulate LC3-II protein and cleaved PARP expression, while downregulating Bcl-2, p-S6K T389, and p-Akt expression [279].

Withaferin A

Withaferin A (Figure 7), a terpenoid phytochemical historically used in Ayurvedic medicine, is derived from *Withania somnifera* and has been purported to possess immunomodulatory, antibacterial, and cardioprotective effects [389,390]. General anticancer activities of withaferin A include induction of apoptosis via p53 and suppression the activity of TASK-3 channels [391,392]. When studied in the context of lung cancer, withaferin A was demonstrated to promote apoptosis and increase oxidative stress in A549 lung cancer cells [280].

7.1.5. Miscellaneous Compounds

Cannabidiol

Cannabidiol (Figure 8) is derived from the plant *Cannabis sativa* and is reported to have several therapeutic benefits, such as anticonvulsant, analgesic, antipsychotic, neuroprotective, anxiolytic, anti-inflammatory, and antioxidant activities [393]. Cannabidiol has been demonstrated to be effective in lung cancer. When 3 μM of cannabidiol was applied to A549 and H460 cells, researchers observed reduced lymphoid trafficking and increased apoptosis [281,282]. In another study, 1–10 μM of cannabidiol was reported to inhibit lymphoid trafficking and enhance COX-2, thereby negatively regulating the growth of lung cancer in A549 and H460 cells [283]. Moreover, a separate study validated these findings by showing that, at a concentration of 3 μM, cannabidiol reduced cell invasion and promoted apoptosis in the A549 cell line [284]. In vivo analysis of cannabidiol demonstrated decreased cell proliferation and migration when cannabidiol at a dose of 5 mg/kg was administered to nude mice with xenograft tumors. The researchers attribute these findings to an observed increase in COX-2, peroxisome proliferator-activated receptor-γ (PPAR-γ), and intercellular adhesion molecule-1 (ICAM-1) expression [283].

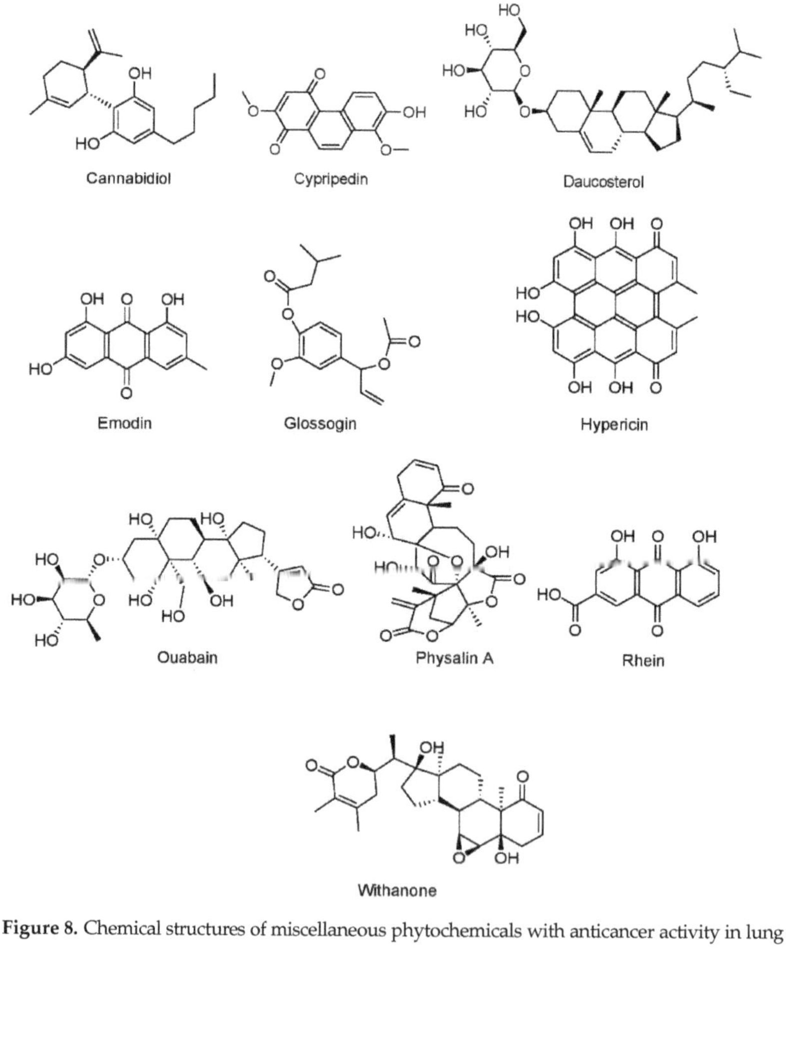

Figure 8. Chemical structures of miscellaneous phytochemicals with anticancer activity in lung cancer.

Cypripedin

Cypripedin (Figure 8) is a phenanthrenequinone derived from the orchid *Dendrobium densiflorum* and has been reported to have antiproliferative, anti-inflammatory, antimicrobial, and antioxidant effects [394]. In lung cancer, cypripedin has been shown to inhibit proliferation of H23 cells at a concentration of 50 μM. The researchers reported these effects to be mediated by inhibiting N-cadherin, vimentin, and the Akt/GSK-3β signaling pathway [285]. In lung cancer cell line H460, 50 μM of cypripedin decreased cell proliferation. The investigators suggested these findings to be mediated by inhibition of Bcl-2 expression [286].

Daucosterol

Daucosterol (Figure 8) is a steroidal saponin derived from *Grewia tiliaefolia* and has several pharmacological activities, such as antidiabetic, antioxidant, hypolipidemic, anticancer, immunomodulatory, anti-inflammatory, and neuroprotective actions [395]. When applied to A549 cells, daucosterol was found to increase apoptosis and inhibit the cell cycle at the G2/M phase. The researchers believe these anticancer effects to be mediated by downregulation of Bcl-2 expression, with concurrent upregulation of Bax and caspase-3 cleavage [268].

Emodin

Emodin (Figure 8) is a natural compound belonging to the anthraquinone family that can be derived from *Polygonum cuspidatum*, *Rheum palmatum*, and *Polygonum multiflorum*; it acts as a tyrosine kinase inhibitor and suppresses tumor growth and cancer cell transformation [396]. Emodin demonstrates anticancer potential against lung neoplasias through its actions on A549 and H1299 cells. Researchers observed that emodin caused endoplasmic reticulum (ER) stress-mediated apoptosis by the tribbles homolog 3 (TRIB3)/NF-κB pathway at concentrations of 20, 40, 60, and 80 μM [287]. Furthermore, te researchers went on to analyze these effects in an in vivo model in nude mice with xenografted tumors, where emodin was again found to initiate ER stress-mediated apoptosis when administrated at a dose of 50 mg/kg [287].

Glossogin

Glossogin (Figure 8) is derived from *Glossogyne tenuifolia* and has shown anticancer activity against breast and liver cancer cell lines [397]. In an in vitro analysis of glossogin against A549 lung cancer cells, researchers demonstrated its ability to decrease cell proliferation at a concentration of 12.5 μg/mL. The investigators attributed these findings to an increase in cytochrome c, caspase-3, caspase-9, and the Bak/Bcl-2 ratio [288].

Hypericin

Hypericin (Figure 8) is an anthraquinone derivative derived from *Hypericum perforatum* and has been shown to possess anti-inflammatory effects and inhibit various oncogenic signaling molecules, ultimately causing reduced angiogenesis, adhesion, and mitochondrial thioredoxin [168]. In an in vivo study, hypericin enhanced siRNA transfection and reduced HIF-1α, resulting in decreased cell proliferation and angiogenesis in a BALB/c nude mouse tumor model at a dose of 0.1 mg/kg [168,311]. Additional research conducted in a W256 tumor rat and mouse model demonstrated the ability of hypericin to initiate apoptosis at a dose of 2 mg/kg. The researchers did not report any mechanism of action [168,312].

Ouabain

Ouabain (Figure 8) is a cardiac glycoside derived from ripe seeds of *Strophanthus gratus* and bark of *Acokanthera ouabaio*, having therapeutic potentials in the management of hypertension, arrhythmia, and heart failure [398,399]. In A549 and H1975 lung cancer cells, ouabain was shown to reduce cell proliferation at a concentration of 25 nM. The researchers believe these results to be mediated by inhibition of JNK and Bcl-2 expression in A549 lung cancer cell lines [289].

Physalin A

Physalin A (Figure 8) is an active withanolide derived from *Physalis alkekengi*. It has several biological activities, such as anticancer, antiparasitic, anti-inflammatory, antimicrobial, antiviral, and antinociceptive effects [400]. In lung cancer, physalin A was shown to decrease cell migration, angiogenesis, migration, and proliferation via the JAK/STAT3 signaling pathway in H292, H358, and H1975 cell lines. Following their in vitro analysis, the researchers evaluated the effects of 40 or 80 mg/kg of physalin A in a xenograft mouse model and again found a reduced JAK/STAT3 signaling pathway, with associated reductions in cell proliferation, migration, invasion, and angiogenesis [290].

Rhein

Rhein (4, 5-dihydroxyanthraquinone-2-carboxylic acid, Figure 8) is an anthraquinone glycoside abundantly present in several plant species including *Rheum palmatum*, *Polygonum multiflorum* Thunb, *Cassia tora*, and *Aloe barbadensis* Miller. Pharmacological properties of rhein include its ability to cause cell cycle arrest and DNA damage to tumor cells in several cancer models [401]. When applied to A549 cells at a concentration of 45 μM, rhein was shown to inhibit cell proliferation, migration, and invasion. The researchers noted these findings to be associated with an increase in G0/G1 phase cell cycle arrest and p53, p21, and Bax expression [291,292]. In another study, rhein caused apoptosis by reduction of p-PI3K, Akt, mTOR, and Bcl-2 expression at a 100 μM concentration in A549 cells [293]. Moreover, rhein was again demonstrated to inhibit cancer cell proliferation, angiogenesis, and metastasis when applied to PC-9, H460, and A549 cell lines at concentrations of 24.59 μM, 52.88 μM, and 23.9 μM, respectively. The researchers attribute these findings to upregulation of G2/M phase cell cycle arrest and decreased STAT3 and Bcl-2 expression [294]. In a follow-up in vivo study, rhein was again shown to reduce the expression of STAT3 and promote G2/M phase cell cycle arrest at a dose of 60 or 100 mg/kg in a xenograft mouse model [294].

Withanone

Withanone (Figure 8) is a steroidal lactone also derived from *Withania somnifera* with an array of therapeutic applications, including anticancer effects [402] and activity against SARS-CoV-2 [403]. In one study utilizing A549 lung cancer cells, withanone was found to decrease cell proliferation, migration, invasion, and metastasis. The researchers noted these findings to be accompanied by reduced expression of CDK2, CDK4, cyclin D and cyclin E, and mortalin and increased p53 and CARF expression [269].

7.2. Clinical Studies

While preclinical studies have sparked interest in phytochemicals as agents against lung cancer, clinical trials are required to validate their effects and change the current practice of medical oncology. Most naturally derived agents, such as vincristine, vinblastine, and camptothecin, against lung cancer represented in clinical studies are FDA approved for at least one form of cancer. Two exceptions, however, are resveratrol and seliciclib. Resveratrol is a polyphenol found in berries, grapes, red wine, and peanuts that has been reported to possess antioxidant, antidiabetic, anti-inflammatory, and anticancer effects [404]. In a clinical trial carried out on 96 lung cancer patients, resveratrol suppressed tumor growth by downregulating Forkhead box C2 (FOXC2) and upregulating miR-520h-mediated PP2A/C expression, thereby causing apoptosis in lung cancer cells [405]. Seliciclib is a natural compound present in radish (*Raphnus sativus* L.). Seliciclib (R-roscovitine), a drug in the family of cyclin-dependent kinases, is reported to be effective in treating cancers, inflammation, neurodegenerative diseases, viral infections, glomerulonephritis, and polycystic kidney disease [406]. In a separate, phase II trial, seliciclib (R-roscovitine) was shown to cause decreased tumor growth in lung cancer cells. The researchers attribute this finding to its role in inhibiting RNA-polymerase-II-dependent transcription, leading to the downregulation of myeloid leukemia 1 (Mcl-1) protein [407].

Although use of camptothecin has not been directly approved by the FDA since its isolation from *Camptotheca acuminata*, several of its analogs have received approval for cancer therapy [408]. In a phase I study on cancer patients, camptothecin was documented to synergize with topoisomerase I and DNA, resulting in hindered reassembly of single-strand DNA by intercalating between its nitrogenous bases, leading to the inhibition of bonds at the sites of nicks, thereby harming the structure of the double-stranded DNA chain. Several vinca alkaloids have been approved by the FDA for cancer treatment. Members of this family, including vincristine, vinblastine, vinorelbine, vindesine, and vinflunine, are derived from the Madagascar periwinkle plant [409] and were shown to prevent the polymerization of microtubules, leading to metaphase arrest and cell death in a phase II clinical trial [410]. Paclitaxel and docetaxel were reported to bind with tubulin and disrupt microtubule dynamics, thereby causing mitotic arrest and cell death [411]. In another phase II clinical study, paclitaxel and docetaxel were documented to have response rates of 21–24% and 28–38%, respectively, in advanced non-small lung cancer cell patients, who were first treated with cisplatin [412]. In another phase II clinical study, paclitaxel was reported to promote G2/M phase cell cycle arrest in 37 patients with stage III lung cancer. Paclitaxel was administrated at a concentration of 225 mg/m^2 for three weeks and although mild hematologic toxicity was observed, adverse events were well tolerated overall [413].

Despite strong support in favor of natural compounds against the development and progression of lung cancer, there is an obvious need for additional clinical trials. Future trials should strive to evaluate the effects of a phytochemical compared to current, first-line treatments. Besides lack of data, other barriers exist before phytochemicals may see widespread use. Taxol, in a phase II clinical study, exhibited cytotoxic symptoms against healthy tissue [414]. Therefore, there is a need to better evaluate the safety profile of phytochemicals, even if their toxicity profiles tend to be better than those of current therapies. Ultimately, the success of these plant-derived anticancer agents as FDA-approved therapies highlights the potential of future drug discovery. The review of the available literature, however, underscores the need for additional studies of underinvestigated compounds.

8. Conclusions and Future Perspectives

Lung cancer is the foremost reason for mortality in cancer patients [7]. Despite current chemotherapeutic options, many patients are left without efficacious treatments and suffer as a result. And for those receiving treatment, they must endure numerous side effects. Accordingly, there is an obvious need for the development of safe and effective pharmacons against lung cancer, and the evidence outlined in this review provides strong rationale for further investigation into phytochemicals as potential chemotherapeutic agents. Previously published reviews on phytochemicals targeting lung cancer involved fewer phytochemicals and were not utterly comprehensive or did not incorporate all types of preclinical and clinical studies. Furthermore, a detailed discussion of the preclinical and clinical studies, and molecular mechanisms outlined therein, was previously lacking. Therefore, this comprehensive review serves to explore the anticancer potential of bioactive compounds in lung cancer, along with their molecular mechanisms, as a critical analysis of currently available in vitro, in vivo, and clinical evidence for their role in mitigating lung cancer.

Phytochemicals are widely reported for their anticancer potential against lung cancer and have been a robust area of research for many years. Several plant metabolites belonging to the class of secondary metabolites such as alkaloids, sulfur-containing compounds, phenolics, and terpenoids are well documented to have antitumor activity or decrease cancer progression. These agents function by modulating various signaling pathways, inducing apoptosis, inhibiting angiogenesis, promoting the disruption of the mitochondrial membrane, and regulating transcription factors and oxidative stress. Several cancer signaling pathways, such as ERK1/2, Akt/mTOR, TGF-β, MAPK, JAK/STAT, NF-κB, and Akt/GSK-3β signaling pathways, have been affected by a range of phytochemicals in various lung cancer models (summarized in Figure 9). Most of the phytochemicals act through complex mechanisms, induce apoptosis and/or inhibit tumor growth, and ultimately play an important role in the cell proliferation and survival. The present review highlights the potential of phytochemicals as promising candidates for cancer prevention and treatment. By targeting multiple cancer hallmarks through various signaling pathways, phytochemicals demonstrate their ability to halt tumor growth and progression. However, further research is needed to fully comprehend the mechanisms and optimize the clinical applications of these natural compounds in cancer therapy.

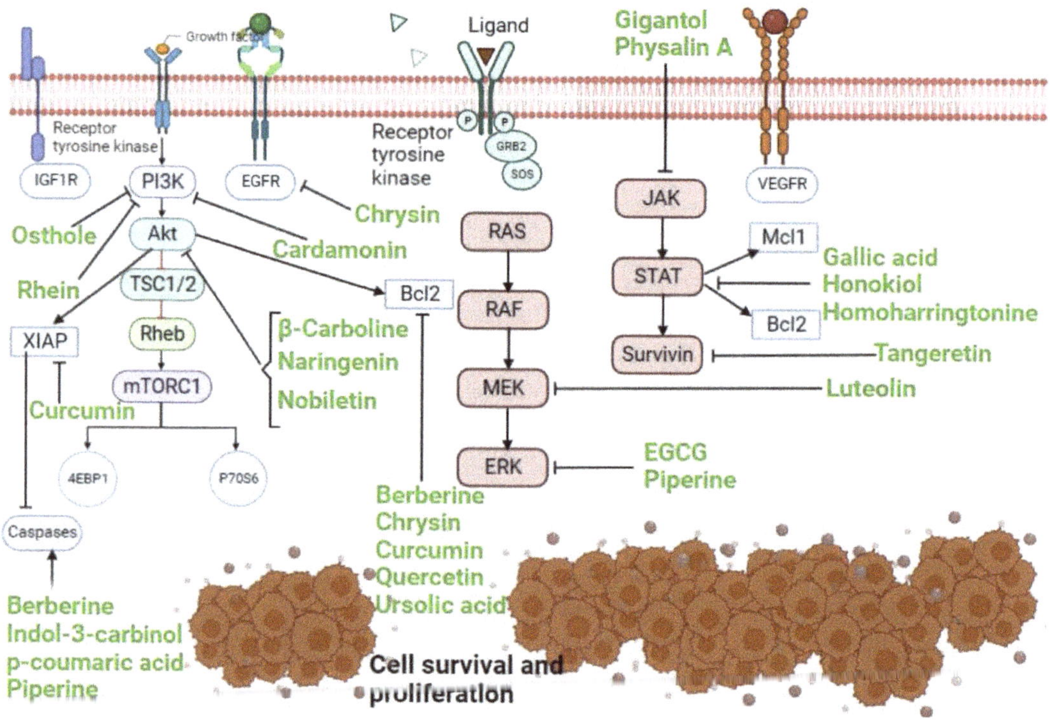

Figure 9. Reported therapeutic targets of select phytochemicals against lung cancer. Binding of ligand to any RTK like EGFR, VEGFR, IGF-1R, HER2, c-MET, or RET results in activation of a multitude of downstream signaling pathways. PI3K/Akt/mTOR pathway incites the activation of effector proteins like 4EBP1 and p70S6K and prosurvival oncogenes including Bcl-2 and XIAP that inhibit the actions of apoptotic caspases. The PI3K/Akt/mTOR pathway also blocks the actions of proapoptotic FOXO. The RAS/RAF/MEK/ERK pathway results in the activation of proto-oncogenes like c-Myc and c-Jun. The JAK/STAT pathway results in the activation of prosurvival oncogenes like Bcl-2, Mcl-1, and survivin. Each of these pathways results in cell survival and proliferation in lung cancer. Signaling molecules and effector proteins of these major pathways of lung cancer serve as targets for phytochemicals. Abbreviations: Bcl-2, B cell lymphoma protein-2; c-MET, c-mesenchymal–epithelial transition factor; 4EBP1, 4E-binding protein 1; EGFR, epidermal growth factor receptor; FOXO, Forkhead box O; HER2, human epidermal growth factor receptor 2; IGF-1R, insulin-like growth factor-1 receptor; Mcl-1, myeloid cell leukemia sequence 1; p70S6K, p70S6 kinase 1; RET, rearranged during transfection; RTK, receptor tyrosine kinase; VEGFR, vascular endothelial growth factor receptor; XIAP, X-linked inhibitor of apoptosis protein (created with BioRender.com, accessed on 28 July 2023).

Notably, the outcomes of the in vitro, in vivo, and clinical studies are promising, but certain limitations are apparent. Numerous preclinical studies had contradictory outcomes, while some studies did not explore the mechanisms of action of the phytochemicals. Furthermore, several phytochemicals were restricted to one type of study (in vitro, in vivo, or clinical). To overcome these limitations, additional preclinical and clinical studies should be conducted to analyze the efficacy of each phytochemical and to explore the potential role of various combinations of phytochemicals in the treatment of lung cancer. Moreover, their potential as adjuvants or complementary agents alongside conventional cancer treatments presents a compelling avenue for future investigation and development of effective anticancer strategies against lung cancer.

Additional research may also address challenges faced by phytochemical-based treatments. The major drawback associated with phytochemicals is their low bioavailability and rapid metabolism in the human body. This may result in reduced effective uptake, causing deficient targeting and undesirable toxicity when consumed in high enough quantities to produce results. To overcome these problems, there is a need to explore a novel delivery system for the effective delivery of plant metabolites. Some phytochemical studies were conducted outside of lung cancer which have observed beneficial results with nanoparticles [415,416]. Moreover, large-scale, well-designed, high-quality, and multicenter randomized clinical studies comparing phytochemicals to first-line treatments are necessary to validate the safety and clinical efficacy of plant metabolites.

In conclusion, numerous phytochemicals exhibit promising outcomes for the prevention and treatment of lung cancer. This review was constructed with hopes that it may open the door for the development of more effective treatments for individuals suffering with lung cancer. It is our anticipation that the information shared in this article will be useful to researchers exploring unique and non-toxic therapeutic avenues for the management of lung cancer. Notably, based on the available literature, several phytochemicals exhibit remarkable and inspiring potential to meet the ever-growing need to prevent and treat lung cancer.

Author Contributions: Conceptualization, D.T.; methodology, N.C. and S.B.; data curation, N.C. and S.B.; writing—original draft preparation, N.C. and S.B.; writing—review and editing, D.T., J.T.B., D.S. and A.B.; supervision, D.T. and A.B.; project administration, A.B. All authors have read and agreed to the published version of the manuscript.

Funding: This research received no external funding.

Conflicts of Interest: The authors declare no conflict of interest.

References

1. Thandra, K.C.; Barsouk, A.; Saginala, K.; Aluru, J.S.; Barsouk, A. Epidemiology of lung cancer. *Wspolczesna Onkol.* **2021**, *25*, 45–52. [CrossRef] [PubMed]
2. de Groot, P.M.; Wu, C.C.; Carter, B.W.; Munden, R.F. The epidemiology of lung cancer. *Transl. Lung Cancer Res.* **2018**, *7*, 220–233. [CrossRef] [PubMed]
3. Davidson, M.R.; Gazdar, A.F.; Clarke, B.E. The pivotal role of pathology in the management of lung cancer. *J. Thorac. Dis.* **2013**, *5* (Suppl. S5), S463–S478. [CrossRef]
4. Nojiri, T.; Hamasaki, T.; Inoue, M.; Shintani, Y.; Takeuchi, Y.; Maeda, H.; Okumura, M. Long Term Impact of Postoperative Complications on Cancer Recurrence Following Lung Cancer Surgery. *Ann. Surg. Oncol.* **2017**, *24*, 1135–1142. [CrossRef] [PubMed]
5. Lemjabbar-Alaoui, H.; Hassan, O.U.I.; Yang, Y.W.; Buchanan, P. Lung cancer: Biology and treatment options. *Biochim. Et Biophys. Acta (BBA)-Rev. Cancer* **2015**, *1856*, 189–210. [CrossRef]
6. Sever, R.; Brugge, J.S. Signal transduction in cancer. *Cold Spring Harb. Perspect. Med.* **2015**, *5*, a006098. [CrossRef] [PubMed]
7. Sung, H.; Ferlay, J.; Siegel, R.L.; Laversanne, M.; Soerjomataram, I.; Jemal, A.; Bray, F. Global Cancer Statistics 2020: GLOBOCAN Estimates of Incidence and Mortality Worldwide for 36 Cancers in 185 Countries. *CA Cancer J. Clin.* **2021**, *71*, 209–249. [CrossRef]
8. Lee, W.H.; Loo, C.Y.; Ghadiri, M.; Leong, C.R.; Young, P.M.; Traini, D. The potential to treat lung cancer via inhalation of repurposed drugs. *Adv. Drug Deliv. Rev.* **2018**, *133*, 107–130. [CrossRef]

9. Rossi, A.; Di Maio, M.; Chiodini, P.; Rudd, R.M.; Okamoto, H.; Skarlos, D.V.; Früh, M.; Qian, W.; Tamura, T.; Samantas, E.; et al. Carboplatin- or cisplatin-based chemotherapy in first-line treatment of small-cell lung cancer: The COCIS meta-analysis of individual patient data. *J. Clin. Oncol.* **2012**, *30*, 1692–1698. [CrossRef]
10. Ban, H.; Kim, K.S.; Oh, I.J.; Yoon, S.H.; Lee, B.; Yu, J.; Kim, S.; Lee, H.S.; Shin, H.J.; Park, C.K.; et al. Efficacy and safety of docetaxel plus oxaliplatin as a first-line chemotherapy in patients with advanced or metastatic non-small cell lung cancer. *Thorac. Cancer* **2014**, *5*, 525–529. [CrossRef]
11. Khan, T.; Ali, M.; Khan, A.; Nisar, P.; Jan, S.A.; Afridi, S.; Shinwari, Z.K. Anticancer plants: A review of the active phytochemicals, applications in animal models, and regulatory aspects. *Biomolecules* **2020**, *10*, 47. [CrossRef]
12. Atanasov, A.G.; Zotchev, S.B.; Dirsch, V.M.; Orhan, I.E.; Banach, M.; Rollinger, J.M.; Barreca, D.; Weckwerth, W.; Bauer, R.; Bayer, E.A.; et al. Natural products in drug discovery: Advances and opportunities. *Nat. Rev. Drug Discov.* **2021**, *20*, 200–216. [CrossRef]
13. Choudhary, N.; Prabhakar, P.K.; Khatik, G.L.; Chamakuri, S.R.; Tewari, D.; Suttee, A. Evaluation of acute toxicity, in-vitro, in-vivo antidiabetic potential of the flavonoid fraction of the plant *Chenopodium album* L. *Pharmacogn. J.* **2021**, *13*, 765–779. [CrossRef]
14. Choudhary, N.; Khatik, G.L.; Sharma, R.; Khurana, N.; Lobo, R.; Bhatt, S.; Tewari, D.; Suttee, A. Ameliorative potential of Operculina turpethum against streptozotocin-induced diabetes in rats: Biochemical and histopathological studies. *3 Biotech* **2021**, *11*, 309. [CrossRef] [PubMed]
15. Dehelean, C.A.; Marcovici, I.; Soica, C.; Mioc, M.; Coricovac, D.; Iurciuc, S.; Cretu, O.M.; Pinzaru, I. Plant-derived anticancer compounds as new perspectives in drug discovery and alternative therapy. *Molecules* **2021**, *26*, 1109. [CrossRef]
16. Wattanathamsan, O.; Hayakawa, Y.; Pongrakhananon, V. Molecular mechanisms of natural compounds in cell death induction and sensitization to chemotherapeutic drugs in lung cancer. *Phyther. Res.* **2019**, *33*, 2531–2547. [CrossRef]
17. Yang, Y.; Li, N.; Wang, T.M.; Di, L. Natural products with activity against lung cancer: A review focusing on the tumor microenvironment. *Int. J. Mol. Sci.* **2021**, *22*, 10827. [CrossRef]
18. Ahmed, B.; Joseph, A.; Das, S.; Roy, S.; Rahaman, S.B.; Akbar, S.; Halder, D.; Ramachandran, A.K. Structure-Activity Relationship Insight of Naturally Occurring Bioactive Molecules and Their Derivatives against Non-Small Cell Lung Cancer: A Comprehensive Review. *Curr. Med. Chem.* **2022**, *29*, 6030–6062. [CrossRef]
19. Heng, W.S.; Kruyt, F.A.E.; Cheah, S.-C. Understanding lung carcinogenesis from a morphostatic perspective: Prevention and therapeutic potential of phytochemicals for targeting cancer stem cells. *Int. J. Mol. Sci.* **2021**, *22*, 5697. [CrossRef]
20. Singh, J.; Luqman, S.; Meena, A. Emerging role of phytochemicals in targeting predictive, prognostic, and diagnostic biomarkers of lung cancer. *Food Chem. Toxicol.* **2020**, *144*, 111592. [CrossRef] [PubMed]
21. Muller, A.G.; Sarker, S.D.; Saleem, I.Y.; Hutcheon, G.A. Delivery of natural phenolic compounds for the potential treatment of lung cancer. *DARU J. Pharm. Sci.* **2019**, *27*, 433–449. [CrossRef] [PubMed]
22. Travis, W.D.; Brambilla, E.; Noguchi, M.; Nicholson, A.G.; Geisinger, K.R.; Yatabe, Y.; Beer, D.G.; Powell, C.A.; Riely, G.J.; Van Schil, P.E.; et al. International association for the study of lung cancer/american thoracic society/european respiratory society international multidisciplinary classification of lung adenocarcinoma. *J. Thorac. Oncol.* **2011**, *6*, 244–285. [CrossRef]
23. Byers, L.A.; Rudin, C.M. Small cell lung cancer: Where do we go from here? *Cancer* **2015**, *121*, 664–672. [CrossRef]
24. Santarpia, M.; Daffinà, M.G.; Karachaliou, N.; González-Cao, M.; Lazzari, C.; Altavilla, G.; Rosell, R. Targeted drugs in small-cell lung cancer. *Transl. Lung Cancer Res.* **2016**, *5*, 51–70. [CrossRef]
25. Wistuba, I.I.; Gazdar, A.F. Lung cancer preneoplasia. *Annu. Rev. Pathol.* **2006**, *1*, 331–348. [CrossRef]
26. Sánchez-Ortega, M.; Carrera, A.C.; Garrido, A. Role of NRF2 in Lung Cancer. *Cells* **2021**, *10*, 1879. [CrossRef] [PubMed]
27. Kadara, H.; Scheet, P.; Wistuba, I.I.; Spira, A.E. Early Events in the Molecular Pathogenesis of Lung Cancer. *Cancer Prev. Res.* **2016**, *9*, 518–527. [CrossRef] [PubMed]
28. Bernhardt, E.B.; Jalal, S.I. Small Cell Lung Cancer. *Cancer Treat. Res.* **2016**, *170*, 301–322. [CrossRef]
29. Kadara, H.; Wistuba, I.I. Field cancerization in non-small cell lung cancer: Implications in disease pathogenesis. *Proc. Am. Thorac. Soc.* **2012**, *9*, 38–42. [CrossRef]
30. Steiling, K.; Ryan, J.; Brody, J.S.; Spira, A. The field of tissue injury in the lung and airway. *Cancer Prev. Res.* **2008**, *1*, 396–403. [CrossRef]
31. Auerbach, O.; Stout, A.P.; Hammond, E.C.; Garfinkel, L. Changes in bronchial epithelium in relation to cigarette smoking and in relation to lung cancer. *N. Engl. J. Med.* **1961**, *265*, 253–267. [CrossRef] [PubMed]
32. Curtius, K.; Wright, N.A.; Graham, T.A. An evolutionary perspective on field cancerization. *Nat. Rev. Cancer* **2018**, *18*, 19–32. [CrossRef] [PubMed]
33. Pirlog, R.; Cismaru, A.; Nutu, A.; Berindan-Neagoe, I. Field Cancerization in NSCLC: A New Perspective on MicroRNAs in Macrophage Polarization. *Int. J. Mol. Sci.* **2021**, *22*, 746. [CrossRef] [PubMed]
34. Saab, S.; Zalzale, H.; Rahal, Z.; Khalifeh, Y.; Sinjab, A.; Kadara, H. Insights Into Lung Cancer Immune-Based Biology, Prevention, and Treatment. *Front. Immunol.* **2020**, *11*, 159. [CrossRef]
35. Chan, B.A.; Hughes, B.G.M. Targeted therapy for non-small cell lung cancer: Current standards and the promise of the future. *Transl. Lung Cancer Res.* **2015**, *4*, 36–54. [CrossRef]
36. Peifer, M.; Fernández-Cuesta, L.; Sos, M.L.; George, J.; Seidel, D.; Kasper, L.H.; Plenker, D.; Leenders, F.; Sun, R.; Zander, T.; et al. Integrative genome analyses identify key somatic driver mutations of small-cell lung cancer. *Nat. Genet.* **2012**, *44*, 1104–1110. [CrossRef]

37. Rudin, C.M.; Durinck, S.; Stawiski, E.W.; Poirier, J.T.; Modrusan, Z.; Shames, D.S.; Bergbower, E.A.; Guan, Y.; Shin, J.; Guillory, J.; et al. Comprehensive genomic analysis identifies SOX2 as a frequently amplified gene in small-cell lung cancer. *Nat. Genet.* **2012**, *44*, 1111–1116. [CrossRef]
38. Wistuba, I.I.; Gazdar, A.F.; Minna, J.D. Molecular genetics of small cell lung carcinoma. *Semin. Oncol.* **2001**, *28*, 3–13. [CrossRef]
39. Yuan, M.; Zhao, Y.; Arkenau, H.-T.; Lao, T.; Chu, L.; Xu, Q. Signal pathways and precision therapy of small-cell lung cancer. *Signal Transduct. Target. Ther.* **2022**, *7*, 187. [CrossRef]
40. Abolfathi, H.; Arabi, M.; Sheikhpour, M. A literature review of microRNA and gene signaling pathways involved in the apoptosis pathway of lung cancer. *Respir. Res.* **2023**, *24*, 55. [CrossRef]
41. Iksen; Pothongsrisit, S.; Pongrakhananon, V. Targeting the PI3K/AKT/mTOR Signaling Pathway in Lung Cancer: An Update Regarding Potential Drugs and Natural Products. *Molecules* **2021**, *26*, 4100. [CrossRef] [PubMed]
42. Alam, M.; Hasan, G.M.; Eldin, S.M.; Adnan, M.; Riaz, M.B.; Islam, A.; Khan, I.; Hassan, M.I. Investigating regulated signaling pathways in therapeutic targeting of non-small cell lung carcinoma. *Biomed. Pharmacother.* **2023**, *161*, 114452. [CrossRef] [PubMed]
43. Henriques, A.F.A.; Barros, P.; Moyer, M.P.; Matos, P.; Jordan, P. Expression of tumor-related Rac1b antagonizes B-Raf-induced senescence in colorectal cells. *Cancer Lett.* **2015**, *369*, 368–375. [CrossRef]
44. Ritt, D.A.; Abreu-Blanco, M.T.; Bindu, L.; Durrant, D.E.; Zhou, M.; Specht, S.I.; Stephen, A.G.; Holderfield, M.; Morrison, D.K. Inhibition of Ras/Raf/MEK/ERK Pathway Signaling by a Stress-Induced Phospho-Regulatory Circuit. *Mol. Cell* **2016**, *64*, 875–887. [CrossRef]
45. Avery, T.Y.; Köhler, N.; Zeiser, R.; Brummer, T.; Ruess, D.A. Onco-immunomodulatory properties of pharmacological interference with RAS-RAF-MEK-ERK pathway hyperactivation. *Front. Oncol.* **2022**, *12*, 931774. [CrossRef]
46. Cristea, S.; Sage, J. Is the Canonical RAF/MEK/ERK Signaling Pathway a Therapeutic Target in SCLC? *J. Thorac. Oncol.* **2016**, *11*, 1233–1241. [CrossRef] [PubMed]
47. Xie, M.; Xu, X.; Fan, Y. KRAS-Mutant Non-Small Cell Lung Cancer: An Emerging Promisingly Treatable Subgroup. *Front. Oncol.* **2021**, *11*, 672612. [CrossRef]
48. Adderley, H.; Blackhall, F.H.; Lindsay, C.R. KRAS-mutant non-small cell lung cancer: Converging small molecules and immune checkpoint inhibition. *EBioMedicine* **2019**, *41*, 711–716. [CrossRef] [PubMed]
49. McCubrey, J.A.; Steelman, L.S.; Chappell, W.H.; Abrams, S.L.; Wong, E.W.T.; Chang, F.; Lehmann, B.; Terrian, D.M.; Milella, M.; Tafuri, A.; et al. Roles of the Raf/MEK/ERK pathway in cell growth, malignant transformation and drug resistance. *Biochim. Biophys. Acta* **2007**, *1773*, 1263–1284. [CrossRef]
50. Chilamakuri, R.; Agarwal, S. Direct Targeting of the Raf-MEK-ERK Signaling Cascade Inhibits Neuroblastoma Growth. *Curr. Oncol.* **2022**, *29*, 6508–6522. [CrossRef]
51. Yan, N.; Guo, S.; Zhang, H.; Zhang, Z.; Shen, S.; Li, X. BRAF-Mutated Non-Small Cell Lung Cancer: Current Treatment Status and Future Perspective. *Front. Oncol.* **2022**, *12*, 863043. [CrossRef] [PubMed]
52. Tan, A.C. Targeting the PI3K/Akt/mTOR pathway in non-small cell lung cancer (NSCLC). *Thorac. Cancer* **2020**, *11*, 511–518. [CrossRef]
53. Papadimitrakopoulou, V. Development of PI3K/AKT/mTOR pathway inhibitors and their application in personalized therapy for non–small-cell lung cancer. *J. Thorac. Oncol.* **2012**, *7*, 1315–1326. [CrossRef] [PubMed]
54. Tsurutani, J.; Fukuoka, J.; Tsurutani, H.; Shih, J.H.; Hewitt, S.M.; Travis, W.D.; Jen, J.; Dennis, P.A. Evaluation of two phosphorylation sites improves the prognostic significance of Akt activation in non-small-cell lung cancer tumors. *J. Clin. Oncol.* **2006**, *24*, 306–314. [CrossRef]
55. Cappuzzo, F.; Ligorio, C.; Jänne, P.A.; Toschi, L.; Rossi, E.; Trisolini, R.; Paioli, D.; Holmes, A.J.; Magrini, E.; Finocchiaro, G.; et al. Prospective study of gefitinib in epidermal growth factor receptor fluorescence in situ hybridization-positive/phospho-Akt-positive or never smoker patients with advanced non-small-cell lung cancer: The ONCOBELL trial. *J. Clin. Oncol.* **2007**, *25*, 2248–2255. [CrossRef] [PubMed]
56. Marsit, C.J.; Zheng, S.; Aldape, K.; Hinds, P.W.; Nelson, H.H.; Wiencke, J.K.; Kelsey, K.T. PTEN expression in non-small-cell lung cancer: Evaluating its relation to tumor characteristics, allelic loss, and epigenetic alteration. *Hum. Pathol.* **2005**, *36*, 768–776. [CrossRef] [PubMed]
57. Soria, J.-C.; Lee, H.-Y.; Lee, J.I.; Wang, L.; Issa, J.-P.; Kemp, B.L.; Liu, D.D.; Kurie, J.M.; Mao, L.; Khuri, F.R. Lack of PTEN expression in non-small cell lung cancer could be related to promoter methylation. *Clin. Cancer Res.* **2002**, *8*, 1178–1184.
58. Okudela, K.; Suzuki, M.; Kageyama, S.; Bunai, T.; Nagura, K.; Igarashi, H.; Takamochi, K.; Suzuki, K.; Yamada, T.; Niwa, H.; et al. PIK3CA mutation and amplification in human lung cancer. *Pathol. Int.* **2007**, *57*, 664–671. [CrossRef]
59. Yamamoto, H.; Shigematsu, H.; Nomura, M.; Lockwood, W.W.; Sato, M.; Okumura, N.; Soh, J.; Suzuki, M.; Wistuba, I.I.; Fong, K.M.; et al. PIK3CA mutations and copy number gains in human lung cancers. *Cancer Res.* **2008**, *68*, 6913–6921. [CrossRef]
60. Kawano, O.; Sasaki, H.; Okuda, K.; Yukiue, H.; Yokoyama, T.; Yano, M.; Fujii, Y. PIK3CA gene amplification in Japanese non-small cell lung cancer. *Lung Cancer* **2007**, *58*, 159–160. [CrossRef] [PubMed]
61. Angulo, B.; Suarez-Gauthier, A.; Lopez-Rios, F.; Medina, P.P.; Conde, E.; Tang, M.; Soler, G.; Lopez-Encuentra, A.; Cigudosa, J.C.; Sanchez-Cespedes, M. Expression signatures in lung cancer reveal a profile for EGFR-mutant tumours and identify selective PIK3CA overexpression by gene amplification. *J. Pathol.* **2008**, *214*, 347–356. [CrossRef]
62. Samuels, Y.; Wang, Z.; Bardelli, A.; Silliman, N.; Ptak, J.; Szabo, S.; Yan, H.; Gazdar, A.; Powell, S.M.; Riggins, G.J. High frequency of mutations of the PIK3CA gene in human cancers. *Science* **2004**, *304*, 554. [CrossRef] [PubMed]

63. Thomas, S.J.; Snowden, J.A.; Zeidler, M.P.; Danson, S.J. The role of JAK/STAT signalling in the pathogenesis, prognosis and treatment of solid tumours. *Br. J. Cancer* **2015**, *113*, 365–371. [CrossRef] [PubMed]
64. Hu, X.; Li, J.; Fu, M.; Zhao, X.; Wang, W. The JAK/STAT signaling pathway: From bench to clinic. *Signal Transduct. Target. Ther.* **2021**, *6*, 402. [CrossRef] [PubMed]
65. Khanna, P.; Chua, P.J.; Bay, B.H.; Baeg, G.H. The JAK/STAT signaling cascade in gastric carcinoma (Review). *Int. J. Oncol.* **2015**, *47*, 1617–1626. [CrossRef]
66. Lu, H.; Wu, S.; Chen, H.; Huang, Y.; Qiu, G.; Liu, L.; Li, Y. Crizotinib induces apoptosis of lung cancer cells through JAK-STAT pathway. *Oncol. Lett.* **2018**, *16*, 5992–5996. [CrossRef]
67. Espert, L.; Dusanter-Fourt, I.; Chelbi-Alix, M.K. Negative regulation of the JAK/STAT: Pathway implication in tumorigenesis. *Bull. Cancer* **2005**, *92*, 845–857.
68. Camiña, N.; Penning, T.M. Genetic and epigenetic regulation of the NRF2-KEAP1 pathway in human lung cancer. *Br. J. Cancer* **2022**, *126*, 1244–1252. [CrossRef]
69. Zhang, D.; Hou, Z.; Aldrich, K.E.; Lockwood, L.; Odom, A.L.; Liby, K.T. A novel NRF2 pathway inhibitor sensitizes keap1-mutant lung cancer cells to chemotherapy. *Mol. Cancer Ther.* **2021**, *20*, 1692–1701. [CrossRef]
70. Tian, Y.; Liu, Q.; Yu, S.; Chu, Q.; Chen, Y.; Wu, K.; Wang, L. NRF2-Driven KEAP1 transcription in human lung cancer. *Mol. Cancer Res.* **2020**, *18*, 1465–1476. [CrossRef]
71. Jaganjac, M.; Milkovic, L.; Sunjic, S.B.; Zarkovic, N. The NRF2, thioredoxin, and glutathione system in tumorigenesis and anticancer therapies. *Antioxidants* **2020**, *9*, 1151. [CrossRef] [PubMed]
72. Silva, M.M.; Rocha, C.R.R.; Kinker, G.S.; Pelegrini, A.L.; Menck, C.F.M. The balance between NRF2/GSH antioxidant mediated pathway and DNA repair modulates cisplatin resistance in lung cancer cells. *Sci. Rep.* **2019**, *9*, 17639. [CrossRef]
73. Ko, E.; Kim, D.; Min, D.W.; Kwon, S.H.; Lee, J.Y. NRF2 regulates cell motility through RhoA–ROCK1 signalling in non-small-cell lung cancer cells. *Sci. Rep.* **2021**, *11*, 1247. [CrossRef] [PubMed]
74. Lignitto, L.; LeBoeuf, S.E.; Homer, H.; Jiang, S.; Askenazi, M.; Karakousi, T.R.; Pass, H.I.; Bhutkar, A.J.; Tsirigos, A.; Ueberheide, B.; et al. NRF2 Activation Promotes Lung Cancer Metastasis by Inhibiting the Degradation of Bach1. *Cell* **2019**, *178*, 316–329.e18. [CrossRef]
75. Gong, M.; Li, Y.; Ye, X.; Zhang, L.; Wang, Z.; Xu, X.; Shen, Y.; Zheng, C. Loss-of-function mutations in KEAP1 drive lung cancer progression via KEAP1/NRF2 pathway activation. *Cell Commun. Signal.* **2020**, *18*, 98. [CrossRef]
76. Zhao, J.; Lin, X.; Meng, D.; Zeng, L.; Zhuang, R.; Huang, S.; Lv, W.; Hu, J. NRF2 Mediates Metabolic Reprogramming in Non-Small Cell Lung Cancer. *Front. Oncol.* **2020**, *10*, 578315. [CrossRef]
77. Qin, W.; Hu, L.; Zhang, X.; Jiang, S.; Li, J.; Zhang, Z.; Wang, X. The Diverse Function of PD-1/PD-L Pathway Beyond Cancer. *Front. Immunol.* **2019**, *10*, 2298. [CrossRef] [PubMed]
78. Han, Y.; Liu, D.; Li, L. PD-1/PD-L1 pathway: Current researches in cancer. *Am. J. Cancer Res.* **2020**, *10*, 727–742. [PubMed]
79. Ghosh, C.; Luong, G.; Sun, Y. A snapshot of the PD-1/PD-L1 pathway. *J. Cancer* **2021**, *12*, 2735–2746. [CrossRef]
80. Ohaegbulam, K.C.; Assal, A.; Lazar-Molnar, E.; Yao, Y.; Zang, X. Human cancer immunotherapy with antibodies to the PD-1 and PD-L1 pathway. *Trends Mol. Med.* **2015**, *21*, 24–33. [CrossRef] [PubMed]
81. Jiang, X.; Wang, J.; Deng, X.; Xiong, F.; Ge, J.; Xiang, B.; Wu, X.; Ma, J.; Zhou, M.; Li, X.; et al. Role of the tumor microenvironment in PD-L1/PD-1-mediated tumor immune escape. *Mol. Cancer* **2019**, *18*, 10. [CrossRef] [PubMed]
82. Rebuzzi, S.E.; Zullo, L.; Rossi, G.; Grassi, M.; Murianni, V.; Tagliamento, M.; Prelaj, A.; Coco, S.; Longo, L.; Dal Bello, M.G.; et al. Novel Emerging Molecular Targets in Non-Small Cell Lung Cancer. *Int. J. Mol. Sci.* **2021**, *22*, 2625. [CrossRef] [PubMed]
83. Dholaria, B.; Hammond, W.; Shreders, A.; Lou, Y. Emerging therapeutic agents for lung cancer. *J. Hematol. Oncol.* **2016**, *9*, 138. [CrossRef]
84. Piperdi, B.; Perez-Soler, R. Role of erlotinib in the treatment of non-small cell lung cancer: Clinical outcomes in wild-type epidermal growth factor receptor patients. *Drugs* **2012**, *72* (Suppl. S1), 11–19. [CrossRef]
85. Nurwidya, F.; Takahashi, F.; Takahashi, K. Gefitinib in the treatment of nonsmall cell lung cancer with activating epidermal growth factor receptor mutation. *J. Nat. Sci. Biol. Med.* **2016**, *7*, 119–123. [CrossRef] [PubMed]
86. Bethune, G.; Bethune, D.; Ridgway, N.; Xu, Z. Epidermal growth factor receptor (EGFR) in lung cancer: An overview and update. *J. Thorac. Dis.* **2010**, *2*, 48–51.
87. Antonicelli, A.; Cafarotti, S.; Indini, A.; Galli, A.; Russo, A.; Cesario, A.; Lococo, F.M.; Russo, P.; Mainini, A.F.; Bonifati, L.G. EGFR-targeted therapy for non-small cell lung cancer: Focus on EGFR oncogenic mutation. *Int. J. Med. Sci.* **2013**, *10*, 320. [CrossRef]
88. Scagliotti, G.; Moro-Sibilot, D.; Kollmeier, J.; Favaretto, A.; Cho, E.K.; Grosch, H.; Kimmich, M.; Girard, N.; Tsai, C.-M.; Hsia, T.-C. A randomized-controlled phase 2 study of the MET antibody emibetuzumab in combination with erlotinib as first-line treatment for EGFR mutation–positive NSCLC patients. *J. Thorac. Oncol.* **2020**, *15*, 80–90. [CrossRef]
89. Boolell, V.; Alamgeer, M.; Watkins, D.N.; Ganju, V. The Evolution of Therapies in Non-Small Cell Lung Cancer. *Cancers* **2015**, *7*, 1815–1846. [CrossRef]
90. Golding, B.; Luu, A.; Jones, R.; Viloria-Petit, A.M. The function and therapeutic targeting of anaplastic lymphoma kinase (ALK) in non-small cell lung cancer (NSCLC). *Mol. Cancer* **2018**, *17*, 52. [CrossRef]

91. Soda, M.; Choi, Y.L.; Enomoto, M.; Takada, S.; Yamashita, Y.; Ishikawa, S.; Fujiwara, S.; Watanabe, H.; Kurashina, K.; Hatanaka, H.; et al. Identification of the transforming EML4-ALK fusion gene in non-small-cell lung cancer. *Nature* **2007**, *448*, 561–566. [CrossRef] [PubMed]
92. Aubry, A.; Galiacy, S.; Allouche, M. Targeting ALK in cancer: Therapeutic potential of proapoptotic peptides. *Cancers* **2019**, *11*, 275. [CrossRef] [PubMed]
93. Heo, H.; Kim, J.-H.; Lim, H.J.; Kim, J.-H.; Kim, M.; Koh, J.; Im, J.-Y.; Kim, B.-K.; Won, M.; Park, J.-H.; et al. DNA methylome and single-cell transcriptome analyses reveal CDA as a potential druggable target for ALK inhibitor–resistant lung cancer therapy. *Exp. Mol. Med.* **2022**, *54*, 1236–1249. [CrossRef] [PubMed]
94. Drilon, A.; Oxnard, G.R.; Tan, D.S.W.; Loong, H.H.F.; Johnson, M.; Gainor, J.; McCoach, C.E.; Gautschi, O.; Besse, B.; Cho, B.C.; et al. Efficacy of Selpercatinib in RET Fusion-Positive Non-Small-Cell Lung Cancer. *N. Engl. J. Med.* **2020**, *383*, 813–824. [CrossRef] [PubMed]
95. Xie, Q.; Yu, Z.; Lu, Y.; Fan, J.; Ni, Y.; Ma, L. microRNA-148a-3p inhibited the proliferation and epithelial-mesenchymal transition progression of non-small-cell lung cancer via modulating Ras/MAPK/Erk signaling. *J. Cell. Physiol.* **2019**, *234*, 12786–12799. [CrossRef]
96. Zhang, Y.; Hu, X. miR-148a promotes cell sensitivity through downregulating SOS2 in radiation-resistant non-small cell lung cancer cells. *Oncol. Lett.* **2022**, *23*, 135. [CrossRef]
97. Yoder, L.H. An overview of lung cancer symptoms, pathophysiology, and treatment. *Medsurg Nurs.* **2006**, *15*, 231.
98. Mornex, F.; Girard, N. Gemcitabine and radiation therapy in non-small cell lung cancer: State of the art. *Ann. Oncol.* **2006**, *17*, 1743–1747. [CrossRef]
99. Sharma, P.; Mehta, M.; Dhanjal, D.S.; Kaur, S.; Gupta, G.; Singh, H.; Thangavelu, L.; Rajeshkumar, S.; Tambuwala, M.; Bakshi, H.A.; et al. Emerging trends in the novel drug delivery approaches for the treatment of lung cancer. *Chem. Biol. Interact.* **2019**, *309*, 108720. [CrossRef]
100. Daffrè, E.; Prieto, M.; Huang, H.; Janet-Vendroux, A.; Blanc, K.; N'Guyen, Y.-L.; Fournel, L.; Alifano, M. Normalized Pulmonary Artery Diameter Predicts Occurrence of Postpneumonectomy Respiratory Failure, ARDS, and Mortality. *Cancers* **2020**, *12*, 1515. [CrossRef]
101. Belluomini, L.; Calvetti, L.; Inno, A.; Pasello, G.; Roca, E.; Vattemi, E.; Veccia, A.; Menis, J.; Pilotto, S. SCLC Treatment in the Immuno-Oncology Era: Current Evidence and Unmet Needs. *Front. Oncol.* **2022**, *12*, 840783. [CrossRef] [PubMed]
102. Yang, S.; Zhang, Z.; Wang, Q. Emerging therapies for small cell lung cancer. *J. Hematol. Oncol.* **2019**, *12*, 47. [CrossRef]
103. Schiller, J.H.; Harrington, D.; Belani, C.P.; Langer, C.; Sandler, A.; Krook, J.; Zhu, J.; Johnson, D.H. Comparison of four chemotherapy regimens for advanced non–small-cell lung cancer. *N. Engl. J. Med.* **2002**, *346*, 92–98. [CrossRef] [PubMed]
104. Wang, Y.; Zou, S.; Zhao, Z.; Liu, P.; Ke, C.; Xu, S. New insights into small-cell lung cancer development and therapy. *Cell Biol. Int.* **2020**, *44*, 1564–1576. [CrossRef]
105. Perez, M.A.S.; Cerqueira, N.; Fernandes, P.A.; Ramos, M.J. Ribonucleotide reductase: A mechanistic portrait of substrate analogues inhibitors. *Curr. Med. Chem.* **2010**, *17*, 2854–2872. [CrossRef] [PubMed]
106. Cerqueira, N.M.; Fernandes, P.A.; Ramos, M.J. Understanding ribonucleotide reductase inactivation by gemcitabine. *Chem. Eur. J.* **2007**, *13*, 8507–8515. [CrossRef]
107. Toschi, L.; Cappuzzo, F. Gemcitabine for the treatment of advanced nonsmall cell lung cancer. *Onco Targets Ther.* **2009**, *2*, 209.
108. Yang, J.; Solimando, D.A., Jr.; Waddell, J.A. Docetaxel and Cisplatin regimen for non-small-cell lung cancer. *Hosp. Pharm.* **2013**, *48*, 550–557. [CrossRef]
109. Gubens, M.A.; Wakelee, H.A. Docetaxel in the treatment of non-small cell lung carcinoma: An update and analysis. *Lung Cancer Targets Ther.* **2010**, *1*, 63.
110. Dasari, S.; Tchounwou, P.B. Cisplatin in cancer therapy: Molecular mechanisms of action. *Eur. J. Pharmacol.* **2014**, *740*, 364–378. [CrossRef]
111. Okamoto, H.; Watanabe, K.; Kunikane, H.; Yokoyama, A.; Kudoh, S.; Asakawa, T.; Shibata, T.; Kunitoh, H.; Tamura, T.; Saijo, N. Randomised phase III trial of carboplatin plus etoposide vs split doses of cisplatin plus etoposide in elderly or poor-risk patients with extensive disease small-cell lung cancer: JCOG 9702. *Br. J. Cancer* **2007**, *97*, 162–169. [CrossRef]
112. Odogwu, L.; Mathieu, L.; Blumenthal, G.; Larkins, E.; Goldberg, K.B.; Griffin, N.; Bijwaard, K.; Lee, E.Y.; Philip, R.; Jiang, X.; et al. FDA Approval Summary: Dabrafenib and Trametinib for the Treatment of Metastatic Non-Small Cell Lung Cancers Harboring BRAF V600E Mutations. *Oncologist* **2018**, *23*, 740–745. [CrossRef]
113. Khunger, A.; Khunger, M.; Velcheti, V. Dabrafenib in combination with trametinib in the treatment of patients with BRAF V600-positive advanced or metastatic non-small cell lung cancer: Clinical evidence and experience. *Ther. Adv. Respir. Dis.* **2018**, *12*, 1753466618767611. [CrossRef] [PubMed]
114. Herbst, R.S.; Giaccone, G.; de Marinis, F.; Reinmuth, N.; Vergnenegre, A.; Barrios, C.H.; Morise, M.; Felip, E.; Andric, Z.; Geater, S. Atezolizumab for first-line treatment of PD-L1–selected patients with NSCLC. *N. Engl. J. Med.* **2020**, *383*, 1328–1339. [CrossRef]
115. Morrissey, K.M.; Marchand, M.; Patel, H.; Zhang, R.; Wu, B.; Chan, H.P.; Mecke, A.; Girish, S.; Jin, J.Y.; Winter, H.R.; et al. Alternative dosing regimens for atezolizumab: An example of model-informed drug development in the postmarketing setting. *Cancer Chemother. Pharmacol.* **2019**, *84*, 1257–1267. [CrossRef]
116. Reck, M.; Rodríguez-Abreu, D.; Robinson, A.G.; Hui, R.; Csőszi, T.; Fülöp, A.; Gottfried, M.; Peled, N.; Tafreshi, A.; Cuffe, S. Pembrolizumab versus chemotherapy for PD-L1–positive non–small-cell lung cancer. *N. Engl. J. Med.* **2016**, *375*, 1823–1833. [CrossRef]

117. Yoo, S.H.; Keam, B.; Kim, M.; Kim, S.H.; Kim, Y.J.; Kim, T.M.; Kim, D.-W.; Lee, J.S.; Heo, D.S. Low-dose nivolumab can be effective in non-small cell lung cancer: Alternative option for financial toxicity. *ESMO Open* **2018**, *3*, e000332. [CrossRef] [PubMed]
118. Sale, M.J.; Cook, S.J. The BH3 mimetic ABT-263 synergizes with the MEK1/2 inhibitor selumetinib/AZD6244 to promote BIM-dependent tumour cell death and inhibit acquired resistance. *Biochem. J.* **2013**, *450*, 285–294. [CrossRef] [PubMed]
119. Imyanitov, E.N.; Levchenko, E.V.; Kuligina, E.S.; Orlov, S.V. Treating non-small cell lung cancer with selumetinib: An up-to-date drug evaluation. *Expert Opin. Pharmacother.* **2020**, *21*, 1943–1953. [CrossRef]
120. Gandhi, L.; Camidge, D.R.; de Oliveira, M.R.; Bonomi, P.; Gandara, D.; Khaira, D.; Hann, C.L.; McKeegan, E.M.; Litvinovich, E.; Hemken, P.M.; et al. Phase I study of Navitoclax (ABT-263), a novel Bcl-2 family inhibitor, in patients with small-cell lung cancer and other solid tumors. *J. Clin. Oncol.* **2011**, *29*, 909–916. [CrossRef]
121. Bradford, D.; Larkins, E.; Mushti, S.L.; Rodriguez, L.; Skinner, A.M.; Helms, W.S.; Price, L.S.L.; Zirkelbach, J.F.; Li, Y.; Liu, J. FDA approval summary: Selpercatinib for the treatment of lung and thyroid cancers with RET gene mutations or fusions. *Clin. Cancer Res.* **2021**, *27*, 2130–2135. [CrossRef]
122. Bebb, D.G.; Agulnik, J.; Albadine, R.; Banerji, S.; Bigras, G.; Butts, C.; Couture, C.; Cutz, J.C.; Desmeules, P.; Ionescu, D.N. Crizotinib inhibition of ROS1-positive tumours in advanced non-small-cell lung cancer: A Canadian perspective. *Curr. Oncol.* **2019**, *26*, 551–557. [CrossRef] [PubMed]
123. Sahu, A.; Prabhash, K.; Noronha, V.; Joshi, A.; Desai, S. Crizotinib: A comprehensive review. *South Asian J. Cancer* **2013**, *2*, 91–97. [CrossRef] [PubMed]
124. Hida, T.; Nokihara, H.; Kondo, M.; Kim, Y.H.; Azuma, K.; Seto, T.; Takiguchi, Y.; Nishio, M.; Yoshioka, H.; Imamura, F. Alectinib versus crizotinib in patients with ALK-positive non-small-cell lung cancer (J-ALEX): An open-label, randomised phase 3 trial. *Lancet* **2017**, *390*, 29–39. [CrossRef]
125. Cho, B.C.; Obermannova, R.; Bearz, A.; McKeage, M.; Kim, D.-W.; Batra, U.; Borra, G.; Orlov, S.; Kim, S.-W.; Geater, S.L. Efficacy and safety of ceritinib (450 mg/d or 600 mg/d) with food versus 750-mg/d fasted in patients with ALK receptor tyrosine kinase (ALK)–positive NSCLC: Primary efficacy results from the ASCEND-8 study. *J. Thorac. Oncol.* **2019**, *14*, 1255–1265. [CrossRef] [PubMed]
126. Shaw, A.T.; Kim, D.-W.; Mehra, R.; Tan, D.S.W.; Felip, E.; Chow, L.Q.M.; Camidge, D.R.; Vansteenkiste, J.; Sharma, S.; De Pas, T. Ceritinib in ALK-rearranged non–small-cell lung cancer. *N. Engl. J. Med.* **2014**, *370*, 1189–1197. [CrossRef]
127. Horn, L.; Wakelee, H.A.; Reckamp, K.L.; Blumenschein, G.R.; Infante, J.R.; Carter, C.A.; Waqar, S.N.; Neal, J.W.; Gockerman, J.P.; Harrow, K. Plasma genotyping of patients enrolled on the expansion phase I/II trial of X-396 in patients (pts) with ALK+ non-small cell lung cancer (NSCLC). *J. Clin. Oncol.* **2016**, *34*, 9056. [CrossRef]
128. Horn, L.; Wang, Z.; Wu, G.; Poddubskaya, E.; Mok, T.; Reck, M.; Wakelee, H.; Chiappori, A.A.; Lee, D.H.; Breder, V.; et al. Ensartinib vs Crizotinib for Patients With Anaplastic Lymphoma Kinase−Positive Non–Small Cell Lung Cancer: A Randomized Clinical Trial. *JAMA Oncol.* **2021**, *7*, 1617–1625. [CrossRef]
129. Horn, L.; Infante, J.R.; Reckamp, K.L.; Blumenschein, G.R.; Leal, T.A.; Waqar, S.N.; Gitlitz, B.J.; Sanborn, R.E.; Whisenant, J.G.; Du, L.; et al. Ensartinib (X-396) in ALK-Positive Non-Small Cell Lung Cancer: Results from a First-in-Human Phase I/II, Multicenter Study. *Clin. Cancer Res.* **2018**, *24*, 2771–2779. [CrossRef]
130. Russo, A.E.; Priolo, D.; Antonelli, G.; Libra, M.; McCubrey, J.A.; Ferraù, F. Bevacizumab in the treatment of NSCLC: Patient selection and perspectives. *Lung Cancer* **2017**, *8*, 259–269. [CrossRef]
131. Reck, M.; von Pawel, J.; Zatloukal, P.; Ramlau, R.; Gorbounova, V.; Hirsh, V.; Leighl, N.; Mezger, J.; Archer, V.; Moore, N.; et al. Overall survival with cisplatin-gemcitabine and bevacizumab or placebo as first-line therapy for nonsquamous non-small-cell lung cancer: Results from a randomised phase III trial (AVAiL). *Ann. Oncol.* **2010**, *21*, 1804–1809. [CrossRef] [PubMed]
132. Vansteenkiste, J.F.; Canon, J.-L.; De Braud, F.; Grossi, F.; De Pas, T.; Gray, J.E.; Su, W.-C.; Felip, E.; Yoshioka, H.; Gridelli, C.; et al. Safety and Efficacy of Buparlisib (BKM120) in Patients with PI3K Pathway-Activated Non-Small Cell Lung Cancer: Results from the Phase II BASALT-1 Study. *J. Thorac. Oncol.* **2015**, *10*, 1319–1327. [CrossRef]
133. McGowan, D.R.; Skwarski, M.; Bradley, K.M.; Campo, L.; Fenwick, J.D.; Gleeson, F.V.; Green, M.; Horne, A.; Maughan, T.S.; McCole, M.G. Buparlisib with thoracic radiotherapy and its effect on tumour hypoxia: A phase I study in patients with advanced non-small cell lung carcinoma. *Eur. J. Cancer* **2019**, *113*, 87–95. [CrossRef]
134. Cochin, V.; Gross-Goupil, M.; Ravaud, A.; Godbert, Y.; Le Moulec, S. Cabozantinib: Mechanism of action, efficacy and indications. *Bull. Cancer* **2017**, *104*, 393–401. [CrossRef]
135. Wang, G.; Gao, J.; Lv, J.; Chen, X.; Wu, J.; Wang, R.; Jiang, J. Effective Treatment with Cabozantinib in an Advanced Non-Small-Cell Lung Cancer Patient Harboring a CD74-ROS1 Fusion: A Case Report. *Onco Targets Ther.* **2020**, *13*, 1171. [CrossRef] [PubMed]
136. Esaki, T.; Hirai, F.; Makiyama, A.; Seto, T.; Bando, H.; Naito, Y.; Yoh, K.; Ishihara, K.; Kakizume, T.; Natsume, K. Phase I dose-escalation study of capmatinib (INC 280) in Japanese patients with advanced solid tumors. *Cancer Sci.* **2019**, *110*, 1340–1351. [CrossRef]
137. Yeo, W.-L.; Riely, G.J.; Yeap, B.Y.; Lau, M.W.; Warner, J.L.; Bodio, K.; Huberman, M.S.; Kris, M.G.; Tenen, D.G.; Pao, W. Erlotinib at a dose of 25 mg daily for non-small cell lung cancers with EGFR mutations. *J. Thorac. Oncol.* **2010**, *5*, 1048–1053. [CrossRef]
138. Wu, Y.-L.; Zhou, C.; Hu, C.-P.; Feng, J.; Lu, S.; Huang, Y.; Li, W.; Hou, M.; Shi, J.H.; Lee, K.Y. Afatinib versus cisplatin plus gemcitabine for first-line treatment of Asian patients with advanced non-small-cell lung cancer harbouring EGFR mutations (LUX-Lung 6): An open-label, randomised phase 3 trial. *Lancet Oncol.* **2014**, *15*, 213–222. [CrossRef]

139. Yang, J.C.-H.; Reckamp, K.L.; Kim, Y.-C.; Novello, S.; Smit, E.F.; Lee, J.-S.; Su, W.-C.; Akerley, W.L.; Blakely, C.M.; Groen, H.J.M.; et al. Efficacy and Safety of Rociletinib Versus Chemotherapy in Patients With EGFR-Mutated NSCLC: The Results of TIGER-3, a Phase 3 Randomized Study. *JTO Clin. Res. Rep.* **2021**, *2*, 100114. [CrossRef]
140. Sequist, L.V.; Soria, J.-C.; Goldman, J.W.; Wakelee, H.A.; Gadgeel, S.M.; Varga, A.; Papadimitrakopoulou, V.; Solomon, B.J.; Oxnard, G.R.; Dziadziuszko, R. Rociletinib in EGFR-mutated non–small-cell lung cancer. *N. Engl. J. Med.* **2015**, *372*, 1700–1709. [CrossRef] [PubMed]
141. Pirker, R.; Filipits, M. Cetuximab in non-small-cell lung cancer. *Transl. Lung Cancer Res.* **2012**, *1*, 54–60. [CrossRef] [PubMed]
142. Becerra, C.; Spira, A.I.; Conkling, P.R.; Richey, S.L.; Hanna, W.T.; Cote, G.M.; Heist, R.S.; Langleben, A.; Laurie, S.A.; Edenfield, W.J. A phase Ib/II study of cancer stemness inhibitor napabucasin (BB608) combined with weekly paclitaxel in advanced non-small cell lung cancer. *J. Clin. Oncol.* **2016**, *34*, 9093. [CrossRef]
143. Li, X.; Wei, Y.; Wei, X. Napabucasin, a novel inhibitor of STAT3, inhibits growth and synergises with doxorubicin in diffuse large B-cell lymphoma. *Cancer Lett.* **2020**, *491*, 146–161. [CrossRef] [PubMed]
144. Olaussen, K.A.; Dunant, A.; Fouret, P.; Brambilla, E.; André, F.; Haddad, V.; Taranchon, E.; Filipits, M.; Pirker, R.; Popper, H.H.; et al. DNA repair by ERCC1 in non-small-cell lung cancer and cisplatin-based adjuvant chemotherapy. *N. Engl. J. Med.* **2006**, *355*, 983–991. [CrossRef] [PubMed]
145. Lord, R.V.N.; Brabender, J.; Gandara, D.; Alberola, V.; Camps, C.; Domine, M.; Cardenal, F.; Sánchez, J.M.; Gumerlock, P.H.; Tarón, M.; et al. Low ERCC1 expression correlates with prolonged survival after cisplatin plus gemcitabine chemotherapy in non-small cell lung cancer. *Clin. Cancer Res.* **2002**, *8*, 2286–2291.
146. de Sousa, G.F.; Wlodarczyk, S.R.; Monteiro, G. Carboplatin: Molecular mechanisms of action associated with chemoresistance. *Braz. J. Pharm. Sci.* **2014**, *50*, 693–701. [CrossRef]
147. Schneider, B.J.; Saxena, A.; Downey, R.J. Surgery for early-stage small cell lung cancer. *J. Natl. Compr. Cancer Netw.* **2011**, *9*, 1132–1139. [CrossRef]
148. Chatterjee, D.; Roy, S.; Hazra, A.; Dasgupta, P.; Ganguly, S.; Das, A.K. Variation of adverse drug reaction profile of platinum-based chemotherapy with body mass index in patients with solid tumors: An observational study. *Indian J. Pharmacal.* **2014**, *46*, 222–224. [CrossRef]
149. Oun, R.; Moussa, Y.E.; Wheate, N.J. The side effects of platinum-based chemotherapy drugs: A review for chemists. *Dalton Trans.* **2018**, *47*, 6645–6653. [CrossRef]
150. Surendiran, A.; Balamurugan, N.; Gunaseelan, K.; Akhtar, S.; Reddy, K.S.; Adithan, C. Adverse drug reaction profile of cisplatin-based chemotherapy regimen in a tertiary care hospital in India: An evaluative study. *Indian J. Pharmacol.* **2010**, *42*, 40–43. [CrossRef]
151. Barlesi, F.; Scherpereel, A.; Rittmeyer, A.; Pazzola, A.; Tur, N.F.; Kim, J.-H.; Ahn, M.-J.; Aerts, J.G.; Gorbunova, V.; Vikström, A.; et al. Randomized phase III trial of maintenance bevacizumab with or without pemetrexed after first-line induction with bevacizumab, cisplatin, and pemetrexed in advanced nonsquamous non-small-cell lung cancer: AVAPERL (MO22089). *J. Clin. Oncol.* **2013**, *31*, 3004–3011. [CrossRef]
152. Barlesi, F.; Scherpereel, A.; Gorbunova, V.; Gervais, R.; Vikström, A.; Chouaid, C.; Chella, A.; Kim, J.H.; Ahn, M.J.; Reck, M.; et al. Maintenance bevacizumab-pemetrexed after first-line cisplatin-pemetrexed-bevacizumab for advanced nonsquamous nonsmall-cell lung cancer: Updated survival analysis of the AVAPERL (MO22089) randomized phase III trial. *Ann. Oncol.* **2014**, *25*, 1044–1052. [CrossRef]
153. Ricciardi, S.; Tomao, S.; de Marinis, F. Efficacy and safety of erlotinib in the treatment of metastatic non-small-cell lung cancer. *Lung Cancer* **2011**, *2*, 1–9. [CrossRef] [PubMed]
154. Maemondo, M.; Inoue, A.; Kobayashi, K.; Sugawara, S.; Oizumi, S.; Isobe, H.; Gemma, A.; Harada, M.; Yoshizawa, H.; Kinoshita, I. Gefitinib or chemotherapy for non–small-cell lung cancer with mutated EGFR. *N. Engl. J. Med.* **2010**, *362*, 2380–2388. [CrossRef] [PubMed]
155. Planchard, D.; Smit, E.F.; Groen, H.J.M.; Mazieres, J.; Besse, B.; Helland, Å.; Giannone, V.; D'Amelio, A.M., Jr.; Zhang, P.; Mookerjee, B. Dabrafenib plus trametinib in patients with previously untreated BRAFV600E-mutant metastatic non-small-cell lung cancer: An open-label, phase 2 trial. *Lancet Oncol.* **2017**, *18*, 1307–1316. [CrossRef] [PubMed]
156. Casaluce, F.; Sgambato, A.; Maione, P.; Sacco, P.C.; Santabarbara, G.; Gridelli, C. Selumetinib for the treatment of non-small cell lung cancer. *Expert Opin. Investig. Drugs* **2017**, *26*, 973–984. [CrossRef] [PubMed]
157. Nakajima, E.C.; Drezner, N.; Li, X.; Mishra-Kalyani, P.S.; Liu, Y.; Zhao, H.; Bi, Y.; Liu, J.; Rahman, A.; Wearne, E.; et al. FDA Approval Summary: Sotorasib for KRAS G12C-Mutated Metastatic NSCLC. *Clin. Cancer Res.* **2022**, *28*, 1482–1486. [CrossRef] [PubMed]
158. Skoulidis, F.; Li, B.T.; Dy, G.K.; Price, T.J.; Falchook, G.S.; Wolf, J.; Italiano, A.; Schuler, M.; Borghaei, H.; Barlesi, F. Sotorasib for lung cancers with KRAS p. G12C mutation. *N. Engl. J. Med.* **2021**, *384*, 2371–2381. [CrossRef]
159. Tie, Y.; Yang, H.; Zhao, R.; Zheng, H.; Yang, D.; Zhao, J.; Liu, M. Safety and efficacy of atezolizumab in the treatment of cancers: A systematic review and pooled-analysis. *Drug Des. Dev. Ther.* **2019**, *13*, 523–538. [CrossRef]
160. Tomasini, P.; Egea, J.; Souquet-Bressand, M.; Greillier, L.; Barlesi, F. Alectinib in the treatment of ALK-positive metastatic non-small cell lung cancer: Clinical trial evidence and experience with a focus on brain metastases. *Ther. Adv. Respir. Dis.* **2019**, *13*, 1753466619831906. [CrossRef]

161. Vuong, H.G.; Nguyen, T.Q.; Nguyen, H.C.; Nguyen, P.T.; Ho, A.T.N.; Hassell, L. Efficacy and safety of crizotinib in the treatment of advanced non-small-cell lung cancer with ROS1 rearrangement or MET alteration: A systematic review and meta-analysis. *Target. Oncol.* **2020**, *15*, 589–598. [CrossRef]
162. Besse, B.; Salgia, R.; Solomon, B.; Shaw, A.; Kim, D.; Schachar, R.; Wilner, K.; Reisman, A.; Bartlett, C.H.; Iyer, S. Visual disturbances in patients (pts) with anaplastic lymphoma kinase (ALK)-positive advanced non-small cell lung cancer (NSCLC) treated with crizotinib. *Ann. Oncol.* **2012**, *23*, ix416. [CrossRef]
163. Schnell, P.; Safferman, A.Z.; Bartlett, C.H.; Tang, Y.; Wilner, K.D. Clinical presentation of hepatotoxicity-associated crizotinib in ALK-positive (ALK+) advanced non-small cell lung cancer (NSCLC). *J. Clin. Oncol.* **2012**, *30*, 7598. [CrossRef]
164. Ou, S.-H.I.; Azada, M.; Dy, J.; Stiber, J.A. Asymptomatic profound sinus bradycardia (heart rate $\leq$ 45) in non-small cell lung cancer patients treated with crizotinib. *J. Thorac. Oncol.* **2011**, *6*, 2135–2137. [CrossRef] [PubMed]
165. Weickhardt, A.J.; Rothman, M.S.; Salian-Mehta, S.; Kiseljak-Vassiliades, K.; Oton, A.B.; Doebele, R.C.; Wierman, M.E.; Camidge, D.R. Rapid-onset hypogonadism secondary to crizotinib use in men with metastatic nonsmall cell lung cancer. *Cancer* **2012**, *118*, 5302–5309. [CrossRef]
166. Song, J.; Fan, X.; Zhao, Z.; Chen, M.; Chen, W.; Wu, F.; Zhang, D.; Chen, L.; Tu, J.; Ji, J. 125I brachytherapy of locally advanced non-small-cell lung cancer after one cycle of first-line chemotherapy: A comparison with best supportive care. *Onco Targets Ther.* **2017**, *10*, 1345. [CrossRef] [PubMed]
167. Hilaris, B.S.; Mastoras, D.A. Contemporary brachytherapy approaches in non–small-cell lung cancer. *J. Surg. Oncol.* **1998**, *69*, 258–264. [CrossRef]
168. Liberati, A.; Altman, D.G.; Tetzlaff, J.; Mulrow, C.; Gøtzsche, P.C.; Ioannidis, J.P.; Clarke, M.; Devereaux, P.J.; Kleijnen, J.; Moher, D. The PRISMA statement for reporting systematic reviews and meta-analyses of studies that evaluate healthcare interventions: Explanation and elaboration. *J. Clin. Epidemiol.* **2009**, *62*, e1–e34. [CrossRef]
169. Page, M.J.; McKenzie, J.E.; Bossuyt, P.M.; Boutron, I.; Hoffmann, T.C.; Mulrow, C.D.; Shamseer, L.; Tetzlaff, J.M.; Akl, E.A.; Brennan, S.E.; et al. The PRISMA 2020 statement: An updated guideline for reporting systematic reviews. *BMJ* **2021**, *372*, n71. [CrossRef] [PubMed]
170. Seca, A.M.L.; Pinto, D.C.G.A. Plant Secondary Metabolites as Anticancer Agents: Successes in Clinical Trials and Therapeutic Application. *Int. J. Mol. Sci.* **2018**, *19*, 263. [CrossRef]
171. Hashem, S.; Ali, T.A.; Akhtar, S.; Nisar, S.; Sageena, G.; Ali, S.; Al-Mannai, S.; Therachiyil, L.; Mir, R.; Elfaki, I.; et al. Targeting cancer signaling pathways by natural products: Exploring promising anti-cancer agents. *Biomed. Pharmacother.* **2022**, *150*, 113054. [CrossRef] [PubMed]
172. Mondal, A.; Gandhi, A.; Fimognari, C.; Atanasov, A.G.; Bishayee, A. Alkaloids for cancer prevention and therapy: Current progress and future perspectives. *Eur. J. Pharmacol.* **2019**, *858*, 172472. [CrossRef]
173. Matsuura, H.N.; Fett-Neto, A.G. *Plant Alkaloids: Main Features, Toxicity, and Mechanisms of Action BT—Plant Toxins*; Gopalakrishnakone, P., Carlini, C.R., Ligabue-Braun, R., Eds.; Springer: Dordrecht, The Netherlands, 2015; pp. 1–15. ISBN 978-94-007-6728-7.
174. Chen, Q.; Peng, W.; Qi, S.; Xu, A. Apoptosis of human highly metastatic lung cancer cell line 95-D induced by acutiaporberine, a novel bisalkaloid derived from Thalictrum acutifolium. *Planta Med.* **2002**, *68*, 550–553. [CrossRef] [PubMed]
175. Abe, A.; Yamada, H.; Moriya, S.; Miyazawa, K. The β-carboline alkaloid harmol induces cell death via autophagy but not apoptosis in human non-small cell lung cancer A549 cells. *Biol. Pharm. Bull.* **2011**, *34*, 1264–1272. [CrossRef]
176. Katiyar, S.K.; Meeran, S.M.; Katiyar, N.; Akhtar, S. P53 cooperates berberine-induced growth inhibition and apoptosis of non-small cell human lung cancer cells in vitro and tumor xenograft growth in vivo. *Mol. Carcinog.* **2009**, *48*, 24–37. [CrossRef] [PubMed]
177. Cao, W.; Liu, Y.; Zhang, R.; Zhang, B.; Wang, T.; Zhu, X.; Mei, L.; Chen, H.; Zhang, H.; Ming, P.; et al. Homoharringtonine induces apoptosis and inhibits STAT3 via IL-6/JAK1/STAT3 signal pathway in Gefitinib-resistant lung cancer cells. *Sci. Rep.* **2015**, *5*, 8477. [CrossRef]
178. Weng, T.Y.; Wu, H.F.; Li, C.Y.; Hung, Y.H.; Chang, Y.W.; Chen, Y.L.; Hsu, H.P.; Chen, Y.H.; Wang, C.Y.; Chang, J.Y.; et al. Homoharringtonine induced immune alteration for an Efficient Anti-tumor Response in Mouse Models of Non-small Cell Lung Adenocarcinoma Expressing Kras Mutation. *Sci. Rep.* **2018**, *8*, 8216. [CrossRef]
179. Lim, H.M.; Park, S.H.; Nam, M.J. Induction of apoptosis in indole-3-carbinol-treated lung cancer H1299 cells via ROS level elevation. *Hum. Exp. Toxicol.* **2021**, *40*, 812–825. [CrossRef]
180. Shao, S.; Zhang, H.; Yuan, C.M.; Zhang, Y.; Cao, M.M.; Zhang, H.Y.; Feng, Y.; Ding, X.; Zhou, Q.; Zhao, Q.; et al. Cytotoxic indole alkaloids from the fruits of Melodinus cochinchinensis. *Phytochemistry* **2015**, *116*, 367–373. [CrossRef]
181. Lin, Y.; Xu, J.; Liao, H.; Li, L.; Pan, L. Piperine induces apoptosis of lung cancer A549 cells via p53-dependent mitochondrial signaling pathway. *Tumor Biol.* **2014**, *35*, 3305–3310. [CrossRef]
182. Marques da Fonseca, L.; Jacques da Silva, L.R.; Santos Dos Reis, J.; Rodrigues da Costa Santos, M.A.; de Sousa Chaves, V.; Monteiro da Costa, K.; Sa-Diniz, J.N.; Freire de Lima, C.G.; Morrot, A.; Nunes Franklim, T.; et al. Piperine Inhibits TGF-β Signaling Pathways and Disrupts EMT-Related Events in Human Lung Adenocarcinoma Cells. *Medicines* **2020**, *7*, 19. [CrossRef]
183. Chen, Y.; Tang, Q.; Xiao, Q.; Yang, L.J.; Hann, S.S. Targeting EP4 downstream c-Jun through ERK1/2-mediated reduction of DNMT1 reveals novel mechanism of solamargine-inhibited growth of lung cancer cells. *J. Cell. Mol. Med.* **2017**, *21*, 222–233. [CrossRef] [PubMed]

184. Mishra, D.P.; Khan, M.A.; Yadav, D.K.; Rawat, A.K.; Singh, R.K.; Ahamad, T.; Hussain, M.K.; Saquib, M.; Khan, M.F. Monoterpene Indole Alkaloids from *Anthocephalus cadamba* Fruits Exhibiting Anticancer Activity in Human Lung Cancer Cell Line H1299. *ChemistrySelect* **2018**, *3*, 8468–8472. [CrossRef]
185. Chien, S.T.; Lin, S.S.; Wang, C.K.; Lee, Y.B.; Chen, K.S.; Fong, Y.; Shih, Y.W. Acacetin inhibits the invasion and migration of human non-small cell lung cancer A549 cells by suppressing the p38α MAPK signaling pathway. *Mol. Cell. Biochem.* **2011**, *350*, 135–148. [CrossRef]
186. Paul, S.; Chakrabarty, S.; Ghosh, S.; Nag, D.; Das, A.; Dastidar, D.G.; Dasgupta, M.; Dutta, N.; Kumari, M.; Pal, M.; et al. Targeting cellular microtubule by phytochemical apocynin exhibits autophagy-mediated apoptosis to inhibit lung carcinoma progression and tumorigenesis. *Phytomedicine* **2020**, *67*, 153152. [CrossRef]
187. Zhang, X.; Ruan, Q.; Zhai, Y.; Lu, D.; Li, C.; Fu, Y.; Zheng, Z.; Song, Y.; Guo, J. Baicalein inhibits non-small-cell lung cancer invasion and metastasis by reducing ezrin tension in inflammation microenvironment. *Cancer Sci.* **2020**, *111*, 3802–3812. [CrossRef]
188. Pinkhien, T.; Petpiroon, N.; Sritularak, B.; Chanvorachote, P. Batatasin III inhibits migration of human lung cancer cells by suppressing epithelial to mesenchymal transition and FAK-AKT signals. *Anticancer Res.* **2017**, *37*, 6281–6289. [CrossRef]
189. Bouzaiene, N.N.; Jaziri, S.K.; Kovacic, H.; Chekir-Ghedira, L.; Ghedira, K.; Luis, J. The effects of caffeic, coumaric and ferulic acids on proliferation, superoxide production, adhesion and migration of human tumor cells in vitro. *Eur. J. Pharmacol.* **2015**, *766*, 99–105. [CrossRef]
190. Wang, Z.; Liu, H.; Hu, Q.; Shi, L.; Lö, M.; Deng, M.; Luo, G. Cardamonin inhibits the progression of oesophageal cancer by inhibiting the PI3K/AKT signalling pathway. *J. Cancer* **2021**, *12*, 3597–3610. [CrossRef] [PubMed]
191. Tang, Y.; Fang, Q.; Shi, D.; Niu, P.; Chen, Y.; Deng, J. MTOR inhibition of cardamonin on antiproliferation of A549 cells is involved in a FKBP12 independent fashion. *Life Sci.* **2014**, *99*, 44–51. [CrossRef]
192. He, W.; Jiang, Y.; Zhang, X.; Zhang, Y.; Ji, H.; Zhang, N. Anticancer cardamonin analogs suppress the activation of NF-kappaB pathway in lung cancer cells. *Mol. Cell. Biochem.* **2014**, *389*, 25–33. [CrossRef]
193. Ramchandani, S.; Naz, I.; Lee, J.H.; Khan, M.R.; Ahn, K.S. An overview of the potential antineoplastic effects of casticin. *Molecules* **2020**, *25*, 1287. [CrossRef]
194. Liu, F.; Cao, X.; Liu, Z.; Guo, H.; Ren, K.; Quan, M.; Zhou, Y.; Xiang, H.; Cao, J. Casticin suppresses self-renewal and invasion of lung cancer stem-like cells from A549 cells through down-regulation of pAkt. *Acta Biochim. Biophys. Sin.* **2014**, *46*, 15–21. [CrossRef]
195. Lakshmi, S.; Suresh, S.; Rahul, B.S.; Saikant, R.; Maya, V.; Gopi, M.; Padmaja, G.; Remani, P. In vitro and in vivo studies of 5,7-dihydroxy flavones isolated from *Alpinia galanga* (L.) against human lung cancer and ascetic lymphoma. *Med. Chem. Res.* **2019**, *28*, 39–51. [CrossRef]
196. Sak, K. Radiosensitizing Potential of Curcumin in Different Cancer Models. *Nutr. Cancer* **2020**, *72*, 1276–1289. [CrossRef]
197. Lin, S.-S.; Huang, H.-P.; Yang, J.-S.; Wu, J.-Y.; Hsai, T.-C.; Lin, C.-C.; Lin, C.-W.; Kuo, C.-L.; Wood, W.G.; Chung, J.-G. DNA damage and endoplasmic reticulum stress mediated curcumin-induced cell cycle arrest and apoptosis in human lung carcinoma A-549 cells through the activation caspases cascade- and mitochondrial-dependent pathway. *Cancer Lett.* **2008**, *272*, 77–90. [CrossRef] [PubMed]
198. Wu, S.H.; Hang, L.W.; Yang, J.S.; Chen, H.Y.; Lin, H.Y.; Chiang, J.H.; Lu, C.C.; Yang, J.L.; Lai, T.Y.; Ko, Y.C.; et al. Curcumin induces apoptosis in human non-small cell lung cancer NCI-H460 cells through ER stress and caspase cascade- and mitochondria-dependent pathways. *Anticancer Res.* **2010**, *30*, 2125–2133.
199. Chen, H.W.; Lee, J.Y.; Huang, J.Y.; Wang, C.C.; Chen, W.J.; Su, S.F.; Huang, C.W.; Ho, C.C.; Chen, J.J.W.; Tsai, M.F.; et al. Curcumin inhibits lung cancer cell invasion and metastasis through the tumor suppressor HLJ1. *Cancer Res.* **2008**, *68*, 7428–7438. [CrossRef]
200. Saha, A.; Kuzuhara, T.; Echigo, N.; Fujii, A.; Suganuma, M.; Fujiki, H. Apoptosis of human lung cancer cells by curcumin mediated through up-regulation of "growth arrest and DNA damage inducible genes 45 and 153". *Biol. Pharm. Bull.* **2010**, *33*, 1291–1299. [CrossRef] [PubMed]
201. Tang, L.; Liu, J.; Zhu, L.; Chen, Q.; Meng, Z.; Sun, L.; Hu, J.; Ni, Z.; Wang, X. Curcumin inhibits growth of human NCI-H292 lung squamous cell carcinoma cells by increasing FOXA2 expression. *Front. Pharmacol.* **2018**, *9*, 60. [CrossRef]
202. Peng, W.; Wu, J.-G.; Jiang, Y.-B.; Liu, Y.-J.; Sun, T.; Wu, N.; Wu, C.-J. Antitumor activity of 4-O-(2″-O-acetyl-6″-O-p-coumaroyl-β-d-glucopyranosyl)-p-coumaric acid against lung cancers via mitochondrial-mediated apoptosis. *Chem. Biol. Interact.* **2015**, *233*, 8–13. [CrossRef] [PubMed]
203. Jeong, H.; Phan, A.N.H.; Choi, J.W. Anti-cancer effects of polyphenolic compounds in epidermal growth factor receptor tyrosine kinase inhibitor-resistant non-small cell lung cancer. *Pharmacogn. Mag.* **2017**, *13*, 595–599. [CrossRef]
204. Zhang, L.; Xie, J.; Gan, R.; Wu, Z.; Luo, H.; Chen, X.; Lu, Y.; Wu, L.; Zheng, D. Synergistic inhibition of lung cancer cells by EGCG and NF-κB inhibitor BAY11-7082. *J. Cancer* **2019**, *10*, 6543–6556. [CrossRef] [PubMed]
205. Forester, S.C.; Lambert, J.D. Synergistic inhibition of lung cancer cell lines by (−)-epigallocatechin-3-gallate in combination with clinically used nitrocatechol inhibitors of catechol-O-methyltransferase. *Carcinogenesis* **2014**, *35*, 365–372. [CrossRef]
206. Shi, J.; Liu, F.; Zhang, W.; Liu, X.; Lin, B.; Tang, X. Epigallocatechin-3-gallate inhibits nicotine-induced migration and invasion by the suppression of angiogenesis and epithelial-mesenchymal transition in non-small cell lung cancer cells. *Oncol. Rep.* **2015**, *33*, 2972–2980. [CrossRef]

207. Huang, J.; Chen, S.; Shi, Y.; Li, C.H.; Wang, X.J.; Li, F.J.; Wang, C.H.; Meng, Q.H.; Zhong, J.N.; Liu, M.; et al. Epigallocatechin gallate from green tea exhibits potent anticancer effects in A-549 non-small lung cancer cells by inducing apoptosis, cell cycle arrest and inhibition of cell migration. *J. BUON* **2017**, *22*, 1422–1427. [PubMed]
208. Datta, S.; Sinha, D. Low dose epigallocatechin-3-gallate revives doxorubicin responsiveness by a redox-sensitive pathway in A549 lung adenocarcinoma cells. *J. Biochem. Mol. Toxicol.* **2022**, *36*, e22999. [CrossRef]
209. Datta, S.; Sinha, D. EGCG maintained NRF2-mediated redox homeostasis and minimized etoposide resistance in lung cancer cells. *J. Funct. Foods* **2019**, *62*, 103553. [CrossRef]
210. Wang, H.; Bian, S.; Yang, C.S. Green tea polyphenol EGCG suppresses lung cancer cell growth through upregulating miR-210 expression caused by stabilizing HIF-1α. *Carcinogenesis* **2011**, *32*, 1881–1889. [CrossRef]
211. Gu, J.J.; Qiao, K.S.; Sun, P.; Chen, P.; Li, Q. Study of EGCG induced apoptosis in lung cancer cells by inhibiting PI3K/Akt signaling pathway. *Eur. Rev. Med. Pharmacol. Sci.* **2018**, *22*, 4557–4563.
212. Amin, A.R.M.R.; Wang, D.; Zhang, H.; Peng, S.; Shin, H.J.C.; Brandes, J.C.; Tighiouart, M.; Khuri, F.R.; Chen, Z.G.; Shin, D.M. Enhanced anti-tumor activity by the combination of the natural compounds (−)-epigallocatechin-3-gallate and luteolin: Potential role of p53. *J. Biol. Chem.* **2010**, *285*, 34557–34565. [CrossRef]
213. Ganguly, C.; Saha, P.; Panda, C.K.; Das, S. Inhibition of growth, induction of apoptosis and alteration of gene expression by tea polyphenols in the highly metastatic human lung cancer cell line NCI-H460. *Asian Pac. J. Cancer Prev.* **2005**, *6*, 326–331. [PubMed]
214. Khan, N.; Afaq, F.; Khusro, F.H.; Mustafa Adhami, V.; Suh, Y.; Mukhtar, H. Dual inhibition of phosphatidylinositol 3-kinase/Akt and mammalian target of rapamycin signaling in human nonsmall cell lung cancer cells by a dietary flavonoid fisetin. *Int. J. Cancer* **2012**, *130*, 1695–1705. [CrossRef] [PubMed]
215. Kang, K.A.; Piao, M.J.; Madduma Hewage, S.R.K.; Ryu, Y.S.; Oh, M.C.; Kwon, T.K.; Chae, S.; Hyun, J.W. Fisetin induces apoptosis and endoplasmic reticulum stress in human non-small cell lung cancer through inhibition of the MAPK signaling pathway. *Tumor Biol.* **2016**, *37*, 9615–9624. [CrossRef] [PubMed]
216. Kang, K.A.; Piao, M.J.; Hyun, J.W. Fisetin induces apoptosis in human nonsmall lung cancer cells via a mitochondria-mediated pathway. *Vitr. Cell. Dev. Biol. Anim.* **2015**, *51*, 300–309. [CrossRef] [PubMed]
217. Zhang, L.; Huang, Y.; Zhuo, W.; Zhu, Y.; Zhu, B.; Chen, Z. Fisetin, a dietary phytochemical, overcomes erlotinib-resistance of lung adenocarcinoma cells through inhibition of MAPK and AKT pathways. *Am. J. Transl. Res.* **2016**, *8*, 4857–4868.
218. You, B.R.; Park, W.H. Gallic acid-induced lung cancer cell death is related to glutathione depletion as well as reactive oxygen species increase. *Toxicol. Vitr.* **2010**, *24*, 1356–1362. [CrossRef]
219. Phan, A.N.; Hua, T.N.; Kim, M.-K.; Vo, V.T.; Choi, J.-W.; Kim, H.-W.; Rho, J.K.; Kim, K.W.; Jeong, Y. Gallic acid inhibition of Src-Stat3 signaling overcomes acquired resistance to EGF receptor tyrosine kinase inhibitors in advanced non-small cell lung cancer. *Oncotarget* **2016**, *7*, 54702–54713. [CrossRef]
220. Shiau, R.-J.; Chen, K.-Y.; Wen, Y.-D.; Chuang, C.-H.; Yeh, S.-L. Genistein and β-carotene enhance the growth-inhibitory effect of trichostatin A in A549 cells. *Eur. J. Nutr.* **2010**, *49*, 19–25. [CrossRef]
221. Gadgeel, S.M.; Ali, S.; Philip, P.A.; Wozniak, A.; Sarkar, F.H. Retraction to: Genistein enhances the effect of epidermal growth factor receptor tyrosine kinase inhibitors and inhibits nuclear factor kappa B in nonsmall cell lung cancer cell lines (Cancer, 10.1002/cncr.24250). *Cancer* **2016**, *122*, 3248. [CrossRef]
222. Zou, H.; Zhan, S.; Cao, K. Apoptotic activity of genistein on human lung adenocarcinoma SPC-A-1 cells and preliminary exploration of its mechanisms using microarray. *Biomed. Pharmacother.* **2008**, *62*, 583–589. [CrossRef] [PubMed]
223. Li, Y.; Ahmed, F.; Ali, S.; Philip, P.A.; Kucuk, O.; Sarkar, F.H. Inactivation of nuclear factor κB by soy isoflavone genistein contributes to increased apoptosis induced by chemotherapeutic agents in human cancer cells. *Cancer Res.* **2005**, *65*, 6934–6942. [CrossRef]
224. Cai, Y.; Hao, Y.; Xu, H.; Chen, K.; Ren, B. Gigantol inhibits cell proliferation and induces apoptosis by regulating DEK in non-small cell lung cancer. *Exp. Ther. Med.* **2021**, *22*, 1317. [CrossRef]
225. Unahabhokha, T.; Chanvorachote, P.; Sritularak, B.; Kitsongsermthon, J.; Pongrakhananon, V. Gigantol Inhibits Epithelial to Mesenchymal Process in Human Lung Cancer Cells. *Evid. Based Complement. Altern. Med.* **2016**, *2016*, 4561674. [CrossRef]
226. Losuwannarak, N.; Maiuthed, A.; Kitkumthorn, N.; Leelahavanichkul, A.; Roytrakul, S.; Chanvorachote, P. Gigantol targets cancer stem cells and destabilizes tumors via the suppression of the PI3K/AKT and JAK/STAT pathways in ectopic lung cancer xenografts. *Cancers* **2019**, *11*, 2032. [CrossRef] [PubMed]
227. Cincin, Z.B.; Unlu, M.; Kiran, B.; Bireller, E.S.; Baran, Y.; Cakmakoglu, B. Anti-proliferative, apoptotic and signal transduction effects of hesperidin in non-small cell lung cancer cells. *Cell. Oncol.* **2015**, *38*, 195–204. [CrossRef]
228. Zhu, J.; Xu, S.; Gao, W.; Feng, J.; Zhao, G. Honokiol induces endoplasmic reticulum stress-mediated apoptosis in human lung cancer cells. *Life Sci.* **2019**, *221*, 204–211. [CrossRef]
229. Rauf, A.; Olatunde, A.; Imran, M.; Alhumaydhi, F.A.; Aljohani, A.S.M.; Khan, S.A.; Uddin, M.S.; Mitra, S.; Emran, T.B.; Khayrullin, M.; et al. Honokiol: A review of its pharmacological potential and therapeutic insights. *Phytomedicine* **2021**, *90*, 153647. [CrossRef]
230. Deng, S.; Zhang, C.F.; Yang, L.; Ma, L. Formylated honokiol analogs showed antitumor activity against lung carcinoma. *Anticancer Drugs* **2019**, *30*, 795–802. [CrossRef]
231. Xiao, H.; Yang, C.S.; Li, S.; Jin, H.; Ho, C.T.; Patel, T. Monodemethylated polymethoxyflavones from sweet orange (*Citrus sinensis*) peel inhibit growth of human lung cancer cells by apoptosis. *Mol. Nutr. Food Res.* **2009**, *53*, 398–406. [CrossRef] [PubMed]

232. Zhao, X.; Dong, W.L.; Gao, Y.D.; Shin, D.S.; Ye, Q.; Su, L.; Jiang, F.; Zhao, B.X.; Miao, J.Y. Novel indolyl-chalcone derivatives inhibit A549 lung cancer cell growth through activating Nrf-2/HO-1 and inducing apoptosis in vitro and in vivo. *Sci. Rep.* **2017**, *7*, 3919. [CrossRef] [PubMed]
233. Ruan, Y.; Hu, K.; Chen, H. Autophagy inhibition enhances isorhamnetin.induced mitochondria.dependent apoptosis in non-small cell lung cancer cells. *Mol. Med. Rep.* **2015**, *12*, 5796–5806. [CrossRef]
234. Zhang, B.Y.; Wang, Y.M.; Gong, H.; Zhao, H.; Lv, X.Y.; Yuan, G.H.; Han, S.R. Isorhamnetin flavonoid synergistically enhances the anticancer activity and apoptosis induction by cis-platin and carboplatin in non-small cell lung carcinoma (NSCLC). *Int. J. Clin. Exp. Pathol.* **2015**, *8*, 25–37.
235. Hang, M.; Zhao, F.; Chen, S.B.; Sun, Q.; Zhang, C.X. Kaempferol modulates the metastasis of human non-small cell lung cancer cells by inhibiting epithelial-mesenchymal transition. *Bangladesh J. Pharmacol.* **2015**, *10*, 267–270. [CrossRef]
236. Jo, E.; Park, S.J.; Choi, Y.S.; Jeon, W.K.; Kim, B.C. Kaempferol Suppresses Transforming Growth Factor-β1-Induced Epithelial-to-Mesenchymal Transition and Migration of A549 Lung Cancer Cells by Inhibiting Akt1-Mediated Phosphorylation of Smad3 at Threonine-179. *Neoplasia* **2015**, *17*, 525–537. [CrossRef] [PubMed]
237. Leung, H.W.C.; Lin, C.J.; Hour, M.J.; Yang, W.H.; Wang, M.Y.; Lee, H.Z. Kaempferol induces apoptosis in human lung non-small carcinoma cells accompanied by an induction of antioxidant enzymes. *Food Chem. Toxicol.* **2007**, *45*, 2005–2013. [CrossRef]
238. Kumar, S.; Prajapati, K.S.; Shuaib, M.; Kushwaha, P.P.; Tuli, H.S.; Singh, A.K. Five-Decade Update on Chemopreventive and Other Pharmacological Potential of Kurarinone: A Natural Flavanone. *Front. Pharmacol.* **2021**, *12*, 737137. [CrossRef]
239. Chung, T.W.; Lin, C.C.; Lin, S.C.; Chan, H.L.; Yang, C.C. Antitumor effect of kurarinone and underlying mechanism in small cell lung carcinoma cells. *Onco Targets Ther.* **2019**, *12*, 6119–6131. [CrossRef]
240. Cai, X.; Ye, T.; Liu, C.; Lu, W.; Lu, M.; Zhang, J.; Wang, M.; Cao, P. Luteolin induced G2 phase cell cycle arrest and apoptosis on non-small cell lung cancer cells. *Toxicol. Vitr.* **2011**, *25*, 1385–1391. [CrossRef]
241. Meng, G.; Chai, K.; Li, X.; Zhu, Y.; Huang, W. Luteolin exerts pro-apoptotic effect and anti-migration effects on A549 lung adenocarcinoma cells through the activation of MEK/ERK signaling pathway. *Chem. Biol. Interact.* **2016**, *257*, 26–34. [CrossRef]
242. Jiang, Z.Q.; Li, M.H.; Qin, Y.M.; Jiang, H.Y.; Zhang, X.; Wu, M.H. Luteolin inhibits tumorigenesis and induces apoptosis of non-small cell lung cancer cells via regulation of microRNA-34a-5p. *Int. J. Mol. Sci.* **2018**, *19*, 447. [CrossRef]
243. Lin, Y.; Shi, R.; Wang, X.; Shen, H.-M. Luteolin, a Flavonoid with Potential for Cancer Prevention and Therapy. *Curr. Cancer Drug Targets* **2008**, *8*, 634–646. [CrossRef] [PubMed]
244. Ma, L.; Peng, H.; Li, K.; Zhao, R.; Li, L.; Yu, Y.; Wang, X.; Han, Z. Luteolin exerts an anticancer effect on NCI-H460 human non-small cell lung cancer cells through the induction of Sirt1-mediated apoptosis. *Mol. Med. Rep.* **2015**, *12*, 4196–4202. [CrossRef]
245. Busaranon, K.; Plaimee, P.; Sritularak, B.; Chanvorachote, P. Moscatilin inhibits epithelial-to-mesenchymal transition and sensitizes anoikis in human lung cancer H460 cells. *J. Nat. Med.* **2016**, *70*, 18–27. [CrossRef]
246. Chang, H.L.; Chang, Y.M.; Lai, S.C.; Chen, K.M.; Wang, K.C.; Chiu, T.T.; Chang, F.H.; Hsu, L.S. Naringenin inhibits migration of lung cancer cells via the inhibition of matrix metalloproteinases-2 and-9. *Exp. Ther. Med.* **2017**, *13*, 739–744. [CrossRef] [PubMed]
247. Shi, X.; Luo, X.; Chen, T.; Guo, W.; Liang, C.; Tang, S.; Mo, J. Naringenin inhibits migration, invasion, induces apoptosis in human lung cancer cells and arrests tumour progression in vitro. *J. Cell. Mol. Med.* **2021**, *25*, 2563–2571. [CrossRef] [PubMed]
248. Moon, J.Y.; Hung, L.V.M.; Unno, T.; Cho, S.K. Nobiletin enhances chemosensitivity to adriamycin through modulation of the Akt/GSK3β/β–catenin/ MYCN/MRP1 signaling pathway in A549 human non-small-cell lung cancer cells. *Nutrients* **2018**, *10*, 1829. [CrossRef]
249. Xu, X.; Zhang, Y.; Qu, D.; Jiang, T.; Li, S. Osthole induces G2/M arrest and apoptosis in lung cancer A549 cells by modulating PI3K/Akt pathway. *J. Exp. Clin. Cancer Res.* **2011**, *30*, 33–37. [CrossRef]
250. Xu, X.M.; Zhang, Y.; Qu, D.; Feng, X.W.; Chen, Y.; Zhao, L. Osthole suppresses migration and invasion of A549 human lung cancer cells through inhibition of matrix metalloproteinase-2 and matrix metallopeptidase-9 in vitro. *Mol. Med. Rep.* **2012**, *6*, 1018–1022. [CrossRef]
251. Shokoohinia, Y.; Jafari, F.; Mohammadi, Z.; Bazvandi, L.; Hosseinzadeh, L.; Chow, N.; Bhattacharyya, P.; Farzaei, M.H.; Farooqi, A.A.; Nabavi, S.M.; et al. Potential anticancer properties of osthol: A comprehensive mechanistic review. *Nutrients* **2018**, *10*, 36. [CrossRef]
252. Feng, H.; Lu, J.J.; Wang, Y.; Pei, L.; Chen, X. Osthole inhibited TGF β-induced epithelial–mesenchymal transition (EMT) by suppressing NF-κB mediated Snail activation in lung cancer A549 cells. *Cell Adhes. Migr.* **2017**, *11*, 464–475. [CrossRef] [PubMed]
253. Ma, L.; Wang, R.; Nan, Y.; Li, W.; Wang, Q.; Jin, F. Phloretin exhibits an anticancer effect and enhances the anticancer ability of cisplatin on non-small cell lung cancer cell lines by regulating expression of apoptotic pathways and matrix metalloproteinases. *Int. J. Oncol.* **2016**, *48*, 843–853. [CrossRef]
254. Min, J.; Li, X.; Huang, K.; Tang, H.; Ding, X.; Qi, C.; Qin, X.; Xu, Z. Phloretin induces apoptosis of non-small cell lung carcinoma A549 cells via JNK1/2 and p38 MAPK pathways. *Oncol. Rep.* **2015**, *34*, 2871–2879. [CrossRef] [PubMed]
255. Zhang, Y.; Zhuang, Z.; Meng, Q.; Jiao, Y.; Xu, J.; Fan, S. Polydatin inhibits growth of lung cancer cells by inducing apoptosis and causing cell cycle arrest. *Oncol. Lett.* **2014**, *7*, 295–301. [CrossRef] [PubMed]
256. Schneider, J.G.; Alosi, J.A.; McDonald, D.E.; McFadden, D.W. Pterostilbene Inhibits Lung Cancer through Induction of Apoptosis1. *J. Surg. Res.* **2010**, *161*, 18–22. [CrossRef] [PubMed]
257. Zheng, S.Y.; Li, Y.; Jiang, D.; Zhao, J.; Ge, J.F. Anticancer effect and apoptosis induction by quercetin in the human lung cancer cell line A-549. *Mol. Med. Rep.* **2012**, *5*, 822–826. [CrossRef] [PubMed]

258. Wang, H.; Zhang, H.; Tang, L.; Chen, H.; Wu, C.; Zhao, M.; Yang, Y.; Chen, X.; Liu, G. Resveratrol inhibits TGF-β1-induced epithelial-to-mesenchymal transition and suppresses lung cancer invasion and metastasis. *Toxicology* **2013**, *303*, 139–146. [CrossRef]
259. Yin, H.T.; Tian, Q.Z.; Guan, L.; Zhou, Y.; Huang, X.E.; Zhang, H. In vitro and in vivo evaluation of the antitumor efficiency of resveratrol against lung cancer. *Asian Pac. J. Cancer Prev.* **2013**, *14*, 1703–1706. [CrossRef]
260. Vejselova, D.; Kutlu, H.M. Inhibitory effects of salicylic acid on A549 human lung adenocarcinoma cell viability. *Turk. J. Biol.* **2015**, *39*, 1–5. [CrossRef]
261. Li, Y.R.; Li, S.; Ho, C.T.; Chang, Y.H.; Tan, K.T.; Chung, T.W.; Wang, B.Y.; Chen, Y.K.; Lin, C.C. Tangeretin derivative, 5-acetyloxy-6,7,8,4′-tetramethoxyflavone induces G2/M arrest, apoptosis and autophagy in human non-small cell lung cancer cells in vitro and in vivo. *Cancer Biol. Ther.* **2016**, *17*, 48–64. [CrossRef]
262. Zheng, C.; Hu, C.; Ma, X.; Peng, C.; Zhang, H.; Qin, L. Cytotoxic phenylpropanoid glycosides from *Fagopyrum tataricum* (L.) Gaertn. *Food Chem.* **2012**, *132*, 433–438. [CrossRef]
263. Pandey, N.; Tyagi, G.; Kaur, P.; Pradhana, S.; Rajam, M.V.; Srivastava, T. Allicin Overcomes Hypoxia Mediated Cisplatin Resistance in Lung Cancer Cells through ROS Mediated Cell Death Pathway and by Suppressing Hypoxia Inducible Factors. *Cell. Physiol. Biochem.* **2020**, *54*, 748–766. [CrossRef]
264. Wang, D.-X.; Zou, Y.-J.; Zhuang, X.-B.; Chen, S.-X.; Lin, Y.; Li, W.-L.; Lin, J.-J.; Lin, Z.-Q. Sulforaphane suppresses EMT and metastasis in human lung cancer through miR-616-5p-mediated GSK3β/β-catenin signaling pathways. *Acta Pharmacol. Sin.* **2017**, *38*, 241–251. [CrossRef]
265. Jiang, L.L.; Zhou, S.J.; Zhang, X.M.; Chen, H.Q.; Liu, W. Sulforaphane suppresses in vitro and in vivo lung tumorigenesis through downregulation of HDAC activity. *Biomed. Pharmacother.* **2016**, *78*, 74–80. [CrossRef]
266. Gao, L.; Cheng, D.; Yang, J.; Wu, R.; Li, W.; Kong, A.N. Sulforaphane epigenetically demethylates the CpG sites of the miR-9-3 promoter and reactivates miR-9-3 expression in human lung cancer A549 cells. *J. Nutr. Biochem.* **2018**, *56*, 109–115. [CrossRef]
267. Garcia, C.; Silva, C.O.; Monteiro, C.M.; Nicolai, M.; Viana, A.; Andrade, J.M.; Barasoain, I.; Stankovic, T.; Quintana, J.; Hernández, I.; et al. Anticancer properties of the abietane diterpene 6, 7-dehydroroyleanone obtained by optimized extraction. *Future Med. Chem.* **2018**, *10*, 1177–1189. [CrossRef]
268. Rajavel, T.; Mohankumar, R.; Archunan, G.; Ruckmani, K.; Devi, K.P. Beta sitosterol and Daucosterol (phytosterols identified in *Grewia tiliaefolia*) perturbs cell cycle and induces apoptotic cell death in A549 cells. *Sci. Rep.* **2017**, *7*, 3418. [CrossRef]
269. Garg, S.; Huifu, H.; Kumari, A.; Sundar, D.; Kaul, S.C.; Wadhwa, R. Induction of Senescence in Cancer Cells by a Novel Combination of Cucurbitacin B and Withanone: Molecular Mechanism and Therapeutic Potential. *J. Gerontol. Ser. A* **2020**, *75*, 1031–1041. [CrossRef]
270. Mu, D.; Zhang, W.; Chu, D.; Liu, T.; Xie, Y.; Fu, E.; Jin, F. The role of calcium, P38 MAPK in dihydroartemisinin-induced apoptosis of lung cancer PC-14 cells. *Cancer Chemother. Pharmacol.* **2008**, *61*, 639–645. [CrossRef]
271. Zhang, B.; Zhang, Z.; Wang, J.; Yang, B.; Zhao, Y.; Rao, Z.; Gao, J. Dihydroartemisinin sensitizes lewis lung carcinoma cells to carboplatin therapy via p38 mitogen-activated protein kinase activation. *Oncol. Lett.* **2018**, *15*, 7531–7536. [CrossRef]
272. Li, Y.; Luan, G.; Guo, P. The inhibitory effect of dihydroartemisinin on non-small cells lung cancer. *Pharmacol. Res. Mod. Chin. Med.* **2021**, *1*, 100006. [CrossRef]
273. Abdullah, N.A.; Md Hashim, N.F.; Ammar, A.; Zakuan, N.M. An insight into the anti-angiogenic and anti-metastatic effects of oridonin: Current knowledge and future potential. *Molecules* **2021**, *26*, 775. [CrossRef] [PubMed]
274. Yang, H.; Gao, Y.; Fan, X.; Liu, X.; Peng, L.; Ci, X. Oridonin sensitizes cisplatin-induced apoptosis via AMPK/Akt/mTOR-dependent autophagosome accumulation in A549 cells. *Front. Oncol.* **2019**, *9*, 769. [CrossRef] [PubMed]
275. Omar, A.; Kalra, R.S.; Putri, J.; Elwakeel, A.; Kaul, S.C.; Wadhwa, R. Soyasapogenol-A targets CARF and results in suppression of tumor growth and metastasis in p53 compromised cancer cells. *Sci. Rep.* **2020**, *10*, 6323. [CrossRef] [PubMed]
276. Attoub, S.; Sperandio, O.; Raza, H.; Arafat, K.; Al-Salam, S.; Al Sultan, M.A.; Al Safi, M.; Takahashi, T.; Adem, A. Thymoquinone as an anticancer agent: Evidence from inhibition of cancer cells viability and invasion in vitro and tumor growth in vivo. *Fundam. Clin. Pharmacol.* **2013**, *27*, 557–569. [CrossRef] [PubMed]
277. Castrejón-Jiménez, N.S.; Leyva-Paredes, K.; Baltierra-Uribe, S.L.; Castillo-Cruz, J.; Campillo-Navarro, M.; Hernández-Pérez, A.D.; Luna-Angulo, A.B.; Chacón-Salinas, R.; Coral-Vázquez, R.M.; Estrada-García, I.; et al. Ursolic and oleanolic acids induce mitophagy in a549 human lung cancer cells. *Molecules* **2019**, *24*, 3444. [CrossRef]
278. Ruan, J.S.; Zhou, H.; Yang, L.; Wang, L.; Jiang, Z.S.; Sun, H.; Wang, S.M. Ursolic acid attenuates TGF-b1-induced epithelial-mesenchymal transition in NSCLC by targeting integrin Avb5/MMPs signaling. *Oncol. Res.* **2019**, *27*, 593–600. [CrossRef] [PubMed]
279. Wang, M.; Yu, H.; Wu, R.; Chen, Z.Y.; Hu, Q.; Zhang, Y.F.; Gao, S.H.; Zhou, G.B. Autophagy inhibition enhances the inhibitory effects of ursolic acid on lung cancer cells. *Int. J. Mol. Med.* **2020**, *46*, 1816–1826. [CrossRef]
280. Liu, X.; Chen, L.; Liang, T.; Tian, X.D.; Liu, Y.; Zhang, T. Withaferin A induces mitochondrial-dependent apoptosis in non-small cell lung cancer cells via generation of reactive oxygen species. *J. BUON* **2017**, *22*, 244–250.
281. Haustein, M.; Ramer, R.; Linnebacher, M.; Manda, K.; Hinz, B. Cannabinoids increase lung cancer cell lysis by lymphokine-activated killer cells via upregulation of ICAM-1. *Biochem. Pharmacol.* **2014**, *92*, 312–325. [CrossRef]

282. Kis, B.; Ifrim, F.C.; Buda, V.; Avram, S.; Pavel, I.Z.; Antal, D.; Paunescu, V.; Dehelean, C.A.; Ardelean, F.; Diaconeasa, Z.; et al. Cannabidiol—From plant to human body: A promising bioactive molecule with multi-target effects in cancer. *Int. J. Mol. Sci.* **2019**, *20*, 5905. [CrossRef] [PubMed]
283. Ramer, R.; Heinemann, K.; Merkord, J.; Rohde, H.; Salamon, A.; Linnebacher, M.; Hinz, B. COX-2 and PPAR-γ confer cannabidiol-induced apoptosis of human lung cancer cells. *Mol. Cancer Ther.* **2013**, *12*, 69–82. [CrossRef] [PubMed]
284. Ramer, R.; Merkord, J.; Rohde, H.; Hinz, B. Cannabidiol inhibits cancer cell invasion via upregulation of tissue inhibitor of matrix metalloproteinases-1. *Biochem. Pharmacol.* **2010**, *79*, 955–966. [CrossRef]
285. Treesuwan, S.; Sritularak, B.; Chanvorachote, P.; Pongrakhananon, V. Cypripedin diminishes an epithelial-to-mesenchymal transition in non-small cell lung cancer cells through suppression of Akt/GSK-3β signalling. *Sci. Rep.* **2018**, *8*, 8009. [CrossRef] [PubMed]
286. Wattanathamsan, O.; Treesuwan, S.; Sritularak, B.; Pongrakhananon, V. Cypripedin, a phenanthrenequinone from Dendrobium densiflorum, sensitizes non-small cell lung cancer H460 cells to cisplatin-mediated apoptosis. *J. Nat. Med.* **2018**, *72*, 503–513. [CrossRef]
287. Su, J.; Yan, Y.; Qu, J.; Xue, X.; Liu, Z.; Cai, H. Emodin induces apoptosis of lung cancer cells through ER stress and the TRIB3/NF-κB pathway. *Oncol. Rep.* **2017**, *37*, 1565–1572. [CrossRef]
288. Hsu, H.F.; Houng, J.Y.; Kuo, C.F.; Tsao, N.; Wu, Y.C. Glossogin, a novel phenylpropanoid from Glossogyne tenuifolia, induced apoptosis in A549 lung cancer cells. *Food Chem. Toxicol.* **2008**, *46*, 3785–3791. [CrossRef]
289. Trenti, A.; Grumati, P.; Cusinato, F.; Orso, G.; Bonaldo, P.; Trevisi, L. Cardiac glycoside ouabain induces autophagic cell death in non-small cell lung cancer cells via a JNK-dependent decrease of Bcl-2. *Biochem. Pharmacol.* **2014**, *89*, 197–209. [CrossRef]
290. Zhu, F.; Dai, C.; Fu, Y.; Loo, J.F.C.; Xia, D.; Gao, S.P.; Ma, Z.; Chen, Z. Physalin A exerts anti-tumor activity in non-small cell lung cancer cell lines by suppressing JAK/STAT3 signaling. *Oncotarget* **2016**, *7*, 9462–9476. [CrossRef]
291. Hsia, T.C.; Yang, J.S.; Chen, G.W.; Chiu, T.H.; Lu, H.F.; Yang, M.D.; Yu, F.S.; Liu, K.C.; Lai, K.C.; Lin, C.C.; et al. The roles of endoplasmic reticulum stress and Ca^{2+} on rhein-induced apoptosis in A-549 human lung cancer cells. *Anticancer Res.* **2009**, *29*, 309–318.
292. Henamayee, S.; Banik, K.; Sailo, B.L.; Shabnam, B.; Harsha, C.; Srilakshmi, S.; Naidu, V.G.M.; Baek, S.H.; Ahn, K.S.; Kunnumakkara, A.B. Therapeutic emergence of rhein as a potential anticancer drug: A review of its molecular targets and anticancer properties. *Molecules* **2020**, *25*, 2278. [CrossRef] [PubMed]
293. Bu, T.; Wang, C.; Jin, H.; Meng, Q.; Huo, X.; Sun, H.; Sun, P.; Wu, J.; Ma, X.; Liu, Z.; et al. Organic anion transporters and PI3K–AKT–mTOR pathway mediate the synergistic anticancer effect of pemetrexed and rhein. *J. Cell. Physiol.* **2020**, *235*, 3309–3319. [CrossRef] [PubMed]
294. Yang, L.; Li, J.; Xu, L.; Lin, S.; Xiang, Y.; Dai, X.; Liang, G.; Huang, X.; Zhu, J.; Zhao, C. Rhein shows potent efficacy against non-small-cell lung cancer through inhibiting the STAT3 pathway. *Cancer Manag. Res.* **2019**, *11*, 1167–1176. [CrossRef]
295. Piechowska, P.; Zawirska-Wojtasiak, R.; Mildner-Szkudlarz, S. Bioactive β-carbolines in food: A review. *Nutrients* **2019**, *11*, 814. [CrossRef]
296. Wang, Y.; Liu, Y.; Du, X.; Ma, H.; Yao, J. The anti-cancer mechanisms of berberine: A review. *Cancer Manag. Res.* **2020**, *12*, 695–702. [CrossRef] [PubMed]
297. Choudhary, N.; Khatik, G.L.; Suttee, A. The possible role of Saponin in Type-II Diabetes—A review. *Curr. Diabetes Rev.* **2020**, *16*, 107–121. [CrossRef]
298. Zhao, T.; Zhang, X.; Zhao, Y.; Zhang, L.; Bai, X.; Zhang, J.; Zhao, X.; Chen, L.; Wang, L.; Cui, L. Pretreatment by evodiamine is neuroprotective in cerebral ischemia: Up-regulated pAkt, pGSK3β, down-regulated NF-κB expression, and ameliorated BBB permeability. *Neurochem. Res.* **2014**, *39*, 1612–1620. [CrossRef]
299. Kobayashi, Y.; Nakano, Y.; Kizaki, M.; Hoshikuma, K.; Yokoo, Y.; Kamiya, T. Capsaicin-like anti-obese activities of evodiamine from fruits of Evodia rutaecarpa, a vanilloid receptor agonist. *Planta Med.* **2001**, *67*, 628–633. [CrossRef]
300. Iwaoka, E.; Wang, S.; Matsuyoshi, N.; Kogure, Y.; Aoki, S.; Yamamoto, S.; Noguchi, K.; Dai, Y. Evodiamine suppresses capsaicin-induced thermal hyperalgesia through activation and subsequent desensitization of the transient receptor potential V1 channels. *J. Nat. Med.* **2016**, *70*, 1–7. [CrossRef]
301. Li, L.; Zhang, C.; Huang, C.; Tian, X.; Sun, W.; Jiang, S. Research Advances in Antitumor Mechanism of Evodiamine. *J. Chem.* **2022**, *2022*, 2784257. [CrossRef]
302. Jiang, Z.B.; Huang, J.M.; Xie, Y.J.; Zhang, Y.Z.; Chang, C.; Lai, H.L.; Wang, W.; Yao, X.J.; Fan, X.X.; Wu, Q.B.; et al. Evodiamine suppresses non-small cell lung cancer by elevating CD8+ T cells and downregulating the MUC1-C/PD-L1 axis. *J. Exp. Clin. Cancer Res.* **2020**, *39*, 249. [CrossRef]
303. Lou, C.; Takahashi, K.; Irimura, T.; Saiki, I.; Hayakawa, Y. Identification of Hirsutine as an anti-metastatic phytochemical by targeting NF-KB activation. *Int. J. Oncol.* **2014**, *45*, 2085–2091. [CrossRef]
304. Zhou, X.; Zhou, R.; Li, Q.; Jie, X.; Hong, J.; Zong, Y.; Dong, X.; Zhang, S.; Li, Z.; Wu, G. Cardamonin inhibits the proliferation and metastasis of non-small-cell lung cancer cells by suppressing the PI3K/Akt/mTOR pathway. *Anticancer Drugs* **2019**, *30*, 241–250. [CrossRef] [PubMed]
305. Zhou, D.H.; Wang, X.; Yang, M.; Shi, X.; Huang, W.; Feng, Q. Combination of low concentration of (−)-epigallocatechin gallate (EGCG) and curcumin strongly suppresses the growth of non-small cell lung cancer in vitro and in vivo through causing cell cycle arrest. *Int. J. Mol. Sci.* **2013**, *14*, 12023–12036. [CrossRef] [PubMed]

306. Mimoto, J.; Kiura, K.; Matsuo, K.; Yoshino, T.; Takata, I.; Ueoka, H.; Kataoka, M.; Harada, M. (−)-Epigallocatechin gallate can prevent cisplatin-induced lung tumorigenesis in A/J mice. *Carcinogenesis* **2000**, *21*, 915–919. [CrossRef]
307. Pan, J.; Lee, Y.; Cheng, G.; Zielonka, J.; Zhang, Q.; Bajzikova, M.; Xiong, D.; Tsaih, S.W.; Hardy, M.; Flister, M.; et al. Mitochondria-Targeted Honokiol Confers a Striking Inhibitory Effect on Lung Cancer via Inhibiting Complex I Activity. *iScience* **2018**, *3*, 192–207. [CrossRef]
308. Chen, Y.; Chen, J.-Q.; Ge, M.-M.; Zhang, Q.; Wang, X.-Q.; Zhu, J.-Y.; Xie, C.-F.; Li, X.-T.; Zhong, C.-Y.; Han, H.-Y. Sulforaphane inhibits epithelial–mesenchymal transition by activating extracellular signal-regulated kinase 5 in lung cancer cells. *J. Nutr. Biochem.* **2019**, *72*, 108219. [CrossRef] [PubMed]
309. He, D.H.; Chen, Y.F.; Zhou, Y.L.; Zhang, S.B.; Hong, M.; Yu, X.; Wei, S.F.; Fan, X.Z.; Li, S.Y.; Wang, Q.; et al. Phytochemical library screening reveals betulinic acid as a novel Skp2-SCF E3 ligase inhibitor in non–small cell lung cancer. *Cancer Sci.* **2021**, *112*, 3218–3232. [CrossRef]
310. Zhang, Y.-Y.; Ren, H.; Yan, Q.-L.; Li, Y.-L.; Liu, Q.; Yao, G.-D.; Song, S.-J. SCP-7, a germacrane-type sesquiterpene lactone derivative, induces ROS-mediated apoptosis in NSCLC cells in vitro and in vivo. *Eur. J. Pharmacol.* **2022**, *925*, 174989. [CrossRef]
311. Li, Y.; Zhang, J.; Wang, B.; Shen, Y.; Ouahab, A. Co-delivery of siRNA and hypericin into cancer cells by hyaluronic acid modified PLGA-PEI nanoparticles. *Drug Dev. Ind. Pharm.* **2016**, *42*, 737–746. [CrossRef]
312. Liu, W.; Zhang, D.; Feng, Y.; Li, Y.; Huang, D.; Jiang, C.; Gao, M.; Peng, F.; Wang, X.; Jing, S.; et al. Biodistribution and anti-tumor efficacy of intratumorally injected necrosis-avid theranostic agent radioiodinated hypericin in rodent tumor models. *J. Drug Target.* **2015**, *23*, 371–379. [CrossRef]
313. Hishiki, T.; Kato, F.; Tajima, S.; Toume, K.; Umezaki, M.; Takasaki, T.; Miura, T. Hirsutine, an indole alkaloid of uncaria rhynchophylla, inhibits late step in dengue virus lifecycle. *Front. Microbiol.* **2017**, *8*, 1674. [CrossRef] [PubMed]
314. Lou, C.; Yokoyama, S.; Saiki, I.; Hayakawa, Y. Selective anticancer activity of hirsutine against HER2-positive breast cancer cells by inducing DNA damage. *Oncol. Rep.* **2015**, *33*, 2072–2076. [CrossRef] [PubMed]
315. Meng, J.; Su, R.; Wang, L.; Yuan, B.; Li, L. Inhibitory effect and mechanism of action (MOA) of hirsutine on the proliferation of T-cell leukemia Jurkat clone E6-1 cells. *PeerJ* **2021**, *9*, e10692. [CrossRef] [PubMed]
316. Dong, H.J.; Wang, Z.H.; Meng, W.; Li, C.C.; Hu, Y.X.; Zhou, L.; Wang, X.J. The natural compound homoharringtonine presents broad antiviral activity in vitro and in vivo. *Viruses* **2018**, *10*, 601. [CrossRef] [PubMed]
317. Wang, L.-B.; Wang, D.-N.; Wu, L.-G.; Cao, J.; Tian, J.-H.; Liu, R.; Ma, R.; Yu, J.-J.; Wang, J.; Huang, Q.; et al. Homoharringtonine inhibited breast cancer cells growth via mir-18a-3p/akt/mtor signaling pathway. *Int. J. Biol. Sci.* **2021**, *17*, 995–1009. [CrossRef]
318. Dadashpour, S.; Emami, S. Indole in the target-based design of anticancer agents: A versatile scaffold with diverse mechanisms. *Eur. J. Med. Chem.* **2018**, *150*, 9–29. [CrossRef]
319. Zhang, Y.; Hu, C. Anticancer activity of bisindole alkaloids derived from natural sources and synthetic bisindole hybrids. *Arch. Pharm.* **2020**, *353*, e2000092. [CrossRef]
320. Stojanović-Radić, Z.; Pejčić, M.; Dimitrijević, M.; Aleksić, A.; Anil Kumar, N.V.; Salehi, B.; Cho, W.C.; Sharifi-Rad, J. Piperine-A Major Principle of Black Pepper: A review of its bioactivity and studies. *Appl. Sci.* **2019**, *9*, 4270. [CrossRef]
321. Fu, R.; Wang, X.; Hu, Y.; Du, H.; Dong, B.; Ao, S.; Zhang, L.; Sun, Z.; Zhang, L.; Lv, G.; et al. Solamargine inhibits gastric cancer progression by regulating the expression of lncNEAT1_2 via the MAPK signaling pathway. *Int. J. Oncol.* **2019**, *54*, 1545–1554. [CrossRef]
322. Dhuguru, J.; Skouta, R. Role of indole scaffolds as pharmacophores in the development of anti-lung cancer agents. *Molecules* **2020**, *25*, 1615. [CrossRef] [PubMed]
323. Cháirez-Ramírez, M.H.; de la Cruz-López, K.G.; García-Carrancá, A. Polyphenols as Antitumor Agents Targeting Key Players in Cancer-Driving Signaling Pathways. *Front. Pharmacol.* **2021**, *12*, 710304. [CrossRef] [PubMed]
324. Zhang, Z.; Li, X.; Sang, S.; McClements, D.J.; Chen, L.; Long, J.; Jiao, A.; Jin, Z.; Qiu, C. Polyphenols as Plant-Based Nutraceuticals: Health Effects, Encapsulation, Nano-Delivery, and Application. *Foods* **2022**, *11*, 2189. [CrossRef]
325. Maiuolo, J.; Gliozzi, M.; Carresi, C.; Musolino, V.; Oppedisano, F.; Scarano, F.; Nucera, S.; Scicchitano, M.; Bosco, F.; Macri, R.; et al. Nutraceuticals and cancer: Potential for natural polyphenols. *Nutrients* **2021**, *13*, 3834. [CrossRef]
326. Singh, S.; Gupta, P.; Meena, A.; Luqman, S. Acacetin, a flavone with diverse therapeutic potential in cancer, inflammation, infections and other metabolic disorders. *Food Chem. Toxicol.* **2020**, *145*, 111708. [CrossRef]
327. Yang, T.; Zang, D.W.; Shan, W.; Guo, A.C.; Wu, J.P.; Wang, Y.J.; Wang, Q. Synthesis and evaluations of novel apocynin derivatives as anti-glioma agents. *Front. Pharmacol.* **2019**, *10*, 951. [CrossRef]
328. Huang, Y.; Tsang, S.Y.; Yao, X.; Chen, Z.Y. Biological properties of baicalein in cardiovascular system. *Curr. Drug Targets Cardiovasc. Haematol. Disord.* **2005**, *5*, 177–184. [CrossRef]
329. Gao, Y.; Snyder, S.A.; Smith, J.N.; Chen, Y.C. Anticancer properties of baicalein: A review. *Med. Chem. Res.* **2016**, *25*, 1515–1523. [CrossRef] [PubMed]
330. Hu, W.P.; Cao, G.D.; Zhu, J.H.; Li, J.Z.; Liu, X.H. Naturally occurring Batatasins and their derivatives as α-glucosidase inhibitors. *RSC Adv.* **2015**, *5*, 82153–82158. [CrossRef]
331. Espíndola, K.M.M.; Ferreira, R.G.; Narvaez, L.E.M.; Rosario, A.C.R.S.; Da Silva, A.H.M.; Silva, A.G.B.; Vieira, A.P.O.; Monteiro, M.C. Chemical and pharmacological aspects of caffeic acid and its activity in hepatocarcinoma. *Front. Oncol.* **2019**, *9*, 541. [CrossRef] [PubMed]

332. Chan, E.W.C.; Wong, S.K.; Chan, H.T. Casticin from Vitex species: A short review on its anticancer and anti-inflammatory properties. *J. Integr. Med.* **2018**, *16*, 147–152. [CrossRef] [PubMed]
333. Talebi, M.; Talebi, M.; Farkhondeh, T.; Simal-Gandara, J.; Kopustinskiene, D.M.; Bernatoniene, J.; Samarghandian, S. Emerging cellular and molecular mechanisms underlying anticancer indications of chrysin. *Cancer Cell Int.* **2021**, *21*, 214. [CrossRef]
334. Tomeh, M.A.; Hadianamrei, R.; Zhao, X. A review of curcumin and its derivatives as anticancer agents. *Int. J. Mol. Sci.* **2019**, *20*, 1033. [CrossRef]
335. Jang, M.G.; Ko, H.C.; Kim, S.J. Effects of p-coumaric acid on microRNA expression profiles in SNU-16 human gastric cancer cells. *Genes Genom.* **2020**, *42*, 817–825. [CrossRef]
336. Aggarwal, V.; Tuli, H.S.; Tania, M.; Srivastava, S.; Ritzer, E.E.; Pandey, A.; Aggarwal, D.; Barwal, T.S.; Jain, A.; Kaur, G.; et al. Molecular mechanisms of action of epigallocatechin gallate in cancer: Recent trends and advancement. *Semin. Cancer Biol.* **2022**, *80*, 256–275. [CrossRef] [PubMed]
337. Chen, B.H.; Hsieh, C.H.; Tsai, S.Y.; Wang, C.Y.; Wang, C.C. Anticancer effects of epigallocatechin-3-gallate nanoemulsion on lung cancer cells through the activation of AMP-activated protein kinase signaling pathway. *Sci. Rep.* **2020**, *10*, 5163. [CrossRef] [PubMed]
338. Gao, J.; Yu, H.; Guo, W.; Kong, Y.; Gu, L.; Li, Q.; Yang, S.; Zhang, Y.; Wang, Y. The anticancer effects of ferulic acid is associated with induction of cell cycle arrest and autophagy in cervical cancer cells. *Cancer Cell Int.* **2018**, *18*, 102. [CrossRef]
339. Gupta, A.; Singh, A.K.; Loka, M.; Pandey, A.K.; Bishayee, A. Ferulic acid-mediated modulation of apoptotic signaling pathways in cancer. *Adv. Protein Chem. Struct. Biol.* **2021**, *125*, 215–257.
340. Sundarraj, K.; Raghunath, A.; Perumal, E. A review on the chemotherapeutic potential of fisetin: In vitro evidences. *Biomed. Pharmacother.* **2018**, *97*, 928–940. [CrossRef]
341. Kahkeshani, N.; Farzaei, F.; Fotouhi, M.; Alavi, S.S.; Bahramsoltani, R.; Naseri, R.; Momtaz, S.; Abbasabadi, Z.; Rahimi, R.; Farzaei, M.H.; et al. Pharmacological effects of gallic acid in health and disease: A mechanistic review. *Iran. J. Basic Med. Sci.* **2019**, *22*, 225–237. [CrossRef]
342. Bhat, S.S.; Prasad, S.K.; Shivamallu, C.; Prasad, K.S.; Syed, A.; Reddy, P.; Cull, C.A.; Amachawadi, R.G. Genistein: A potent anti-breast cancer agent. *Curr. Issues Mol. Biol.* **2021**, *43*, 1502–1517. [CrossRef] [PubMed]
343. Yu, S.; Wang, Z.; Su, Z.; Song, J.; Zhou, L.; Sun, Q.; Liu, S.; Li, S.; Li, Y.; Wang, M.; et al. Gigantol inhibits Wnt/β-catenin signaling and exhibits anticancer activity in breast cancer cells. *BMC Complement. Altern. Med.* **2018**, *18*, 59. [CrossRef]
344. Yap, K.M.; Sekar, M.; Wu, Y.S.; Gan, S.H.; Rani, N.N.I.M.; Seow, L.J.; Subramaniyan, V.; Fuloria, N.K.; Fuloria, S.; Lum, P.T. Hesperidin and its aglycone hesperetin in breast cancer therapy: A review of recent developments and future prospects. *Saudi J. Biol. Sci.* **2021**, *28*, 6730–6747. [CrossRef]
345. Ong, C.P.; Lee, W.L.; Tang, Y.Q.; Yap, W.H. Honokiol: A review of its anticancer potential and mechanisms. *Cancers* **2019**, *12*, 48. [CrossRef]
346. Gong, G.; Guan, Y.Y.; Zhang, Z.L.; Rahman, K.; Wang, S.J.; Zhou, S.; Luan, X.; Zhang, H. Isorhamnetin: A review of pharmacological effects. *Biomed. Pharmacother.* **2020**, *128*, 110301. [CrossRef] [PubMed]
347. Younas, M.; Hano, C.; Giglioli-Guivarc'H, N.; Abbasi, B.H. Mechanistic evaluation of phytochemicals in breast cancer remedy: Current understanding and future perspectives. *RSC Adv.* **2018**, *8*, 29714–29744. [CrossRef] [PubMed]
348. Nishikawa, S.; Inoue, Y.; Hori, Y.; Miyajima, C.; Morishita, D.; Ohoka, N.; Hida, S.; Makino, T.; Hayashi, H. Anti-inflammatory activity of kurarinone involves induction of ho-1 via the keap1/NRF2 pathway. *Antioxidants* **2020**, *9*, 842. [CrossRef]
349. Taheri, Y.; Sharifi-Rad, J.; Antika, G.; Yilmaz, Y.B.; Tumer, T.B.; Abuhamdah, S.; Chandra, S.; Saklani, S.; Kiliç, C.S.; Sestito, S.; et al. Paving Luteolin Therapeutic Potentialities and Agro-Food-Pharma Applications: Emphasis on in vivo Pharmacological Effects and Bioavailability Traits. *Oxid. Med. Cell. Longev.* **2021**, *2021*, 1987588. [CrossRef]
350. Choudhary, N.; Tewari, D.; Nabavi, S.F.; Kashani, H.R.K.; Lorigooini, Z.; Filosa, R.; Khan, F.B.; Masoudian, N.; Nabavi, S.M. Plant based food bioactives: A boon or bane for neurological disorders. *Crit. Rev. Food Sci. Nutr.* **2022**. [CrossRef]
351. Yu, C.L.; Weng, M.S.; Chen, W.C.; Chien, K.T.; Chi, C.W.; Chung, C.H.; Huang, C.W.; Wang, P.C.; Chen, C.C.; Tsai, A.C.; et al. Moscatilin inhibits metastatic behavior of human hepatocellular carcinoma cells: A crucial role of upa suppression via akt/nf-κb-dependent pathway. *Int. J. Mol. Sci.* **2021**, *22*, 2930. [CrossRef]
352. Choi, J.; Lee, D.H.; Jang, H.; Park, S.Y.; Seol, J.W. Naringenin exerts anticancer effects by inducing tumor cell death and inhibiting angiogenesis in malignant melanoma. *Int. J. Med. Sci.* **2020**, *17*, 3049–3057. [CrossRef] [PubMed]
353. Ashrafizadeh, M.; Zarrabi, A.; Saberifar, S.; Hashemi, F.; Hushmandi, K.; Hashemi, F.; Moghadam, E.R.; Mohammadinejad, R.; Najafi, M.; Garg, M. Nobiletin in cancer therapy: How this plant derived-natural compound targets various oncogene and onco-suppressor pathways. *Biomedicines* **2020**, *8*, 110. [CrossRef] [PubMed]
354. Sun, M.; Sun, M.; Zhang, J. Osthole: An overview of its sources, biological activities, and modification development. *Med. Chem. Res.* **2021**, *30*, 1767–1794. [CrossRef] [PubMed]
355. Mariadoss, A.V.A.; Vinyagam, R.; Rajamanickam, V.; Sankaran, V.; Venkatesan, S.; David, E. Pharmacological Aspects and Potential Use of Phloretin: A Systemic Review. *Mini-Rev. Med. Chem.* **2019**, *19*, 1060–1067. [CrossRef]
356. Zhao, G.; Yang, L.; Zhong, W.; Hu, Y.; Tan, Y.; Ren, Z.; Ban, Q.; Yang, C.S.; Wang, Y.; Wang, Z. Polydatin, A Glycoside of Resveratrol, Is Better Than Resveratrol in Alleviating Non-alcoholic Fatty Liver Disease in Mice Fed a High-Fructose Diet. *Front. Nutr.* **2022**, *9*, 857879. [CrossRef]

357. Gao, Z.; Gao, W.; Zeng, S.L.; Li, P.; Liu, E.H. Chemical structures, bioactivities and molecular mechanisms of citrus polymethoxyflavones. *J. Funct. Foods* **2018**, *40*, 498–509. [CrossRef]
358. Ma, Z.; Zhang, X.; Xu, L.; Liu, D.; Di, S.; Li, W.; Zhang, J.; Zhang, H.; Li, X.; Han, J.; et al. Pterostilbene: Mechanisms of its action as oncostatic agent in cell models and in vivo studies. *Pharmacol. Res.* **2019**, *145*, 104265. [CrossRef]
359. Lucarini, M.; Durazzo, E.B.; Tzvetkov, N.T.; Jóźwik, M.S.; Strzałkowska, N.; Horbańczuk, A.G. Quercetin: Total-scale literature landscape analysis of a valuable nutraceutical with numerous potential applications in the promotion of human and animal health—A review. *Anim. Sci. Pap. Rep.* **2021**, *39*, 199–212.
360. Khan, F.; Niaz, K.; Maqbool, F.; Hassan, F.I.; Abdollahi, M.; Venkata, K.C.N.; Nabavi, S.M.; Bishayee, A. Molecular Targets Underlying the Anticancer Effects of Quercetin: An Update. *Nutrients* **2016**, *8*, 529. [CrossRef]
361. Yang, D.; Wang, T.; Long, M.; Li, P. Quercetin: Its Main Pharmacological Activity and Potential Application in Clinical Medicine. *Oxid. Med. Cell. Longev.* **2020**, *2020*, 8825387. [CrossRef]
362. Varoni, E.M.; Lo Faro, A.F.; Sharifi-Rad, J.; Iriti, M. Anticancer Molecular Mechanisms of Resveratrol. *Front. Nutr.* **2016**, *3*, 8. [CrossRef] [PubMed]
363. Ko, J.-H.; Sethi, G.; Um, J.-Y.; Shanmugam, M.K.; Arfuso, F.; Kumar, A.P.; Bishayee, A.; Ahn, K.S. The Role of Resveratrol in Cancer Therapy. *Int. J. Mol. Sci.* **2017**, *18*, 2589. [CrossRef] [PubMed]
364. Bishayee, A. Cancer prevention and treatment with resveratrol: From rodent studies to clinical trials. *Cancer Prev. Res.* **2009**, *2*, 409–418. [CrossRef] [PubMed]
365. Vender, R.B.; Andriessen, A.; Barankin, B.; Freiman, A.; Kyritsis, D.; Mistos, L.M.; Salsberg, J.; Amar, L. Cohort Using a Ceramides Containing Cleanser and Cream with Salicylic Acid for Dry, Flaking, and Scaling Skin Conditions. *J. Drugs Dermatol.* **2019**, *18*, 80–85.
366. Ashrafizadeh, M.; Ahmadi, Z.; Mohammadinejad, R.; Afshar, E.G. Tangeretin: A mechanistic review of its pharmacological and therapeutic effects. *J. Basic Clin. Physiol. Pharmacol.* **2020**, *31*, 20190191. [CrossRef]
367. Jing, R.; Li, H.Q.; Hu, C.L.; Jiang, Y.P.; Qin, L.P.; Zheng, C.J. Phytochemical and pharmacological profiles of three Fagopyrum buckwheats. *Int. J. Mol. Sci.* **2016**, *17*, 589. [CrossRef]
368. Lu, Y.; Zhang, M.; Huang, D. Dietary Organosulfur-Containing Compounds and Their Health-Promotion Mechanisms. *Annu. Rev. Food Sci. Technol.* **2022**, *13*, 287–313. [CrossRef]
369. Miekus, N.; Marszałek, K.; Podlacha, M.; Iqbal, A.; Puchalski, C.; Swiergiel, A.H. Health Benefits of Plant-Derived Sulfur Compounds, Glucosinolates, and Organosulfur Compounds. *Molecules* **2020**, *25*, 3804. [CrossRef]
370. Ruhee, R.T.; Roberts, L.A.; Ma, S.; Suzuki, K. Organosulfur Compounds: A Review of Their Anti-inflammatory Effects in Human Health. *Front. Nutr.* **2020**, *7*, 64. [CrossRef] [PubMed]
371. De Greef, D.; Barton, E.M.; Sandberg, E.N.; Croley, C.R.; Pumarol, J.; Wong, T.L.; Das, N.; Bishayee, A. Anticancer potential of garlic and its bioactive constituents: A systematic and comprehensive review. *Semin. Cancer Biol.* **2021**, *73*, 219–264. [CrossRef]
372. Kaiser, A.E.; Baniasadi, M.; Giansiracusa, D.; Giansiracusa, M.; Garcia, M.; Fryda, Z.; Wong, T.L.; Bishayee, A. Sulforaphane: A Broccoli Bioactive Phytocompound with Cancer Preventive Potential. *Cancers* **2021**, *13*, 4796. [CrossRef] [PubMed]
373. Salehi, B.; Zucca, P.; Orhan, I.E.; Azzini, E.; Adetunji, C.O.; Mohammed, S.A.; Banerjee, S.K.; Sharopov, F.; Rigano, D.; Sharifi-Rad, J.; et al. Allicin and health: A comprehensive review. *Trends Food Sci. Technol.* **2019**, *86*, 502–516. [CrossRef]
374. Kamal, M.M.; Akter, S.; Lin, C.N.; Nazzal, S. Sulforaphane as an anticancer molecule: Mechanisms of action, synergistic effects, enhancement of drug safety, and delivery systems. *Arch. Pharm. Res.* **2020**, *43*, 371–384. [CrossRef] [PubMed]
375. Thoppil, R.J.; Bishayee, A. Terpenoids as potential chemopreventive and therapeutic agents in liver cancer. *World J. Hepatol.* **2011**, *3*, 228–249. [CrossRef]
376. González, M.A. Aromatic abietane diterpenoids: Their biological activity and synthesis. *Nat. Prod. Rep.* **2015**, *32*, 684–704. [CrossRef]
377. Alvarez-Sala, A.; Attanzio, A.; Tesoriere, L.; Garcia-Llatas, G.; Barberá, R.; Cilla, A. Apoptotic effect of a phytosterol-ingredient and its main phytosterol (β-sitosterol) in human cancer cell lines. *Int. J. Food Sci. Nutr.* **2019**, *70*, 323–334. [CrossRef]
378. Jiang, W.; Li, X.; Dong, S.; Zhou, W. Betulinic acid in the treatment of tumour diseases: Application and research progress. *Biomed. Pharmacother.* **2021**, *142*, 111990. [CrossRef]
379. Jing, S.; Zou, H.; Wu, Z.; Ren, L.; Zhang, T.; Zhang, J.; Wei, Z. Cucurbitacins: Bioactivities and synergistic effect with small-molecule drugs. *J. Funct. Foods* **2020**, *72*, 104042. [CrossRef]
380. Yu, R.; Jin, G.; Fujimoto, M. Dihydroartemisinin: A Potential Drug for the Treatment of Malignancies and Inflammatory Diseases. *Front. Oncol.* **2021**, *11*, 722331. [CrossRef]
381. Bajalia, E.M.; Azzouz, F.B.; Chism, D.A.; Giansiracusa, D.M.; Wong, C.G.; Plaskett, K.N.; Bishayee, A. Phytochemicals for the Prevention and Treatment of Renal Cell Carcinoma: Preclinical and Clinical Evidence and Molecular Mechanisms. *Cancers* **2022**, *14*, 3278. [CrossRef]
382. Gao, Y.; Nie, Z.; Cao, H.; Huang, D.; Chen, M.; Xiang, Y.; Yu, X.; Zhang, S. Scabertopin Derived from Elephantopus scaber L. Mediates Necroptosis by Inducing Reactive Oxygen Species Production in Bladder Cancer in vitro. *Cancers* **2022**, *14*, 5976. [CrossRef]
383. Peng, L.; Liu, A.; Shen, Y.; Xu, H.Z.; Yang, S.Z.; Ying, X.Z.; Liao, W.; Liu, H.X.; Lin, Z.Q.; Chen, Q.Y.; et al. Antitumor and anti-angiogenesis effects of thymoquinone on osteosarcoma through the NF-κB pathway. *Oncol. Rep.* **2013**, *29*, 571–578. [CrossRef] [PubMed]

384. Begum, S.; Mannan, A. A Review on Nigella sativa: A Marvel Herb. *J. Drug Deliv. Ther.* **2020**, *10*, 213–219. [CrossRef]
385. Shanmugam, M.K.; Arfuso, F.; Kumar, A.P.; Wang, L.; Goh, B.C.; Ahn, K.S.; Bishayee, A.; Sethi, G. Modulation of diverse oncogenic transcription factors by thymoquinone, an essential oil compound isolated from the seeds of Nigella sativa Linn. *Pharmacol. Res.* **2018**, *129*, 357–364. [CrossRef] [PubMed]
386. Alhmied, F.; Alammar, A.; Alsultan, B.; Alshehri, M.; Pottoo, F.H. Molecular Mechanisms of Thymoquinone as Anticancer Agent. *Comb. Chem. High Throughput Screen.* **2020**, *24*, 1644–1653. [CrossRef] [PubMed]
387. Shanmugam, M.K.; Dai, X.; Kumar, A.P.; Tan, B.K.H.; Sethi, G.; Bishayee, A. Ursolic acid in cancer prevention and treatment: Molecular targets, pharmacokinetics and clinical studies. *Biochem. Pharmacol.* **2013**, *85*, 1579–1587. [CrossRef]
388. Mlala, S.; Oyedeji, A.O.; Gondwe, M.; Oyedeji, O.O. Ursolic Acid and Its Derivatives as Bioactive Agents. *Molecules* **2019**, *24*, 2751. [CrossRef] [PubMed]
389. Atteeq, M. Evaluating anticancer properties of Withaferin A—A potent phytochemical. *Front. Pharmacol.* **2022**, *13*, 975320. [CrossRef]
390. Kumar, S.; Mathew, S.O.; Aharwal, R.P.; Tulli, H.S.; Mohan, C.D.; Sethi, G.; Ahn, K.S.; Webber, K.; Sandhu, S.S.; Bishayee, A. Withaferin A: A Pleiotropic Anticancer Agent from the Indian Medicinal Plant *Withania somnifera* (L.) Dunal. *Pharmaceuticals* **2023**, *16*, 160. [CrossRef] [PubMed]
391. Lee, I.C.; Choi, B.Y. Withaferin-A—A natural anticancer agent with pleitropic mechanisms of action. *Int. J. Mol. Sci.* **2016**, *17*, 290. [CrossRef]
392. Zúñiga, R.; Concha, G.; Cayo, A.; Cikutović-Molina, R.; Arevalo, B.; González, W.; Catalán, M.A.; Zúñiga, L. Withaferin A suppresses breast cancer cell proliferation by inhibition of the two-pore domain potassium (K2P9) channel TASK-3. *Biomed. Pharmacother.* **2020**, *129*, 110383. [CrossRef] [PubMed]
393. Stasiłowicz, A.; Tomala, A.; Podolak, I.; Cielecka-Piontek, J. *Cannabis sativa* L. As a natural drug meeting the criteria of a multitarget approach to treatment. *Int. J. Mol. Sci.* **2021**, *22*, 778. [CrossRef] [PubMed]
394. Vasas, A. Phenanthrenes from Orchidaceae and Their Biological Activities. In *Orchids Phytochemistry, Biology and Horticulture*; Merillon, J.M., Kodja, H., Eds.; Reference Series in Phytochemistry; Springer: Cham, Switzerland, 2021; pp. 1–41.
395. El Omari, N.; Jaouadi, I.; Lahyaoui, M.; Benali, T.; Taha, D.; Bakrim, S.; El Menyiy, N.; El Kamari, F.; Zengin, G.; Bangar, S.P.; et al. Natural Sources, Pharmacological Properties, and Health Benefits of Daucosterol: Versatility of Actions. *Appl. Sci.* **2022**, *12*, 5779. [CrossRef]
396. Li, Q.; Gao, J.; Pang, X.; Chen, A.; Wang, Y. Molecular Mechanisms of Action of Emodin: As an Anti-Cardiovascular Disease Drug. *Front. Pharmacol.* **2020**, *11*, 559607. [CrossRef]
397. Hsu, H.F.; Houng, J.Y.; Chang, C.L.; Wu, C.C.; Chang, F.R.; Wu, Y.C. Antioxidant activity, cytotoxicity, and DNA information of Glossogyne tenuifolia. *J. Agric. Food Chem.* **2005**, *53*, 6117–6125. [CrossRef]
398. Osborn, H.M.I.; Evans, P.G.; Gemmell, N.; Osborne, S.D. Carbohydrate-based therapeutics. *J. Pharm. Pharmacol.* **2010**, *56*, 691–702. [CrossRef]
399. Wu, J.; Li, D.; Du, L.; Baldawi, M.; Gable, M.E.; Askari, A.; Liu, L. Ouabain prevents pathological cardiac hypertrophy and heart failure through activation of phosphoinositide 3-kinase α in mouse. *Cell Biosci.* **2015**, *5*, 64. [CrossRef]
400. Meira, C.S.; Soares, J.W.C.; dos Reis, B.P.Z.C.; Pacheco, L.V.; Santos, I.P.; Silva, D.K.C.; de Lacerda, J.C.; Daltro, S.R.T.; Guimarães, E.T.; Soares, M.B.P. Therapeutic Applications of Physalins: Powerful Natural Weapons. *Front. Pharmacol.* **2022**, *13*, 864714. [CrossRef]
401. Zhang, H.; Yi, J.K.; Huang, H.; Park, S.; Park, S.; Kwon, W.; Kim, E.; Jang, S.; Kim, S.Y.; Choi, S.K.; et al. Rhein suppresses colorectal cancer cell growth by inhibiting the mtor pathway in vitro and in vivo. *Cancers* **2021**, *13*, 2176. [CrossRef]
402. Wadegaonkar, V.P.; Wadegaonkar, P.A. Withanone as an inhibitor of survivin: A potential drug candidate for cancer therapy. *J. Biotechnol.* **2013**, *168*, 229–233. [CrossRef]
403. Balkrishna, A.; Pokhrel, S.; Singh, H.; Joshi, M.; Mulay, V.P.; Haldar, S.; Varshney, A. Withanone from *Withania somnifera* attenuates SARS-CoV-2 rbd and host ace2 interactions to rescue spike protein induced pathologies in humanized zebrafish model. *Drug Des. Devel. Ther.* **2021**, *15*, 1111–1133. [CrossRef]
404. Koushki, M.; Amiri-Dashatan, N.; Ahmadi, N.; Abbaszadeh, H.A.; Rezaei-Tavirani, M. Resveratrol: A miraculous natural compound for diseases treatment. *Food Sci. Nutr.* **2018**, *6*, 2473–2490. [CrossRef] [PubMed]
405. Yu, Y.H.; Chen, H.A.; Chen, P.S.; Cheng, Y.J.; Hsu, W.H.; Chang, Y.W.; Chen, Y.H.; Jan, Y.; Hsiao, M.; Chang, T.Y.; et al. MiR-520h-mediated FOXC2 regulation is critical for inhibition of lung cancer progression by resveratrol. *Oncogene* **2013**, *32*, 431–443. [CrossRef] [PubMed]
406. Cicenas, J.; Kalyan, K.; Sorokinas, A.; Stankunas, E.; Levy, J.; Meskinyte, I.; Stankevicius, V.; Kaupinis, A.; Valius, M. Roscovitine in cancer and other diseases. *Ann. Transl. Med.* **2015**, *3*, 135. [PubMed]
407. MacCallum, D.E.; Melville, J.; Frame, S.; Watt, K.; Anderson, S.; Gianella-Borradori, A.; Lane, D.P.; Green, S.R. Seliciclib (CYC202, R-Roscovitine) induces cell death in multiple myeloma cells by inhibition of RNA polymerase II-dependent transcription and down-regulation of Mcl-1. *Cancer Res.* **2005**, *65*, 5399–5407. [CrossRef]
408. Li, F.; Jiang, T.; Li, Q.; Ling, X. Camptothecin (CPT) and its derivatives are known to target topoisomerase I (Top1) as their mechanism of action: Did we miss something in CPT analogue molecular targets for treating human disease such as cancer? *Am. J. Cancer Res.* **2017**, *7*, 2350–2394.
409. Moudi, M.; Go, R.; Yien, C.Y.S.; Nazre, M. Vinca alkaloids. *Int. J. Prev. Med.* **2013**, *4*, 1131–1135.

410. Mazumder, K.; Aktar, A.; Roy, P.; Biswas, B.; Hossain, M.E.; Sarkar, K.K.; Bachar, S.C.; Ahmed, F.; Monjur-Al-hossain, A.S.M.; Fukase, K. A Review on Mechanistic Insight of Plant Derived Anticancer Bioactive Phytocompounds and Their Structure Activity Relationship. *Molecules* **2022**, *27*, 3036. [CrossRef]
411. Mann, J.; Yang, N.; Montpetit, R.; Kirschenman, R.; Lemieux, H.; Goping, I.S. BAD sensitizes breast cancer cells to docetaxel with increased mitotic arrest and necroptosis. *Sci. Rep.* **2020**, *10*, 355. [CrossRef] [PubMed]
412. Francis, P.A.; Kris, M.G.; Rigas, J.R.; Grant, S.C.; Miller, V.A. Paclitaxel (Taxol) and Docetaxel (Taxotere): Active chemotherapeutic agents in lung cancer. *Lung Cancer* **1995**, *12*, S163–S172. [CrossRef]
413. Gatzemeier, U.; Heckmayr, M.; Neuhauss, R.; Schlüter, I.; Pawel, J.V.; Wagner, H.; Dreps, A. Phase II study with paclitaxel for the treatment of advanced inoperable non-small cell lung cancer. *Lung Cancer* **1995**, *12*, S101–S106. [CrossRef] [PubMed]
414. Murphy, W.K.; Fossella, F.V.; Winn, R.J.; Shin, D.M.; Hynes, H.E.; Gross, H.M.; Davilla, E.; Leimert, J.; Dhingra, H.; Raber, M.N.; et al. Phase II study of taxol in patients with untreated advanced non-small-cell lung cancer. *J. Natl. Cancer Inst.* **1993**, *85*, 384–388. [CrossRef] [PubMed]
415. Sharma, A.; Shambhwani, D.; Pandey, S.; Singh, J.; Lalhlenmawia, H.; Kumarasamy, M.; Singh, S.K.; Chellappan, D.K.; Gupta, G.; Prasher, P.; et al. Advances in Lung Cancer Treatment Using Nanomedicines. *ACS Omega* **2022**, *8*, 10–41. [CrossRef]
416. Wei, Z.; Zou, H.; Liu, G.; Song, C.; Tang, C.; Chen, S.; Zhang, G.; Ran, J.; Wang, Y.; Yin, X. Peroxidase-mimicking evodiamine/indocyanine green nanoliposomes for multimodal imaging-guided theranostics for oral squamous cell carcinoma. *Bioact. Mater.* **2021**, *6*, 2144–2157. [CrossRef] [PubMed]

cancers MDPI

Review

Potential of Synthetic and Natural Compounds as Novel Histone Deacetylase Inhibitors for the Treatment of Hematological Malignancies

Dilipkumar Pal [1], Khushboo Raj [1], Shyam Sundar Nandi [2], Surajit Sinha [3], Abhishek Mishra [4], Arijit Mondal [5], Ricardo Lagoa [6], Jack T. Burcher [7] and Anupam Bishayee [7,*]

1 Department of Pharmaceutical Sciences, Guru Ghasidas Vishwavidyalaya (A Central University), Bilaspur 495 009, India
2 Department of Biotechnology, Indian Council for Medical Research-National Institute of Virology, Mumbai 400 012, India
3 Department of Cancer Biology, Memorial Sloan Kettering Cancer Center, New York, NY 10065, USA
4 Aurobindo Pharma, Durham, NC 27703, USA
5 Department of Pharmaceutical Chemistry, M.R. College of Pharmaceutical Sciences and Research, Balisha 743 234, India
6 Associate Laboratory in Chemical Engineering, Polytechnic Institute of Leiria, Morro do Lena, Alto do Vieiro, 2411-901 Leiria, Portugal
7 College of Osteopathic Medicine, Lake Erie College of Osteopathic Medicine, Bradenton, FL 34211, USA
* Correspondence: abishayee@lecom.edu or abishayee@gmail.com

Simple Summary: Histone deacetylases (HDACs) are epigenetic regulators that influence chromatin structure and gene transcription, but also the function of non-histone targets like chaperones and proteins participating in the DNA damage response. Histone modifications are implicated in cancer and HDAC inhibitors (HDACis) can be useful to treat hematological malignancies, including leukemia, B-cell lymphoma, virus-associated tumors, and multiple myeloma. Several HDACis were approved for clinical use and others are showing promising results, especially as adjuvants to conventional treatments. In addition to synthetic inhibitors, this work discusses the potential of phytocompounds, such as chrysin and oleacein as well as marine-derived agents, such as halenaquinone and xestoquinone, as therapeutic agents against hematological cancers.

Abstract: Histone deacetylases (HDACs) and histone acetyltransferases (HATs) are enzymes that remove or add acetyl groups to lysine residues of histones, respectively. Histone deacetylation causes DNA to more snugly encircle histones and decreases gene expression, whereas acetylation has the opposite effect. Through these small alterations in chemical structure, HATs and HDACs regulate DNA expression. Recent research indicates histone deacetylase inhibitors (HDACis) may be used to treat malignancies, including leukemia, B-cell lymphoma, virus-associated tumors, and multiple myeloma. These data suggest that HDACis may boost the production of immune-related molecules, resulting in the growth of CD8-positive T-cells and the recognition of nonreactive tumor cells by the immune system, thereby diminishing tumor immunity. The argument for employing epigenetic drugs in the treatment of acute myeloid leukemia (AML) patients is supported by evidence that both epigenetic changes and mutations in the epigenetic machinery contribute to AML etiology. Although hypomethylating drugs have been licensed for use in AML, additional epigenetic inhibitors, such as HDACis, are now being tested in humans. Preclinical studies evaluating the efficacy of HDACis against AML have shown the ability of specific agents, such as anobinostat, vorinostat, and tricostatin A, to induce growth arrest, apoptosis, autophagy and cell death. However, these inhibitors do not seem to be successful as monotherapies, but instead achieve results when used in conjunction with other medications. In this article, we discuss the mounting evidence that HDACis promote extensive histone acetylation, as well as substantial increases in reactive oxygen species and DNA damage in hematological malignant cells. We also evaluate the potential of various natural product-based HDACis as therapeutic agents to combat hematological malignancies.

Keywords: leukemia; multiple myeloma; DNA damage; HDAC inhibitors; oxidative stress; chromatin remodeling; natural agents

1. Introduction

Approximately 1% of the DNA sequences within the human genome are responsible for coding the 20,000–25,000 genes of functional protein products. Noncoding DNA serves as binding sites for transcription factors, which contributes to a transcriptome that is many times larger than the number of genes. Still, further diversification of the proteome occurs by post-translational modifications (PTMs) of amino acid side chains. Most PTMs are considered to be dynamic in nature, meaning that an individual protein may be found in one of many different states and have the freedom to flow through each of them [1]. The α-amino side chain of lysine, for example, is the focus of many PTMs through alkylation or acylation processes. In contrast to acylation, which adds carbon to proteins and results in neutral or negatively charged side chains [2], alkylation augments the lysine side chain while maintaining its positive charge within a normal pH. Two PTMs, methylation and acetylation, occur in histone proteins, which contain a lysine-rich N-terminal, and play a major role in chromatin remodeling and management of binding partners to influence transcription [3,4]. For this reason, modifiers of lysine acetylation enzymes and agents promoting their elimination have become prime candidates for small molecule therapeutic development.

Lysine acetylation was originally identified in the early 1960s when scientists noticed large amounts of PTMs in histones [5]. Soon afterwards, enzymes that catalyze the forward acetylation process and the reverse deacetylation reaction were found and named histone acetyltransferases (HATs) and histone deacetylases (HDACs), respectively [5]. As epigenetic regulators, HDACs control histone tail length, chromatin structure, protein-DNA interactions, and gene transcription. Additionally, proteins other than histones are the targets for HATs and HDACs. These include chaperone proteins, transcription factors, hormone receptors, signaling mediators, and other proteins implicated in the DNA damage response [6]. Given their extensive role in genetic regulation, it is unsurprising that histone modifications are implicated in numerous pathophysiologic states [6]. Many of these changes are observed in hematological malignancies and may be remedied, in part, by HDACis [7]. For example, the following changes are observed in lymphomas and leukemias:

1. Cancer cells express changes in the global pattern of acetylation
2. Levels of HDACs are increased in lymphoma cells
3. HDACs are abnormally attracted to the promoter of a target gene, where they suppress transcription and prevent differentiation, thereby contributing to the generation of acute promyelocytic leukemia.

Epigenetics refers to a multitude of changes in gene expression not involving modifications of the underlying DNA sequence [8,9]. As mentioned previously, lysine acetylation is a key histone chemical change necessary for epigenetic gene expression. HATs and HDACs are targets for cancer treatment because of their roles in reversibly regulating histone acetylation. HDACs' inhibitors (HDACis) are a large and varied family of compounds found throughout nature and as synthetic products. Many different agents are being studied for their potential as HDACis; n-butyrate was the first to be recognized as the agent responsible for the accumulation of hyper-acetylated histone within the nucleus. Later, it was shown that HDACs might be inhibited in two more ways: irreversibly by trapoxin A and reversibly by trichostatin A (TSA). Inhibition of HDAC activity is the biochemical mechanism through which HDACis raise histone acetylation levels [10]. Several proteins associated with cancer development, apoptosis, cell cycle regulation, angiogenesis, and cell invasion are all targets of HDACs. HDACis have been demonstrated to support cell cycle arrest and induce apoptosis by triggering both the intrinsic and the extrinsic apoptotic pathways. HDACis may cause differentiation and/or death by blocking the cell cycle during the G1/S or G2/M transition. Moreover, their increased expression of p21WAF1/CIP1 (a cyclin-dependent kinase (CDK) inhibitor) causes cell cycle arrest at the G1/S phase [11].

The primary focus of this review is on the role of HDACis, including those derived naturally from plants, in the treatment of hematological cancers. Hematological cancers, also known as blood cancers, are a diverse group of malignancies that affect the production and functions of blood cells [12]. These cancers include leukemia, lymphoma, multiple myeloma, and other related conditions. HDACis, a form of chemotherapy, have been used in the treatment of hematological cancers. While they have shown promise in improving survival rates, they can also cause significant side effects [13].

One common side effect of HDAC inhibitors in the treatment of hematological cancers is myelosuppression, which is a reduction in the production of blood cells. This can lead to anemia, neutropenia, and thrombocytopenia, which can increase the risk of infections, bleeding, and other complications. Other side effects include fatigue, gastrointestinal symptoms, cardiac toxicity, and neuropathy [13].

As an alternative, natural compounds have been explored as potential therapies for hematological cancers. Some of these compounds have been shown to possess anticancer properties without the toxic side effects associated with traditional agents. For example, curcumin, which is found in turmeric, has been shown to induce apoptosis (cell death) in leukemia and lymphoma cells. Resveratrol, another phytochemical that is found in grapes, has been shown to inhibit the growth of multiple myeloma cells [14].

Other natural compounds that have shown promise in preclinical studies for the treatment of hematological cancers include green tea polyphenols, gingerol, quercetin, and luteolin. While more research is needed to determine the effectiveness of these compounds in humans, they offer a potential avenue for the development of safer and more effective treatments for hematological cancers [15].

It has also been hypothesized that dysregulated epigenetic enzymes and the resulting aberrant epigenetic modifications are intimately connected to tumor development and progression. The comprehensive mechanisms of action, categorization, and association of HDACs with various diseases, such as prostate, breast, and ovarian cancer have been previously studied [12,16]. In breast cancer cells, histone modifications may aid in maintaining genome integrity, DNA repair, transcription, and chromatin modulation [17]. After noticing their presence in a variety of medicines, Hieu et al. [18] created quinazolin-4(3H)-one-based HDACis. Sixteen synthetic compounds were evaluated against HDACs and cancer cells. The most potent HDACis had a half maximal inhibitory concentration (IC_{50}) value of 90 nM, whereas the same molecule had an IC_{50} value of 810 nM against human prostate cancer PC-3 cells. Twelve agents containing hydroxyacetamide and triazole moieties were evaluated against HDACs and MCF-7 cells in a study published by Saha et al. [19]. Some of the designer drugs were hybrids of coumarin and vorinostat and were found to inhibit the expression of the tumor suppressor p53 and increase p21 in prostate and breast cancer models [20].

Epigallocatechin gallate (EGCG), a natural flavonoid found in green tea, has powerful anticancer activities through epigenetic processes, including histone modification [21]. In human colon cancer cell lines, 48 and 72 h treatment with 50 to 150 μM of EGCG was shown to decrease the levels of HDAC1-3 [22]. Notably, HDAC1 expression was less responsive, but EGCG downregulated protein levels of HDAC2 and 3 by more than 50% at a concentration of 100 μM [22]. EGCG (40 μM) and pEGCG (20 μM), a pro-drug of EGCG, significantly suppressed the growth of MDA-MB 231 and MCF-7 breast cancer cells [23].

Apigenin (4′,5,7-trihydroxyflavone) is another flavonoid derived from various natural sources. In PC-3 cells, the flavone was found to function as an HDACi at concentrations of 20–40 μM. Researchers found the treatment of cell lines to result in 41% and 62% suppression of HDAC activity, with the most profound effects seen in HDAC1 and HDAC3.

Furthermore, apigenin promoted acetylation of histone H3 (more than 7-fold) and, less markedly, of H4 globally, while also centering the hyperacetylation of H3 in the p21 WAF1 promoter [24].

Although the impact of epigenetic modification in hematologic malignancies, including leukemia, lymphoma, and multiple myeloma, has been shown, few studies have fully examined the role of HDACis in this context [25,26]. Histone acetylation is an essential mediator of hematopoiesis that is closely tied to malignancy. This review aims to describe the physiologic effects of HDACis and their regulatory role in the development of blood cancers.

2. Classification of HDACs and Inhibitors

The 18 HDACs found in humans are organized into four classes based on their cellular locations, enzyme activity, and similarity to HDACs present in yeast (Table 1). Based on their chemical structures and enzymatic activity, HDACis are often divided into five categories: benzamides, aliphatic acids, cyclic tetrapeptides, hydroximates, and electrophilic ketones. HDACis may target one or more particular HDAC isoforms (HDAC isoform selective inhibitors) or all HDAC isoforms (pan-inhibitors).

Zinc-dependent HDACis have a structure comprised of three domains: (i) a surface recognition unit, or "cap group", (ii) a zinc-binding domain, (iii) a linker domain which connects the previous domains. HDACi selectivity is determined by the cap and linker domains, which participate in the ligand-enzyme interactions; the zinc-binding domain inhibits HDACis activity by binding to the zinc ion. The majority of human HDACs are zinc-dependent metalloenzymes, known individually as HDAC1 through HDAC11. These enzymes use water as a nucleophile to hydrolyze the amide bond [27]. The acyl group is transferred to the C2 position of the ribose sugar by the remaining seven HDACs, referred to as sirtuins (individually as sirtuins 1–7), which use NAD+ as a cofactor. Although members of both enzyme families carry out the identical chemical process of acyllysine cleavage, this discussion will be focused on zinc-dependent HDACs present in classes I, II, and IV (Table 1). HDACis may be categorized into different types based on their chemical structures and cancer specificity (Table 2).

Table 1. Classification of HDACs with their cellular locations and physiological functions.

Class	HDAC	Localization	% Similarity to Human (Nucleic Acid/Amino Acid)	Associated Cancer(s)	Physiological Functions
I	HDAC 1	Nucleus	90.8/99.4	Prostate, gastric, colorectal, pancreas, and esophageal	Cell survival and proliferation
	HDAC 2	Nucleus	91.1/98.6	Colorectal, gastric, cervical dysplasia, and invasive carcinoma	Cell proliferation; insulin resistance
	HDAC 3	Nucleus	92.5/99.6	Lung, prostate, and colon	Cell survival and proliferation
	HDAC 8	Nucleus	90.9/96.3	Poor outcomes in pediatric neuroblastoma	Cell proliferation

Table 1. *Cont.*

Class	HDAC	Localization	% Similarity to Human (Nucleic Acid/Amino Acid)	Associated Cancer(s)	Physiological Functions
IIa	HDAC 4	Nucleus/cytoplasm	86.3/94.2	Breast	Regulation of skeletogenesis and gluconeogenesis
	HDAC 5	Nucleus/cytoplasm	91.1/95.6	Colon, AML, and poor outcomes in lung cancer	Cardiovascular growth and function; gluconeogenesis; cardiac myocyte and endothelial cell function
	HDAC 7	Nucleus/cytoplasm	86.8/90.3	Colon	Thymocyte differentiations; endothelial function; gluconeogenesis; homologous recombination
	HDAC 9	Nucleus/cytoplasm	90.394.8	Medulloblastoma and astrocytoma	Thymocyte differentiation; cardiovascular growth and function
IIb	HDAC 6	Cytoplasm	81.1/78.7	Ovarian and AML	Cell motility; control of cytoskeletal dynamics
	HDAC 10	Cytoplasm	78.1/76.4	Hepatocellular carcinoma	Homologous recombination; autophagy-mediated cell survival
IV	HDAC 11	Nucleus/cytoplasm	87.3/91.9	Breast	Immunomodulators DNA replications
III	SIRT1	Nucleus	Not available	AML, colon, prostate, skin, and BCLL	Aging; redox regulation; cell survival; autoimmune system regulation
	SIRT2	Cytoplasm	Not available	Glioma	Cell survival-cell migration and invasion
	SIRT3	Nucleus/Mitochondria	Not available	Breast, prostate, head and neck, and glioblastoma	Urea cycle; redox balance; ATP regulation; metabolism; apoptosis; cell signaling
	SIRT4	Mitochondria	Not available	Breast	Energy metabolism; ATP regulation; metabolism; apoptosis; cell signaling
	SIRT5	Mitochondria	Not available	Pancreas and breast	Urea cycle; energy metabolism; ATP regulation; metabolism; apoptosis; cell signaling
	SIRT6	Nucleus	Not available	Colon and breast	Metabolism
	SIRT7	Nucleus	Not available	Breast	Apoptosis

Abbreviations: AML, acute myeloid leukemia; ATP, adenosine triphosphate; BCLL, B-cell chronic lymphocytic leukemia; HDAC, histone deacetylase; SIRT, sirtuin.

Table 2. Different classes of HDAC inhibitors with their cancer specificity.

Class	HDACis	Target	Structure	Associated Cancer(s)	References
Hydroxamates	SAHA (vorinostat)	HDAC1-11	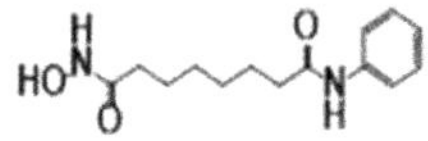	Glioblastoma multiforme and brain metastasis	[28]
	Panobinostat	HDAC1-11	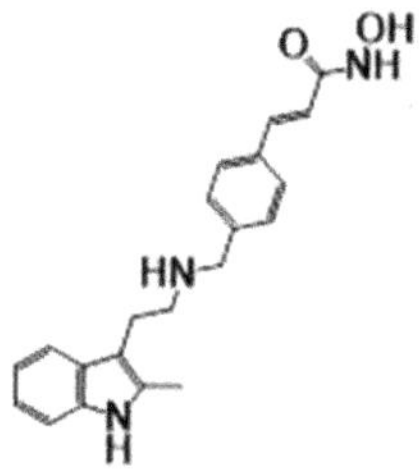	Small cell lung cancer, myelofibrosis, and cutaneous T-cell lymphoma	[29,30]
	Belinostat	HDAC1-11	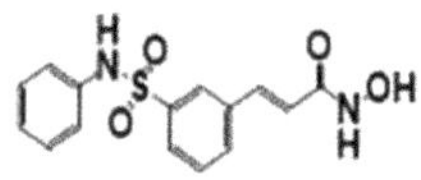	Thymic epithelial tumor and ovarian cancer	[31]
	Trichostatin	HDAC1-11	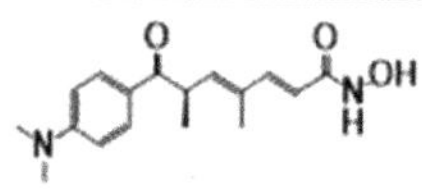	Colon and breast	[32,33]
Aliphatic acids	Pivanex	HDAC1-9	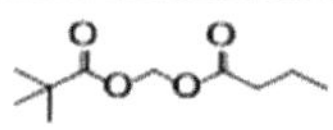	Liver carcinoma, Lung carcinoma and melanoma	[34]
	Valproic acid	HDAC1-9	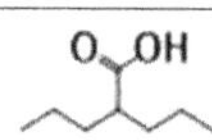	Prostate, breast and melanoma	[35]
Benzamides	Entinostat	HDAC1-3	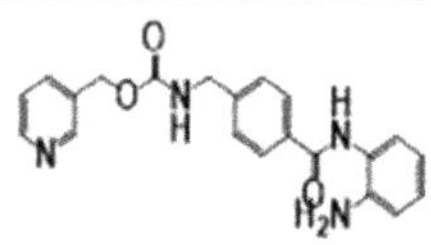	Breast cancer and advanced solid tumors	[36]
Electrophilic ketone	Triflurometհyl Ketones	HDAC4-9	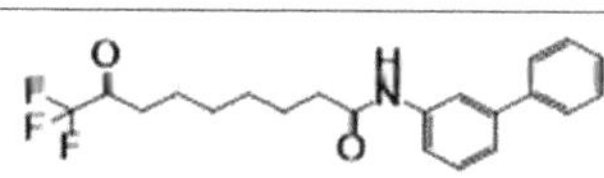	Prostate cancer	[37]
Cyclic tetrapeptides	Romidepsin	HDAC1-2	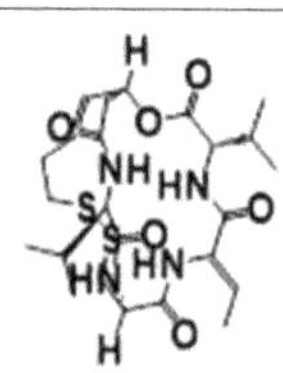	Thyroid, ovarian, pancreatic and breast cancer	[38]
Sirtuin inhibitors	Cambinol	SIRT1	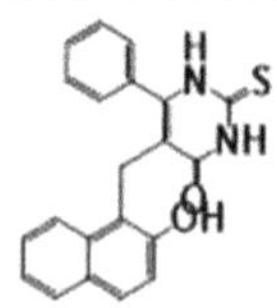	Sarcomas and lymphomas	[39]

Abbreviations: HDAC, histone deacetylase; SAHA, suberoylanilide hydroxamic acid; SIRT, sirtuin.

3. Induction of DNA Damage by HDAC Inhibitors

Bakkenist et al. [40] suggested that the DNA damage response (DDR) can be activated independently of DNA double-strand breaks (DSBs). Their work showed that the activation of ataxia-telangiectasia mutated (ATM) kinase, the first step in the cellular response to ionizing radiation (IR), did not need direct binding to DNA DSB but rather was the consequence of alterations in chromatin structure. Other studies have shown evidence that HDACis may generate significant DNA damage, including DSBs, by increasing reactive oxygen species and oxidative stress and/or variant histone H2AX phosphorylation of serine, gH2AX, which is associated with DSBs (Figure 1) [41]. New studies have also demonstrated that modifications to chromatin may directly or indirectly result in DNA damage. This suggests the mechanisms responsible for chromatin remodeling and DNA damage signaling are intrinsically related [42].

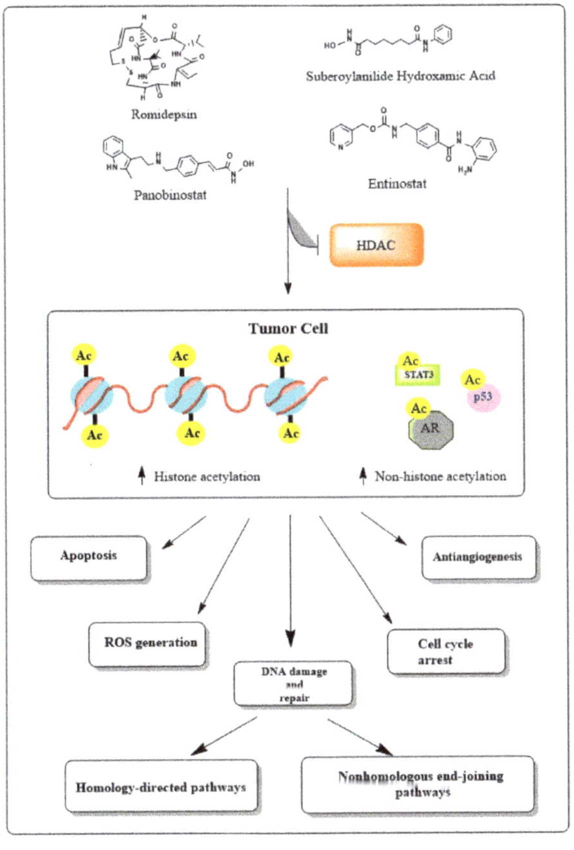

Figure 1. Schematic representation of methods of HDAC inhibition, inducing DNA damage.

Researchers have demonstrated that the application of HDACis to leukemic cells led to the acetylation of histone and prompt production of gH2AX [43]. After 24 h, the acute myeloid leukemia (AML) cell line HL-60 and healthy peripheral blood lymphocytes stimulated with IL-2 (PBL) were exposed to different concentrations of apicidin or TSA. Phosphorylation of H2AX emerged at 3 min, peaked at 30 min, and remained evident at 24 h following TSA (300 nM) treatment in HL-60 cells, but disappeared several hours following treatment in normal PBL. During this transition, acetylation of histone H4 increased on chromatin fibers in both HL-60 and PBL. Myeloid leukemia cell lines K562 and NB4 and primary cells from individuals with AML showed identical outcomes, highlighting the significance of these findings [44–46].

Investigators also found that TSA exposure to HL-60 cells led to enhanced phosphorylation of ATM. After 10 min, phosphorylation was at its highest and gradually decreased over the next 8 h. It is now well-established that induction of apoptosis is a primary mechanism of HDACis anticancer actions in leukemic cells, and all of the HDACis have been found to trigger apoptotic processes [47–53]. It was also observed that, by enhancing histone acetylation, activation of gH2AX and ATM phosphorylation occurred long after the initiation of apoptosis, supported by activation of caspase-3 and also poly(ADP-ribose)polymerase1 (PARP1) in HL-60 cells as early as 4 h after HDACis treatment. However, HDACis still produced early and long-lasting DNA damage, evidenced by gH2AX, when HL-60 and NB4 (AML stage M2 and M3) cells were pretreated with a pan-caspase inhibitor, which effectively blocked endogenous caspase activity [54]. Therefore, it seems that HDACis-dependent induction of DNA damage does not follow apoptosis but rather it occurs before. Moreover, trypan blue exclusion assays revealed that cell death was suppressed in cells pretreated with the caspase inhibitor and then treated with HDACis [55]. All of these studies help to conclude that HDACis selectively induce DNA damage and activate the DDR in neoplastic cells, which in turn leads to apoptotic processes [56].

When compared to other HDACis, such as sodium butyrate or trichostatin A, depsipeptide (FR901228 or FK228) is a stronger inhibitor of class I HDACs. This makes it a potential anticancer drug for both mono- and polytherapy. Depsipeptide exhibits additional biological effects through a variety of modes of action, beyond promoting histone acetylation. Non-histone proteins HSP90 and p53 are acetylated when exposed to depsipeptide. Nucleoside analogues, such as cytarabine and 5-aza-2-deoxycytidine (or 5-aza-CdR), work in tandem with depsipeptide to stimulate transcription and cause apoptosis [57–59].

Apoptosis presumably results from limited repair of DNA damage caused by 5-aza-CdR. In addition, depsipeptide has been shown to be a DNA demethylating agent, an observation that has broadened the scope of its research. The method by which depsipeptide kills human cancer cells may be deduced from these data. Almost all HDACis cause a dramatic upregulation of p21, a protein that causes G1 cell cycle arrest when sufficiently accumulated. It was previously observed that depsipeptide stimulates p21 expression through the elaboration of p53 pathways. Specifically, p53 acetylation at K373/382 may induce p53 trans-activity and expression of p21 in cells treated with depsipeptide. Other HDACis, including TSA, can only promote p53 acetylation in conjunction with nicotinamide (a class III HDACis) or ionizing radiation [60–62].

4. DNA Double-Strand Breaks

In mammalian cells, DSBs are a very harmful form of DNA damage. Due to the loss of duplex integrity, DSBs are more difficult to repair than other kinds of DNA damage and are often lethal for the cell. Ataxia-telangiectasia, a cancer-prone, radiation-sensitive human illness, is caused by pathogenic ATM variants, a protein pivotal role in the activation of cell cycle checkpoints following DSBs. Important for bringing ATM to DSBs, the complex of MRE11-RAD50-NBS1 (MRN) causes ATM to autophosphorylate, changing it from a dimer to a functional monomer. After activation, ATM phosphorylates MRN and subsequent effector proteins to prompt G1/S, intra-S and G2/M cell cycle checkpoints [63]. The activation of these checkpoints improves cell survival and genomic integrity, because it offers more time for DNA damage repair before it may be duplicated or passed on to daughter cells. Emerging data suggests that ATM not only participates in these DSB pathways, but also facilitates repair of DSBs in G0 and G2 cells. There are two major types of mechanisms for repairing DSBs, known as homology-directed repair (HRR) and nonhomologous end-joining (NHEJ) [64].

4.1. Homology-Directed Repair

HRR describes the repair of DSBs associated with replication. Occurring in the S and G2 phases, this repair process uses a template of identical DNA segments obtained from the sister chromatid, a repair pathway often error-free. The first step of HRR is the resection of the DSB using the human MRN complex and CtIP. Then, various accessory proteins, including BRCA2, hRad52, XRCC2, and XRCC3, help recruit hRad51 and assemble it into a nucleoprotein filament. Ultimately, two identical sister chromatids are produced when hRad51 nucleoprotein filaments are recruited and assembled [65].

4.2. Nonhomologous End-Joining

The NHEJ mechanism of DSBs repair begins with a ring-shaped protein complex called the Ku70/Ku86 heterodimer. This complex shields the damaged DNA ends from degradation by binding tightly to them. Following recognition of damaged DNA by the Ku heterodimer, DNA PK and other proteins are recruited. DNA PK undergoes a conformational change to produce active DNA protein kinase (PK), which recruits DNA ligase IV/XRCC4. This ligase completes the repair by connecting the DNA ends. Microhomologies, small complementary sequences present at the break point, are thought to aid in aligning the ends during DNA PK-dependent NHEJ. Larger deletions and chromosomal translocations may be produced by using an alternative form of NHEJ. When compared to DNA PK-mediated NHEJ, the alternative route is characterized by greater deletions and insertions, augmented microhomology regions and more chromosomal translocations. A variety of proteins involved in alternative NHEJ (PARP1, complex MRN, DNA ligase IIIa/XRCC1) are upregulated in malignant cells, though their effects in this context are poorly characterized [66].

5. Downregulation of DSB Repair

The implications of HDACis are greater than that of histone modification alone. Vorinostat (or SAHA) has been demonstrated to upregulate and maintain gH2AX expression in prostate and lung cancer cells by reducing the expression of MRE11 and HRR factor RAD50. In addition to RAD50, vorinostat was reported to reduce the NHEJ proteins Ku70 and Ku80 in melanoma, while NaB has been shown to downregulate Ku80, Ku70, and DNA PK [67]. Additional genes downregulated in AML cells by HDACis MS275 and LAQ824 include RAD50, BRCA1, CHK2, EXO1, and Ku80. Researchers started by looking at the genes involved in DNA repair and found that RAD51, BLM, CHK1, and BRCA1 were all downregulated in prostate cancer cells following SAHA and valproic acid treatment. Immunofluorescence analysis of DSB repair efficiency indicated that not only the expression of RAD51 and BRCA1 decreased, but also the correct targeting of the DNA repairing points was affected. In accordance, it was observed higher DNA damage, determined by the comet test and the development of gH2AX sites, and a reduction in DSB repair efficiency. E2F transcription factor 1 (E2F1), an established activator of CHK1, RAD51 and BRCA1 gene expression, was also found to be suppressed by HDACis. Researchers utilized chromatin immunoprecipitation experiments to verify that E2F1 recruitment to the promoters of CHK1, RAD51, and BRCA1 was compromised in the presence of HDACis [68].

6. Phenomenon of Chromatin Remodeling

Chromatin remodeling has been implicated in DNA damage repair by many independent trials. After DSBs are induced, gH2AX is activated and localized to the damaged sites. gH2AX stimulates the recruitment of MDC1 to DNA DSBs, which attaches ATM to the chromatin by means of NBS1 activation. The MRN complex aids in preparing the damaged sites to repair, whereas CK2 phosphorylation of MDC1 coordinates subsequent modifications to chromatin. When gH2AX is modified, MDC1 triggers the recruitment of the NuA4 complex, which includes the HIV1 HAT Tat interacting protein 60 kDa (TIP60-p400). TIP60, a HAT, acetylates histones H2A and H4K16, which loosens the chromatin and makes it easier for DNA repair proteins to reach sites of DNA damage [69].

Sharma et al. [70] demonstrated that the development of IR-induced gH2Ax is reliant on MOF activity, but its removal is under the control of TIP60. Application of HAT inhibitor anacardic acid to IR-treated lung cancer cells resulted in a reduced recruitment of Ku70 and Ku80 NHEJ proteins, presumably due to silencing or suppression of P300/CBP. The significance of chromatin relaxation in the DNA repair response is further emphasized by the fact that the SWI/SNF chromatin remodeling complex, which is known to enhance NHEJ through the local relaxing of chromatin, is not recruited after treatment with a HAT inhibitor [71].

7. Hematological Cancers

Hematological cancers are those that affect the blood, bone marrow, and lymph nodes. Depending on the kind of cell of origin, they are designated as leukemia, lymphoma, or myeloma (Figure 2). The immune system interconnects these three forms of cancer, and a sickness that affects one often impacts the others [72].

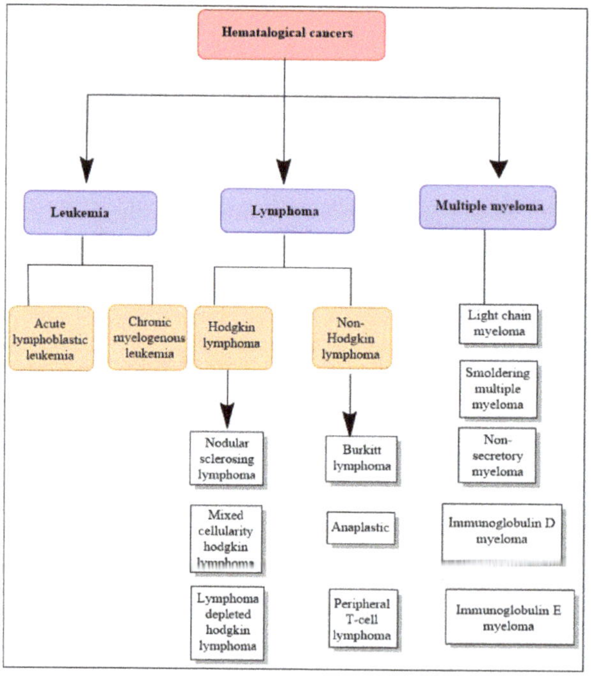

Figure 2. Schematic representation of the diversity of hematological cancers, with interrelated types and their subtypes displayed.

8. Role of HDAC Inhibitors in Hematological Cancers

8.1. Acute Myeloid Leukemia

AML is a clonal illness defined by the accumulation of poorly differentiated (immature) myeloid cells in the peripheral blood and bone marrow due to uncontrolled replication. AML is a type of adult acute leukemia, the most prevalent, showing a median age of onset of 70 years. Although survival metrics have increased in recent years, additional pharmacological options are needed to improve long-term survival rates. Survival is substantially worse in older patients, which is compounded by AML's late age of onset [73].

Despite substantial progress in our understanding of the genetics surrounding its pathogenesis, treatment of AML has remained relatively consistent for the last four decades and consists of conventional chemotherapy and allogeneic hematopoietic stem cell transplantation. In recent years, the United States Food and Drug Administration (FDA) has approved novel medications for AML, including ivosidenib, ozogamicin, gemtuzumab, venetoclax, enasidenib, glasdegib, midostaurin, and glitertinib, summarized in Table 3.

Table 3. Various HDAC inhibitors as drugs used for the treatment of AML and their mechanisms of action.

Classifications	Drug Name	Role in Treatment of AML	References
Hydroximates	Trichostatin A	Inhibits the pathway for DNA repair (NHEJ). Acetylation of repair factors and trapping of PARP1 at DNA double-strand brakes in chromatin, inducing leukemic toxicity. Possible synergistic effect of TSA with an inhibitor of PARP1.	[32,33]
	Vorinostat	Apoptosis and inhibition of cell growth. Increases differentiation induced by retinoic acid in acute promyelocytic leukemia cells. Induction of double-strand breaks and oxidative DNA damage.	[28]
	Panobinostat	Promotes apoptosis and inhibition of cell growth.	[29,30]
	Belinostat	Promotes cell cycle arrest, inhibits cell proliferation, and induces apoptosis.	[31]
Benzamides	Entinostat	Induces growth arrest and apoptosis. Downregulates antiapoptotic molecules BCL-2 and MCL-1, increases p21, and induces acetylation of H3.	[36]
Cyclic peptides	Romidepsin	Promotes apoptosis of chemo-resistant malignant cells and reversed their gene expression profile.	[38]
	Apicidin	Induces selective changes in P21WAF1/Cip1 and gelsolin gene expression, which control cell cycle and cell morphology.	[38]
Aliphatic acids	Valproic acid	Induces differentiation and inhibits proliferation and apoptosis of AML cells. No clinical effect when used as a single-agent therapy for AML. Synergistic effects with ATRA, decitabine, gemtuzumab ozogamicin, curcumin, hydroxyurea, 6-mercaptopurine, dasatinib, bortezomib, cytarabine	[35]

Abbreviations: AML, acute myeloid leukemia; BCL-2, B-cell leukemia/lymphoma 2 protein; MCL-1, myeloid cell leukemia-1; NHEJ, nonhomologous end-joining; PARP1, poly (ADP-ribose) polymerase 1; TSA, trichostatin.

Historically, AML was believed to be a hereditary illness; however, a number of studies have been reinforcing the contribution of epigenetic alterations in the disease. DNA methylation and histone modification are well-studied epigenetic changes linked with chromatin structure and gene expression. Epigenetic regulatory enzymes responsible for DNA and histone modifications are implicated in the pathogenesis of hematological malignancies. In fact, most of these enzymes have been proven to be unregulated or otherwise altered in many malignancies, especially in AML [74]. Encouraged by the findings that epigenetic alterations can be reversed, epigenetic medicines have attracted great interest in the development of AML therapies [75]. HDACis promote histone acetylation, which leads to the expression of repressed genes and ultimately triggers differentiation, apoptosis, cell cycle arrest and cancer cell death through epigenetic or non-epigenetic means [76]. These results are especially promising in patients unsuitable for intense chemotherapy. Unfortunately, additional research is required before HDACis may be used as monotherapeutic agents against AML. In clinical studies, however, combination tactics with a range of anticancer medications are demonstrating strong antileukemic activity by augmenting the efficacy of traditional AML pharmacons [77]. Various mechanisms of action of HDACis in hematological cancers are depicted in Figure 3, and the HDACis landscape as it pertains to AML is summarized below.

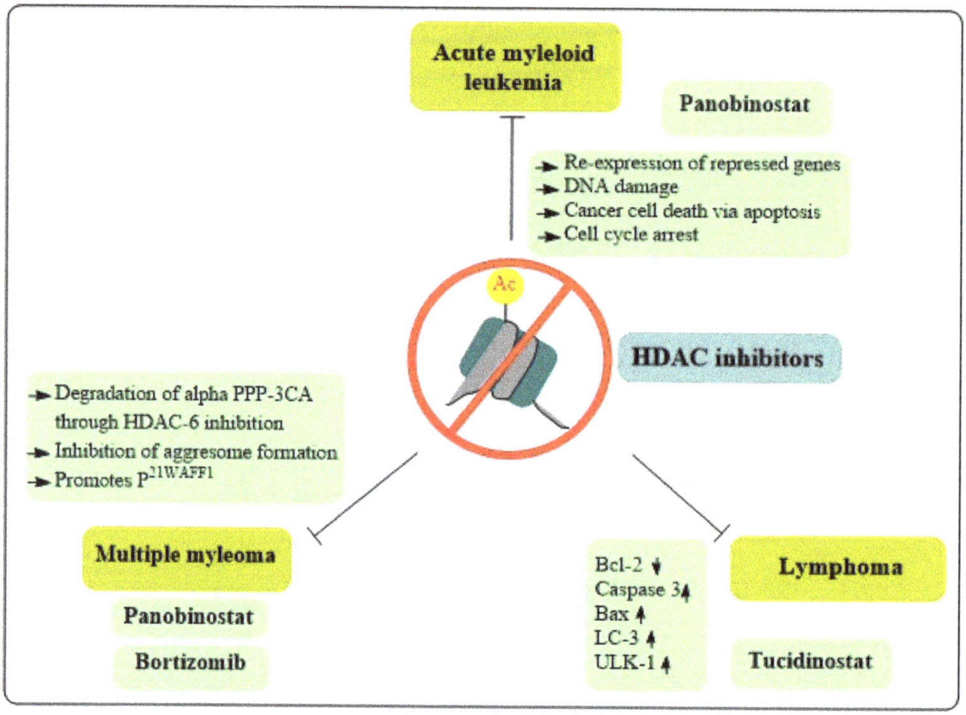

Figure 3. A summary of various mechanisms of action utilized by HDAC inhibitors in hematological cancers: disrupting tumor cell proliferation and survival through multiple mechanisms, including inducing DNA damage and affecting cell cycle progression.

In a study utilizing AML cells, researchers observed the effects of the new HDACi panobinostat (LBH589) in conjunction with doxorubicin [78] All AML cell lines studied, and patient-derived AML primary cells, showed a strong response to panobinostat (IC_{50} 20 nM). Panobinostat also enhanced the efficacy of doxorubicin and other first-line treatments for AML. Gene expression profiling analysis revealed that the application of panobinostat plus doxorubicin had a unique effect on the expression of 588 genes. Specifically, combination treatment upregulated Bax, and, most notably, Bad, which led to caspase-dependent apoptosis in AML cells via mitochondrial outer membrane permeabilization and cytochrome c translocation. The drug combination strongly activated a DNA damage response, suggesting it may generate DSBs and cause cell death. Continued research is important to optimize the pharmacological potential of panobinostat, alone or in conjunction with doxorubicin against AML [79]. Other reports implicated the interference with HSP90's chaperone function in panobinostat's antileukemia activity. C-X-C-chemokine receptor type 4 (CXCR4) is a receptor for stromal cell-derived factor 1, and a marker of poor prognosis when found in excess in leukemic cells. CXCR4 is also a client protein of HSP90. Application of panobinostat to AML cells was determined to induce HSP90 acetylation and diminish CXCR4 levels, possibly by inhibiting CXCR4-HSP90 interaction. Panobinostat was also found to be therapeutic in the treatment of mice harboring t(8;21) translocations via proteasomal degradation of AML1-ETO9a, the spliced variant of the t(8;21)-generated fusion protein known to induce leukemia [80].

8.2. Lymphomas

Lymphoma describes several forms of blood cancer with similar symptoms to leukemia, but with distinct etiology. Leukemia develops in the bone marrow and other blood-forming tissues, while lymphoma begins in the lymphatic system. The lymphatic system, which includes the bone marrow, spleen and lymph nodes, is a part of the immune system that assists in the defense against infection [81].

The two most common subtypes of lymphoma are Hodgkin's (HL) and non-Hodgkin's (NHL). The first is considered to be the more aggressive form and is defined histologically by large B-cells with "owl's eyes" called Reed-Sternberg cells. NHL is up to nine times more common and has over 60 variants. Two groups of NHL are considered: B-cell lymphomas and natural killer/T-cell lymphomas. Also important for therapeutic management is to categorize NHL because some forms are more aggressive [82].

HDACis may play a therapeutic role in manipulating epigenetic and non-epigenetic events involved in lymphomagenesis, including the regulation of cytokines. Cutaneous T-cell lymphoma (CTCL), a subtype of NHL, is characterized by a high affinity IL-2 receptor in up to 30% of patients which may be compromised by HDACis. Additionally, HDAC1 and HDAC6 overexpression has been observed in CTCL, which results in increased production of IL-15—a critical mediator of inflammation in CTCL [83,84].

Peripheral T-cell lymphoma, another NHL subtype, was shown to be responsive to Tucidinostat, an HDACis which causes cell death in malignant cells by downregulating Bcl-2 and upregulating caspase-3 and Bax. HDACis were identified to influence the expression of key genes in CTCL cells. The Ras Homolog Family Member B (RhoB) is a tumor suppressor gene associated with different cancers. The combination of HDACi with conventional chemotherapy such as romidepsin, plus azacytidine, a demethylating agent, induces RhoB and apoptotic death, providing an effective treatment option for peripheral T-cell lymphoma [85].

T-cell malignancies are dysfunctional due to another self-consuming mechanism akin to apoptosis. In addition to deacetylating lysine residues on histones, HDACs regulate a range of cytosolic proteins with diverse biological roles, including autophagy. Vorinostat, a pan-HDACi, upregulated the autophagic factor LC3, blocking the mammalian target of rapamycin (mTOR), resulting in the initiation of the canonical route of autophagosome formation by ULK1 [86]. HDACis and associated autophagy are mandatory for cellular survival, therefore the use of HDACis seems to be a logical therapy for T-cell lymphomas. The primary action of HDACis may be to interfere with histone and chromatin remodeling, although acetylation of histone and other proteins can also induce DNA modifications, alter the expression of oncogenes or disregulate apoptosis and autophagy responses. Because these processes are potential targets in T-cell malignancies, they underline the importance of HDACis in cancer development and prognosis [87].

Cambinol is an inhibitor of the NAD-dependent deacetylase activity of human SIRT1 and SIRT2 and exhibited activity against Burkitt lymphoma. During genotoxic stress, cambinol inhibits SIRT1 activity, resulting in hyperacetylation of critical stress response proteins and encouraging cell cycle arrest. Hyperacetylation of B-cell lymphoma 6 (BCL6) and p53 accompanied apoptosis in BCL6-positive Burkitt lymphoma cells treated with cambinol alone. Cambinol's anticancer action in Burkitt lymphoma might be achieved by a combination of BCL6 inactivation and checkpoint activation since acetylation inactivates BCL6 and promotes p53 and additional checkpoint signaling pathways. Moreover, cambinol decreased the development of model Burkitt lymphoma xenografts and was well tolerated by mice [88]. Other small molecule inhibitors sirtinol and M15, structural analogues of substituted β-naphthols, were discovered using high-throughput phenotypic screening in yeast [89]. Sirtinol was found to silence yeast Sir2 in vitro and in vivo, as well as human SIRT2 in vitro, but not HDAC1. Splitomicin, a compound structurally related to sirtinol, was discovered by a chemical screen of yeast cells and was found to inhibit the Sir2 deacetylase activity [90]. The deacetylation of key regulatory proteins BCL6 and p53 by NAD-dependent HDACs like SIRT1 has been linked to cell adaptations to cancer and stress.

8.3. Multiple Myeloma

Multiple myeloma (MM) is a hematological malignancy characterized by monoclonal plasma cells, most frequently producing IgG or IgA. Of the 1,278,362 new cases of leukemia, lymphoma, and MM in 2020 globally, 176,404 (14%) were MM. Greater rates of incidence and mortality were associated with higher levels of human development, income, frequency of inactivity, excess body weight, obesity, and diabetes. Global trends point towards an increase in MM incidence on a global level. Those at highest risk include men and individuals 50 years and older. Fortunately, mortality attributable to MM is decreasing, especially in women. Still, treatment availability and options should be improved to address the increasing incidence of multiple myeloma [91]. Autologous stem cell transplantation and innovative therapies, such as bortezomib (a proteasome inhibitor) and immunomodulatory medicines (lenalidomide, pomalidomide, thalidomide), have augmented the survival of MM patients. Numerous instances of relapsed myeloma have been documented, necessitating the development of novel medicines to treat these patients [92].

Multiple preclinical studies have shown the effectiveness of HDACis in the treatment of MM. The HDACis vorinostat promotes p21WAF1 in myeloma cells by altering the methylation and acetylation of core histones, and by reducing DNase I enzyme accessibility in promoter regions. By suppressing interleukin-6 release from MM-bound bone marrow stromal cells, vorinostat was also able to overturn cell adhesion-mediated drug resistance [93]. Additionally, MM cells pretreated with bortezomib were more susceptible to the apoptosis and mitochondrial dysfunction caused by vorinostat. Indeed, this combination was effective against MM cells resistant to both dexamethasone and doxorubicin [93].

The proteosome regulates the cell proteome clearing cytotoxic ubiquitinated proteins not correctly folded. MM cells generate an abundance of proteins, including immunoglobulins, and some misfolded/unfolded proteins, which impair cell functioning [94]. Relying on the proteasomal removal of harmful proteins, malignant cells are more vulnerable to mechanisms of proteasomal inhibition compared to healthy cells. When amounts of ubiquitinated misfolded/unfolded proteins exceed the proteasome's destruction capabilities, these proteins collect aggresomes form. Aggresomes are microtubule-based pericentriolar structures, often generated in response to the excess of misfolded/unfolded proteins. The transport of aggresomes and capture of cytotoxic proteins is mediated by HDAC6. Therefore, inhibition of HDAC6 can hinder cells from properly forming aggresomes and prevent them from eliminating protein aggregates [95]. Bortezomib is a known inhibitor of the proteasomal chymotrypsin activity. Normally, bortezomib treatment stimulates aggresome development in MM cells. When combined with panobinostat, another pan-HDAC inhibitor, the treatment promoted apoptosis via a synergistic mechanism by preventing protein degradation. This may partially explain the synergistic effect of bortezomib and panobinostat in multiple myeloma patients [96].

The protein phosphatase 3 or calcineurin is another target of panobinostat. It is a calcium-dependent serine/threonine protein phosphatase and panobinostat induces degradation of its catalytic subunit α (PPP3CA). The phosphatase dephosphorylates NFATc1 and the subsequent translocation of cytoplasmatic NFATc1 to the nucleus is critical for the activation of T-cells [97]. Cyclosporine A and FK506, are commonly used immunosuppressives that function by blocking PPP3CA and calcineurin B. Calcineurin activation has been demonstrated to contribute to the maintenance of T-cell acute lymphoblastic leukemia in a mouse model. B-cell functionality is also linked to calcineurin activity. One study determined that CD138+ cells obtained from patients with advanced MM contained high levels of PPP3CA. This finding suggests a relationship between MM pathogenesis and PPP3CA (Figure 4). Interestingly, PPP3CA acted as a client protein of HSP90 in MM cells [98].

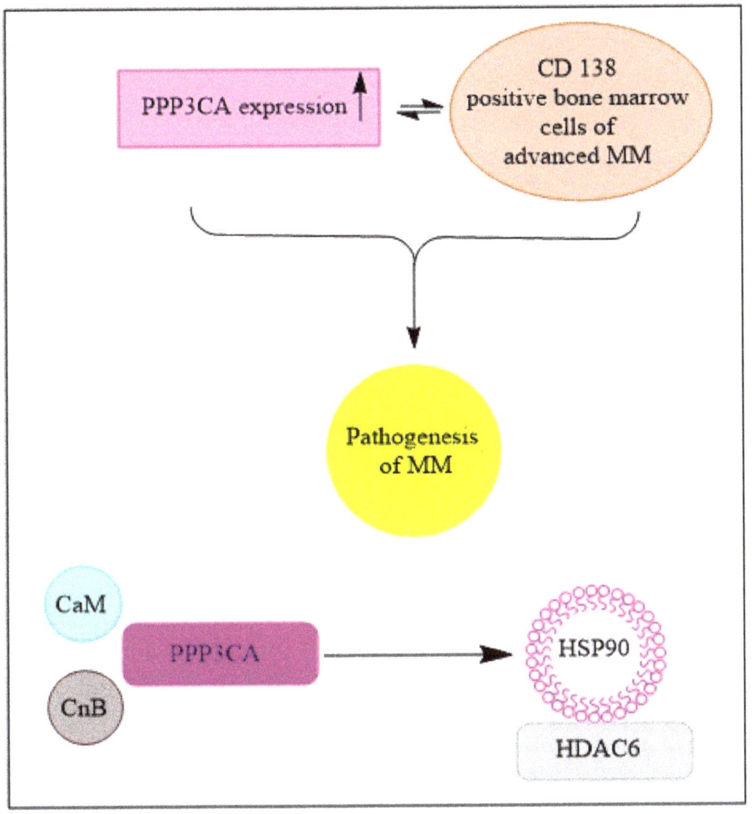

Figure 4. Schematic diagram indicating relationship of PPP3CA and pathogenesis of multiple myeloma before treatment.

Ricolinostat (or ACY-1215) is an orally active hydroxamate and was the first selective inhibitor of HDAC6 in clinical trials [98]. Therapy with ricolinostat prompted the destruction of PPP3CA by dissociation with HSP90, indicating panobinostat may reduce levels of PPP3CA by abolishing HSP90's chaperone function. Moreover, PPP3CA was vital for MM cell growth. While no changes in PPP3CA levels were observed following FK506 treatment, application of this compound with panobinostat did result in the reduction of PPP3CA levels, as well as growth inhibition in preclinical trials. Cotreatment is believed to result in PPP3CA loss via interference with calcineurin B function, which is usually responsible for its protection [99].

A combination of panobinostat with dexamethasone and bortezomib seemed efficacious in patients harboring bortezomib-resistant disease (Figure 5). A review of many patients with MM showed that those with bortezomib-resistant disease had very high levels of PPP3CA. In practice, bortezomib caused inhibition of HDAC6 and reduced expression of PPP3CA. Furthermore, combination therapy with panobinostat plus bortezomib synergistically reduced the viability of MM cells. So, both panobinostat and bortezomib target PPP3CA and the antimyeloma effects of their combination may result from the synergistic PPP3CA reduction, besides aggresome inhibition by bortezomib [98]. Ricolinostat also demonstrated reasonable effectiveness against relapsed MM combined with dexamethasone and lenalidomide proteasome inhibitor [98].

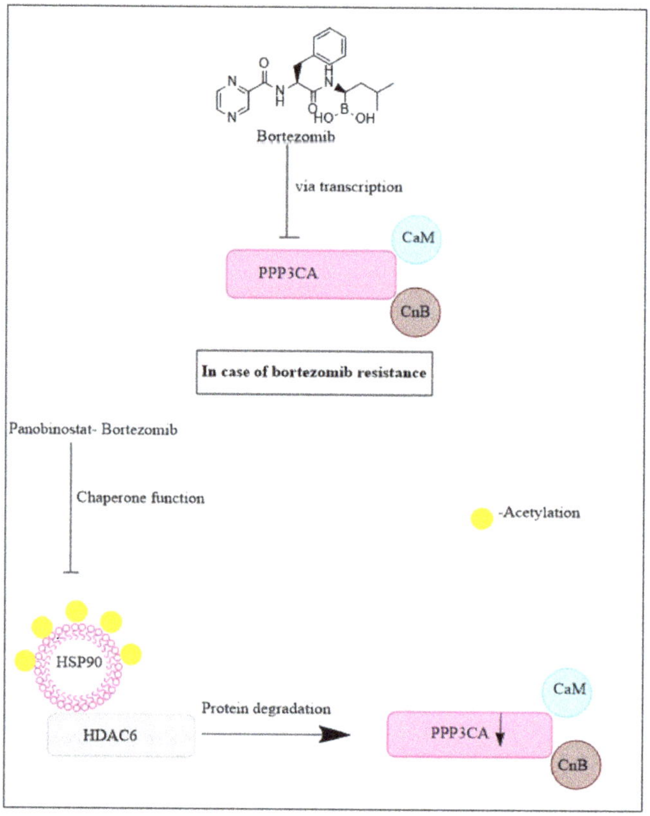

Figure 5. Schematic diagram of mechanism of action of panobinostat and bortezomib against multiple myeloma.

9. Development of HDAC Inhibitors for Hematological Cancer Treatment

All approved HDACis are presently being tested in clinical trials for the treatment of additional cancer settings, alone or combined in adjuvant regimens. Numerous advancements have been achieved in the treatment of solid neoplasms, such as brain and pulmonary cancers, as well as hematological malignancies like AML and B-cell lymphoma. Vorinostat is the subject of nearly 60 active clinical trials, including three phase 3 trials evaluating drug combinations in glioma (NCT01236560), multiple myeloma (NCT01554852), and acute lymphoblastic leukemia and lymphoma (NCT01312818). Tucidinostat could be found in more than 50 studies at ClinicalTrials.gov with various hematological malignancies. Panobinostat is the subject of over 20 trials, including one phase 3 trial aiming at the treatment of AML and myelodysplastic syndromes [99].

Researchers have discovered 22 HDACis that entered clinical trials against different cancers (Table 4). The hydroxamate family is the more represented (11 compounds), but diverse non-hydroxamate drugs are also investigated. Most of these medicines are now being evaluated for hematological cancers, although their effectiveness and safety profiles differ. The creation of isozyme-selective inhibitors is one of the most intriguing areas of research. In the phase 1b study with Epstein–Barr virus (EBV)-associated lymphomas, the HDAC9-selective medication nanatinostat showed promising results, with an overall response rate of 53% and 29% of patients achieving a complete response. In this trial, HDACis appear to work by sensitizing EBV-positive lymphoma cells to nucleoside antiviral drugs like ganciclovir [100].

Table 4. HDAC inhibitors of hydroxamate and non-hydroxamate families in different clinical trials.

Hydroxamate Family			Non-Hydroxamate Family		
Drug Name	**Investigated Malignancy**	**Clinical Trial Phase**	**Drug Name**	**Investigated Malignancy**	**Clinical Trial Phase**
Abexinostat	Skin cancers, non-small lung cancer, mantle cell lymphoma, acute myeloid leukemia	Phase-3	Tacedinaline	Solid and hematological cancers	Phase 3
Fimepinostat	lymphomas, brain tumors	Phase1/2	Entinostat	Gynecological cancers, CNS tumors, pancreatic cancer, non-small lung cancer	Phase 2
Quisinostat	JNJ26481585 ovarian cancer, non-small lung cancer	Phase 2	Domatinostat	Cutaneous T-cell lymphoma	Phase1
Ricolinostat	ACY-1215 lymphomas, Breast cancer, gynecological cancers	Phase 2	Givinostat	Polycythemia vera	Phase 2
Trichostatin A	Hematological cancers	Phase 1	KA2507	Melanoma	Phase 1
Nanatinostat	VRx-3996, EBV-associated cancers	Phase 1	Mocetinostat	Leiomyosarcoma and melanoma	Phase 2
CG200745	Myelodysplastic syndrome, pancreatic cancer	Phase1/2	OBP-801	Lung cancer	Phase 1a
Pracinostat	Prostate cancer, sarcoma, myelofibrosis, myelodysplastic syndrome	Phase 3	AR-42	Sarcoma and meningioma	Phase1
Resminostat	Pancreatic cancer, non-small lung cancer, colorectal carcinoma, Hodgkin's lymphoma	Phase 2	Pivanex	Melanoma and lymphoblastic leukemia	Phase 2
CUDC-101	Advanced solid tumors	Phase 1	Givinostat	Polycythemia vera	Phase 2
MPT0E028	Advanced solid tumors	Phase 1			

Abbreviations: CNS, central nervous system; EBV, Epstein-Barr virus.

10. Natural Products as HDAC Inhibitors in Hematological Malignancies

10.1. Pure Compounds

10.1.1. Berberine

Berberine (Figure 6), an isoquinoline alkaloid isolated from the plant *Berberis aristata*, has been studied in depth for its anticancer effects in various malignancies [101–103]. Berberine was also demonstrated to hinder cancer spread by inhibiting transferase activity. It has been hypothesized that berberine acts by inhibiting HDAC proteins [102]. Initially, molecular docking investigations were conducted using Glide (Schrodinger) and Sitemap (Schrodinger) was used to forecast the live website. The ligands of berberine exhibited a strong affinity for the HDAC family (PDB IDs 2VQM, 3C10, 3C5K, 3SFF, 3MAX, 4A69, and 4BKX). Recent research indicates the probable molecular target of berberine utilizing the Connectivity Map (CMap) database and a gene expression signature-based method. It is hypothesized that berberine might inhibit protein synthesis, HDACs, and Akt/mTOR pathways, which was highly correlated with in silico predictions (Table 5) [103]. Despite preliminary findings, there is currently no reliable evidence of berberine's underlying molecular mechanism for tumor targeting [103].

10.1.2. Chrysin

The flavonoid chrysin (Figure 6) occurs in propolis, *Oroxylum indicum* and *Pelargonium crispum*, and has shown potential antitumor action against melanoma and leukemia [104,105]. Research suggests chrysin acts as an epigenetic modulator by inhibiting specific HDACs. Chrysin, at a concentration of 40 μM, inhibited HDAC8 activity, and also decreased the protein levels of HDAC8 and HDAC2 in vitro. Chrysin was tested on

HDAC1-11 and found to selectively inhibit these two isoenzymes as well. Based on the EC_{50} values, chrysin is a more potent inhibitor of HDAC8 than of HDAC2 (40.2 μM versus 129.0 μM). Chrysin has also demonstrated anticancer action against blood malignancies. Chrysin's antiproliferative action on leukemic cells followed a concentration-dependent pattern. Chrysin caused apoptosis through the mitochondrial route in peripheral blood cells isolated from patients with chronic lymphocytic leukemia. Importantly, fibroblasts and epithelial cells were resistant to the cytotoxicity generated by chrysin [106,107].

10.1.3. Cowaxanthone and Cowain

Garcinia fusca Pierre, also known as "Madan-Paa" or "Mak-Mong", is a member of the Clusiaceae family and native to northeastern Thailand and other southeast Asian nations. Traditional applications of *G. fusca* include uses for blood circulation enhancement, as an expectorant, or as therapy for coughs, indigestion, constipation, and pyrexia [108]. Two active chemicals isolated from *G. fusca* have been evaluated for their therapeutic potential in the context of hematological malignancies. Cowaxanthone (Figure 6), one of the xanthone families derived from *G. fusca*, displayed anticancer properties by inducing apoptosis in leukemic T-cells via downregulation of HDACs activity [109]. However, cowaxanthone was less hazardous to normal Vero cells. Cowanin (Figure 6) is a xanthone isolated from the stem bark of *G. fusca*. Cowanin has been shown to inhibit the growth of a variety of cancer cells, including those derived from lung, breast, oral, and liver cancers, in addition to leukemic HPB-ALL cells [109]. Moreover, cowanin has been purported to suppress the Notch signaling system, which is characteristically overactive in hematologic cancers. Cowanin's activity as an HDACis is supported by its stimulation of cancer cell death in Jurkat cells (human T-cell lymphoma) via apoptosis and autophagy [110]. Thus, cowanin shows promise as an anticancer drug, and its mechanism merits further study.

10.1.4. Curcumin

Curcumin (diferuloylmethane, Figure 6), a lipid-soluble polyphenol derived from the *Curcuma longa* rhizome, is possibly one of the most studied natural anticancer agents [111,112]. The chemo preventive activity of curcumin, in part, is due to its role in epigenetics. In leukemic cells, curcumin inhibits HDAC4 and HDAC6 [113]. Moreover, it increased histone acetylation at the promoter of the gene of the proapoptotic protein Bax, in association with activity inhibition and decreased expression of different HDACs. Despite these findings and its proven applications in other cancer models, curcumin has been understudied in the context of hematological malignancies.

10.1.5. Cyclostellettamines

Cyclostellettamines are pyridine alkaloids that have been isolated from marine sponges (e.g., genus *Stelletta* and *Xestospongia*). Figure 6 presents the structures of cyclostellettamines A and G, as well as dehydrocyclostellettamines D and E. The ability of these compounds to inhibit the histone deacetylase activity was tested with K562 cell preparations and IC_{50} values were measured in the interval of 17–80 μM [114]. When tested against leukemia cells, these compounds exerted moderate cytotoxic effects [115].

10.1.6. Ginsenoside 20(s)-Rh2

Ginseng, an herbal medicinal from the genus *Panax*, has numerous pharmacological activities. Ginsenosides are triterpene saponins, regarded as the primary active components present in the roots and rhizomes of various *Panax* plants [116]. Specifically, ginsenosides have displayed anticancer, anti-inflammatory, antioxidative, and vasorelaxant properties [117]. Among the diversity of ginsenosides, 20(s)-Rh2 (Figure 6) was demonstrated to induce cell cycle arrest and apoptosis of a variety of human cancer cells. Recent research demonstrates that 20(s)-Rh2 can improve the response of human leukemia cells to conventional therapies and reduce cell proliferation. Researchers postulate these results to be due to upregulation of mitochondria-mediated apoptosis, as well as immunomodulatory effects [117].

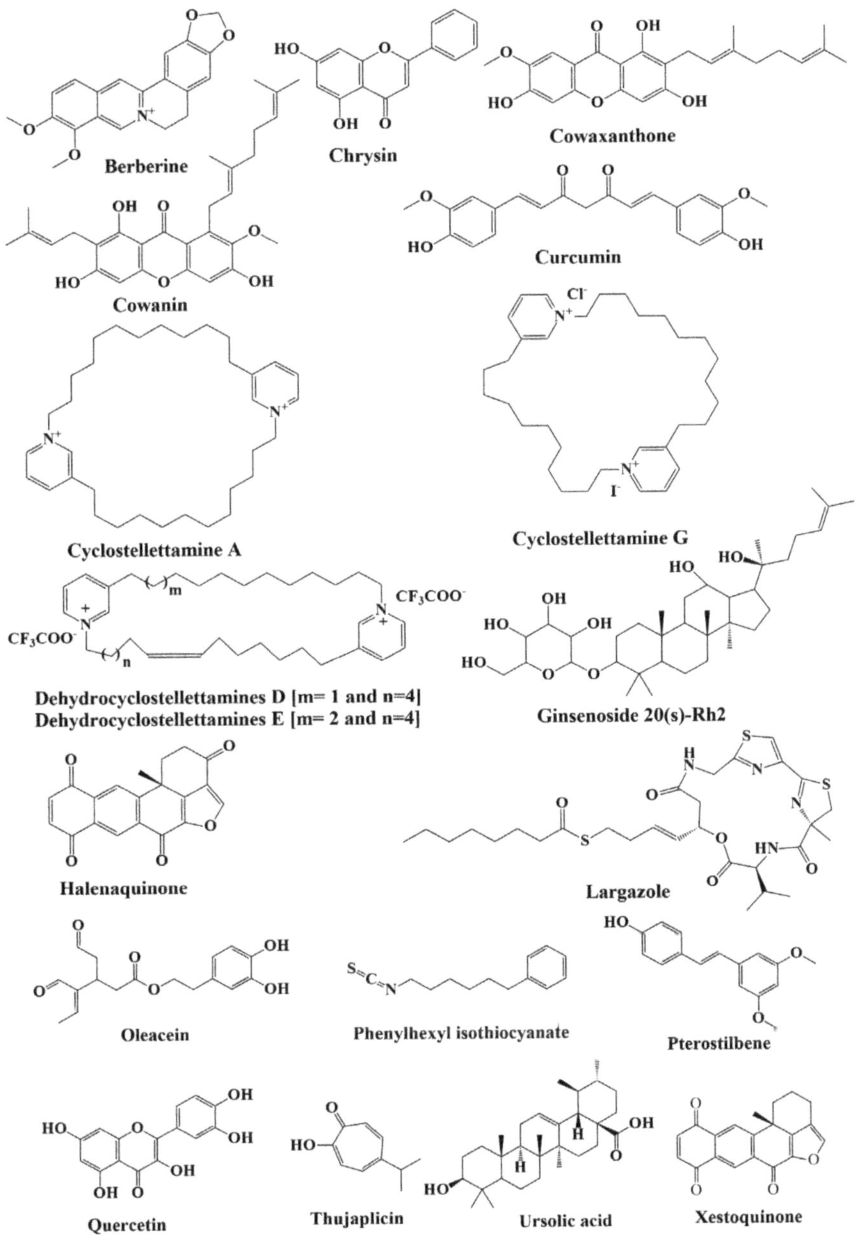

Figure 6. Chemical structure of natural compounds acting as HDAC inhibitors for hematological cancers.

Chen et al. [118] examined the 20(s)-Rh2 actions in K562 and KG-1a cultured cells using immunoblotting to determine levels of protein expression. In association with cell cycle arrest (G0/G1 phase) and apoptosis, the ginsenoside reduced proliferation-related proteins (Bcl-2, ERK, cyclin D1, and p-ERK), and augmented pro-apoptotic factors (activated caspase-3, Bax, JNK and p-JNK, p38 and p-p38). Moreover, 20(s)-Rh2 inhibited HDAC1, 2 and 6, while increasing the acetylation of histone H3 and HAT activity. In summary, 20(s)-Rh2 slowed the proliferation of leukemia cell models while modulating HDACs activity, histone acetylation, and critical cell fate proteins. These effects have been validated in a follow-up in vivo study utilizing naked mice carrying K562. The authors found that rodents treated with 20(s)-Rh2 had smaller xenografted tumors.

10.1.7. Halenaquinones

Halenaquinone (Figure 6), a polycyclic quinone-type metabolite produced by *Xestospongia vansoesti* and *Paracheilinus alfiani*, has been shown to inhibit pan-HDACs and DNA replication via suppression of topoisomerase II production. Anticancer effects of halenaquinone have been observed against Molt-4 leukemia cells, in which experimental results showed reduced cell viability and induction of apoptosis following ROS-induced mitochondrial dysfunction [119]. Researchers attribute these findings to upregulation of Bax, cytochrome c and hexokinase I release, and activation of caspases, with concomitant downregulation of Bid, Bcl-2, cytosolic hexokinase II, p-Akt, tensin homolog, phosphatase, phosphoinositide-dependent kinase-1, and glycogen synthase kinase-3β. Notably, halenaquinone showed a strong in vivo antileukemic impact in mouse xenograft experiments, decreasing the tumor mass and volume without altering the overall body mass of the mice [120].

10.1.8. Largazole

The cyclic depsipeptide largazole (Figure 6) was extracted from Key Largo (Florida) marine cyanobacterium of the genus Symploca in 2008 [121]. The synthesis of largazole and its C7-substituted analogues (4c-d), and the evaluation of these compounds in NB4 leukemia cells, was reported by Souto et al. [121]. The largazole analogues inhibited HDAC1 and 4 recombinant enzymes, which are models of class I and class II HDACs. These compounds were found to possess nanomolar potency against HDAC1. In addition, they exhibited potent apoptosis-inducing action in the NB4 cells, whereas were incapable of inducing their differentiation into mature granulocytes. After treating the leukemia cells with the compounds, increased levels of acetylated tubulin and $p21^{WAF1/CIP1}$ were observed, besides higher global acetylation of H3.

10.1.9. Oleacein

The secoiridoid oleacein (Figure 6) is a polyphenol richly present in *Olea europaea* (common olive). This compound was demonstrated to modulate cancer cells through alterations in proliferation, apoptosis, and differentiation in several different models, including colon, breast, prostate, and skin cancers. Reports indicate that oleacein regulates epigenetic mechanisms in diverse myeloma cell models, namely NCI-H929, RPMI-8226, U266, MM1s, and JJN3. Showing micromolar IC_{50} values, oleacein diminished the viability of myeloma cells in 48-h incubations [122].

Safety assays of oleacein with healthy human peripheral blood mononuclear cells (PBMC) revealed no toxicity. Unlike the positive controls, TSA and SAHA, oleacein had no effect on the HDAC activity of JJN3 nuclear extracts. However, it downregulated the expression of several HDACs and increased histone and tubulin acetylation, without changes in the global DNA methylome [123].

10.1.10. Phenylhexyl Isothiocyanate

Isothiocyanates found in plants and synthesized phenylhexyl isothiocyanate (PHI, Figure 6) inhibit carcinogen-induced tumor formation in rodents [124]. Ma et al. [124]

found that the chemopreventive isothiocyanates can modulate the growth, upregulating $p21^{WAF1}$ inhibitor and suppressing the activity of CDK, important cell cycle regulators in cancer cells. In this study, it was observed that PHI exposure of HL-60 leukemia cells caused cell cycle arrest at G1 and induction of apoptosis.

Researchers investigated the mechanism by which PHI suppressed the proliferation of cancer cells, ultimately attributing this phenomenon to its role as an HDACis. In addition, PHI decreased the HDAC expression and raised the amount of the acetyltransferase p300, causing an increase in acetylated histone accumulation. PHI also led to particular alterations to histone methylation, suggestive of favorable transcriptional activity. Chromatin immunoprecipitation assay revealed increased p21 DNA in the hyperacetylated histones from the PHI-exposed cells. This finding indicates chromatin unfolding leads to heightened access of the transcriptional elements to the location of the p21 promoter, resulting in the activation of cell cycle inhibitors. Apoptosis of HL-60 cells triggered by PHI was modulated by caspase-9 and Bcl-2, but normal PBMC or those obtained from the bone marrow were not susceptible to the compound. Therefore, PHI may act selectively on cancer cells [124].

10.1.11. Pterostilbene

Another polyphenol, pterostilbene is a stilbenoid (Figure 6) found primarily in blueberries, grapes, and wood. Pterostilbene is a natural dimethylated analog of resveratrol possessing greater liposolubility and bioavailability, making it possibly a more effective anticarcinogenic molecule [125]. Pterostilbene induces apoptosis in diverse malignancies—bladder, breast, colon, lung, pancreatic, and stomach cancers, as well as leukemia cells [126,127]. Naturally-derived resveratrol analogues, pterostilbene and 3′-hydroxypterostilbene have been shown to be efficient apoptosis-inducing drugs in multiple-drug resistance (MDR) and BCR-ABL-expressing leukemia cells. Different in vitro analysis in bortezomib resistance cell line H929R underscores their significance in the treatment of resistant hematologic malignancies through cell cycle arrest, autophagy, and apoptosis [127].

10.1.12. Quercetin

Quercetin (Figure 6) is a flavonol present in many plants, including various fruits, vegetables, and grains as well as leaves and seeds with red apples, onions, parsley, and sage are popular foods containing substantial levels of quercetin [128]. Alvarez et al. [129] explored the molecular processes behind quercetin's anticancer actions by analyzing its impact on DNA methylation and histone modification. This research was conducted in vivo utilizing mice with human AML tumor xenografts and in vitro on HL-60 and U937 cells. Incubations with quercetin significantly down-regulated the expression of DNMT1 and DNMT3a, an effect partially reliant on STAT-3. Class I HDACs were likewise downregulated by the therapy. Additionally, co-treatment with quercetin plus the proteasome inhibitor MG132 reduced the loss of class I HDACs in comparison to quercetin alone, demonstrating that quercetin promoted HDACs degradation by proteasomes. The methylation of the proapoptotic BCL2L11 and DAPK1 genes was decreased by quercetin in a concentration- and time-dependent manner. In addition, treatment of cells with the flavonoid, for 48 h, buildup acetylated H3 and H4 in the promoters of BNIP3L, BAX, BCL2L11, DAPK1, APAF-1, and BNIP3L. In accordance, treatment with quercetin substantially enhanced the transcription of each of these genes. The accumulation of H3ac and H4ac at the promoters of genes implicated in apoptosis, resulting in their increased expression, may contribute to accelerated apoptosis induced by quercetin, according to the findings.

10.1.13. Thujaplicin

Thujaplicins (Figure 6) are naturally occurring substances generated from tropolone, a toxin produced by the agricultural pathogen *Burkholderia plantarii*. Recently, Ononye et al. [130] revealed that some tropolones potently and specifically target HDACs and impede the proliferation of hematological cell lines. A naturally occurring non-benzenoid aromatic containing a metal-directing tropone unit comprises the tropolone nucleus.

Tropolones show an antiproliferative effect on Jurkat cells in a way unique from vorinostat, a pan-HDAC inhibitor. While both agents cause apoptosis in this cell line, it seems that the tropolones function via a smaller selection of biological processes. Specifically, compared to vorinostat, tropolones had a lesser impact on histone hyperacetylation and do not seem to increase the expression of p21. Vorinostat appears to activate an extrinsic mechanism of apoptosis; the tropolones do not, although both enhance the activity of caspase-3 and caspase-7. Both tropolones and vorinostat seem to increase the expression of perforin, which may be associated with cell maturation and, perhaps, caspase-3 activation. Overall, the more restricted activation of apoptosis by tropolones compared to pan-HDAC inhibitors may enable the creation of more targeted anti-leukemia therapies. In this sense, the tropolone nucleus is well-suited for producing HDAC inhibitors with specific cellular effects, which may lead to the development of drugs with unique therapeutic properties.

10.1.14. Ursolic Acid

There are several plants and foods that contain ursolic acid (Figure 6), a pentacyclic triterpenoid [131]. Some natural sources of ursolic acid include rosemary (*Rosmarinus officinalis*), ginseng (*Panax ginseng*), plum (*Prunus domestica*), pear, apple peel, and cranberry. Its potential for both cancer prevention and treatment has been investigated. Studies on ursolic acid have focused on its potential to inhibit HDAC proteins; HDAC1-3 and 6-8 were shown to be significantly downregulated by this bioactive chemical, beginning at a concentration of 2.5 μM (a non-toxic concentration) [132]. Moreover, in leukocytes, ursolic acid counteracted HDAC1 and HDAC3 induction.

10.1.15. Xestoquinone

The polycyclic quinone-type metabolite termed xestoquinone (Figure 6) is also a marine drug isolated from sponges of the *Xestospongia* and *Petrosia* genus, and has been shown to have an anticancer potential [133].

The cytotoxic effects of xestoquinone on various hematological cancer cell lines have been investigated in preclinical trials. In one study, cell growth was inhibited by the compound with low-micromolar IC_{50} values. Additionally, topoisomerase I and II activity were reduced by 50% and 30%, respectively, at concentrations of 0.235 and 0.094 μM in the cell-free system. Researchers purport xestoquinone's lethal action on Molt-4 cells to be caused by the activation of many distinct apoptotic pathways, such as the death-receptor pathway. Pretreatment of these cells with N-acetyl cysteine alleviated the loss of mitochondrial membrane potential, decreased apoptosis, and maintained topoisomerase I and II expressions. In another study, xestoquinone (1 μg/g) effectively inhibited leukemia cancer cell development in a nude mouse xenograft model, decreasing it by 31.2% relative to the solvent control [115]. These results warrant further investigation into xestoquinone as a potential antileukemic agent capable of targeting cancer cells via numerous pathways [115].

10.2. Plant Products and Extracts

10.2.1. *Antrodia camphorate*

Due to its antioxidant properties, the plant *Antrodia camphorata* is widely used in herbal medicine in Taiwan. The capacity of *A. camphorata* to induce apoptotic cell death in a leukemia model was investigated by Yang et al. [134]. Using the HL-60 cell line, the authors observed a decrease in cell viability, accompanied by chromatin condensation and internucleosomal DNA fragmentation indicative of apoptosis, following treatment with 20–80 μg/mL A. camphorate extract. Researchers also note an increase in cytochrome c release, caspase-3 activation, and the proteolytic cleavage of PARP. An uptick in *A. camphorata*-induced apoptosis coincided with a decrease in Bcl-2, a powerful inhibitor of cell death, and upregulation of Bax [135]. Accordingly, *A. camphorata* may possess anticancer potential, and so further studies are warranted to elucidate its role against hematological malignancies. In support of these findings, follow-up in vivo analysis in which investigators observed delayed tumor volume in a xenograft mice model treated with 80 or 120 mg/kg *A. camphorata* extract. Tissue analysis confirmed these results to be mediated by increased cell cycle arrest [135].

10.2.2. *Feijoa sellowiana*

Feijoa sellowiana Berg. (Myrtaceae) is a bushy evergreen shrub native to South America that has adapted well to the Mediterranean climate. *F. sellowiana* grows all over the Mediterranean and is widely consumed as a food source. *F. sellowiana* also contains high levels of bioflavonoids or vitamin P-active polyphenols, including catechin, leucoanthocyanins, flavonols, proanthocyanidins, and naphthoquinones [136]. It was reported that the acetonic extract of *F. sellowiana* selectively inhibited the growth of hematological cancer cells when applied to malignant cells and healthy myeloid progenitors. Flavone (2-phenyl-4H-chromen-4-one) was determined to be the active component in the *F. sellowiana* acetonic extract through fractionation, purification, and analysis. Flavone induces apoptosis in human myeloid leukemia cells, which is accompanied by caspase activation and increased expression of p16, p21, and TRAIL. The use of ex vivo myeloid leukemia blasts confirms the ability of both the full acetonic *F. sellowiana* extract and its derived flavone to induce apoptosis. In myeloid leukemia patient blasts and in other cell models, the apoptotic inducing action of *F. sellowiana* extract and flavone is accompanied by HDAC inhibition and associated rise in acetylation of histone and other proteins. These findings demonstrated for the first time that the apoptotic active principle of *F. sellowiana* is flavone, whose effects are at least in part attributable to its impact on acetylation status. These findings support the hypothesis that its epigenetic pro-apoptotic regulation in hematological cancers is dependent on HDAC inhibition [136].

10.2.3. Olive Oil

Mutations in somatic cells are crucial to cancer development and progression. Environmental and endogenous genotoxic chemicals induce genetic changes. Reactive oxygen species, which are produced in all aerobic organisms as metabolic byproducts and also as bactericidal agents in phagocytic cells, are likely to be the most important endogenously produced genotoxic chemicals [137]. Thus, oxidative stress has been linked to several degenerative disorders, including cancer.

Due to their antioxidant properties, small phenolic chemicals in olive oil are thought to prevent cancer. The impact of olive oil bioactives on DNA damage by H_2O_2 incubation of human PBMC and leukemia HL-60 cells has been examined previously [138]. Hydroxytyrosol and a combination of polyphenols derived from olive oil and olive mill residues decreased DNA damage at concentrations of 1 μM. With 10 μM hydroxytyrosol, 93% viability of HL-60 cells and 88% of PBMC cells were protected. In both types of cells, the dialdehydic version of elenoic acid coupled with hydroxytyrosol exhibited a comparable protective effect. Other isolated substances, like tyrosol, oleuropein and verbascoside similarly attenuated the DNA damage. Overall, these data imply that olive oil and its bioactive constituents can be useful in preventing the starting phase of carcinogenesis in vivo, since the quantities necessary to prevent oxidative DNA damage are readily attained with typical olive oil consumption [138].

Table 5. Natural anticancer HDAC inhibitors in hematological cancers.

Active Constituents	Source	Mechanism(s) of Action	References
Berberine	*Berberis aristate*	Inhibited protein synthesis, HDACs, and Akt/mTOR pathways	[101–103]
Chrysin	*Oroxylum indicum* and *Pelargonium crispum*	Derepressed the epigenetically silenced genes and inhibited HDAC8 both directly and indirectly by reducing its protein concentration	[104]

Table 5. *Cont.*

Active Constituents	Source	Mechanism(s) of Action	References
Cowaxanthone and Cowain	*Garcinia fusca*	Induced apoptosis and autophagy in leukemic T-cells	[109,110]
Curcumin	*Curcuma longa*	Increased histone acetylation on gene promoters of the proapoptotic BAX gene due to inhibition of HDAC1, HDAC3, and HDAC8 activity and expression in leukemic cells	[113]
Cyclostellettamine G and dehydrocyclostellettamines D and E	*Haliclona* and *Xestospongia*	Induced apoptosis	[114,115]
Ginsenoside 20(s)-Rh2	*Panax ginseng*	Induced apoptosis	[118]
Halenaquinone	*Xestospongia vansoesti* and *Paracheilinus alfiani*	Induced apoptosis	[120]
Hydroxytyrosol [3,4-dyhydroxyphenyl-ethanol (3,4-DHPEA)]	Virgin olive oil and olive mill wastewater	Induced DNA damage	[138]
Largazole	*Symploca* sp.	Induced apoptosis	[121]
Oleacein	*Olea europaea*	Exhibited epigenetic modulation in multiple myeloma cells	[122]
Phenylhexyl isothiocyanate	Cruciferous vegetables	Promoted G1 arrest and apoptosis	[124]
Pterostilbene	Blueberries and grapes	Cell cycle arrest, autophagy	[127]
Quercetin	Apples, onions, parsley, and sage	Induced apoptosis	[129]
Thujaplicin	Troplone	Promoted cell cycle arrest and induced apoptosis	[130]
Ursolic acid	*Panax ginseng*, *Rosmarinus officinalis*, and *Prunus domestica*	Promoted cell cycle arrest and induced apoptosis	[132]
Xestoquinone	*Petrosia* sp.	Induced apoptosis	[115]
Acetonic extract and flavone	*Feijoa sellowiana*	Induced apoptosis	[136]
Antrodia camphorate	*Antrodia camphorate*	Induced apoptosis	[135]

Abbreviations: HDAC, histone deacetylase; mTOR, mammalian target of rapamycin.

11. Conclusions

Epigenetic changes carried out by HDAC proteins are implicated in carcinogenesis and metastasis of hematological malignancies. Some HDACis are approved for the treatment of hematological malignancies, and many others are currently being investigated for their anticancer effects as monotherapies or adjuvant agents. HDACis have demonstrated effectiveness in AML, CTCLs, and MM by various mechanisms. These anticancer effects are broad in nature and are not limited to changes in acetylation status. Multiple preclinical studies demonstrate the role of HDACis as regulators of the cell cycle and agents of apoptosis. Current data most strongly supports the use of HDACis as adjuvants to conventional treatments. One study, for example, demonstrated the efficacy of panobinostat for therapy of refractory MM when used in combination with bortezomib and dexamethasone—even after a failed response to bortezomib monotherapy. The success of synthetic HDACis has fostered an interest in naturally occurring alternatives. Phytochemical HDACis, such as chrysin, oleacein, quercetin, as well as marine-derived HDACis halenaquinone and xestoquinone are being investigated as potential drugs against hematological cancers. Importantly, phytochemicals are generally less toxic compared to conventional chemotherapy, but their efficacy may be limited by bioavailability. Despite preliminary encouraging results, further studies are required to investigate the exact role HDACis play against hematological malignancies. Additionally, expanded in vivo research is required to elucidate the safety profiles and pharmacokinetics of these bioactive compounds before more robust clinical trials can ensue.

Author Contributions: Conceptualization, D.P.; methodology, D.P. and A.B.; investigation, D.P. and K.R.; data curation, D.P. and K.R.; writing—original draft preparation, D.P., K.R., S.S.N., S.S., A.M. (Abhishek Mishra) and A.B.; writing—review and editing, D.P., R.L., J.T.B. and A.B.; visualization, D.P. and A.M. (Arijit Mondal), supervision, A.B.; project administration, A.B. All authors have read and agreed to the published version of the manuscript.

Funding: This research received no external funding.

Institutional Review Board Statement: Not applicable.

Informed Consent Statement: Not applicable.

Conflicts of Interest: The authors declare no conflict of interest.

References

1. Adams, H.; Fritzsche, F.R.; Dirnhofer, S.; Kristiansen, G.; Tzankov, A. Class I histone deacetylases 1, 2 and 3 are highly expressed in classical Hodgkin's lymphoma. *Expert Opin. Ther. Targets* **2010**, *14*, 577–584. [CrossRef] [PubMed]
2. Nikolova, T.; Kiweler, N.; Krämer, O.H. Interstrand crosslink repair as a target for HDAC inhibition. *Trends Pharmacol. Sci.* **2017**, *38*, 822–836. [CrossRef] [PubMed]
3. Li, Y.; Seto, E. HDACs and HDAC inhibitors in cancer development and therapy. *Cold Spring Harb. Perspect. Med.* **2016**, *6*, a026831. [CrossRef] [PubMed]
4. Lu, H.; Bai, L.; Zhou, Y.; Lu, Y.; Jiang, Z.; Shi, J. Recent study of dual HDAC/PARP inhibitor for the treatment of tumor. *Curr. Top Med. Chem.* **2019**, *19*, 1041–1050. [CrossRef] [PubMed]
5. Narita, T.; Weinert, B.T.; Choudhary, C. Functions and Mechanisms of Non-Histone Protein Acetylation. *Nat. Rev. Mol. Cell Biol.* **2019**, *20*, 156–174. [CrossRef] [PubMed]
6. Robert, C.; Rassool, F.V. HDAC inhibitors: Roles of DNA damage and repair. *Adv. Cancer Res.* **2012**, *116*, 87–129.
7. Butler, L.M.; Zhou, X.; Xu, W.S.; Scher, H.I.; Rifkind, R.A.; Marks, P.A.; Richon, V.M. The histone deacetylase inhibitor SAHA arrests cancer cell growth, up-regulates thioredoxin-binding protein-2, and down-regulates thioredoxin. *Proc. Natl. Acad. Sci. USA* **2002**, *99*, 11700–11707. [CrossRef]
8. Singh, A.K.; Bishayee, A.; Pandey, A.K. Targeting histone deacetylases with natural and synthetic agents: An emerging anti-cancer strategy. *Nutrients* **2018**, *10*, 731. [CrossRef]
9. Bouyahya, A.; El Hachlafi, N.; Aanniz, T.; Bourais, I.; Mechchate, H.; Benali, T.; Shariati, M.A.; Burkov, P.; Lorenzo, J.M.; Wilairatana, P.; et al. Natural Bioactive Compounds Targeting Histone Deacetylases in Human Cancers: Recent Updates. *Molecules* **2022**, *27*, 2568. [CrossRef]
10. Ruzic, D.; Djoković, N.; Srdić-Rajić, T.; Echeverria, C.; Nikolic, K.; Santibanez, J.F. Targeting histone deacetylases: Opportunities for cancer treatment and chemoprevention. *Pharmaceutics* **2022**, *14*, 209. [CrossRef]
11. De Felice, F.; Tombolini, V.; Marampon, F.; Musella, A.; Marchetti, C. Defective DNA repair mechanisms in prostate cancer: Impact of olaparib. *Drug Des Devel Ther.* **2017**, *11*, 547–552. [CrossRef] [PubMed]
12. Hu, D.; Shilatifard, A. Epigenetics of hematopoiesis and hematological malignancies. *Genes Dev.* **2016**, *30*, 2021–2041. [CrossRef] [PubMed]
13. Yang, Y.; Liu, Q.; Wang, X.; Gou, S. Design, synthesis, and biological evaluation of novel HDAC inhibitors with a 3-(benzazol-2-yl) quinoxaline framework. *Bioorg. Med. Chem.* **2023**, *88*, 129305. [CrossRef] [PubMed]
14. Huang, M.; Lu, J.J.; Ding, J. Natural products in cancer therapy: Past, present and future. *Nat. Prod. Bioprospect.* **2021**, *11*, 5–13. [CrossRef]
15. Lecumberri, E.; Dupertuis, Y.M.; Miralbell, R.; Pichard, C. Green tea polyphenol epigallocatechin-3-gallate (EGCG) as adjuvant in cancer therapy. *Clin. Nutr.* **2013**, *32*, 894–903. [CrossRef]
16. Pramanik, S.D.; Kumar Halder, A.; Mukherjee, U.; Kumar, D.; Dey, Y.N. Potential of histone deacetylase inhibitors in the control and regulation of prostate, breast and ovarian cancer. *Front. Chem.* **2022**, *10*, 847. [CrossRef]
17. Feng, J.; Meng, X. Histone modification and histone modification-targeted anti-cancer drugs in breast cancer: Fundamentals and beyond. *Front. Pharmacol.* **2022**, *13*, 946811. [CrossRef]
18. Hieu, D.T.; Anh, D.T.; Tuan, N.M.; Hai, P.T.; Kim, J.; Kang, J.S.; Vu, T.K.; Dung, P.T.; Han, S.B.; Nam, N.H.; et al. Design, synthesis and evaluation of novel N-hydroxybenzamides/N-hydroxypropenamides incorporating quinazolin-4 (3H)-ones as histone deacetylase inhibitors and antitumor agents. *Bioorg. Chem.* **2018**, *76*, 258–267. [CrossRef]
19. Saha, S.; Pal, D.; Kumar, S. Design, synthesis and antiproliferative activity of hydroxyacetamide derivatives against HeLa cervical carcinoma cell and breast cancer cell line. *Trop. J. Pharm. Res.* **2016**, *15*, 1401–1411. [CrossRef]

20. García, S.; Mercado-Sánchez, I.; Bahena, L.; Alcaraz, Y.; García-Revilla, M.A.; Robles, J.; Santos-Martínez, N.; Ordaz-Rosado, D.; García-Becerra, R.; Vazquez, M.A. Design of fluorescent coumarin-hydroxamic acid derivatives as inhibitors of HDACs: Syn-thesis, anti-proliferative evaluation and docking studies. *Molecules* **2020**, *25*, 5134. [CrossRef]
21. Moseley, V.R.; Morris, J.; Knackstedt, R.W.; Wargovich, M.J. Green Tea Polyphenol Epigallocatechin 3-Gallate, Contributes to the Degradation of DNMT3A and HDAC3 in HCT 116 Human Colon Cancer Cells. *Anticancer Res.* **2013**, *33*, 5325–5333. [PubMed]
22. Meeran, S.M.; Patel, S.N.; Chan, T.-H.; Tollefsbol, T.O. A Novel Prodrug of Epigallocatechin-3-Gallate: Differential Epigenetic HTERT Repression in Human Breast Cancer Cells. *Cancer Prev. Res.* **2011**, *4*, 1243–1254. [CrossRef] [PubMed]
23. Pandey, M.; Kaur, P.; Shukla, S.; Abbas, A.; Fu, P.; Gupta, S. Plant Flavone Apigenin Inhibits HDAC and Remodels Chromatin to Induce Growth Arrest and Apoptosis in Human Prostate Cancer Cells: In Vitro and in Vivo Study. *Mol. Carcinog.* **2012**, *51*, 952–962. [CrossRef] [PubMed]
24. Zeng, H.; Huang, P.; Wang, X.; Wu, J.; Wu, M.; Huang, J. Galangin-Induced down-Regulation of BACE1 by Epigenetic Mechanisms in SH-SY5Y Cells. *Neuroscience* **2015**, *294*, 172–181. [CrossRef] [PubMed]
25. Dimopoulos, K.; Grønbæk, K. Epigenetic therapy in hematological cancers. *Apmis* **2019**, *127*, 316–328. [CrossRef] [PubMed]
26. Fernández-Serrano, M.; Winkler, R.; Santos, J.C.; Le Pannérer, M.M.; Buschbeck, M.; Roué, G. Histone modifications and their targeting in lymphoid malignancies. *Int. J. Mol. Sci.* **2022**, *23*, 253. [CrossRef]
27. Rathinavelu, A.; Natarajan, U. HDAC inhibition in cancer. In *Epigenetics in Organ Specific Disorders*; Academic Press: Cambridge, MA, USA, 2023; pp. 63–97.
28. Andrade, M.B. The Role of Epigenetics in Glioblastoma—A Meta Analysis. 2020. Available online: https://repositorio-aberto.up.pt/bitstream/10216/130224/2/429915.pdf (accessed on 29 April 2023).
29. Wang, L.; Syn, N.L.; Subhash, V.V.; Any, Y.; Thuya, W.L.; Cheow, E.S.; Kong, L.; Yu, F.; Peethala, P.C.; Wong, A.L.; et al. Pan-HDAC inhibition by panobino-stat medi-ates chemosensi-tization to carboplatin in non-small cell lung cancer via at-tenuation of EGFR signaling. *Cancer Lett.* **2018**, *417*, 152–160. [CrossRef]
30. Khot, A.; Dickinson, M.; Prince, H.M. Panobinostat in lymphoid and myeloid malignancies. *Expert Opin. Investig. Drugs* **2013**, *22*, 1211–1223. [CrossRef]
31. Giaccone, G.; Rajan, A.; Berman, A.; Kelly, R.J.; Szabo, E.; Lopez-Chavez, A.; Trepel, J.; Lee, M.J.; Cao, L.; Espinoza-Delgado, I.; et al. Phase II study of belinostat in patients with recurrent or refractory advanced thymic epithelial tumors. *Clin. Oncol.* **2011**, *29*, 2052. [CrossRef]
32. Tavakoli-Yaraki, M.; Karami-Tehrani, F.; Salimi, V.; Sirati-Sabet, M. Induction of apoptosis by Trichostatin A in human breast cancer cell lines: Involvement of 15-Lox-1. *Tumor Biol.* **2013**, *34*, 241–249. [CrossRef]
33. Liu, Y.; He, G.; Wang, Y.; Guan, X.; Pang, X.; Zhang, B. MCM-2 is a therapeutic target of Trichostatin A in colon cancer cells. *Toxicol. Lett.* **2013**, *221*, 23–30. [CrossRef] [PubMed]
34. Reid, T.; Valone, F.; Lipera, W.; Irwin, D.; Paroly, W.; Natale, R.; Sreedharan, S.; Keer, H.; Lum, B.; Scappaticci, F.; et al. Phase II trial of the histone deacetylase inhibitor pivaloyloxymethyl butyrate (Pivanex, AN-9) in advanced non-small cell lung cancer. *Clin. Lung Cancer* **2004**, *45*, 381–386. [CrossRef] [PubMed]
35. McIntyre, J.; Moral, M.A.; Bozzo, J. Combination therapy with valproic acid in cancer: Initial clinical approach. *Drugs Future* **2007**, *32*, 45. [CrossRef]
36. Connolly, R.M.; Rudek, M.A.; Piekarz, R. Entinostat: A promising treatment option for patients with advanced breast cancer. *Future Oncol.* **2017**, *13*, 1137–1148. [CrossRef]
37. Saito, Y.; Mizokami, A.; Izumi, K.; Naito, R.; Goto, M.; Nakagawa-Goto, K. α-Trifluoromethyl chalcones as potent anticancer agents for androgen receptor-independent prostate cancer. *Molecules* **2021**, *26*, 2812. [CrossRef] [PubMed]
38. Slingerland, M.; Guchelaar, H.J.; Gelderblom, H. Histone deacetylase inhibitors: An overview of the clinical studies in solid tumors. *Anticancer. Drugs* **2014**, *25*, 140–149. [CrossRef]
39. Jang, K.Y.; Hwang, S.H.; Kwon, K.S.; Kim, K.R.; Choi, H.N.; Lee, N.R.; Kwak, J.Y.; Park, B.H.; Park, H.S.; Chung, M.J.; et al. SIRT1 expression is associated with poor prognosis of diffuse large B-cell lymphoma. *Am. J. Surg. Pathol.* **2008**, *32*, 1523–1531. [CrossRef]
40. Bakkenist, C.J.; Kastan, M.B. DNA damage activates ATM through intermolecular autophosphorylation and dimer dissocia-tion. *Nature* **2003**, *421*, 499–506. [CrossRef]
41. Gaymes, T.J.; Padua, R.A.; Pla, M.; Orr, S.; Omidvar, N.; Chomienne, C.; Mufti, G.J.; Rassool, F.V. Histone deacetylase inhibitors (HDI) cause DNA damage in leukemia cells: A mechanism for leukemia-specific HDI-dependent apoptosis? *Mol. Cancer* **2006**, *4*, 563–573. [CrossRef]
42. Lukas, J.; Lukas, C.; Bartek, J. More than just a focus: The chromatin response to DNA damage and its role in genome integrity maintenance. *Nat. Cell Biol.* **2011**, *13*, 1161–1169. [CrossRef]
43. Daśko, M.; de Pascual-Teresa, B.; Ortín, I.; Ramos, A. HDAC inhibitors: Innovative strategies for their design and applications. *Molecules* **2022**, *27*, 715. [CrossRef] [PubMed]
44. Misteli, T.; Soutoglou, E. The emerging role of nuclear architecture in DNA repair and genome maintenance. *Nat. Rev. Mol. Cell Biol.* **2009**, *10*, 243–254. [CrossRef] [PubMed]
45. Shanmugam, G.; Rakshit, S.; Sarkar, K. HDAC inhibitors: Targets for tumor therapy, immune modulation and lung diseases. *Transl. Oncol.* **2022**, *16*, 101312. [CrossRef]
46. Lanzi, C.; Cassinelli, G. Combinatorial strategies to potentiate the efficacy of HDAC inhibitors in fusion-positive sarcomas. *Biochem. Pharmacol.* **2022**, *198*, 114944. [CrossRef] [PubMed]

47. Ito, A.; Kawaguchi, Y.; Lai, C.H.; Kovacs, J.J.; Higashimoto, Y.; Appella, E.; Yao, T.P. MDM2–HDAC1-mediated deacetylation of p53 is required for its degradation. *EMBO J.* **2002**, *21*, 6236–6245. [CrossRef]
48. Johnstone, R.W. Histone-deacetylase inhibitors: Novel drugs for the treatment of cancer. *Nat. Rev. Drug Discov.* **2002**, *1*, 287–299. [CrossRef]
49. Jiang, X.; Sun, Y.; Chen, S.; Roy, K.; Price, B.D. The FATC domains of PIKK proteins are functionally equivalent and participate in the Tip60-dependent activation of DNA-PKcs and ATM. *J. Biol. Chem.* **2006**, *281*, 15741–15746. [CrossRef]
50. Lee, S.F.; Pervaiz, S. Assessment of oxidative stress-induced DNA damage by immunoflourescent analysis of 8-oxodG. *Methods Cell Biol.* **2011**, *103*, 99–113.
51. Dasmahapatra, G.; Lembersky, D.; Son, M.P.; Attkisson, E.; Dent, P.; Fisher, R.I.; Friedberg, J.W.; Grant, S. Carfilzomib Interacts Synergistically with Histone Deacetylase Inhibitors in Mantle Cell Lymphoma Cells In Vitro and In VivoCarfilzomib and Vorinostat in Mantle Cells. *Mol. Cancer Ther.* **2011**, *10*, 1686–1697. [CrossRef]
52. McClure, J.J.; Li, X.; Chou, C.J. Advances and Challenges of HDAC inhibitors in cancer therapeutics. *Adv. Cancer Res.* **2018**, *138*, 183–211.
53. Dai, Y.; Rahmani, M.; Dent, P.; Grant, S. Blockade of histone deacetylase inhibitor-induced RelA/p65 acetylation and NF-κB activation potentiates apoptosis in leukemia cells through a process mediated by oxidative damage, XIAP downregulation, and c-Jun N-terminal kinase 1 activation. *Mol. Cell. Biol.* **2005**, *25*, 5429–5444. [CrossRef] [PubMed]
54. Huertas, P.; Jackson, S.P. Human CtIP mediates cell cycle control of DNA end resection and double strand break repair. *J. Biol. Chem.* **2009**, *284*, 9558–9565. [CrossRef] [PubMed]
55. Cui, H.; Hong, Q.; Wei, R.; Li, H.; Wan, C.; Chen, X.; Zhao, S.; Bu, H.; Zhang, B.; Yang, D.; et al. Design and synthesis of HDAC inhibitors to enhance the therapeutic effect of diffuse large B-cell lymphoma by improving metabolic stability and pharmacokinetic characteristics. *Eur. J. Med. Chem.* **2022**, *22*, 114049. [CrossRef] [PubMed]
56. Ho, T.C.; Chan, A.H.; Ganesan, A. Thirty years of HDAC inhibitors: 2020 insight and hindsight. *J. Med. Chem.* **2020**, *63*, 12460–12484. [CrossRef] [PubMed]
57. Zhao, C.; Dong, H.; Xu, Q.; Zhang, Y. Histone deacetylase (HDAC) inhibitors in cancer: A patent review (2017-present). *Expert Opin. Ther. Pat.* **2020**, *30*, 263–274. [CrossRef] [PubMed]
58. Rahman, M.M.; Kukita, A.; Kukita, T.; Shobuike, T.; Nakamura, T.; Kohashi, O. Two histone deacetylase inhibitors, trichostatin A and sodium butyrate, suppress differentiation into osteoclasts but not into macrophages. *Blood J. Am. Soc. Hematol.* **2003**, *101*, 3451–3459. [CrossRef]
59. Chang, J.; Varghese, D.S.; Gillam, M.C.; Peyton, M.; Modi, B.; Schiltz, R.L.; Girard, L.; Martinez, E.D. Differential response of cancer cells to HDAC inhibitors trichostatin A and depsipeptide. *BJC* **2012**, *106*, 116–125. [CrossRef]
60. Schäker-Hübner, L.; Haschemi, R.; Büch, T.; Kraft, F.B.; Brumme, B.; Schöler, A.; Jenke, R.; Meiler, J.; Aigner, A.; Bendas, G.; et al. Balancing Histone Deacetylase (HDAC) Inhibition and Drug-likeness: Biological and Physicochemical Evaluation of Class I Selective HDAC Inhibitors. *Chem. Med. Chem.* **2022**, *17*, e202100755. [CrossRef]
61. Basile, V.; Mantovani, R.; Imbriano, C. DNA damage promotes histone deacetylase 4 nuclear localization and repression of G2/M promoters, via p53 C-terminal lysines. *J. Biol. Chem.* **2006**, *281*, 2347–2357. [CrossRef]
62. Bolden, J.E.; Peart, M.J.; Johnstone, R.W. Anticancer activities of histone deacetylase inhibitors. *Nat. Rev. Drug Discov.* **2006**, *5*, 769–784. [CrossRef]
63. Kutil, Z.; Novakova, Z.; Meleshin, M.; Mikesova, J.; Schutkowski, M.; Barinka, C. Histone deacetylase 11 is a fatty-acid deac-ylase. *ACS Chem. Biol.* **2018**, *13*, 685–693. [CrossRef] [PubMed]
64. Walker, J.R.; Corpina, R.A.; Goldberg, J. Structure of the Ku heterodimer bound to DNA and its implications for double-strand break repair. *Nature* **2001**, *412*, 607–614. [CrossRef] [PubMed]
65. Gottlieb, T.M.; Jackson, S.P. The DNA-dependent protein kinase: Requirement for DNA ends and association with Ku antigen. *Cell* **1993**, *72*, 131–142. [CrossRef] [PubMed]
66. Karagiannis, T.C.; Kn, H.; El-Osta, A. The epigenetic modifier, valproic acid, enhances radiation sensitivity. *Epigenetics* **2006**, *1*, 131–137. [CrossRef]
67. Lee, J.H.; Choy, M.L.; Ngo, L.; Foster, S.S.; Marks, P.A. Histone deacetylase inhibitor induces DNA damage, which normal but nottransformed cells can repair. *Proc. Natl. Acad. Sci. USA* **2010**, *107*, 14639–14644. [CrossRef]
68. Kachhap, S.K.; Rosmus, N.; Collis, S.J.; Kortenhorst, M.S.; Wissing, M.D.; Hedayati, M.; Shabbeer, S.; Mendonca, J.; Deangelis, J.; Marchionni, L.; et al. Downregulation of homologous recombination DNA repair genes by HDAC inhibition in prostate cancer is mediated through the E2F1 transcription factor. *PLoS ONE* **2010**, *5*, e11208. [CrossRef]
69. Sun, Y.; Jiang, X.; Price, B.D. Tip60: Connecting chromatin to DNA damage signaling. *Cell Cycle* **2010**, *9*, 930–936. [CrossRef]
70. Sharma, G.G.; So, S.; Gupta, A.; Kumar, R.; Cayrou, C.; Avvakumov, N.; Bhadra, U.; Pandita, R.K.; Porteus, M.H.; Chen, D.J.; et al. MOF and histone H4 acetylation at lysine 16 are critical for DNA damage response and double-strand break repair. *Mol. Cell. Biol.* **2010**, *30*, 3582–3595. [CrossRef]
71. Polo, S.E.; Kaidi, A.; Baskcomb, L.; Galanty, Y.; Jackson, S.P. Regulation of DNA-damage responses and cell-cycle progression by the chromatin remodelling factor CHD4. *EMBOJ* **2010**, *29*, 3130–3139. [CrossRef]
72. Petruccelli, L.A.; Dupéré-Richer, D.; Pettersson, F.; Retrouvey, H.; Skoulikas, S.; Miller, W.H., Jr. Vorinostat induces reactive oxygen species and DNA damage in acute myeloid leukemia cells. *PLoS ONE* **2011**, *6*, e20987. [CrossRef]

73. Sartori, A.A.; Lukas, C.; Coates, J.; Mistrik, M.; Fu, S.; Bartek, J.; Baer, R.; Lukas, J.; Jackson, S.P. Human CtIP promotes DNA end resection. *Nature* **2007**, *450*, 509–514. [CrossRef] [PubMed]
74. Tsai, H.C.; Li, H.; Van Neste, L.; Cai, Y.; Robert, C.; Rassool, F.V.; Shin, J.J.; Harbom, K.M.; Beaty, R.; Pappou, E.; et al. Transient low doses of DNA-demethylating agents exert durable antitumor effects on hematological and epithelial tumor cells. *Cancer Cell* **2012**, *21*, 430–446. [CrossRef] [PubMed]
75. Shao, Y.; Sun, Y. Epigenetic regulators as promising targets in acute myeloid leukemia therapy. *Signal Transduct. Target The.r* **2020**, *5*, 1–20.
76. Lawson, M.; Uciechowska, U.; Schemies, J.; Rumpf, T.; Jung, M.; Sippl, W. Inhibitors to understand molecular mechanisms of NAD+-dependent deacetylases (sirtuins). *Biochim. Et Biophys. Acta (BBA)-Gene Regul. Mech.* **2010**, *1799*, 726–739. [CrossRef]
77. San José-Enériz, E.; Gimenez-Camino, N.; Agirre, X.; Prosper, F. HDAC inhibitors in acute myeloid leukemia. *Cancers* **2019**, *11*, 1794. [CrossRef] [PubMed]
78. Maiso, P.; Colado, E.; Ocio, E.M.; Garayoa, M.; Martin, J.; Atadja, P.; Pandiella, A.; San-Miguel, J.F. The synergy of panobinostat plus doxorubicin in acute myeloid leukemia suggests a role for HDAC inhibitors in the control of DNA repair. *Leukemia* **2009**, *23*, 2265–2274. [CrossRef] [PubMed]
79. Ramaiah, M.J.; Tangutur, A.D.; Manyam, R.R. Epigenetic modulation and understanding of HDAC inhibitors in cancer therapy. *Life Sci.* **2021**, *277*, 119504. [CrossRef] [PubMed]
80. Wang, J.; Hoshino, T.; Redner, R.L.; Kajigaya, S.; Liu, J.M. ETO, fusion partner in t(8;21) acute myeloid leukemia, represses transcription by interaction with the human N-CoR/mSin3/HDAC1 complex. *Proc. Natl. Acad. Sci. USA* **1998**, *95*, 10860–10865. [CrossRef] [PubMed]
81. Zullo, K.M.; Guo, Y.; Cooke, L.; Jirau-Serrano, X.; Mangone, M.; Scotto, L.; Amengual, J.E.; Mao, Y.; Nandakumar, R.; Cremers, S.; et al. Aurora A Kinase Inhibition Selectively Synergizes with Histone Deacetylase Inhibitor through Cytokinesis Failure in T-cell LymphomaAlisertib Synergizes with Romidepsin in TCL. *Clin. Cancer Res.* **2015**, *21*, 4097–4109. [CrossRef]
82. Palomero, T.; Couronne, L.; Khiabanian, H. Recurrent mutations in epigenetic regulators, RHOA and FYN kinase in peripheral T cell lymphomas. *Nat. Genet.* **2014**, *46*, 166–170. [CrossRef]
83. Vader, G.; Lens, S.M. The Aurora kinase family in cell division and cancer. *Biochim. Biophys. Acta* **2008**, *1786*, 60–72. [CrossRef] [PubMed]
84. Marchi, E.; Zullo, K.M.; Amengual, J.E. The combination of hypomethylating agents and histone deacetylase inhibitors produce marked synergy in preclinical models of T-cell lymphoma. *Br. J. Haematol.* **2015**, *171*, 215–226. [CrossRef] [PubMed]
85. Grant, C.; Rahman, F.; Piekarz, R.; Peer, C.; Frye, R.; Robey, R.W.; Gardner, E.R.; Figg, W.D.; Bates, S.E. Romidepsin: A new therapy for cutaneous T-cell lymphoma and a potential therapy for solid tumors. *Expert Rev. Anticancer Ther.* **2010**, *10*, 997–1008. [CrossRef]
86. Patra, S.; Praharaj, P.P.; Klionsky, D.J.; Bhutia, S.K. Vorinostat in autophagic cell death: A critical insight into autopha-gy-mediated,-associated and-dependent cell death for cancer prevention. *Drug Discov. Today* **2022**, *27*, 269–279. [CrossRef] [PubMed]
87. Mrakovcic, M.; Bohner, L.; Hanisch, M.; Fröhlich, L.F. Epigenetic targeting of autophagy via HDAC inhibition in tumor cells: Role of p53. *Int. J. Mol. Sci.* **2018**, *19*, 3952. [CrossRef]
88. Heltweg, B.; Gatbonton, T.; Schuler, A.D.; Posakony, J.; Li, H.; Goehle, S.; Kollipara, R.; DePinho, R.A.; Gu, Y.; Simon, J.A.; et al. Antitumor activity of a small-molecule inhibitor of human silent information regulator 2 enzymes. *Cancer Res.* **2006**, *66*, 4368–4377. [CrossRef]
89. Grozinger, C.M.; Chao, E.D.; Blackwell, H.E.; Moazed, D.; Schreiber, S.L. Identification of a class of small molecule inhibitors of the sirtuin family of NAD-dependent deacetylases by phenotypic screening. *J. Biol. Chem.* **2001**, *276*, 38837–38843. [CrossRef]
90. Bedalov, A.; Gatbonton, T.; Irvine, W.P.; Gottschling, D.E.; Simon, J.A. Identification of a small molecule inhibitor of Sir2p. *Proc Natl. Acad. Sci. USA* **2001**, *98*, 15113–15118. [CrossRef]
91. Huang, J.; Chan, S.C.; Lok, V.; Zhang, L.; Lucero-Prisno, D.E.; Xu, W.; Zheng, Z.J.; Elcarte, E.; Withers, M.; Wong, M.C. The epidemiological landscape of multiple myeloma: A global cancer registry estimate of disease burden, risk factors, and temporal trends. *Lancet Haematol.* **2022**, *9*, e670–e677. [CrossRef]
92. Pei, X.Y.; Dai, Y.; Grant, S. Synergistic induction of oxidative injury and apoptosis in human multiple myeloma cells by the proteasome inhibitor bortezomib and histone deacetylase inhibitors. *Clin. Cancer Res.* **2004**, *10*, 3839–3852. [CrossRef]
93. Duvic, M.; Dimopoulos, M. The safety profile of vorinostat (suberoylanilide hydroxamic acid) in hematologic malignancies: A review of clinical studies. *Cancer Treat. Rev.* **2016**, *43*, 58–66. [CrossRef] [PubMed]
94. Mitsiades, N.; Mitsiades, C.S.; Richardson, P.G. Molecular sequelae of histone deacetylase inhibition in human malignant B cells. *Blood* **2003**, *101*, 4055–4062. [CrossRef] [PubMed]
95. Kawaguchi, Y.; Kovacs, J.J.; McLaurin, A.; Vance, J.M.; Ito, A.; Yao, T.P. The deacetylase HDAC6 regulates aggresome formation and cell viability in response to misfolded protein stress. *Cell* **2003**, *115*, 727–738. [CrossRef] [PubMed]
96. Vogl, D.T.; Raje, N.; Jagannath, S.; Richardson, P.; Hari, P.; Orlowski, R.; Supko, J.G.; Tamang, D.; Yang, M.; Jones, S.S.; et al. Ricolinostat, the First Selective Histone Deacetylase 6 Inhibitor, in Combination with Bortezomib and Dexamethasone for Relapsed or Refractory Multiple MyelomaRicolinostat, Bortezomib, and Dexamethasone for Mye-loma. *Clin. Cancer Res.* **2017**, *23*, 3307–3315. [CrossRef]

97. Amengual, J.E.; Lue, J.K.; Ma, H.; Lichtenstein, R.; Shah, B.; Cremers, S.; Jones, S.; Sawas, A. First-in-Class Selective HDAC6 Inhibitor (ACY-1215) Has a Highly Favorable Safety Profile in Patients with Relapsed and Refractory Lymphoma. *J. Oncol.* **2021**, *26*, 184-e366. [CrossRef] [PubMed]
98. Imai, Y.; Ohta, E.; Takeda, S.; Sunamura, S.; Ishibashi, M.; Tamura, H.; Wang, Y.H.; Deguchi, A.; Tanaka, J.; Maru, Y.; et al. Histone deacetylase inhibitor panobinostat induces calcineurin degradation in multiple myeloma. *JCI Insight* **2016**, *1*, e85061. [CrossRef]
99. Di Bello, E.; Noce, B.; Fioravanti, R.; Mai, A. Current HDAC Inhibitors in Clinical Trials. *Chimia* **2022**, *76*, 448. [CrossRef]
100. Ghosh, S.K.; Perrine, S.P.; Williams, R.M.; Faller, D.V. Histone deacetylaseinhibitors are potent inducers of gene expression in latent EBVand sensitize lymphoma cells to nucleoside antiviral agents. *Blood* **2012**, *119*, 1008–1017. [CrossRef]
101. Park, S.H.; Sung, J.H.; Chung, N. Berberine diminishes side population and down regulates stem cell-associated genes in the pancreatic cancer cell lines PANC-1 and MIA sssPaCa-2. Mol. *Mol. Cell. Biochem.* **2014**, *394*, 209–215. [CrossRef]
102. Wang, Z.; Liu, Y.; Xue, Y.; Hu, H.; Ye, J.; Li, X.; Lu, Z.; Meng, F.; Liang, S. Berberine Acts as a Putative Epigenetic Modulator by Affecting the Histone Code. *Toxicol. In Vitro* **2016**, *36*, 10–17. [CrossRef]
103. Li, C.; Su, R.; Wang, X.; Huang, G.; Liu, Y.; Yang, J.; Yin, Z.; Gu, C.; Fei, J. Discovery of the oncogenic MDM2, a direct binding target of berberine and a potential therapeutic, in multiple myeloma. *Funct. Integr. Genom.* **2022**, *22*, 1031–1041. [CrossRef] [PubMed]
104. Moghadam, E.R.; Ang, H.L.; Asnaf, S.E.; Zabolian, A.; Saleki, H.; Yavari, M.; Esmaeili, H.; Zarrabi, A.; Ashrafizadeh, M.; Kumar, A.P. Broad-spectrum preclinical antitumor activity of chrysin: Current trends and future perspectives. *Biomolecules* **2020**, *10*, 1374. [CrossRef] [PubMed]
105. Talebi, M.; Farkhondeh, T.; Simal-Gandara, J.; Kopustinskiene, D.M.; Bernatoniene, J.; Pourbagher-Shahri, A.M.; Sa-marghandian, S. Promising protective effects of chrysin in cardiometabolic diseases. *Curr. Drug Targets* **2022**, *23*, 458–470. [CrossRef] [PubMed]
106. Ganai, S.A.; Sheikh, F.A.; Baba, Z.A. Plant flavone Chrysin as an emerging histone deacetylase inhibitor for prosperous epigenetic-based anticancer therapy. *Phytother. Res.* **2021**, *35*, 823–834. [CrossRef]
107. Ganai, S.A. Designing isoform-selective inhibitors against classical HDACs for effective anticancer therapy: Insight and perspectives from in Silico. *Curr. Drug Targets* **2018**, *19*, 815–824. [CrossRef] [PubMed]
108. Murthy, H.N.; Yadav, G.G. Chemistry and Biological Activities of Garcinia Resin. In *Gums, Resins and Latexes of Plant Origin: Chemistry, Biological Activities and Uses*; Springer International Publishing: Cham, Switzerland, 2021; pp. 1–38.
109. Punpai, S.; Saenkham, A.; Jarintanan, F.; Jongrungruangchok, S.; Choowongkomon, K.; Suksamrarn, S.; Tanechpongtamb, W. HDAC inhibitor cowanin extracted from *G. fusca* induces apoptosis and autophagy via inhibition of the PI3K/Akt/mTOR pathways in Jurkat cells. *Biomed. Pharmacother* **2022**, *147*, 112577. [CrossRef]
110. Wahyuni, F.S.; Shaari, K.; Stanslas, J.; Lajis, N.H.; Hamidi, D. Cytotoxic properties and complete nuclear magnetic resonance assignment of isolated xanthones from the root of *Garcinia cowa* Roxb. *Pharmacogn. Mag.* **2016**, *12* (Suppl. 1), S52.
111. Kasi, P.D.; Tamilselvam, R.; Skalicka-Woźniak, K.; Nabavi, S.F.; Daglia, M.; Bishayee, A.; Pazoki-Toroudi, H.; Nabavi, S.M. Molecular targets of curcumin for cancer therapy: An updated review. *Tumor Biol.* **2016**, *37*, 13017–13028. [CrossRef]
112. Arslan, A.K.; Uzunhisarcıklı, E.; Yerer, M.B.; Bishayee, A. The golden spice curcumin in cancer: A perspective on finalized clinical trials during the last 10 years. *J. Cancer Ther.* **2022**, *18*, 19–26.
113. Liu, H.L.; Chen, Y.; Cui, G.H.; Zhou, J.F. Curcumin, a potent anti-tumor reagent, is a novel histone deacetylase inhibitor regulating B-NHL cell line Raji proliferation. *Acta Pharmacol. Sin.* **2005**, *26*, 603–609. [CrossRef]
114. Oku, N.; Nagai, K.; Shindoh, N.; Terada, Y.; van Soest, R.W.; Matsunaga, S.; Fusetani, N. Three new cyclostellettamines, which inhibit histone deacetylase, from a marine sponge of the genus Xestospongia. *Bioorg. Med. Chem. Lett.* **2004**, *14*, 2617–2620. [CrossRef] [PubMed]
115. Wang, K.C.; Lu, M.C.; Hsu, K.C.; El-Shazly, M.; Shih, S.P.; Lien, S.T.; Kuo, F.W.; Yang, S.C.; Chen, C.L.; Yang, Y.C. The an-tileukemic effect of xestoquinone, a marine-derived polycyclic quinone-type metabolite, is mediated through ros-induced inhibition of hsp-90. *Molecules* **2021**, *26*, 7037. [CrossRef] [PubMed]
116. Liu, Z.H.; Li, J.; Xia, J.; Jiang, R.; Zuo, G.W.; Li, X.P.; Chen, Y.; Xiong, W.; Chen, D.L. Ginsenoside 20 (s)-Rh2 as potent natural histone deacetylase inhibitors suppressing the growth of human leukemia cells. *Chem. Biol. Interact.* **2015**, *242*, 227–234. [CrossRef] [PubMed]
117. Kim, J.H. Pharmacological and medical applications of Panax ginseng and ginsenosides: A review for use in cardiovascular diseases. *JGR* **2018**, *42*, 264–269. [CrossRef] [PubMed]
118. Chen, C.; Sun, S.; Fang, W.; Jin, J. 20(S)-Ginsenoside Rh2 induces apoptosis and differentiation of K562 leukemia cells. *J. Ethnopharmacol.* **2016**, *194*, 126–133.
119. Shih, S.P.; Lee, M.G.; El-Shazly, M.; Juan, Y.S.; Wen, Z.H.; Du, Y.C.; Su, J.H.; Sung, P.J.; Chen, Y.C.; Yang, J.C. Tackling the Cytotoxic Effect of a Marine Polycyclic Quinone-Type Metabolite: Halenaquinone Induces Molt 4 Cells Apoptosis via Oxi-dative Stress Combined with the Inhibition of HDAC and Topoisomerase Activities. *Mar. Drugs* **2015**, *13*, 3132–3153. [CrossRef]
120. Luparello, C.; Mauro, M.; Arizza, V.; Vazzana, M. Histone deacetylase inhibitors from marine invertebrates. *Biology* **2020**, *9*, 429. [CrossRef]
121. Souto, J.A.; Vaz, E.; Lepore, I.; Pöppler, A.C.; Franci, G.; Alvarez, R.; Altucci, L.; de Lera, A.R. Synthesis and biological characterization of the histone deacetylase inhibitor largazole and C7-modified analogues. *J. Med. Chem.* **2010**, *53*, 4654–4667. [CrossRef]

122. Emma, M.R.; Augello, G.D.; Stefano, V.; Azzolina, A.; Giannitrapani, L.; Montalto, G.; Cervello, M.; Cusimano, A. Potential uses of olive oil secoiridoids for the prevention and treatment of cancer: A narrative review of preclinical studies. *Int. J. Mol. Sci.* **2021**, *22*, 1234. [CrossRef]
123. Juli, G.; Oliverio, M.; Bellizzi, D.; Gallo Cantafio, M.E.; Grillone, K.; Passarino, G.; Colica, C.; Nardi, M.; Rossi, M.; Procopio, A.; et al. Anti-tumor activity and epigenetic impact of the polyphenol oleacein in multiple myeloma. *Cancers* **2019**, *11*, 990. [CrossRef]
124. Ma, X.; Fang, Y.; Beklemisheva, A.; Dai, W.; Feng, J.; Ahmed, T.; Liu, D.; Chiao, J.W. Phenylhexyl isothiocyanate inhibits histone deacetylases and remodels chromatins to induce growth arrest in human leukemia cells. *Int. J. Oncol.* **2006**, *28*, 1287–1293. [CrossRef] [PubMed]
125. Chen, G.; Xu, Z.; Chang, G.; Hou, J.; Hu, L.; Zhang, Y.; Yu, D.; Li, B.; Chang, S.; Xie, Y.; et al. The blueberry component pterostilbene has potent anti-myeloma activity in bortezomib-resistant cells. *Oncol. Rep.* **2017**, *38*, 488–496. [CrossRef] [PubMed]
126. Chen, R.J.; Ho, C.T.; Wang, Y.J. Pterostilbene induces autophagy and apoptosis in sensitive and chemoresistant human bladder cancer cells. *Mol. Nutr. Food Res.* **2010**, *54*, 1819–1832. [CrossRef] [PubMed]
127. McCormack, D.; McFadden, D. Pterostilbene and cancer: Current review. *J. Surg Res.* **2012**, *173*, e53–e61. [CrossRef] [PubMed]
128. Maurya, P.K. Health benefits of quercetin in age-related diseases. *Molecules* **2022**, *27*, 2498.
129. Alvarez, M.C.; Maso, V.; Torello, C.O.; Ferro, K.P.; Saad, S.T. The polyphenol quercetin induces cell death in leukemia by targeting epigenetic regulators of pro-apoptotic genes. *Clin. Epigenetics* **2018**, *10*, 139. [CrossRef] [PubMed]
130. Ononye, S.N.; VanHeyst, M.D.; Giardina, C.; Wright, D.L.; Anderson, A.C. Studies on the antiproliferative effects of tropolone derivatives in Jurkat T-lymphocyte cells. *Bioorg. Med. Chem.* **2014**, *22*, 2188–2193. [CrossRef]
131. Shanmugam, M.K.; Dai, X.; Kumar, A.P.; Tan, B.K.; Sethi, G.; Bishayee, A. Ursolic acid in cancer prevention and treatment: Molecular targets, pharmacokinetics and clinical studies. *Biochem. Pharmacol.* **2013**, *85*, 1579–1587. [CrossRef]
132. Zhang, C.; Wang, C.; Li, W.; Wu, R.; Guo, Y.; Cheng, D.; Yang, Y.; Androulakis, I.P.; Kong, A.N. Pharmacokinetics and Pharmacodynamics of the Triterpenoid Ursolic Acid in Regulating the Antioxidant, Anti-Inflammatory, and Epigenetic Gene Responses in Rat Leukocytes. *Mol. Pharm.* **2017**, *14*, 3709–3717. [CrossRef]
133. Dung, D.T.; Hang, D.T.; Yen, P.H.; Quang, T.H.; Nhiem, N.X.; Tai, B.H.; Minh, C.V.; Kim, Y.C.; Kim, D.C.; Oh, H.; et al. Macrocyclic bis-quinolizidine alkaloids from Xestospongia muta. *Nat. Prod. Res.* **2019**, *33*, 400–406. [CrossRef]
134. Yang, H.L.; Kumar, K.S.; Kuo, Y.T.; Chang, H.C.; Liao, J.W.; Hsu, L.S.; Hseu, Y.C. *Antrodia camphorata* induces G 1 cell-cycle arrest in human premyelocytic leukemia (HL-60) cells and suppresses tumor growth in athymic nude mice. *Food Funct.* **2014**, *5*, 2278–2288. [CrossRef] [PubMed]
135. Hseu, Y.C.; Yang, H.L.; Lai, Y.C.; Lin, J.G.; Chen, G.W.; Chang, Y.H. Induction of apoptosis by *Antrodia camphorata* in human premyelocytic leukemia HL-60 cells. *Nutr. Cancer* **2004**, *48*, 189–197. [CrossRef] [PubMed]
136. Bontempo, P.; Mita, L.; Miceli, M.; Doto, A.; Nebbioso, A.; De Bellis, F.; Conte, M.; Minichiello, A.; Manzo, F.; Carafa, V.; et al. *Feijoa sellowiana* derived natural Flavone exerts anti-cancer action displaying HDAC inhibitory activities. *Int. J. Biochem.* **2007**, *39*, 1902–1914. [CrossRef]
137. Gawlik-Dziki, U.; Świeca, M.; Dziki, D. Comparison of Phenolic Acids Profile and Antioxidant Potential of Six Varieties of Spelt (*Triticum spelta* L.). *J. Agric. Food Chem.* **2012**, *60*, 4603–4612. [CrossRef] [PubMed]
138. Fabiani, R.; Rosignoli, P.; De Bartolomeo, A.; Fuccelli, R.; Servili, M.; Montedoro, G.F.; Morozzi, G. Oxidative DNA damage is prevented by extracts of olive oil, hydroxytyrosol, and other olive phenolic compounds in human blood mononuclear cells and HL60 cells. *J. Nutr.* **2008**, *138*, 1411–1416. [CrossRef] [PubMed]

cancers

MDPI

Systematic Review

Camptothecin and Its Derivatives from Traditional Chinese Medicine in Combination with Anticancer Therapy Regimens: A Systematic Review and Meta-Analysis

Paul O. Odeniran [1], Paradise Madlala [2], Nompumelelo P. Mkhwanazi [2,*] and Mahmoud E. S. Soliman [3,*]

1 Department of Veterinary Parasitology and Entomology, University of Ibadan, Ibadan 200001, Nigeria; drpaulekode@gmail.com

2 HIV Pathogenesis Programme, School of Laboratory Medicine and Medical Science, The Doris Duke Medical Research Institute, University of KwaZulu-Natal, Durban 4000, South Africa

3 Molecular Bio-Computation and Drug Design Lab, School of Health Sciences, University of Kwazulu-Natal, Durban 4000, South Africa

* Correspondence: mkhwanazi@ukzn.ac.za (N.P.M.); soliman@ukzn.ac.za (M.E.S.S.); Tel.: +27-312604072 (N.P.M.); +27-312608019 (M.E.S.S.)

Simple Summary: This study aims to systematically assess the efficacy and safety of camptothecin derivative-based drug combinations, such as irinotecan and topotecan, in treating various cancers, including non-small cell lung cancer (NSCLC), colorectal cancer, oesophageal/gastric cancer, and small cell lung cancer. By reviewing phase II and III clinical trials, the research focused on comparing objective response rates (RR), survival outcomes, and toxicity profiles across different chemotherapy regimens. Findings highlight that irinotecan combined with cisplatin showed superior RR and progression-free survival in NSCLC, while bevacizumab-irinotecan combinations demonstrated better outcomes in colorectal cancer. The results from this meta-analysis may inform clinical decision-making, guiding oncologists toward more effective treatment combinations for different cancer types and improving patient outcomes.

Abstract: Background/Objectives: Camptothecin (CPT) and its derivatives, irinotecan and topotecan, are integral components of cancer chemotherapy, often used in combination therapies. This meta-analysis evaluates the efficacy of CPT-based combination treatments in cancer patients. **Methods**: We systematically searched the literature database using the Preferred Reporting Items for Systematic Reviews and Meta-Analyses checklist for articles published between 2000 and 2022. Published studies were retrieved through an electronic search on the Web of Science, PubMed, and Google Scholar databases. A total of 138 studies were downloaded and examined, and 71 eligible studies were selected for meta-analysis after excluding studies that did not meet the inclusion criteria. **Results**: Ultimately, a total of 71 studies were included in the analysis, comprising non-small cell lung cancer (NSCLC), colorectal cancer (COLRC), oesophageal/gastric cancer (O/GC), and small cell lung cancer (SCLC). For NSCLC, the objective response rate (RR) was 31.8% (95% CI: 27.3–37.1%, $p = 0.025$), with irinotecan plus cisplatin showing significantly higher efficacy compared to other irinotecan-based combinations. In COLRC, irinotecan and 5-fluorouracil/leucovorin plus bevacizumab demonstrated superior efficacy with a RR of 44% (95% CI: 34–58, $p < 0.001$) and minimal haematological toxicity. In O/GC, irinotecan-based combinations showed an average RR of 43% (95% CI: 27–70, $p < 0.001$) and average overall survival (OS) and progression-free survival (PFS) rates of 10.2 and 5.5 months, respectively. For SCLC, irinotecan-based combinations had a higher control response than topotecan-based ones, while the latter exhibited higher rates of stable and progressive disease. The overall RR for SCLC was 45% (95% CI: 34.3–60.2, $p < 0.001$). **Conclusions**: The existing evidence underscored the potential of CPT-based combination therapy in various cancers. Among the various combinations discussed in this analysis, irinotecan plus cisplatin demonstrated the highest objective RR in 12 trials focused on NSCLC. This study provides valuable insights into potential treatment strategies for various types of cancer, emphasising the importance of personalised and tailored approaches to maximise efficacy and minimise adverse effects.

Keywords: anticancer drugs; camptothecin derivatives; objective response; meta-analysis; combinational therapy

1. Introduction

Globally, cancer remains a significant health challenge, with nearly 10.0 million deaths and an estimated 19.3 million new cases reported in 2020 [1]. Female breast cancer ranks as the most diagnosed cancer, accounting for approximately 2.3 million new cases (11.7%), followed closely by lung (11.4%), colorectal (10.0%), prostate (7.3%), and stomach (5.6%) cancers. Despite advancements in treatment, lung cancer continues to be the leading cause of cancer-related deaths, claiming nearly 1.8 million lives (18%), followed by colorectal (9.4%), liver (8.3%), stomach (7.7%), and female breast (6.9%) cancers. Projections suggest a significant rise in cancer cases by 2040, with an anticipated 28.4 million new cases globally, representing a 47% increase from 2020 [1]. In 2020, lung cancer accounted for 2.21 million new cases and resulted in 1.8 million deaths globally. The age-standardised incidence rate stood at 22.4 per 100,000 individuals, with a higher incidence among males (31.5 per 100,000) than females (14.6 per 100,000). Similarly, the age-standardised mortality rates were 18.0 per 100,000 overall, with males experiencing a higher mortality rate (25.9 per 100,000) compared to females (11.2 per 100,000) [2]. This meta-analysis investigates the effective treatment combinations for different cancer types using camptothecin (CPT) and its derivatives from traditional Chinese medicine (TCM).

The utilisation of complementary and alternative medicines (CAMs) among cancer patients has increased in popularity. Notably, studies indicate that approximately one-third of individuals diagnosed with cancer incorporate CAMs into their treatment regimen [3]. Over the past five decades, extensive clinical research has highlighted the potential benefits of TCM in cancer therapy. Evidence suggests that TCM may reduce treatment-related toxicity, enhance the effectiveness of radiotherapy and chemotherapy, prolong survival in advanced cancer patients, and aid in preventing and managing recurrence and metastasis [4]. Given its widespread use, further research is imperative to elucidate TCM's clinical efficacy and safety profile in cancer management.

Camptothecin, derived from *Camptotheca acuminata*, a tree native to China and a recognised traditional Chinese medicine, garnered interest in cancer treatment research in the late 1950s and mid to late 1960s [5]. Despite its potent anticancer properties, CPT's unpredictable pharmacological behaviour and adverse effects (AEs) hampered its clinical success. Efforts to enhance CPT's pharmacological profile and reduce side effects led to the development of semi-synthetic and synthetic analogues [6]. Topotecan and irinotecan, the first Food and Drug Administration-approved analogues, are now widely used in chemotherapy. Irinotecan is indicated for metastatic colorectal carcinoma, while topotecan serves as a second-line treatment for ovarian and small cell lung cancer [6]. The incorporation of front-line chemotherapy in cancer treatment strategies has expanded, particularly for advanced disease stages, through multimodal approaches [7]. Numerous clinical trials spanning five decades have explored CPT derivatives in cancer treatment. Previous studies have focused on the pharmacological profile, clinical evaluations, structural modifications, and therapeutic efficacy of CPT and its various forms [8–10]. However, no study has conducted a detailed, case-by-case clinical analysis of CPT analogues to thoroughly assess their combinational efficacy and identify the most suitable options for specific cancer therapies. This comprehensive meta-analysis aims to systematically assess the efficacy and safety of CPT derivative-based combinations in clinical trial settings, offering insights into their role in cancer therapy and the best choices at clinicians' disposal.

2. Methods

2.1. Literature Searches

The study adhered to the Preferred Reporting Items for Systematic Reviews and Meta-Analyses criteria (PRISMA) [11] to ensure comprehensive inclusion of relevant data. A systematic literature search was conducted across multiple databases, including Web of Science, PubMed, and Google Scholar. Key search terms such as "camptothecin", "irinotecan", "topotecan", "response rate", "cancer", "colorectal", "gastric," "oesophagus", "small cell", "non-small cell", "lung cancer", and "stomach" were employed.

Only studies published between January 2000 and December 2022 were considered, and inclusion criteria stipulated that articles must have full texts or abstracts available in English. Trials must be completed within the specified timeframe, objective response rates (RR) must be reported, clear details on the chemotherapeutic regimen must be provided, and a sample size of at least 10 must be used for statistical analysis. Articles lacking these characteristics were excluded from the study. The systematic review followed the recommendations of the PRISMA in Table S1 (Prisma 2020 checklist). The protocol has not been registered.

2.2. Quality of the Studies

The risk of bias within the included studies was assessed using a quality evaluation checklist based on criteria earlier outlined [12]. Each item was rated as yes, no, or uncertain and graded on a scale from 1 to 10. The checklist covered the following topics: clarity of study objectives, mention of therapy duration, documentation of gender distribution, mention of previous treatment, disclosure of sample size and RR, evaluation of progression-free and patient survival times, specification of substance class, division of examined subjects into subgroups, accurate description of therapy duration, and mention of patients' performance status. These criteria were employed to systematically assess the quality and potential biases within the selected studies.

2.3. Data Extraction

Study characteristics (first author's name, year of publication, impact factor, response rate, including control response (CR), partial response (PR), stable disease (SD), and progression disease (PD)); median age, prior therapies, toxicity effects, survival time, progression-free survival, performance status, and overall survival time (Supplementary File S1) were all noted.

2.4. Statistical Analysis

To evaluate the efficacy of cancer chemotherapy, the primary outcome measure utilised was the objective RR, presented alongside its corresponding 95% confidence interval (95% CI). All descriptive analyses employed 95% confidence intervals, while the raw data were processed in Microsoft Excel. In certain instances, standard deviation (StD) and standard error of the mean (SEM) were also examined. The objective response encompasses control and partial response, whereas the disease control rate incorporates control response, partial response, and stable disease. These metrics provide valuable insights into the effectiveness of cancer chemotherapeutic interventions. The response rate from each trial was combined using the Microsoft Excel meta-analysis program METAXL version 3.1 [13,14]. The quality effects model computed the estimated response rate and 95% confidence intervals (CI). According to this model's quality ratings, research is ranked according to its quality and sample size [13]. Prevalence information was taken from various sub-group analyses. I2 (degree of inconsistency) was used to evaluate heterogeneity in the study (Cochran's Q). According to Barendregt and Doi [14], the I2 values of 25%, 50%, and 75% indicated low, moderate, and high degrees of heterogeneity, respectively. Both Doi plots and funnel plots were used to evaluate the risk of bias. According to Barendregt and Doi [14], a Luis Frya-Kanamori (LFK) score greater than 2 denotes significant asymmetry (publication bias). Plotting the z-score versus double arcs in the prevalence of the analysed publications yields the LFK index. The total number of sampled population ($n - 1$), where "n" is the sample population, is denoted by the degree of freedom (df) in the text.

3. Results

3.1. Meta-Analysis Trial Flow

The literature database searches yielded 2257 articles, including references from relevant studies (Figure 1). After diligent observation, 1051 studies were removed as they were unrelated to the subject being considered. Thereafter, 1019 articles were excluded based on screening titles and abstracts from the initial 1206 records. Additionally, 49 duplicate studies were identified. Upon review of the full texts of the remaining articles, 67 did not meet the inclusion criteria out of the 138 downloaded. Ultimately, 71 studies were included in the analysis, comprising 23 for NSCLC, 14 for colorectal cancer (COLRC), 5 for oesophageal/gastric cancer (O/GC), and 29 for SCLC.

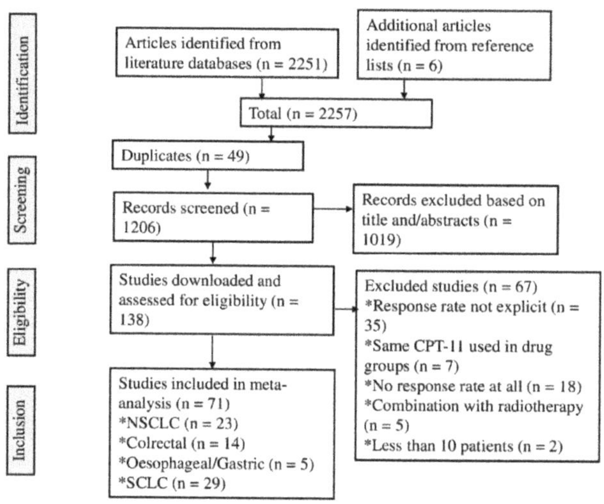

Figure 1. Flow diagram on the exclusion and inclusion of articles in a systematic approach for the camptothecin derivative-based combinations on some specific cancer treatments.

Non-Small Cell Lung Cancer (NSCLC) Analysis with Irinotecan-Based Combinations

The objective response rate in studies focusing on non-small cell lung cancer was determined to be 31.8% (n = 23 studies), based on 1092 individuals assessed for response (Figure 2). The overall pooled control response rates for CR, PR, SD, and PD were calculated as follows: CR = 0.15 (StD = 0.6708, SEM = 0.15), PR = 13.6 (StD = 10.84, SEM = 2.42), SD = 18.3 (StD = 10.70, SEM = 2.52), and PD = 13 (StD = 9.35, SEM = 2.20), respectively (Figure 3). The overall analysis revealed heterogeneity among the studies (RR = 31.8%, 95% CI: 27.3–37.1%, I2 = 40.8%, Cochran's Q = 35.5, p = 0.025, df = 21, Q-index = 15.0).

3.2. NSCLC Study Analyses

The average median age across the studies examined was 62 years (df = 19). The one-year overall survival rate (OS), as observed in four studies, was determined to be 22.2% (17.1–28.1). Evaluating the overall statuses of the examined studies based on the Eastern Cooperative Oncology Group Performance Status (ECOG), the results were as follows: ECOG 0 = 30.0% (95% CI: 26.3–33.9, StD = 0.1276, SEM = 0.0191); ECOG 1 = 60.0% (95% CI: 55.9–64.1, StD = 0.1419, SEM = 0.020); and ECOG 2 = 12.2% (95% CI: 9.9–14.8, StD = 0.074, SEM = 0.0119). Patients with an ECOG status of IIIB (24.7%) showed significantly lower rates compared to those with IV status (74.5%) ($\chi^2 = 507.5$; $p < 0.0001$). Recurrent patients accounted for 0.8% of the total. The median survival time estimated across 20 studies was

10.5 months, while the average progression-free survival time, evaluable in 15 studies, was 4.9 months. Toxicity reports were limited to patients experiencing grade III and IV AEs. The observed AEs and their respective percentages (with 95% CI and sample sizes) were as follows: nausea (13.5%, 95% CI: 11.1–16.2, n = 98/727, df = 14), diarrhoea (15.6%, 95% CI: 13.2–18.3, n = 129/826, df = 16), neutropenia (39.3%, 95% CI: 35.9–42.8, n = 311/791, df = 17), anaemia (12.2%, 95% CI: 9.9–14.7, n = 92/755, df = 16), leukopenia (22.0%, 95% CI: 18.1–26.4, n = 91/413, df = 7), anorexia (25.0%, 95% CI: 16.4–35.4, n = 22/88, df = 1), thrombocytopenia (12.1%, 95% CI: 9.8–14.7, n = 87/718, df = 14), fatigue (8.1%, 95% CI: 5.4–11.4, n = 27/335, df = 6), and vomiting (9.9%, 95% CI: 5.4–16.4, n = 13/131, df = 2).

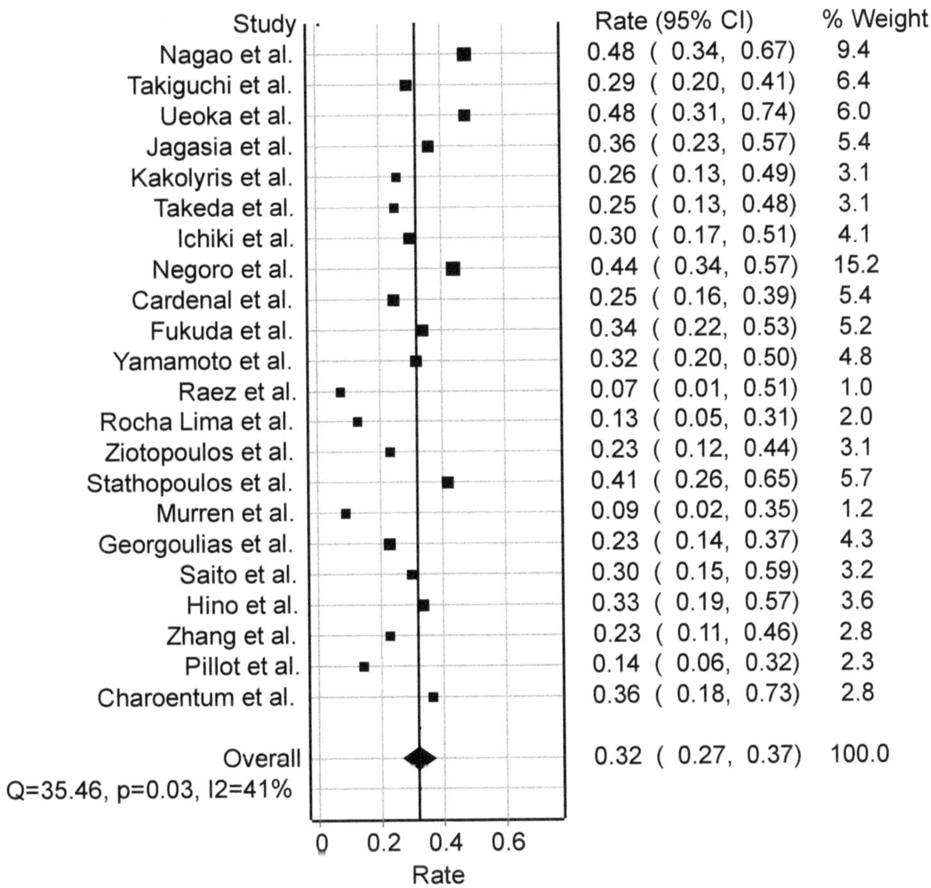

Figure 2. Forest plot of studies on NSCLC among 1092 patients (Georgoulias [7], Nagao [15], Takiguchi [16], Ueoka [17], Jagasia [18], Kakolyris [19], Takeda [20], Ichiki [21], Negoro [22], Cardenal [23], Fukuda [24], Yamamoto [25], Raez [26], Rocha Lima [27], Ziotopoulos [28], Stathopoulos [29], Murren [30], Saito [31], Hino [32], Zhang [33], Pillot [34], Charoentum [35]). Abbreviations: NSCLC, non-small cell lung cancer; Q, measure of heterogeneity; p, p-value; I2, degree of inconsistency; CI, confidence interval.

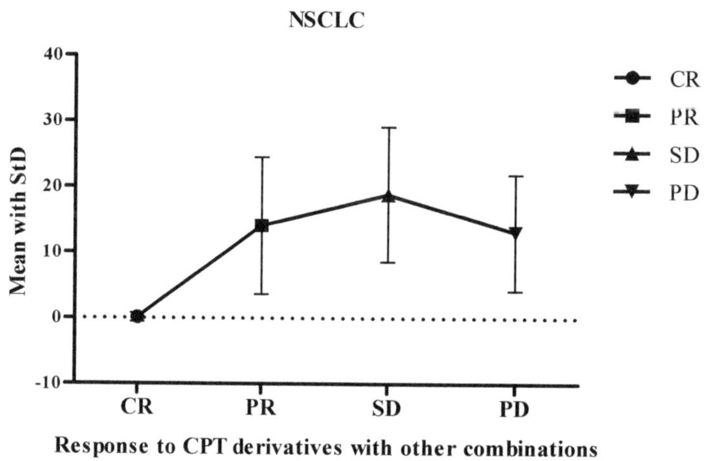

Figure 3. Responses to irinotecan combinations against NSCLC from patient metadata. Abbreviations: CPT, camptothecin; CR, control response; NSCLC, non-small cell lung cancer; PD, progressive disease; PR, partial response; SD, stable disease; StD, standard deviation.

3.3. Irinotecan Drug Combinations and Responses

More studies were observed investigating the combination of irinotecan plus cisplatin against NSCLC compared to other drug combinations, as shown in Table 1. The average objective response rate was also higher in the irinotecan plus cisplatin combination compared to other combinations. The RR analysis indicated that irinotecan plus cisplatin had a significantly higher response rate compared to combinations such as irinotecan plus gemcitabine, irinotecan plus docetaxel, and irinotecan plus carboplatin, but not significantly different ($p > 0.05$) from others like irinotecan plus paclitaxel and irinotecan plus ifosfamide. The median age of patients during chemotherapy was statistically similar across all combinations and did not appear to affect the efficacy of the drugs. Survival analysis revealed that irinotecan plus gemcitabine and irinotecan plus paclitaxel had the lowest OS compared to other irinotecan combinations in the studies that reported higher OS, while irinotecan plus docetaxel exhibited the highest OS. Additionally, progression-free survival (PFS) was notably higher for irinotecan plus cisplatin and irinotecan plus carboplatin than other combinations.

Table 1. Irinotecan-based combinations of chemotherapeutic effects on NSCLC patients.

Combinational Therapy	No. of Studies	Patients Investigated	Average RR%	Average DCR%	Median Age	OS	PFS
IRI + CIS	12	693	34.1	66.8	61	10.5	5.5
IRI + CAR	3	137	25.6	72.3	65	10.6	5.5
IRI + DOC	3	110	25.5	61.8	61	10.8	3.5
IRI + PAC	2	69	30.4	66.7	62	9.2	4.4
IRI + GEM	1	39	12.8	71.8	63	8	3.5
IRI + IFO	1	44	29.5	88.6	65	12.5	5.3

Abbreviations: NSCLC, non-small cell lung cancer; IRI, irinotecan; CIS, cisplastin; CAR, carboplatin; DOC, docetaxel; PAC, paclitaxel; GEM, gemcitabine; IFO, ifosfamide; OS, overall survival rate; PFS, progression-free survival rate.

3.4. Drug Toxicity Among Patients in Grades III and IV

For all irinotecan combinations used against NSCLC, neutropenia is the most severe drug toxicity observed in all the irinotecan-based combinations (Table 2). The low toxicity observed in irinotecan *plus* ifosfamide could be due to only one study examined in that group.

Table 2. Non-haematologic and haematologic responses to irinotecan-based combinations on NSCLC patients.

Combinational Therapy	Toxicity (%)					
	Nausea	Diarrhoea	Anaemia	Neutropenia	Leucopenia	Thrombo
IRI + CIS	19.6	19.6	10.5	37.9	17.2	9.7
IRI + CAR	10.1	7.9	27.3	63.3	35.1	33.1
IRI + DOC	0.0	16.9	3.8	26.4	N/A	0.0
IRI + PAC	1.3	7.6	7.6	20.3	N/A	1.8
IRI + GEM	17.9	N/A	5.1	25.6	12.8	2.6
IRI + IFO	0.0	6.8	4.5	38.6	27.3	0.0

Abbreviations: NSCLC, non-small cell lung cancer; IRI, irinotecan; CIS, cisplastin; CAR, carboplatin; DOC, docetaxel; PAC, paclitaxel; GEM, gemcitabine; IFO, ifosfamide; thrombo, thrombocytopenia.

3.5. Colorectal Cancer

The objective response rate of camptothecin derivatives with or without other drugs against COLRC demonstrates a pooled rate of 44% (95%CI: 34–58) (Figure 4), encompassing 2018 patients. However, the analysis indicates significant heterogeneity between studies (Q = 129.2; p = 0.001; I2 = 90%). The breakdown of response categories reveals a CR of 4.0% (95%CI: 3.2–5.0), PR at 35.4% (95%CI: 33.3–37.6), SD at 30.6% (95%CI: 28.5–32.8), and PD at 20.5% (95%CI: 18.6–22.4). The median age of the examined studies is 63 years. The OS stands at 19.1 months, while PFS is estimated at 10.1 months across the studies. Notably, approximately 49.1% (95CI: 46.0–52.2) of patients exhibit metastases at one site, 34.6% (95%CI: 30.8–38.4) at two sites, and 18.4% (95%CI: 15.5–21.5) at more than two sites. Considering the performance status of patients, ECOG 0 is reported in 66.1% (95%CI: 63.4–68.7, n = 9 studies), ECOG 1 in 36.9% (95%CI: 33.9–40.0, n = 8 studies), and ECOG 2 in 4.5% (95%CI: 3.1–6.4, n = 6 studies).

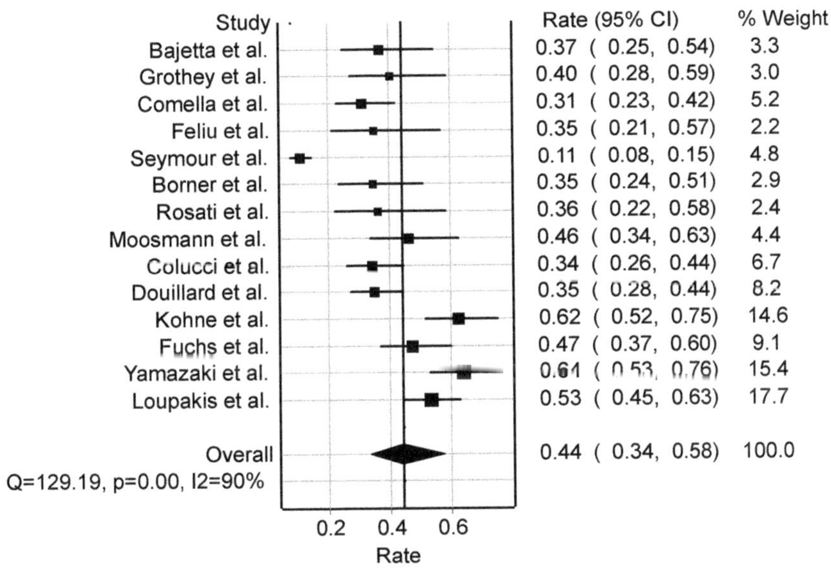

Figure 4. Forest plot of studies on COLRC among 2018 patients using camptothecin-based derivatives with other drugs (Bajetta [36], Grothey [37], Comella [38], Feliu [39], Seymour [40], Borner [41], Rosati [42], Moosmann [43], Colucci [44], Douillard [45], Kohne [46], Fuchs [47], Yamazaki [48], Loupakis [49]). Abbreviations: COLRC, colorectal cancer; Q, measure of heterogeneity; p, p-value; I2, degree of inconsistency; CI, confidence interval.

3.6. Irinotecan-Based Combinations Response

Most studies focused on folinic acid (also known as leucovorin, calcium folinate, or FA), fluorouracil (also known as 5FU), and irinotecan (FOLFIRI) combinations for the treatment of COLRC. Notably, combining bevacizumab with irinotecan and 5-fluorouracil/leucovorin (FOLFIRI) demonstrated significantly higher OS, PFS, RR, and disease control rate (DCR) comparable safety profiles (Table 3). Among irinotecan-based regimens for first-line metastatic COLRC, an infusion schedule of fluorouracil (FU) should be preferred.

Table 3. Irinotecan-based combinations' chemotherapeutic effects on COLRC patients.

Combinational Therapy	No. of Studies	Patients Investigated	Average RR%	Average DCR%	Median Age	OS	PFS
FOLFIRI	4	686	44.5	74.5	61	18.7	7.5
CAPIRI	3	189	37.0	73.0	74	14	7.5
BEVFOLFIRI	2	441	57.6	88.0	61	28.6	10.9

Abbreviations: COLRC, colorectal cancer; FOLFIRI, folinic acid + fluorouracil + irinotecan; CAPIRI, capecitabine + irinotecan; BEVFOLFIRI, bevacizumab + folinic acid + fluorouracil + irinotecan; DCR, disease control rate; OS, overall survival rate; PFS, progression-free survival rate.

3.7. Drug Toxicity

The toxicity was only for grade III and IV patients, with severity signs of anaemia, neutropenia, and leucopenia, most pronounced with patients treated with BEVFOLFIRI. Diarrhoea and vomiting were most severe with CAPIRI (Table 4). In all the analyses, AEs between FOLFIRI and CAPIRI were comparable, as patients' reactions were similar.

Table 4. Non-haematologic and haematologic responses to irinotecan-based combinations on COLRC patients.

	Toxicity (%)					
	Nausea	Diarrhoea	Anaemia	Neutropenia	Leukopaenia	Vomiting
FOLFIRI	3.8	13.7	1.3	20.4	5.0	5.0
CAPIRI	N/A	28.7	6.4	16.4	N/A	6.4
BEVFOLFIRI	4.7	9.8	45.1	31.4	11.3	3.8
	Common treatment plans across studies					
FOLFIRI	FA 500 mg/m^2 as a 2 h infusion and FU 2.6 g/m^2 by intravenous 24 h infusion, irinotecan 80 mg/m^2					
CAPIRI	Irinotecan 80 mg/m^2 i.v. days 1 and 8 and capecitabine 1000 mg/m^2 orally b.i.d. days 1–14; q21d					
BEVFOLFIRI	Bevacizumab (5 mg/kg) followed by FOLFIRI (irinotecan 150–180 mg/m^2; leucovorin 200 mg/m^2; i.v. bolus of fluorouracil 400 mg/m^2, continuous infusion of fluorouracil 2400 mg/m^2)					

Abbreviations: COLRC, colorectal cancer; FOLFIRI, folinic acid + fluorouracil + irinotecan; CAPIRI, capecitabine + irinotecan; BEVFOLFIRI, bevacizumab + folinic acid + fluorouracil + irinotecan.

3.8. Oesophageal/Gastric Cancer

The pooled rate from six studies on the effect of irinotecan-based chemotherapy with other drug combinations revealed a response rate of 43% (95%CI: 27–70) among 355 patients (Figure 5). The most common regimen across studies is FOLFIRI (LV 200 mg/m^2 i.v. followed by FU 400 mg/m^2–600 mg/m^2 i.v. on days 1 and 2 every 14 days plus irinotecan 180 mg/m^2). The study showed heterogeneity (Q = 24.6, p < 0.0001, I2 = 84%) (Figure 5). Observed responses across studies include CR = 2.2%, PR = 36.2%, SD = 27.0%, and PD = 20.5%. The overall median age was 63.4 years in the five studies. A total of 16.8% of 137 patients have prior surgical resection before chemotherapy. Based on performance status, ECOG 0 = 70.6%, ECOG 1 = 27.2%, and ECOG 2 = 2.2%. The median survival time was 10.2 months, while progression-free survival time was 5.5 months. Based on metastatic sites, patients with one organ metastatic sites were 39.7% (95%CI: 33.8–45.8), and two organs were 39.0% (95%CI: 33.1–45.1). while greater than two organs were 21.3% (95%CI: 17.0–26.8). Effects of toxicity were reported in nausea 10.3% (95%CI: 7.4–14.0), diarrhoea

22.4% (95%CI: 18.1–27.0), stomatitis 4.7% (95%CI: 2.4–8.0), anaemia 12.1 (95%CI: 8.7–16.2), neutropenia 26.3% (95%CI: 21.8–31.1), leukopaenia 14.6% (95%CI: 10.1–20.0), anorexia 5.6% (95%CI: 3.2–9.0), and vomiting 7.8% (95%CI: 3.5–14.9).

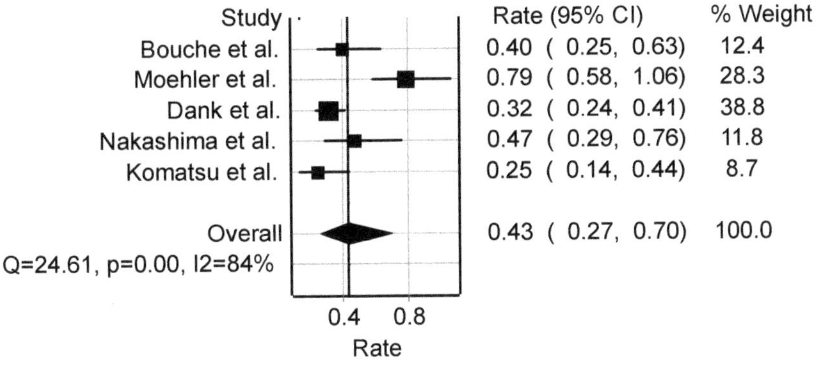

Figure 5. Forest plot of studies conducted on oesophageal/gastric cancer (Bouche [50], Moehler [51], Dank [52], Nakashima [53], Komatsu [54]). Abbreviations: Q, measure of heterogeneity; *p*, *p*-value; I2, degree of inconsistency; CI, confidence interval.

3.9. Small Cell Lung Cancer (SCLC)

From 2002 to 2022, the chemotherapeutic treatment of small cell lung cancer (SCLC) predominantly involved two major camptothecin-based drugs: irinotecan and topotecan, either administered alone or in combination with other drugs. A forest plot analysis revealed a pooled overall response rate of 45.4% (95%CI: 34.3–60.2) across 28 studies involving 2704 patients (Figure 6). However, notable asymmetry and heterogeneity were observed among the studies (Q = 309.4, $p < 0.001$, I2 = 91%) (Figure 6). Specifically, the SCLC analysis indicated control response rates of 4.0% (95%CI: 3.3–4.9), partial response rates of 32.7% (95%CI: 30.8–34.8), stable disease rates of 24.3% (95%CI: 22.5–26.1), and progressive disease rates of 16.0% (95%CI: 15.0–17.6). The median age across all 29 studies encompassing 2704 patients was 64 years. Performance status assessed by the Eastern Cooperative Oncology Group (ECOG) revealed ECOG 0 at 27.2% (95%CI: 25.0–29.6), ECOG 1 at 64.3% (95%CI: 61.8–66.8), and ECOG 2 at 8.8% (95%CI: 7.4–10.4). The median survival time across all SCLC studies was 8.9 months, with a progression-free survival of 4.5 months. Notably, 46.4% (95%CI: 42.5–50.3) of patients had undergone prior radiotherapy, while surgical resection was reported in 14.9% (95%CI: 10.6–20.1) from two studies. The analysis of toxicity revealed varying incidences, including nausea (7.5%), diarrhoea (10.6%), anaemia (22.8%), neutropenia (51.0%), leukopenia (41.7%), anorexia (3.1%), thrombocytopenia (32.0%), fatigue (15.2%), and vomiting (5.1%).

3.10. Comparison of Topotecan-Based Combinations with Irinotecan-Based Combinations Against SCLC from 29 Studies Analysed

A total of 14 and 16 studies investigated the efficacy of topotecan and irinotecan-based combinations in chemotherapy for SCLC. The average response rate was significantly higher in studies utilising irinotecan than those employing topotecan. However, there was no significant difference in the DCR. The median age was comparable between the two groups. Overall survival rate and PFS were higher in irinotecan-based combinations. Drug response analysis revealed a higher control response in irinotecan-based combinations compared to topotecan, although the difference was not significant. Additionally, partial response was significantly higher in irinotecan-based combinations than topotecan (Table 5). Conversely, topotecan-based combinations exhibited a higher rate of stable disease and progressive disease, statistically significant compared to irinotecan-based combinations. Toxicity analysis indicated that irinotecan-based combinations had a greater impact on non-haematological parameters such as anaemia and diarrhoea, while topotecan-based combinations showed higher effects on haematological parameters.

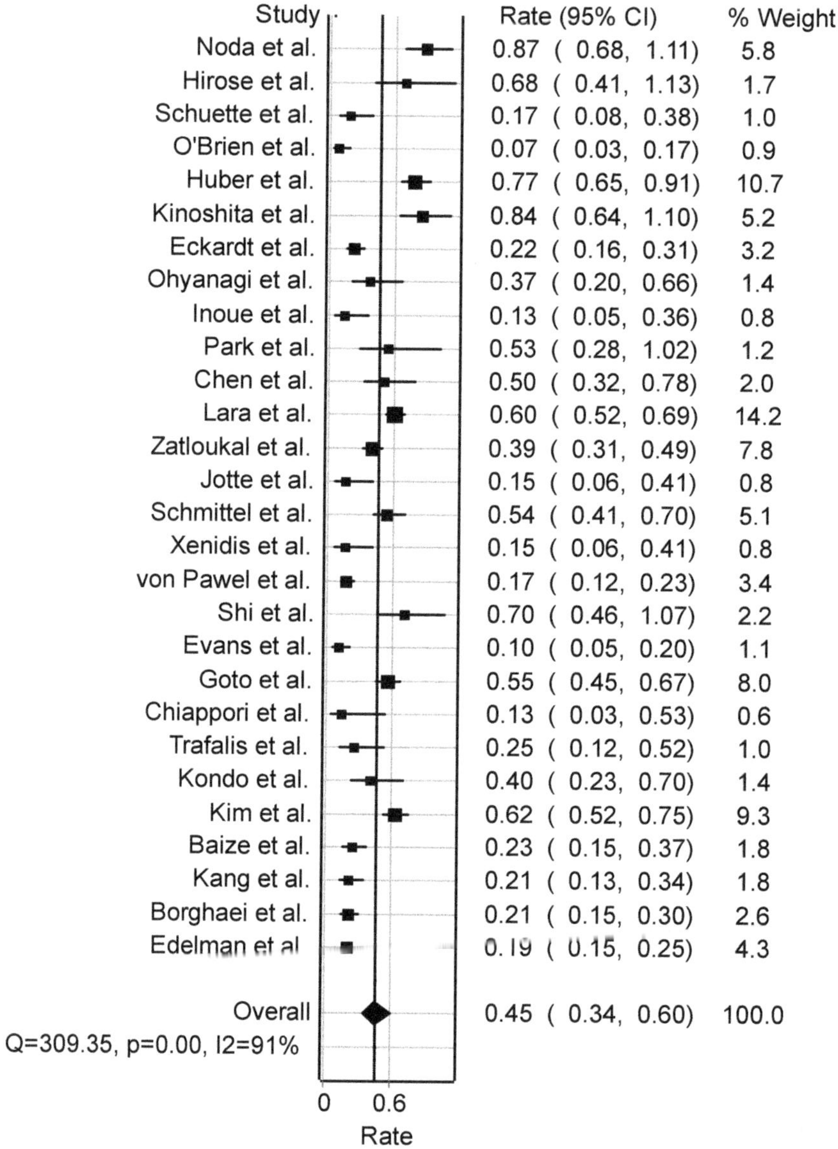

Figure 6. Forest plot of studies on SCLC patients (Noda [55], Hirose [56], Schuette [57], O'Brien [58], Huber [59], Kinoshita [60], Eckardt [61], Ohyanagi [62], Inoue [63], Park [64], Chen [65], Lara [66], Zatloukal [67], Jotte [68], Schmittel [69], Xenidis [70], von Pawel [71], Shi [72], Evans [73], Goto [74], Chiappori [75], Trafalis [76], Kondo [77], Kim [78], Baize [79], Kang [80], Borghaei [81], Edelman [82]). Abbreviations: SCLC, small cell lung cancer; Q, measure of heterogeneity; *p*, *p*-value; I2, degree of inconsistency; CI, confidence interval.

Table 5. Comparison of camptothecin derivative-based combinations on SCLC patients.

Camptothecin Derivatives with/Without Other Drugs Class Against SCLC								
Drug of Interest	**No of Studies**	**Patients Investigated**	**Average RR%, X^2, p**		**Average DCR%**	**Median Age (Yrs)**	**PFS (Months)**	**OS (Months)**
Topotecan combination	14	1251	26.8	177.2, $p < 0.00$	64.5	63	3.8	7.0
Irinotecan combination	16	1453	52.0 *		74.5	64	5.0	10.3

Responses (%, X^2, p_{value})							
	CR	PR		SD		PD	
Topotecan combination	3.7	25.0	126.8, $p < 0.00$	32.9 *	14.8, $p < 0.00$	25.8 *	87.8, $p < 0.00$
Irinotecan combination	5.5	50.3 *		24.4		10.6	

Toxicity (%, X^2, p_{value})											
	Nausea		Diarrhoea		Anaemia		Neutropenia		Leukopaenia	THROMB	
Topotecan combination	1.5	37.7, $p < 0.00$	1.9	66.5, $p < 0.00$	27.2 *	13.6, $p < 0.00$	67.4 *	115.8, $p < 0.00$	45.1	39.4 *	20.9, $p < 0.00$
Irinotecan combination	10.0 *		14.5 *		20.1		42.8		39.7	24.7	

* $p < 0.001$. Abbreviations: SCLC, small cell lung cancer; p, p value; X^2, chi-square; THROMB, thrombocytopenia; RR, response rate; DCR, disease control rate; PFS, progression-free survival rate; CR, control response; PR, partial response; SD, stable disease; PD, progressive disease.

3.11. Sensitivity Test on Analysis

For sensitivity tests of each MetaXL analysis, the stability and dependability of the processed articles were assessed. The Doi plot (LFK index) used for sensitivity analysis eliminated any chance of major bias in the study. NSCLC provides an LFK index of −3.17, colorectal cancer analysis shows −2.07, O/GC LFK index is −0.30, and SCLC analysis LFK index shows −4.95. All except O/GC analysis show major asymmetry.

4. Discussion

The meta-analysis focused on phase II and III studies investigating the efficacy of irinotecan and topotecan in combination with other drugs (such as cisplatin, carboplatin, fluorouracil, etc.) across four cancer types (SCLC, NSCLC, COLRC, and O/GC), with a total cohort of 6169 patients.

Irinotecan-based regimens, augmented with additional medications, predominated in the treatment of NSCLC, yielding an average RR of 32%. However, the CR rate was notably low, with less than 0.2% reported across 23 studies. Notably, irinotecan administration has been linked to suboptimal CR outcomes, particularly in patients classified as grade IV [26,30,34]. The analysis underscored the significant incidence of severe AEs, encompassing haematologic and non-haematologic manifestations commonly associated with CPT chemotherapies [82,83]. Irinotecan plus cisplatin had the best OS and PFS time, which could be why more studies were conducted on this combination for NSCLC. The analysis revealed that irinotecan plus cisplatin demonstrated the highest objective RR among the combinations studied in 12 trials focused on NSCLC (Table 1). While irinotecan plus ifosfamide exhibited the highest DCR%, its relatively low RR% might deter its widespread use. Notably, the chemotherapy regimen comprising irinotecan plus cisplatin consistently outperformed other combinational regimens across multiple parameters, including objective response rate, median time to tumour progression, median survival time, and 1-year survival in the studies analysed for NSCLC. This suggests that the irinotecan plus cisplatin combination may be the preferred treatment option among the examined regimens.

In studies involving metastatic COLRC patients, phase III randomised trials indicated improved PFS with CPT derivative-based combination therapies. Notably, CAPIRI and FOLFIRI emerged as the most frequently utilised drugs, according to literature databases. Compared to other combination therapies, BEVFOLFIRI exhibited superior OS and PFS. However, inconsistencies in OS and PFS observed in studies focusing on FOLFIRI may be attributed to data from phase II trials [47]. Overall, no significant difference was observed in the RR and DCR between FOLFIRI and CAPIRI. The enhanced outcomes associated with

BEVFOLFIRI may be attributed to including Bevacizumab, a monoclonal antibody known for inhibiting the formation of blood vessels crucial for cancer growth. Additionally, the higher dose of irinotecan (150–180 mg/m^2) in BEVFOLFIRI compared to other regimens may contribute to its efficacy. Notably, severe AEs such as anaemia and neutropenia were more pronounced with BEVFOLFIRI, while CAPIRI was associated with more severe diarrhoea compared to previous medication options. The high proportion of patients with an ECOG performance status of zero (66.1%) suggests that a more intensive treatment regimen may be feasible without compromising patient selection criteria. Overall survival notably improved, underscoring the importance of incorporating irinotecan into the treatment regimen. Esteemed guidelines and established data advocate for a maintenance phase and continuum of care for individuals grappling with metastatic colorectal cancer [84–86].

The reviewed trials demonstrated objective response rates (RR) falling within the reported range (25–79%) for phase II and III investigations in O/GC. While one study encompassed both stomach and oesophageal cancer, four studies focused solely on gastric cancer. These irinotecan-based combinations show promise, as evidenced by the average OS and PFS rates of 10.2 and 5.5 months, respectively. A detailed examination reveals a low CR rate with a moderately robust partial response, consistent with prior research findings [87–89]. With oncologists prioritising the extension of meaningful survival, consideration of treatment-related toxicity is imperative. Patients with shorter survival times and/or disease progression often experience a diminished quality of life, potentially impacting the reliability of the LFK index analyses due to varying RR reports across sub-groups. Irinotecan, etoposide, and 5-FU/LV exhibited safety profiles commensurate with the observed toxicities in this trial overall. Notably, the FOLFIRI combination demonstrated minimal and acceptable incidences of haematological toxicity, rendering it well tolerated. Gastrointestinal toxicity, a known side effect of FOLFIRI therapy, may necessitate hospitalisation and immediate medical attention [45]. However, overall toxicity reports may be lower compared to other studies, possibly attributable to the inclusion of studies employing weekly irinotecan (80 mg/m^2) alongside an AIO-based regimen of 24 h high-dose 5-FU (2300 mg/m^2) preceded by 2 h LV 500 mg/m^2, with 44% of patients experiencing grade III/IV [45].

In small cell lung cancer (SCLC) studies, irinotecan-based combinations demonstrated significantly longer overall survival than topotecan-based combinations. These trials primarily enrolled patients with relapsed SCLC, predominantly with favourable Eastern Cooperative Oncology Group (ECOG) statuses. Predominantly phase II cases with substantial objective response rates underscore the efficacy of salvage chemotherapy with irinotecan. Notably, other parameters, including disease control rate, were comparable, suggesting both combinations as viable options. The heightened AEs on haematological parameters observed with topotecan could be linked to the prevalent topotecan dose of 1.5 mg/m^2 in most patients, representing an overdose, particularly in relapsed SCLC patients, thereby depleting bone marrow reserves. This study revealed significantly higher levels of anaemia, neutropenia, and leucopenia than irinotecan-based combinations. Notably, some authors have explored trials employing lower dose ranges of 1.0–1.25 mg/m^2 [59]. Irinotecan-based combinations were predominantly paired with cisplatin, etoposide, carboplatin, and bevacizumab. However, cisplatin-based combinations emerged as the most frequently observed and demonstrated superior efficacy compared to topotecan-based combinations. Additionally, the overall toxicity profile favoured irinotecan-based combinations. These findings align with previous meta-analyses suggesting that topotecan-based therapy does not outperform other agents in relapsed SCLC. However, weak evidence indicates its inferiority to platinum-based combinations in sensitive diseases [90]. Previous research has shown that the irinotecan and cisplatin combination was unsuccessful in phase III trials conducted in SCLC patients from the USA, Canada, the Republic of Korea, and Australia [66,78,91]. The study's limitations included missing data in some studies, preventing a comprehensive analysis. For example, the impact of pharmacogenetics on treatment outcomes and specific details regarding first-line treatments were not available in cases where the studies only reported on second-line treatments. Advances in targeted drug delivery systems—particularly those employing nanotechnology and sophisticated combinational formulations—offer promising solutions to longstanding challenges with CPT bioavailability and delivery. Despite these obstacles, CPT derivatives show immense promise as cancer therapies due to their strong cytotoxic effects on cancer cells. Extensive efforts have been devoted to optimising CPT derivatives through structural modifications to gain mechanistic insights, developing innovative targeted delivery systems to enhance CPT's pharmacological properties, and overcoming existing limitations [9,10]. This meta-analysis offers critical insights into irinotecan-based chemotherapy, highlighting considerable efficacy in NSCLC with an objective response rate of 31.8% across 23 studies. Irinotecan combined with cisplatin consistently demonstrated superior response rates compared to alternative drug pairings, supporting its preferential use for NSCLC. Despite significant heterogeneity and asymmetry across studies, the results affirm irinotecan's efficacy in improving progression-free survival, particularly with combinations involving cisplatin and carboplatin. However, elevated toxicity, especially neutropenia, necessitates cautious clinical application. For COLRC and SCLC, irinotecan with bevacizumab and fluorouracil showed optimal survival benefits, but toxicity risks remain a significant challenge. Likewise, the combination therapy of irinotecan with folinic acid and fluorouracil proved most effective for treating O/GC. This review explains the need for tailored therapeutic strategies to balance efficacy and safety across cancer types.

5. Conclusions

In conclusion, trials involving camptothecin derivative-based combinations are ongoing and remain the standard treatment regime for cancer therapy. The future of cancer treatment is poised for significant advancements through several emerging trends. Genomic, proteomic, and pharmacogenomic innovations will enable personalised treatments based on individual tumours' genetic and molecular profiles. Immunotherapy and the application of artificial intelligence and machine learning in analysing large datasets from clinical trials and genetic studies will enhance treatment precision. Liquid biopsies will improve early detection and real-time monitoring of cancer progression. Clustered, regularly interspaced short palindromic repeats and other gene-editing technologies hold promise for correcting cancer-driving mutations. Combination therapies, integrating modalities like chemotherapy, immunotherapy, and radiation, are expected to improve treatment efficacy. Additionally, advancements in nanotechnology, telemedicine, stem cell research, preventive oncology, and lifestyle interventions will contribute to more effective and comprehensive cancer care.

Supplementary Materials: The following supporting information can be downloaded at https://www.mdpi.com/article/10.3390/cancers16223802/s1, Table S1: Prisma 2020 checklist; File S1: Total number of references used. Reference [92] is cited in the Supplementary Materials.

Author Contributions: Conceptualization, M.E.S.S. and P.O.O.; methodology, P.O.O.; software, M.E.S.S.; validation, M.E.S.S., P.O.O. and N.P.M.; formal analysis, P.O.O.; investigation P.O.O.; resources, P.O.O.; data curation, P.O.O.; writing—original draft preparation, P.O.O.; writing—review and editing, N.P.M., P.M., M.E.S.S. and P.O.O.; supervision, M.E.S.S.; project administration, P.O.O.; funding acquisition, M.E.S.S. and N.P.M. All authors have read and agreed to the published version of the manuscript.

Funding: The APC was funded by the University of KwaZulu-Natal Research Office.

Data Availability Statement: The datasets generated during and/or analysed during the current study are available from the corresponding author upon reasonable request.

Acknowledgments: We would like to acknowledge our administration staff and all the personnel that was involved in this study.

Conflicts of Interest: The authors declare no conflict of interest.

References

1. Sung, H.; Ferlay, J.; Siegel, R.L.; Laversanne, M.; Soerjomataram, I.; Jemal, A.; Bray, F. Global Cancer Statistics 2020: GLOBOCAN Estimates of Incidence and Mortality Worldwide for 36 Cancers in 185 Countries. *CA Cancer J. Clin.* **2021**, *71*, 209–249. [CrossRef] [PubMed]
2. Sharma, R. Mapping of global, regional and national incidence, mortality and mortality-to-incidence ratio of lung cancer in 2020 and 2050. *Int. J. Clin. Oncol.* **2022**, *27*, 665. [CrossRef] [PubMed]
3. Sanford, N.N.; Sher, D.J.; Ahn, C.; Aizer, A.A.; Mahal, B.A. Prevalence and Nondisclosure of Complementary and Alternative Medicine Use in Patients with Cancer and Cancer Survivors in the United States. *JAMA Oncol.* **2019**, *5*, 735–737. [CrossRef] [PubMed]
4. Liu, J.; Wang, S.; Zhang, Y.; Fan, H.T.; Lin, H.S. Traditional Chinese medicine and cancer: History, present situation, and development. *Thorac. Cancer* **2015**, *6*, 561. [CrossRef] [PubMed]
5. Schultz, A.G. Camptothecin. *Chem. Rev.* **1973**, *73*, 385–405. [CrossRef]
6. Legarza, K.; Yang, L.X. Novel Camptothecin Derivatives. *In Vivo* **2005**, *19*, 283–292.
7. Georgoulias, V.; Agelidou, A.; Kouroussis, A.; Samonis, N.; Kakolyris, H.; Tsiafaki, I.; Vardakis, V.; Souglakos, J. Second-line treatment with irinotecan plus cisplatin vs cisplatin of patients with advanced non-small-cell lung cancer pretreated with taxanes and gemcitabine: A multicenter randomised phase II study. *Br. J. Cancer* **2005**, *93*, 763–769. [CrossRef]
8. Kamle, M.; Pandhi, S.; Mishra, S.; Barua, S.; Kurian, A.; Mahato, D.K.; Rasane, P.; Büsselberg, D.; Kumar, P.; Calina, D.; et al. Camptothecin and its derivatives: Advancements, mechanisms and clinical potential in cancer therapy. *Med. Oncol.* **2024**, *41*, 263. [CrossRef]
9. Chen, Z.; Liu, M.; Wang, N.; Xiao, W.; Shi, J. Unleashing the Potential of Camptothecin: Exploring Innovative Strategies for Structural Modification and Therapeutic Advancements. *J. Med. Chem.* **2024**, *67*, 3244–3273; Erratum in *J. Med. Chem.* **2024**, *67*, 9772. [CrossRef]
10. Ghanbari-Movahed, M.; Kaceli, T.; Mondal, A.; Farzaei, M.H.; Bishayee, A. Recent Advances in Improved Anticancer Efficacies of Camptothecin Nano-Formulations: A Systematic Review. *Biomedicines* **2021**, *9*, 480. [CrossRef]
11. Moher, D.; Liberati, A.; Tetzlaff, J.; Altman, D.G. Preferred reporting items for systematic reviews and meta-analyses: The PRISMA statement. *J. Clin. Epidemiol.* **2009**, *62*, 1006–1012. [CrossRef]
12. Hoy, D.; Brooks, P.; Woolf, A.; Blyth, F.; March, L.; Bain, P.; Williams, E.; Smith, T.L. Assessing risk of bias in prevalence studies: Modification of an existing tool and evidence of interrater agreement. *J. Clin. Epidemiol.* **2012**, *65*, 934–939. [CrossRef]
13. Barendregt, J.J.; Doi, S.A.; Lee, Y.Y.; Norman, R.E.; Vos, T. Meta-analysis of prevalence. *J. Epidemiol. Community Health* **2013**, *67*, 974–978. [CrossRef] [PubMed]
14. Barendregt, J.J.; Doi, S.A. MetaXL User Guide. 2015. Available online: www.epigear.com (accessed on 7 August 2023).
15. Nagao, K.; Saito, H.; Mori, S.; Yamazaki, T.; Inoue, M.; Matsui, T. A phase II study of irinotecan combined with cisplatin in non-small cell lung cancer. CPT-11 Lung Cancer Study Group. *Gan Kagaku Ryoho* **2000**, *27*, 413–421.
16. Takiguchi, Y.; Ohta, H.; Hirata, K.; Morita, S.; Kawahara, T. The final results of a randomized phase III trial comparing irinotecan (CPT-11) and cisplatin (CDDP) with vindesine (VDS) and CDDP in advanced non-small cell lung cancer (NSCLC). *Lung Cancer* **2000**, *1* (Suppl. 1), 28–29. [CrossRef]
17. Ueoka, H.; Kiura, Y.; Tabata, T.; Takigawa, M.; Segawa, S.; Kamei, S.; Hiraki, T.; Harada, M. Fractionated administration of irinotecan and cisplatin for treatment of non-small-cell lung cancer: A phase II study of Okayama Lung Cancer Study Group. *Br. J. Cancer* **2001**, *85*, 9–13. [CrossRef] [PubMed]
18. Jagasia, M.H.; Langer, C.J.; Johnson, D.H.; Yunus, F.; Rodgers, J.S.; Schlabach, L.L.; Cohen, A.G.; Shyr, Y.; Carbone, D.P.; Devore, R.F. Weekly irinotecan and cisplatin in advanced non-small cell lung cancer: A multicenter phase II study. *Clin. Cancer Res.* **2001**, *7*, 68–73.
19. Kakolyris, S.; Kouroussis, C.; Souglakos, J.; Agelaki, S.; Kalbakis, K.; Vardakis, N.; Vamvakas, L.; Georgoulias, V. Cisplatin and Irinotecan (CPT-11) as Second-Line Treatment in Patients with Advanced Non-Small Cell Lung Cancer. *Lung Cancer* **2001**, *34*, 71–76. [CrossRef]
20. Takeda, K.; Takifuji, N.; Uejima, H.; Yoshimura, N.; Terakawa, K.; Negoro, S. Phase II Study of Irinotecan and Carboplatin for Advanced Non-Small Cell Lung Cancer. *Lung Cancer* **2002**, *38*, 303–308. [CrossRef]
21. Ichiki, M.; Hanada, M.; Sasaki, K.; Yoshida, M.; Koike, T.; Tanaka, Y.; Nishi, Y.; Motoyoshi, Y.; Umehara, T. Phase II study of irinotecan and ifosfamide in patients with advanced non-small cell lung cancer. *Oncology* **2003**, *64*, 306–311. [CrossRef]
22. Negoro, S.; Masuda, Y.; Takada, M.; Katakami, K.; Kudoh, H.; Sawa, H.; Matsui, H.; Fukuoka, M. Randomised phase III trial of irinotecan combined with cisplatin for advanced non-small-cell lung cancer. *Br. J. Cancer* **2003**, *88*, 335–341. [CrossRef] [PubMed]
23. Cardenal, F.; Domine, M.; Massutí, B.; Carrato, A.; Felip, E.; Garrido, P.; Juan, O.; Artal, A.; Barneto, I.; Lopez-Vivanco, G.; et al. Three-Week Schedule of Irinotecan and Cisplatin in Advanced Non-Small Cell Lung Cancer: A Multicentre Phase II Study. *Lung Cancer* **2003**, *39*, 201–207. [CrossRef]
24. Fukuda, M.; Kudoh, Y.; Nakabayashi, H.; Shimoyama, H.; Hishida, K.; Fukuoka, T.; Ohe, T. Phase II study of irinotecan combined with carboplatin in previously untreated non-small-cell lung cancer. *Cancer Chemother. Pharmacol.* **2004**, *54*, 573–577. [CrossRef]
25. Yamamoto, N.; Nakagawa, K.; Nishiwaki, K.; Yoshimori, K.; Aokage, H.; Hanada, S.; Mitsuoka, T.; Eguchi, K. Randomised phase II study of docetaxel/cisplatin vs docetaxel/irinotecan in advanced non-small-cell lung cancer: A West Japan Thoracic Oncology Group Study (WJTOG9803). *Br. J. Cancer* **2004**, *90*, 87–92. [CrossRef] [PubMed]

26. Raez, L.E.; Rosado, M.F.; Santos, E.S.; Reis, I.M. Irinotecan and docetaxel as first line chemotherapy in patients with stage IIIB/IV non-small cell lung cancer—Experience from a prematurely closed phase II study. *Lung Cancer* **2004**, *45*, 131–132. [CrossRef]
27. Lima, C.M.S.R.; Herndon, L.; Kosty, D.R.; Green, G.P.; Eckardt, L.A.; Richards, S.; Crawford, R.; Hensing, D. Randomized phase II trial of gemcitabine plus irinotecan or docetaxel in stage IIIB or stage IV NSCLC. *Ann. Oncol.* **2004**, *15*, 410–418. [CrossRef] [PubMed]
28. Ziotopoulos, P.; Kouvatseas, A.; Samantas, N.; Pavlidis, P.; Kalofonos, E.; Fountzilas, G. Front-line treatment of advanced non-small cell lung cancer with irinotecan and docetaxel: A multicentre phase II study. *Lung Cancer* **2005**, *50*, 115–122. [CrossRef]
29. Stathopoulos, G.P.; Veslemes, D.; Georgatou, I.; Koutantos, A.; Malamos, S.; Kostouros, V. Front-line paclitaxel and irinotecan combination chemotherapy in advanced non-small-cell lung cancer: A phase I-II trial. *Br. J. Cancer* **2005**, *93*, 1106–1111. [CrossRef]
30. Murren, J.R.; Kao, F.T.; Bodkin, D.; Heald, J.P. Evaluation of irinotecan plus paclitaxel in patients with advanced non-small cell lung cancer. *Cancer Biol. Ther.* **2005**, *4*, 1311–1315. [CrossRef]
31. Saito, H.; Takada, M.; Ichinose, S.; Kato, T.; Mori, K.; Tanimoto, H.; Eguchi, K. Phase II study of 3-week scheduling of irinotecan in combination with cisplatin in patients with advanced nonsmall-cell lung cancer. *Am. J. Clin. Oncol. Cancer Clin. Trials* **2006**, *29*, 503–507. [CrossRef]
32. Hino, M.; Kobayashi, K.; Yoshimura, A.; Takeda, Y.; Hisakatsu, S.; Yoneda, S.; Gemma, A.; Moriya, H.; Kudoh, S.; Group, E.J.C. Weekly administration of irinotecan (CPT $_{-11}$) plus cisplatin for non-small cell lung cancer. *Anticancer Res.* **2006**, *26*, 4697–4704. [PubMed]
33. Zhang, X.R.; Zhu, Y.Z.; Xiu, Q.Y.; Han, F.C.; Liu, D.Q.; Chu, D.T. Irinotecan plus cisplatin for the treatment of advanced non-small cell lung cancer. *Chin. J. Oncol.* **2006**, *28*, 777–779.
34. Pillot, G.A.; Souquet, F.; Guy, C.; Dumontet, C. A Phase II Study of Irinotecan and Carboplatin in Advanced Non-small Cell Lung Cancer with Pharmacogenomic Analysis: Final Report. *J. Thorac. Oncol.* **2006**, *1*, 972–978. [CrossRef]
35. Charoentum, C.; Thongprasert, S.; Chewasakulyong, B.; Euathrongchit, J.; Sorraritchingchai, S.; Munprakan, S. Phase II Study of Cisplatin Combined to Irinotecan Administered Alternatingly with Docetaxel in Advanced Non-Small Cell Lung Cancer. *J. Med. Assoc. Thail.* **2007**, *90*, 2506–2512.
36. Bajetta, E.; Di Bartolomeo, L.; Mariani, P.; Buzzoni, A.; Beretta, M.; Ferrario, M.; Di Leo, S.; Vullo, S.L. Uracil/ftorafur/leucovorin combined with irinotecan (TEGAFIRI) or oxaliplatin (TEGAFOX) as first-line treatment for metastatic colorectal cancer patients: Results of randomised phase II study. *Br. J. Cancer* **2007**, *96*, 439–444. [CrossRef]
37. Grothey, A.; Jordan, K.; Kellner, O.; Constantin, C.; Dietrich, G.; Kroening, H.; Mantovani, L.; Schlichting, C.; Forstbauer, H.; Schmoll, H.J. Capecitabine plus irinotecan (CAPIRI) vs capecitabine plus oxaliplatin (CAPOX) as first-line therapy of advanced colorectal cancer (ACRC): Updated results of a randomized phase II trial. *Eur. J. Cancer* **2003**, *1*, S90–S91. [CrossRef]
38. Comella, P.; Casaretti, S.; Sandomenico, A.; Avallone, E.; Franco, F.; Monfardini, P.D.; Massidda, F. Oxaliplatin plus high-dose folinic acid and 5-fluorouracil i.v. bolus (OXAFAFU) versus irinotecan plus high-dose folinic acid and 5-fluorouracil i.v. bolus (IRIFAFU) in patients with metastatic colorectal carcinoma: A Southern Italy Cooperative Oncology Group phase III trial. *Ann. Oncol.* **2005**, *16*, 878–886. [CrossRef]
39. Feliu, J.; Escudero, A.; Llosa, I.; Baron, L.G.; Carrato, M.A.; Nistal, A. Phase II randomised trial of raltitrexed-oxaliplatin vs raltitrexed-irinotecan as first-line treatment in advanced colorectal cancer. *Br. J. Cancer* **2005**, *93*, 1230–1235. [CrossRef]
40. Seymour, M.T.; Thompson, J.R.; Wasan, T.; Middleton, A.P.; Brewster, R.S.; Shepherd, C.J.; Stenning, J. Different strategies of sequential and combination chemotherapy for patients with poor prognosis advanced colorectal cancer (MRC FOCUS): A randomised controlled trial. *Lancet* **2007**, *370*, 143–152. [CrossRef]
41. Borner, M.M.; Koeberle, S.; von Moos, M.; Saletti, M.; Cathomas, P.; Caspar, A. A randomized phase II trial of capecitabine and two different schedules of irinotecan in first-line treatment of metastatic colorectal cancer: Efficacy, quality-of-life and toxicity. *Ann. Oncol.* **2005**, *16*, 282–288. [CrossRef]
42. Rosati, G.; Cordio, F.; Bordonaro, C.; Bavetta, G.A.; Ferrara, F.; Russo, S.; Barbarino, A. Capecitabine in combination with oxaliplatin or irinotecan in elderly patients with advanced colorectal cancer: Results of a randomized phase II study. *Ann. Oncol.* **2009**, *21*, 781–786. [CrossRef]
43. Moosmann, N.; Heinemann, C.; Laubender, H.; Bokemeyer, G.; Schöberl, T.M.; von Weikersthal, A.F. Cetuximab plus capecitabine and irinotecan compared with cetuximab plus capecitabine and oxaliplatin as first-line treatment for patients with metastatic colorectal cancer: AIO KRK-0104—A randomized trial of the German AIO CRC study group. *J. Clin. Oncol.* **2011**, *29*, 1050–1058. [CrossRef] [PubMed]
44. Colucci, G.; Gebbia, A.; Paoletti, R.; Giuliani, P.; Biganzoli, G.G.; Rabitti, P.; Pancera, L. Phase III randomized trial of FOLFIRI versus FOLFOX4 in the treatment of advanced colorectal cancer: A Multicenter Study of the Gruppo Oncologico Dell'Italia Meridionale. *J. Clin. Oncol.* **2005**, *23*, 4866–4875. [CrossRef]
45. Douillard, J.Y.; Cunningham, D.; Roth, A.D.; Navarro, M.; James, R.D.; Karasek, P.; Jandik, P.; Iveson, T.; Carmichael, P.J.; Alakl, M. Irinotecan combined with fluorouracil compared with fluorouracil alone as first-line treatment for metastatic colorectal cancer: A multicentre randomised trial. *Lancet* **2000**, *355*, 1041–1047. [CrossRef] [PubMed]
46. Köhne, C.H.; Greil, R.; Wils, G.; Bodoky, F.; Keilholz, W.; Burkitt, P.; Kerr, D.J. Phase III study of weekly high-dose infusional fluorouracil plus folinic acid with or without irinotecan in patients with metastatic colorectal cancer: European Organisation for Research and Treatment of Cancer Gastrointestinal Group Study 40986. *J. Clin. Oncol.* **2005**, *23*, 4856–4865. [CrossRef]

47. Fuchs, C.S.; Goldberg, R.B.; Sargent, R.J.; Meyerhardt, M.; Zhu, T.L.; Hecht, M. Randomized, controlled trial of irinotecan plus infusional, bolus, or oral fluoropyrimidines in first-line treatment of metastatic colorectal cancer: Results from the BICC-C study. *J. Clin. Oncol.* **2007**, *25*, 4779–4786. [CrossRef]
48. Yamazaki, K.; Nagase, M.; Suzuki, T.; Ando, S.; Hayashi, Y.; Fujimoto, T.; Nishimura, H. Randomized phase III study of bevacizumab plus FOLFIRI and bevacizumab plus mFOLFOX6 as first-line treatment for patients with metastatic colorectal cancer (WJOG4407G). *Ann. Oncol.* **2016**, *27*, 1539–1546. [CrossRef]
49. Loupakis, F.; Cremolini, G.; Masi, M.; Lonardi, A.; Zagonel, S.; Salvatore, P.; Falcone, A. Initial Therapy with FOLFOXIRI and Bevacizumab for Metastatic Colorectal Cancer. *N. Engl. J. Med.* **2014**, *371*, 1609–1618. [CrossRef]
50. Bouché, O.; Bondoux, P.Y.; Brouquet, C.; Sobrin, J.M.; Saint-Aubert, E.; Louvet, P.C. Randomized multicenter phase II trial of a biweekly regimen of fluorouracil and leucovorin (LV5FU2), LV5FU2 plus cisplatin, or LV5FU2 plus irinotecan in patients with previously untreated metastatic gastric cancer: A Fédération Francophone de Cancérologie Digestive Group Study-FFCD 9803. *J. Clin. Oncol.* **2004**, *22*, 4319–4328. [CrossRef]
51. Moehler, M.; Siebler, A.; Hoehler, F.; Kaiser, R. Randomised phase II evaluation of irinotecan plus high-dose 5-fluorouracil and leucovorin (ILF) vs 5-fluorouracil, leucovorin, and etoposide (ELF) in untreated metastatic gastric cancer. *Br. J. Cancer* **2005**, *92*, 2122–2128. [CrossRef]
52. Dank, M.; Zitt, M.; Mai, A.; Greil, G.; Samonigg, W. Randomized phase III study comparing irinotecan combined with 5-fluorouracil and folinic acid to cisplatin combined with 5-fluorouracil in chemotherapy naive patients with advanced adenocarcinoma of the stomach or esophagogastric junction. *Ann. Oncol.* **2008**, *19*, 1450–1457. [CrossRef] [PubMed]
53. Nakashima, K.; Takinami, Y.; Akai, S.; Iizuka, T.; Tsumura, T.; Saito, T.; Nishio, N. Irinotecan plus cisplatin therapy and S-1 plus cisplatin therapy for advanced or recurrent gastric cancer in a single institution. *Jpn. J. Clin. Oncol.* **2008**, *38*, 810–815. [CrossRef] [PubMed]
54. Komatsu, Y.; Doki, K.; Takahashi, S.; Nakayama, S.; Mori, M.; Fujiwara, T.; Oda, M. Randomized phase II trial of first-line treatment with tailored irinotecan plus S-1 therapy versus S-1 monotherapy for advanced or recurrent gastric carcinoma (JFMC31-0301). *Anti-Cancer Drugs* **2011**, *22*, 576–583. [CrossRef] [PubMed]
55. Noda, K.; Nishiwaki, M.; Kawahara, H.; Sato, Y.; Komuta, T.; Yokoyama, T. Irinotecan plus cisplastin compared with etoposide plus cisplastin for extensive small-cell lung cancer. *N. Engl. J. Med.* **2002**, *346*, 85–91. [CrossRef]
56. Hirose, T.; Tamiya, K.; Segawa, M.; Nakano, K.; Nishizawa, H.; Miura, T. Phase II study of irinotecan and carboplatin in patients with the refractory or relapsed small cell lung cancer. *Lung Cancer* **2003**, *40*, 333–338. [CrossRef]
57. Schuette, W.; Meisel, C.E.; Seeber, P.; Gross, J. Phase II trial of gemcitabine/irinotecan in refractory or relapsed small-cell lung cancer. *Clin. Lung Cancer* **2005**, *7*, 133–137. [CrossRef]
58. O'Brien, M.E.R.; Szczesna, D.; Burtin, H.J.; Stawicka, J.; Leyes, C.; Kordyjal, P.; Kropf, F. Phase III trial comparing supportive care alone with supportive care with oral topotecan in patients with relapsed small-cell lung cancer. *J. Clin. Oncol.* **2006**, *24*, 5441–5447. [CrossRef]
59. Huber, R.M.; Reck, A.; von Pawel, U.; Thomas, K.; Gauler, M.; Spengler, F.; Stahel, R.H. Efficacy of a toxicity-adjusted topotecan therapy in recurrent small cell lung cancer. *Eur. Respir. J.* **2006**, *27*, 1183–1189. [CrossRef]
60. Kinoshita, A.; Eguchi, H.; Tokoro, Y.; Ishikawa, K.; Mase, T.; Takemoto, H.; Yoshida, M. Phase II study of irinotecan combined with carboplatin in previously untreated small-cell lung cancer. *Br. J. Cancer* **2006**, *94*, 1267–1271. [CrossRef]
61. Eckardt, J.R.; von Pawel, M.; Pujol, A.; Enns, H.; Stelmakh, R.; O'Brien, A.F.; Meehan, W.A. Phase III study of oral compared with intravenous topotecan as second-line therapy in small-cell lung cancer. *J. Clin. Oncol.* **2007**, *25*, 2086–2092. [CrossRef]
62. Ohyanagi, F.; Yokoyama, M.; Nakazawa, M.; Hino, K.; Kobayashi, M.; Sakuma, T.; Minami, K. Phase II trial of gemcitabine and irinotecan in previously treated patients with small-cell lung cancer. *Cancer Chemother. Pharmacol.* **2008**, *61*, 503–508. [CrossRef] [PubMed]
63. Inoue, A.; Takahashi, M.; Fujiwara, N.; Arai, S.; Sugiyama, H.; Tanaka, H.; Fujita, T. Randomized phase II trial comparing amrubicin with topotecan in patients with previously treated small-cell lung cancer: North Japan lung cancer study group trial 0402. *J. Clin. Oncol.* **2008**, *26*, 5401–5406. [CrossRef]
64. Park, S.H.; Lee, M.; Son, K.; Kim, H.; Kim, J. Salvage treatment with topotecan in patients with irinotecan-refractory small cell lung cancer. *Cancer Chemother. Pharmacol.* **2008**, *62*, 1009–1014. [CrossRef] [PubMed]
65. Chen, G.; Tashkin, A.H.; Ryder, C.C. Phase II Trial of Irinotecan and Carboplatin for Extensive or Relapsed Small-Cell Lung Cancer. *J. Clin. Oncol.* **2009**, *27*, 1401. [CrossRef] [PubMed]
66. Lara, P.N.; Chansky, S.; Davies, R.A.; Gumerlock, R.H.; Mack, H.E.T.; Pham, K. Phase III trial of irinotecan/cisplatin compared with etoposide/cisplatin in extensive-stage small-cell lung cancer: Clinical and pharmacogenomic results from SWOG S0124. *J. Clin. Oncol.* **2009**, *27*, 2530–2535. [CrossRef]
67. Zatloukal, P.; Spicka, M.R.; Hainz, P.; Sedlák, J.; Pavlik, F.; Zemanová, B. A multicenter international randomized phase III study comparing cisplatin in combination with irinotecan or etoposide in previously untreated small-cell lung cancer patients with extensive disease. *Ann. Oncol.* **2010**, *21*, 1810–1816. [CrossRef] [PubMed]
68. Jotte, R.; von Pawel, L.; Spicer, R.; Zimmermann, M.; Guns, K. Randomized phase II trial of single-agent amrubicin or topotecan as second-line treatment in patients with small-cell lung cancer sensitive to first-line platinum-based chemotherapy. *J. Clin. Oncol.* **2011**, *29*, 287–293. [CrossRef]
69. Schmittel, A.; Sebastian, M.; von Weikersthal, L.F.; Martus, P.; Gauler, T.C.; Kaufmann, C.; Hortig, P.; Fischer, J.R.; Link, H.; Binder, D.; et al. Arbeitsgemeinschaft Internistische Onkologie Thoracic Oncology Study Group. A German multicenter, randomized phase III trial comparing irinotecan-carboplatin with etoposide-carboplatin as first-line therapy for extensive-disease small-cell lung cancer. *Ann. Oncol.* **2011**, *22*, 1798–1804. [CrossRef]

70. Xenidis, N.; Zografos, E.; Koukourakis, G.; Koumakis, C.; Fountzilas, T.; Tsavaris, S. A multicenter phase II study of pegylated liposomal doxorubicin in combination with irinotecan as second-line treatment of patients with refractory small-cell lung cancer. *Cancer Chemother. Pharmacol.* **2011**, *68*, 63–68. [CrossRef]
71. Von Pawel, J.; Gervais, R.; Eckardt, M.; Spira, G.; Harvey, A.; von Dehn, T. Randomized phase III trial of Amrubicin versus topotecan as second-line treatment for patients with small-cell lung cancer. *J. Clin. Oncol.* **2014**, *32*, 4012–4018. [CrossRef]
72. Shi, Y.; Hu, Y.; Hu, X.; Li, X.; Lin, L.; Han, X. Cisplatin combined with irinotecan or etoposide for untreated extensive-stage small cell lung cancer: A multicenter randomized controlled clinical trial. *Thorac. Cancer* **2015**, *6*, 785–791. [CrossRef] [PubMed]
73. Evans, T.L.; Cho, M.N.; Shih, M.; McCusker, C.; Hanna, D.W. Cabazitaxel versus topotecan in patients with small-cell lung cancer with progressive disease during or after first-line platinum-based chemotherapy. *J. Thorac. Oncol.* **2015**, *10*, 1221–1228. [CrossRef] [PubMed]
74. Goto, K.; Ohe, Y.; Sekine, M.; Kunitoh, H.; Saito, M.; Takada, N.; Nishiwaki, T. Combined chemotherapy with cisplatin, etoposide, and irinotecan versus topotecan alone as second-line treatment for patients with sensitive relapsed small-cell lung cancer (JCOG0605): A multicentre, open-label, randomised phase 3 trial. *Lancet Oncol.* **2016**, *17*, 1147–1157. [CrossRef]
75. Chiappori, A.A.; Otterson, J.A.; Dowlati, T.; Shah, S.; Goff, J.E.; Govindan, A.R. A Randomized Phase II Study of Linsitinib (OSI-906) Versus Topotecan in Patients with Relapsed Small-Cell Lung Cancer. *Oncologist* **2016**, *21*, 1163. [CrossRef]
76. Trafalis, D.T.; Alifieris, C.; Stathopoulos, G.P.; Sitaras, N. Phase II study of bevacizumab plus irinotecan on the treatment of relapsed resistant small cell lung cancer. *Cancer Chemother. Pharmacol.* **2016**, *77*, 713–722. [CrossRef]
77. Kondo, R.; Watanabe, K.; Sato, M.; Matsuo, N. A Phase II Study of Irinotecan for Patients with Previously Treated Small-Cell Lung Cancer. *Oncology* **2018**, *94*, 223–232. [CrossRef]
78. Kim, D.W.; Kim, S.K.; Shin, J.S.; Lee, C.H.; Kim, S.W.; Park, J.H.; Ahn, H.S. Randomized phase III trial of irinotecan plus cisplatin versus etoposide plus cisplatin in chemotherapy-naïve Korean patients with extensive-disease small cell lung cancer. *Cancer Res. Treat.* **2019**, *51*, 119–127. [CrossRef]
79. Baize, N.; Monnet, C.; Voisin, B.F.; Daniel, F.; Leonce, A.; Cortot, A. Carboplatin plus etoposide versus topotecan as second-line treatment for patients with sensitive relapsed small-cell lung cancer: An open-label, multicentre, randomised, phase 3 trial. *Lancet Oncol.* **2020**, *21*, 1224–1233. [CrossRef]
80. Kang, J.H.; Lee, M.W.; Oh, J.H.; Ryu, J.S. A randomised phase 2b study comparing the efficacy and safety of belotecan vs. topotecan as monotherapy for sensitive-relapsed small-cell lung cancer. *Br. J. Cancer* **2021**, *124*, 713–720. [CrossRef]
81. Borghaei, H.; Paz-Ares, N.; Horn, C.; Baas, P.; Reck, M.; Spigel, D. OA12.05 Phase 1 Updated Exploration and First Expansion Data for DLL3-targeted T-cell Engager Tarlatamab in Small Cell Lung Cancer. *J. Thorac. Oncol.* **2022**, *17*, S33. [CrossRef]
82. Edelman, M.J.; Pang, S.S.; Kotsakis, J.A.; Gralla, R.J.; Reck, M.; Kerrigan, J. Randomized phase 3 study of the anti-disialoganglioside antibody dinutuximab and irinotecan vs irinotecan or topotecan for second-line treatment of small cell lung cancer. *Lung Cancer* **2022**, *166*, 135–142. [CrossRef] [PubMed]
83. Hermes, A.; Gatzemeier, D.; Koschel, C.; Bauer, T.; Wilke, U.; Beyer, H. Irinotecan plus carboplatin versus oral etoposide plus carboplatin in extensive small-cell lung cancer: A randomized phase III trial. *J. Clin. Oncol.* **2008**, *26*, 4261–4267. [CrossRef] [PubMed]
84. Goldberg, R.M.; Alberts, M.S.; Venook, J.; Haller, N.; Rothenberg, C.K. The continuum of care: A paradigm for the management of metastatic colorectal cancer. *Oncologist* **2007**, *12*, 38–50. [CrossRef]
85. Schmoll, H.J.; Van Cutsem, E.; Stein, K.; Valentini, J.; Nordlinger, P.C. ESMO Consensus Guidelines for management of patients with colon and rectal cancer. A personalized approach to clinical decision making. *Ann. Oncol.* **2012**, *23*, 2479–2516. [CrossRef]
86. Ikoma, N.; Raghav, K.; Chang, G. An Update on Randomized Clinical Trials in Metastatic Colorectal Carcinoma. *Surg. Oncol. Clin. N. Am.* **2017**, *26*, 667–687. [CrossRef]
87. Zeng, C.; Zhou, H.; Wei, Y.; Wang, L.Y.; Xie, H.; Yao, W.X. Chemotherapy with or without irinotecan in patients with advanced or recurrent gastric cancer: A meta-analysis of randomized controlled trials. *Chin. Med. J. (Engl.)* **2014**, *127*, 951–956. [CrossRef]
88. Nishikawa, K.; Aoyama, T.; Fukuda, H.; Kawano, S.; Nakamura, Y. Meta-analysis of biweekly irinotecan plus cisplatin versus irinotecan alone as second-line treatment for advanced gastric cancer. *Ann. Oncol.* **2018**, *29*, VIII228. [CrossRef]
89. Cho, Y.H.; Yoon, S.Y.; Kim, S.N. Irinotecan Monotherapy Versus Irinotecan-Based Combination as Second-Line Chemotherapy in Advanced Gastric Cancer: A Meta-Analysis. *Cancer Res. Treat.* **2016**, *49*, 255–262. [CrossRef]
90. Petrelli, F.; Ghidini, A.; Luciani, A. Topotecan or other agents as second-line therapy for relapsed small-cell lung cancer: A meta-analysis of randomized studies. *Mol. Clin. Oncol.* **2021**, *15*, 1–7. [CrossRef]
91. Hanna, N.; Einhorn, S.B.; Crowley, S.O.; Shibles, J.G.; Blackburn, R.W.; Brown, J.N. Randomized phase III trial comparing irinotecan/cisplatin with etoposide/cisplatin in patients with previously untreated extensive-stage disease small-cell lung cancer. *J. Clin. Oncol.* **2006**, *24*, 2038–2043. [CrossRef]
92. Page, M.J.; McKenzie, J.E.; Bossuyt, P.M.; Boutron, I.; Hoffmann, T.C.; Mulrow, C.D.; Shamseer, L.; Tetzlaff, J.M.; Akl, E.A.; Brennan, S.E.; et al. The PRISMA 2020 statement: An updated guideline for reporting systematic reviews. *BMJ* **2021**, *372*, n71. [CrossRef] [PubMed]

MDPI AG
Grosspeteranlage 5
4052 Basel
Switzerland
Tel.: +41 61 683 77 34

Cancers Editorial Office
E-mail: cancers@mdpi.com
www.mdpi.com/journal/cancers

www.ingramcontent.com/pod-product-compliance
Lightning Source LLC
Chambersburg PA
CBHW061620220926
51850CB00005B/559
* 9 7 8 3 7 2 5 8 5 2 7 7 2 *